Promoting Human Wellness

PROMOTING HUMAN WELLNESS

NEW FRONTIERS FOR RESEARCH, PRACTICE, AND POLICY

Edited by
Margaret Schneider Jamner
and Daniel Stokols

University of California Press
Published in Collaboration with the California Wellness Foundation
and the Office of Health Affairs of the University of California
Berkeley   Los Angeles   London

University of California Press
Berkeley and Los Angeles, California

University of California Press, Ltd.
London, England

Library of Congress Cataloging-in-Publication Data

Promoting human wellness : new frontiers for
research, practice, and policy / edited by Margaret
Schneider Jamner and Daniel Stokols.
      p.   cm.
   Includes bibliographical references and index.
   ISBN 0-520-22608-9 (cloth : alk. paper) —
ISBN 0-520-22609-7 (paper : alk. paper)
   1. Health promotion.   2. Health promotion—
Social aspects.   I. Jamner, Margaret Schneider.
II. Stokols, Daniel.
RA427.8.P7665   2000
613—dc21
                              99-087690

Printed in the United States of America
08 07 06 05 04 03 02 01 00 99
10 9 8 7 6 5 4 3 2 1

The paper used in this publication meets the
minimum requirements of ANSI/NISO Z39.48-1992
(R 1997) ∞.

Contents

Foreword

On behalf of the University of California, we are proud to offer this collection of essays and Wellness Papers in the new *Promoting Human Wellness* text. This volume represents the fruits of a collaborative vision shared by The California Wellness Foundation (TCWF) and the University of California. Since 1991, Wellness Award Lectures have been published annually as policy analyses of varied elements of health promotion and disease prevention, emanating from a selection of the most innovative work of University of California faculty. In 1997, we accepted an invitation from the University of California Press to expand that vision into a text on human wellness, augmented by invited contributions from national experts who have written original papers on the state of women's health, AIDS prevention developments, and wellness promotion evaluation strategies.

The original Wellness Award topics and authors were chosen as a result of an annual university-wide call for abstracts and blinded peer review of submissions. The abstracts were screened for scholarly excellence and applicability to a wide array of health promotion and disease prevention issues. A distinguished university-wide multidisciplinary committee of deans, faculty, and other academic personnel reviewed the submissions and selected each year's awardees. With the addition of invited essays, we have created a collection that brings into focus the major human health issues facing our nation today.

Our partnership with TCWF, which began in 1995, was intended to further faculty scholarship in response to critical public health problems facing families and communities in California. Among the concerns that the lectures have addressed have been the growth of violence in society, workplace hazards, teen pregnancy, socioeconomic disparities, aging and health promotion, environmental health planning, and other problems that might respond to thoughtful policy realignment and a community health approach.

Free public lectures based on these papers were delivered at University of California campuses each October. In 1997, the papers included proposed solutions to or analyses of different aspects of the problem of violence in our society, particularly gang proliferation and domestic violence recognition; a review that raises significant policy questions for occupational health in the agricultural workplace; an evaluation of a multiyear TCWF Violence Prevention Initiative and its impact on community-based gun ordinances throughout California; and an analysis of *The Wellness Guide* Program, also supported by a grant from TCWF.

An important theme has emerged in several of these papers, namely, that empowerment of communities and individuals is a core prerequisite of good physical and mental health. The related concepts of resilience and self-determination have long been known to contribute to the individual's ability to thrive and grow. As a society, we need to revisit this premise and strive to imbue our community organizations and health and social service programs with the necessary resources and tools that empower individuals and families to recognize and build on their own strengths.

The goal of our Wellness Lectures Program has been to inform the ongoing health policy reform process and to contribute to a more humane future for California and the nation. We believe that the Wellness Award Lectures papers meet that challenge. Our intent is to raise questions in a thoughtful and provocative way among a new generation of health professionals, bioethicists, and social scientists—those who will help shape the humanity and texture of American society in the coming millennium. We hope that these papers will find their way into the classrooms of schools of medicine, nursing, public health, social work, and bioethics as well as college courses in women's studies, ethnic studies, psychology, sociology, economics, and social ecology. We hope that the book will be of interest to health professionals, policy makers, researchers, and students in the field of wellness promotion.

Cornelius L. Hopper, M.D.
Vice President—Health Affairs

Irene Bronston, M.P.H.
Coordinator, Wellness Lectures Program

University of California Office of the President
January 2000

Acknowledgments

The editors would like to thank Roger Greaves, former CEO, Health Net, Gary L. Yates, President and CEO of The California Wellness Foundation (TCWF), and the University of California Office of Health Affairs for support of the UC Wellness Lecture Series and this volume. We would also like to thank the members of the editorial review board, including Lester Breslow, M.D., M.P.H.; Joyce Lashof, M.D.; Sheldon Margen, M.D., M.P.H.; and Mary Walshok, Ph.D., for their valuable contributions to the selection and review of the chapters to be included in this volume. A number of individuals deserve our gratitude for their efforts both on the Lecture Series and with the book project. These include Irene Bronston, M.P.H., Coordinator, TCWF/UC Wellness Lectures Program; Adele Amodeo, M.P.H., Coordinator, UC Health Policy and Legislation; Cornelius Hopper, M.D., UC Vice President of Health Affairs; and Don Prial, Public Relations Counsel. Finally, we would like to thank the following individuals for their comments and suggestions on draft manuscripts: Virginia Alhuesen, Ph.D.; Elaine Alpert, M.D.; Lisa Berkman, Ph.D.; Claire Brindis, M.D.; Ross Conner, Ph.D.; Jeannie Gazzaniga, Ph.D.; Joyce C. Lashof, M.D.; Shari MacMahan, Ph.D.; Lauri Pasch, Ph.D.; Arthur Rubel, Ph.D.; Norman Schneider, Ph.D.; Sora Park Tanjasiri, Ph.D.; Tammy Tengs, Ph.D.; Dawn Upchurch, Ph.D.; and Stewart Wolf, M.D.

Margaret Schneider Jamner

INTRODUCTION

New Frontiers for Research, Practice, and Policy

Wellness promotion, as this volume demonstrates, is at a critical juncture as we enter the new millennium. We have gained an appreciation for the complexity of the task and are beginning to develop methods for identifying the most effective strategies for improving the health-related quality of life among Americans. Moreover, we have expanded our sphere of influence to encompass not only the immediate causes of morbidity and mortality but also the more fundamental determinants that reside in the political, social, and physical environments. This volume illustrates the potential for promoting human wellness that has been generated by these developments. Future success in realizing this potential relies on recognizing that elements that are often encountered as barriers to health promotion (e.g., political agendas, idiosyncratic populations) can and must be embraced and incorporated into the methods that guide wellness research and practice. Only by employing these elements to serve the ends of wellness promotion will we sustain the current momentum toward creating a nation that supports and facilitates optimal health.

The chapters in this volume offer compelling evidence for the complex web of interrelated influences that operate dynamically to determine health and wellness. Regardless of the specific disease or disability being examined, it is clear that one must consider the likelihood that health status may be affected by variables at many levels, including (but certainly not limited to) the human genome, individual health behavior and psychological attributes, medical care, and the physical and social environments. Moreover, each level has the potential to interact with factors from other dimensions. As described by Leonard Duhl (1996), "It is as if there were a ball of interconnected strands that could be picked up at any point, and a relationship to all other issues, institutions, people, and places would exist" (p. 259).

The multidimensional model that could be constructed to depict any specific health problem threatens to be overwhelming in its complexity. Nevertheless, conceptualizing wellness promotion from a systems perspective may turn out to be a requirement for effective intervention (Wandersman et al., 1996). It is important, therefore, to note that work presented in these pages also provides testimony that adopting a systems approach to wellness does not preclude elegant solutions to health problems and, in fact, may simplify matters by identifying optimally effective leverage points for intervention. In order to realize the potential within the systems approach for identifying parsimonious pathways to promoting health, it is crucial that health researchers, health practitioners, and policy makers maintain an exceptionally broad vision of the range of activities and targets that may fall within the health promotion mandate. It is equally important that wellness professionals address explicitly the nonscientific forces bearing on the translation of wellness knowledge into effective action.

Public health, the parent discipline to wellness promotion, has been said to permeate "through all the social, environmental, and other activities of populations" (Holland, 1997, p. 1645). Likewise, although the promotion of human wellness is often identified with orchestrating a change in lifestyle, such individual modifications "usually require some combination of educational, organizational, economic, and environmental interventions in support of change in both behavior and conditions of living" (Green et al., 1997, p. 125). Appropriate targets for change in the pursuit of enhanced health and wellness for a population therefore include elements within the individual, the social milieu, the physical environment, the medical care system, the economy, and the political arena. This point is vividly illustrated by the chapters in this volume, several of which present impressive evidence of the powerful force for change that results from directly addressing contextual factors.

WELLNESS PROMOTION AND THE POLITICAL CONTEXT

A number of the authors featured in this volume argue that the influence of the political context on human wellness deserves greater attention. In particular, the politicization of health-related issues often results in a markedly skewed allocation of resources with respect to research. Strohman (chapter 5), for example, opines that the share of research funds devoted to mapping the human genome is grossly out of proportion to the health benefits that this project is likely to deliver. His work suggests that far greater salutary outcomes might be expected to accrue to the population if sufficient funds were directed to mapping out the ways in which genes interact with their immediate (i.e., organismic) and distal (i.e., extraorganismic) environments to determine phenotypic expression. It is in the interest of the goals of health promotion that scientists make a concerted effort toward educating political decision makers regarding the connection that proposed health research initiatives have to the objective of improving the health of the population.

This advice should not be interpreted as a condemnation of basic research, whose relationship to the human condition may at times be obscure or difficult to discern. Basic research is and will continue to be of great importance since expanding our understanding of the mechanics of our world can serve us in many unforeseen and significant ways. Nevertheless, in a society characterized by limited resources for research, the way in which these resources are distributed should be continually reassessed in order to determine whether adjustments in the allocation are likely to result in greater health returns.

Another instance of value-driven political agendas leading to inequitable resource allocation is the greater emphasis placed on men, as compared to women, in health research. As discussed by Stanton et al. (chapter 22), the historical view of the female as the lesser "deviation" from the male norm has contributed to the disproportionate attention paid to men in health research. The nominal representation of women in the sciences and politics in the past also has helped maintain the illusion that important research questions could be adequately addressed through research on men only. Villablanca (chapter 23) reaffirms this pattern in the case of heart disease. Although coronary heart disease is the leading cause of death for both men and women, the latter have been largely excluded until recently from most heart disease prevention trials. In the last decade, a shift toward greater recognition of the health needs of women has occurred and has led to attempts at establishing greater gender equity in research. This new movement has fueled the Women's Health Initiative, which will yield a wealth of data concerning the factors that influence the health and wellness of women. Wellness professionals would do well to note this apparently successful culmination to years of campaigning for gender equity in research. Results of the current wave of health research directed at women's issues will provide valuable scientific information useful in promoting women's health. In order to continue the momentum toward a more equitable health research agenda at the national level, wellness professionals must find effective ways to supply their expertise to the political decision-making process.

Values-laden political priorities also play a large role in determining the allocation of resources among interventions designed to improve or enhance health. Hofmann (chapter 20) eloquently lays out the argument for providing teens with complete information concerning contraception, yet recent federal legislation provides funds for school-based sex education that teaches abstinence-only pregnancy prevention. Given the strength of the evidence against the utility of the abstinence-only approach, it appears that this legislation is based not on scientific knowledge but rather on the values of individuals, lobbyists, and organized voter groups expressed as political will. Similarly, Waldo and Coates (chapter 24) describe the failure of HIV prevention programs and attribute this lack of success to a political climate that, for example, blocks widespread use of needle exchange despite ample evidence that allowing drug users to receive sterile syringes in exchange for used needles reduces HIV transmission without increasing drug use. A resolution issued in 1998 by the Presidential Advisory Council on HIV/AIDS (American Public Health Association, 1998) rebuked the president and the secretary of health and human services for failing to remove the ban on using federal funds for needle exchange programs and stated that "tragically, we must conclude that it is a lack of political will, not scientific evidence, that is creating this failure to act."

The persistence of the "agrarian myth" (a pervasive belief in the salutary conditions of agricultural occupations) in the face of data concerning the health problems of agricultural workers represents another case of an area in which policy and legislation have lagged behind available scientific information. As explained by Schenker (chapter 21), current health and safety legislation designed to protect farmers and farm laborers in the United States is notably insufficient. For example, Schenker notes that rollover protectors for tractors have been legislated in Europe but not in the United States, even though they essentially eliminate rollover fatalities. These examples demonstrate that successful wellness promotion requires engaging the political process in a data-based evaluation of funding and legislative priorities and pushing for policies that have the greatest likelihood for improving national health status by addressing the actual needs of the nation's constituent populations.

The theorem that the political context plays a large role as a force affecting how public health knowledge is translated into preventive action is generally acknowledged in the field of public health. In the first chapter of the 1997 edition of the *Oxford Textbook of Public Health*, Detels and Breslow state, "What can be done will be determined by the scientific knowledge and resources available. What is done will be determined by the social and political commitments existing at the particular time and place" (p. 3). One model of this process, proposed by Richmond and Kotelchuck (1983), posits three factors that contribute to the shaping of health policy: knowledge base, political will, and a social strategy. According to Richmond and Kotelchuck, the knowledge base refers to "the scientific and administrative data base upon which to make decisions." Thus, epidemiologic research, needs assessments, clinical trials, and other forms of intervention evaluations all contribute to this knowledge base that may be used to inform health policy decisions. How or even whether this information is used, however, depends greatly on the political climate.

In discussing the Richmond and Kotelchuck model, Atwood et al. (1997) address the example of preventive priorities in the United States with respect to tobacco control. They point out that, because of a lack of political will, the proportion of resources currently allocated to preventing tobacco use does not correspond to the magnitude of the toll that tobacco takes on human health. These authors suggest that public health researchers should pay greater attention to how their work may be used to shape health policy and should consider this issue as integral to the research planning process. Planning a research agenda with findings that will be useful in shaping health policy is certainly one way to increase the social validity of public health research (Geller, 1991), yet it would be unnecessarily restrictive to confine the spectrum of public health research to one that speaks directly to policy issues.

More to the point, the authors in this volume demonstrate that wellness professionals need not remain detached from the political arena; rather, they may be able to dramatically impact community health by mobilizing political will. In fact, it has been suggested that "one of health education's major supportive functions is to enhance self-confidence and provide the variety of skills needed by individuals and their communities to influence the policy-making process" (Tones, 1997,

p. 785). The enormous potential for enhancing the impact of wellness promotion activities through shaping political will is illustrated in the interventions described by Minkler and Wallack in this volume. At the neighborhood level, Minkler (chapter 13) demonstrates that residents of a high-crime neighborhood can be successfully mobilized to lobby for increased police protection and consequently create an environment that facilitates improved health behavior. Although the connection between community crime levels and individual health habits has not been clearly established, there is an intuitive link between, for example, a fear of walking in one's neighborhood and the likelihood of walking for exercise. Moreover, as the chapter by Sanders-Phillips (chapter 11) shows, there is evidence suggesting that being exposed to violence in one's community may induce negative psychological states (e.g., depression, hopelessness, ennui) that act as barriers to the establishment of a healthful lifestyle. The Violence Prevention Initiative (VPI) detailed by Wallack (chapter 19) offers a model of what can be accomplished via advocacy of public policy solutions to public health problems. The tools employed by the VPI toward the goal of reducing the widespread and easy availability of handguns to youth have included savvy use of a scientific and applied database, mobilization of a broad range of constituencies, and strategic use of the mass media. Coordination of these elements has resulted in a number of tangible results, including the passage of numerous local gun-control ordinances and statewide legislation (approved by the California State Legislature but later defeated by governor's veto) banning the sale and distribution of Saturday Night Specials.

The programs described by Minkler and Wallack are unique not only because they appear to succeed but also because they squarely address community-level issues that interfere with the "response-ability" of individuals to remain healthy. It is interesting to note that both of these programs are focused on violence. Whereas the VPI (Wallack) targets primarily potential perpetrators and victims of gun violence, the Tenderloin project (Minkler) addresses the indirect effects of living within a climate characterized by the threat of violence. Both programs, however, address the problem of violence through political influence exerted by members of the community. Together, these programs demonstrate that the future success of health promotion relies on a willingness both to tackle social problems that may in the past have been considered outside the domain of public health and to enlist political strategies in the process.

The focus on violence may reflect the growing concern of the American public with the problem of violent crime, a concern that has led to such legislative developments as the "three strikes" law in California. It may be, therefore, that part of the success of these efforts should be attributed to a preexisting political climate that was hospitable to antiviolence innovations. In this way, then, these programs exemplify how programmatic outcomes may be enhanced when the political climate is not hostile to the intent of the intervention. Recent California gun-related legislative action in the wake of shooting incidents in school and day-care settings further demonstrates that when the political will is galvanized by immediate events, health-promoting legislation may be enacted quite rapidly.

WELLNESS PROMOTION
AND INNOVATIVE METHODOLOGY

In addition to mobilizing political will, another strategy with great potential for enhancing the translation of scientific expertise into wellness promotion is a greater reliance on nontraditional methods in both community and clinical settings. This point is made explicitly by Syme (chapter 4), who contrasts the success of *The Wellness Guide,* an intervention tool heavily influenced by qualitative research methods, with large-scale interventions such as MRFIT that were developed using a "top-down" methodology (i.e., expert driven). The idea that purveyors of health information should become familiar with the beliefs, attitudes, knowledge, and perceived needs of the populations they seek to reach is embodied in the tenets of social marketing (Novelli, 1990). Syme extends this approach to incorporate a consumer-driven perspective to selecting not only the method of intervention delivery but also the intervention content. Thus, the *Guide* that was eventually developed to meet the community's needs actually contained relatively little "health" information. Evaluation of the *Guide* suggests that it was used by the recipients and resulted in significant cognitive and behavioral changes with implications for health. Similarly, the program described by Minkler (chapter 13) evolved as it did because elderly residents of an inner-city neighborhood were given the opportunity to shape the program. As a result, the investigator's resources were directed toward assisting the residents in their efforts to reduce the threat of crime in their neighborhood. Although these programs do not conform to the traditional view of a health promotion intervention, they succeeded in the sense that they were embraced by the target communities, resulted in tangible improvements, and facilitated beneficial behavior changes. These success stories offer considerable fuel to the imperative for wellness promotion professionals to step outside the boundaries of traditional public health paradigms and engage in greater attempts to obtain relevant information from the members of the communities that they seek to serve and to do so quite early during program development.

Innovative methods also can play an important role in program evaluation. Strong program evaluations are critical to the growth of community-based health promotion because they can both identify programs that work and provide clues about the reasons that some programs fail. Birckmayer and Weiss (chapter 7) provide a number of examples in their discussion of theory-based evaluation (TBE), in which the use of process evaluation contributes substantially to the interpretation of program evaluation results. Unlike traditional outcomes-only evaluations, documenting program activities in a process evaluation can permit evaluators to distinguish cases in which an intervention fails because of inadequate theory from cases in which an intervention fails because of inadequate program implementation. Since program evaluation remains a linchpin of wellness promotion, it is paramount that future interventions include this type of approach in order to facilitate effective program development.

Ganiats and Sieber (chapter 12), in their discussion of the complexity involved in attaching monetary values to future health outcomes, offer additional evidence in support of using nontraditional methodology in program evaluation. Policy analysts typically assign a numeric discounting rate to both dollars and health in conducting a standard cost-effectiveness analysis. Unfortunately, since most health promotion programs expend dollars in the present for health outcomes in the future, programs tend to fare poorly in these analyses. As Ganiats and Sieber point out, the value that an individual might place on a future health outcome can vary considerably, depending on personal characteristics and circumstances. Only through careful and population-specific studies is it possible to obtain useful estimates concerning how future health outcomes should be valued for a particular program. These authors suggest, therefore, that the qualitative dimension of time preferences with respect to future health outcomes needs to be better understood in order to permit useful comparisons of cost-effectiveness across programs.

Wellness promotion in the clinical setting also stands to gain from incorporating methods that transcend the traditional medical model. Slavin and Wilkes (chapter 17) address this topic from the perspective of the training provided to physicians. In describing their innovative doctoring curriculum, they emphasize the value of a person-centered diagnostic approach in which physicians consider social facets of patients' health problems. They give the example of detecting domestic violence through patient-centered interviewing techniques and mobilizing community resources to address not only the immediate injury but also the potential for future injury. A person-centered (rather than a disease-centered) approach to medical treatment decisions also is encouraged by Duxbury (chapter 15), who reviews the pros and cons of screening for prostate cancer. The high probability for false positives in prostate cancer screening and the likelihood that quality of life will diminish following surgical intervention combine to argue against the ultimate benefit of screening to the patient. This conclusion rests, however, on the qualitative assessment of alternative treatment outcomes. In a broader discussion of health promotion strategies for the elderly, Beck (chapter 16) also favors a person-centered approach. Specifically, he describes a comprehensive preventive assessment for the elderly that takes into account physical, social, and medical resources and yields a prioritized set of recommendations. These recommendations go far beyond the typical physicians' advice and may include suggestions such as reducing or eliminating a medication, enrolling in a class at a community college, or installing shower rails for the handicapped.

Unlike the traditional biomedical model, which tends to reduce patients to a disease entity and focuses on isolating and eliminating the disease, the patient-centered approach put forth by these authors seeks to optimize functioning and well-being. In order to successfully achieve this goal, clinicians must include qualitative assessment methods in their diagnostic procedures and, similarly, must consider the impact of treatment on the patient as a whole being. This method of evaluating alternatives for patient treatment has been formalized in the General Health Policy Model (GHPM) described by Kaplan (chapter 3). The GHPM uses a standard metric, quality-adjusted life years (QALYs), to compare intervention strategies. Quality-adjusted life years are based on "the current life expectancy adjusted for diminished quality of life associated with dysfunctional states and the duration of stay in each state" (p. 50). A key component of the GHPM is generated by individuals drawn from the general population who rate various health outcomes according to their relative importance. In other words, laypersons assign relative values to a series of health outcomes in order to quantify their feelings about various states of disability. Consequently, treatment decisions based on the GHPM are informed by the qualitative dimension of alternative outcomes. All the innovative approaches described by Slavin and Wilkes, Beck, Duxbury, and Kaplan consider the impact of medical intervention on the patient as a functioning person (rather than as a host to a disease) as a factor in treatment decisions. This humanistic framework offers great potential for maximizing patients' health in the face of disease. The future of wellness promotion as an aspect of medical care relies on the institutionalization of these types of innovative approaches in clinical settings.

A MODEL INTERVENTION

The various interventions reported by Syme, Minkler, and Wallack, described previously, illustrate what may be accomplished when program planners are receptive to input from the target community and are willing to engage in activities outside the parameters of what has traditionally been considered health promotion. Similarly, The Smokers' Helpline, a smoking cessation program detailed by Zhu and Anderson (chapter 14), represents a novel intervention that is based on extensive qualitative study of the target population. In addition, the Smokers' Helpline has achieved a unique hybridization of the clinical approach with the public health approach to give rise to a highly efficacious—and effective—program.

The Helpline is unusual in several ways. The menu of services offered to smokers who call the Helpline is one key element to the marriage between a population-based reach (the public health approach) and intensive one-on-one treatment (the clinical approach). Also critical is the proactive strategy in which Helpline counselors follow up on initial calls rather than waiting for smokers to call back to begin counseling. A third component that distinguishes the Helpline is the scheduling of counseling sessions such that more sessions occur during the time with the greatest probability of relapse. The availability of counseling in several languages contributes as well to the Helpline's success. Ultimately, of course, dissemination of the Helpline's toll-free numbers is critical and has been accomplished by including the numbers in ads funded by the Tobacco Control Section of the California Department of Health and by establishing partnerships with primary care physicians.

Although not explicitly, the Smokers' Helpline also acts as a model of a health promotion intervention that works within the political context to further its effectiveness. As explained by Zhu and Anderson, the Helpline was funded through the monies generated by Proposition 99, the California Tobacco Tax Initiative. This proposition was an expression of Californians' support for interventions that would reduce the health threat of tobacco use. Unlike the effort to restrict public smoking, however, the Helpline has not encountered organized political resistance. Very likely, this tacit acceptance stems from the congruence between the conservative point of view that individuals should take responsibility for their own health and behavior and the Helpline's focus on assisting smokers in their own attempts to quit. Even the tobacco industry would be hard-pressed to muster an argument against providing smokers with assistance toward quitting. Consequently, the Helpline has enjoyed a sort of political immunity that has provided room for its growth and success.

WELLNESS PROMOTION
AND INTERVENTION LEVERAGE POINTS

A number of the chapters presented in this volume exemplify an approach to promoting human wellness based on the strategy of identifying high-impact leverage points for intervention. In this approach to health promotion, the goal is to identify and make use of "certain behaviors, social roles, and situational conditions [that] can exert a disproportionate influence on personal and collective well-being" (Stokols, 1996, p. 291). East (chapter 8) identifies one such high-impact leverage point in her discussion of the increased risk for pregnancy among younger sisters of childbearing teens. Specifically, she explains how both the indirect effect generated by sisters' shared family and community environment and the direct effect on younger sisters of having an older sister with a child (e.g., orientation to child-rearing, witnessing of social status attributed to the older sister) combine to place younger sisters of childbearing teens at elevated risk for teen pregnancy. East's research points to the potential impact on teen pregnancy rates that might be brought about through interventions targeting these younger sisters of childbearing teens.

In a somewhat different approach to identifying potential leverage points for health promotion, Guendelman (chapter 9) identifies attributes that may bring about desirable birth outcomes among immigrant mothers. She first describes a paradox wherein immigrants from Mexico and Southeast Asia experience more favorable birth outcomes than would be expected on the basis of their socioeconomic status. She posits that these surprising findings may reflect health-promoting cultural factors, including salutary dietary habits, strong social cohesion, and relatively low substance abuse. Guendelman's approach suggests that wellness promotion should focus not only on intervening to reduce risk factors for disease but also on encouraging attributes associated with more positive health outcomes.

Like Guendelman, Roach (chapter 10) employs an analysis of epidemiologic data to explore an issue of inequity in health outcomes. In this case, the focus is on disentangling the influence of race from that of environmental and behavioral factors associated with race. Through his examination of differential cancer mortality in Blacks versus Whites, Roach calls into question the medical community's adherence to certain disease categorization systems that may mask differences in the extent of disease on diagnosis by a physician. Roach's scrutiny of the data suggests that, by using a grouping scheme that does not differentiate finely enough between stages of cancers, researchers and clinicians may be overlooking the underlying reasons for greater cancer mortality among Blacks. The implication of Roach's argument is that identification of effective leverage points for ameliorating the cancer epidemic will require altering current clinical diagnostic categories and looking beyond race to modifiable variables that may increase the risk of dying from cancer. The more general lesson to be taken from Roach's argument is that clinical diagnostic categories may artificially obscure important differences between patients and that these differences may provide clues for primary or secondary disease prevention.

Another technique for promoting wellness through identifying critical leverage points is to specify a particular context within which individuals may be affected by an intervention and then design a program for that context. Nader offers an example of this strategy in his description of the school-based CATCH intervention (chapter 18). Schools often have been put forth as locales within which children may be reached and effectively influenced to enhance their health. Nader adds to this traditional perspective the proposition that partnerships between universities and schools yield mutually beneficial avenues for promoting children's health. Such partnerships can offer valuable field experience to university students, supply meaningful data to university-based researchers, and bring about positive changes in behavior among schoolchildren. Thus, the partnership between the university and schools may be a potent leverage point both for improving community health directly and for enhancing the education of individuals who will be in a position to influence community health at the conclusion of their training.

CONCLUSIONS

Whether addressing the question of who should be targeted, what to target, or where an intervention should be delivered, identifying optimal leverage points should be a priority in wellness promotion. It has been suggested, for example, that the primary task for those interested in promoting human wellness is to "set up the conditions that optimize health . . . [including] such naively elementary ideas as abolishing war, meeting basic needs (not wants) and redistributing the wealth of the planet" (Duhl, 1996, p. 261). More specifically, Syme (chapter 4) states that the most critical factors related to health are problems of inequity and that, therefore, all available energy should be devoted toward minimizing the unequal distributions of resources within the society of the United States. This goal is perhaps so daunting to most individuals that it may induce a sense of helplessness. In fact, however, there are many specific instances of inequity in American society that appear more vulnerable to influence when viewed independently. Access to health care services is one issue frequently mentioned in discussions of inequity and health. Many factors contribute to the fact that some people have greater and easier access to health care than others. Lack of insurance, transportation, child care, or language skills are but a few of the barriers that can prevent individuals from receiving health care. These impediments are very real and quite prevalent. Nevertheless, one example in this volume— the Smokers' Helpline—demonstrates a program in which all these problems have been minimized. The smoking cessation program is funded through cigarette tax dollars, thus eliminating the need for health insurance. The program is administered via telephone, which does away with the need for transportation or child care. Finally, the service is available in several languages to accommodate non-English speakers and allow some tailoring to specific cross-cultural concerns, such as issues of confidentiality. It would be naive to suggest that similarly elegant solutions could be found for the great host of health care services that are available to some and not to others. Still, it is encouraging to note that in at least one case technology, legislation, and innovative programming have been synthesized into a service that is available free of charge to the great majority of California residents.

The present volume aims to stimulate progressive action in the well-ness field that speaks to the several themes outlined in this introduction (i.e., consideration of the political context and mobilization of political will, deployment of nontraditional assessment and intervention strategies, and identification and appropriate exploitation of high-impact leverage points). There are a number of specific topic areas both within and outside the sphere of traditional public health that are not covered in this collection and that have clear implications for health. For example, there are dramatic contrasts in the quality of schooling provided to the nation's youth. Since education level is quite strongly predictive of various health behaviors as well as of overall health status, it would be appropriate for those interested in improving the health of Americans to turn attention toward equalizing educational opportunities. Other areas that are not featured in this volume include work-site health promotion, unintentional injuries (e.g., vehicular accidents), and substance abuse. The reader should bear in mind that this volume is not intended to be a comprehensive review of the wellness field; rather, it attempts to motivate innovation within the field by drawing attention to topics that have received inadequate attention by wellness researchers and practitioners until now.

This introduction has attempted to highlight some of these previously underemphasized themes. The necessity of adopting a systems perspective toward wellness promotion, the value added by innovative assessment strategies, and the utility of considering political influences as a force in health promotion are acknowledged in these pages by physicians, sociologists, psychologists, biomedical researchers, and those whose training is grounded in the field of public health. That so many disparate disciplines find common ground with regard to wellness promotion is further evidence that the complex web that defines the field reaches into multiple academic domains and requires an interdisciplinary effort to understand the relevant issues and devise appropriately elegant solutions. It should therefore not be surprising that the varied works presented here do in fact share a great deal of overlap in terms of the underlying messages regarding using a multifactorial approach to wellness, examining wellness issues in context, and targeting intervention points that are maximally effective. With these tenets as guidelines, the future of human wellness promotion promises to be replete with innovative solutions to old problems, with rapid responses to new problems, and with greater synergy between existing strategies for coping with ongoing problems. The current trajectory of the field thus holds great potential for improving the health of our nation and its constituent populations.

REFERENCES

American Public Health Association. (1998). AIDS panel chastises administration for inaction on needle exchange. *The Nation's Health,* April, 1.

Atwood, K., Colditz, G. A., and Kawachi, I. (1997). From public health science to prevention policy: Placing science in its social and political contexts. *American Journal of Public Health* 87, 1603–1606.

Detels, R., and Breslow, L. (1997). Current scope and concerns in public health. In R. Detels, W. Holland, J. McEwen, and G. S. Omenn, eds., *Oxford Textbook of Public Health.* Pp. 3–17. New York: Oxford University Press.

Duhl, L. J. (1996). An ecohistory of health: The role of "Healthy Cities." *American Journal of Health Promotion* 10, 258–261.

Geller, E. S. (1991). Where's the validity in social validity? *Journal of Applied Behavior Analysis* 24, 189–204.

Green, L., Simons-Morton, D., and Potvin, L. (1997). Education and life-style determinants of health and disease. In R. Detels, W. Holland, J. McEwen, and G. S. Omenn, eds., *Oxford Textbook of Public Health.* Pp. 125–137. New York: Oxford University Press.

Holland, W. W. (1997). Overview of politics and strategies. In R. Detels, W. Holland, J. McEwen, and G. S. Omenn, eds., *Oxford Textbook of Public Health.* Pp. 239–243. New York: Oxford University Press.

Novelli, W. D. (1990). Applying social marketing to health promotion and disease prevention. In K. Glanz, F. M. Lewis, and B. Rimer, eds., *Health Behavior and Health Education: Theory, Research and Practice.* Pp. 342–369. San Francisco: Jossey-Bass.

Richmond, J. B., and Kotelchuck, M. (1983). Political influences: Rethinking national health policy. In C. McGuire, R. Foley, A. Gorr, et al., eds., *Handbook of Health Professions Education.* Pp. 386–404. San Francisco: Jossey-Bass.

Stokols, D. (1996). Translating social ecological theory into guidelines for community health promotion. *American Journal of Health Promotion* 10, 282–298.

Tones, K. (1997). Health education, behavior change, and the public health. In R. Detels, W. Holland, J. McEwen, and G. S. Omenn, eds., *Oxford Textbook of Public Health.* Pp. 783–814. New York: Oxford University Press.

Wandersman, A., Valois, R., Ochs, L., et al. (1996). Toward a social ecology of community coalitions. *American Journal of Health Promotion* 10, 299–307.

PART ONE

NEW DIRECTIONS
IN HUMAN WELLNESS PROMOTION

The chapters in part 1 introduce a trend toward innovation in the field of human wellness and present both general paradigms and specific examples of the multidimensional and person-centered perspective on wellness promotion. Stokols (chapter 1) describes an emerging paradigm of wellness promotion, traces the societal developments that have prompted greater interest in wellness promotion since the 1970s, and highlights the challenge and value of developing broader-gauged and more comprehensive wellness promotion strategies for the future. Breslow (chapter 2) continues this line of argument and focuses specifically on the need to incorporate the social context as a factor in wellness promotion planning and intervention. Strohman (chapter 5) expands the discussion in an unusual direction with his examination of the role of genetics in human wellness. He argues for a greater appreciation of the complex interrelationships between the genome and both micro- and macroenvironments in the determination of phenotypic expressions related to health. Finally, Kaplan (chapter 3) and Syme (chapter 4) provide concrete examples of the types of programs that can emerge from a more integrative paradigm of wellness. Kaplan describes an alternative model for evaluating medical interventions based on "quality of life years," that is, treatment outcome in terms of both extending the duration of life and improving the quality of life. Kaplan's General Health Policy Model yields a different order of priorities for medical procedures than the traditional approach of valuing interventions solely in terms of effect on longevity. This alternative system of prioritizing reflects the effect of medical intervention on quality of life and suggests that population health status might be enhanced if resources were shifted away from procedure-based reimbursement toward primary prevention. Finally, Syme focuses on community-based wellness interventions and follows a synopsis of noted failures in this area with more encouraging information about several successes employing nontraditional approaches. In particular, he presents initial findings from a theory-based evaluation of *The Wellness Guide,* a printed community resource guide distributed to mothers on the Women, Infants, and Children (WIC) program. These and other data provide fuel for his advice that wellness professionals "should learn from the mistakes of the past . . . to be creative and inventive enough to become experts in the role of not being experts." Thus, as a whole, part 1 functions as a rallying call to the wellness field to step outside the lines of traditional wellness programming and think creatively about new means for promoting human wellness at both the individual and the community level.

Daniel Stokols

THE SOCIAL ECOLOGICAL
PARADIGM OF WELLNESS PROMOTION

INTRODUCTION

Prior to the 1970s, efforts to improve individual and population health focused almost entirely on the medical treatment of disease. The concepts of health promotion and wellness were little known, and financial investment in preventive health care was quite limited, accounting for only 2.5% of the nation's annual health care expenditures during the early 1970s (Brennan, 1982).

Less than three decades later, societal commitment to disease prevention strategies has increased dramatically. Local, state, and federal governments have enacted public policies designed to curtail individuals' use of tobacco products, protect workers' safety, and reduce driving-related injuries and fatalities (Breslow and Johnson, 1993; Pertschuk and Shopland, 1989; Wells et al., 1997; Williams et al., 1983). Businesses and managed care organizations have invested substantial funds toward the development and implementation of disease prevention programs (Fielding and Piserchia, 1989; Satcher and Hull, 1995; U.S. Public Health Service, 1992, 1993). In 1996, the U.S. Food and Drug Administration successfully imposed regulatory constraints on the sale and distribution of cigarettes and smokeless tobacco products to minors (U.S. Food and Drug Administration, 1996). It is likely that even more stringent regulatory constraints on the production and sale of tobacco products will be enacted at state and federal levels during the coming years (*Newsweek*, 1998).

The burgeoning interest in disease prevention and health promotion over the past 30 years has been prompted by several societal develop-ments and concerns. During the 1960s, the U.S. surgeon general's re-ports on smoking and health and the health consequences of smoking (U.S. Public Health Service, 1964, 1967) gave official, widespread recog-nition to the fact that a behavioral factor, cigarette smoking, is a cause of cancer and other serious diseases. Additional evidence for the links between smoking behavior and lung cancer was presented in the *Surgeon General's Report on Health Promotion and Disease Prevention* (U.S. Public Health Service, 1979), which declared that "cigarette smok-ing is the single most important preventable cause of death" (p. 7). In recent years, other developments—including the exponential rise in national health expenditures, growing concerns about the deficiencies of the medical care system, heated debates about health care reform, evidence for the health and financial benefits of disease prevention programs, and growing use of unconventional or "alternative" medical therapies among both physicians and the lay public—brought the con-cepts of wellness and health promotion programming to the forefront of the national agenda (Breslow and Johnson, 1993; Eisenberg et al., 1993; Fielding and Halfon, 1994; Fries et al., 1993; Satcher and Hull, 1995; Schauffler, 1993; Weiss, 1991).

Several scientific studies have documented the substantial health ben-efits and financial savings associated with disease prevention and health promotion programs (DeJoy and Wilson, 1995; O'Donnell and Harris, 1994; Pelletier, 1996; Stokols et al., 1995). Effective wellness promotion strategies include employee health risk appraisal, counseling, and life-style change programs (Erfurt et al., 1991; Fries et al., 1994), cultural change strategies within organizational settings (Allen and Allen, 1986; Bellingham, 1990), and the provision of clinical preventive services to enhance maternal and child health (Thompson et al., 1995; U.S. Pre-ventive Services Task Force, 1989). A mid-decade review of progress to-ward meeting the *Healthy People 2000* goals in the United States found substantial reductions in adult use of tobacco products and in alcohol-related automobile deaths and moderate gains in the proportion of adults exercising regularly and eating less fatty diets (McGinnis and Lee, 1995). Also, the proportion of workplaces providing health pro-motion programs for their employees increased significantly between the mid-1980s and early 1990s (U.S. Department of Health and Human Services, 1992).

Although many health promotion programs have been effective, oth-ers have failed or achieved only limited success. For example, although employers have made substantial efforts to bring their workplaces into compliance with state and federal regulations aimed at reducing occupational injuries and illnesses, the adverse health and economic impacts of work-related conditions continue to be enormous. In 1995, occupational injuries accounted for $121 billion in lost wages and administrative and health care costs (Rosenstock, Olenac, and Wagner, 1998). Moreover, even the best-designed work-site health promotion programs reach only a small proportion of the total workforce. Participants in these programs tend to be healthier, better paid, more educated, and more motivated to change their health habits than nonparticipants (DeJoy and Wilson, 1995; O'Donnell and Harris, 1994). Further, lifestyle-change programs that focus narrowly on modifying specific health behaviors often neglect the contextual circumstances that lead to high relapse and attrition rates once the interventions have ended (Marlatt and Gordon, 1985; Prochaska et al., 1992). In addition, certain health risks such as exposure to community violence, obesity, teen pregnancy, substance abuse, financial barriers to medical and preventive services, and lack of adequate health insurance remain "segmented in pockets of heightened prevalence" (Fisher, 1995), particularly among low-income and minority groups in the population (Adler et al., 1994; Fontanarosa, 1995; Margen and Lashof, this volume's afterword; McGinnis and Lee, 1995; Satcher and Hull, 1995).

To improve the health of vulnerable populations and reduce the self-selection biases and attrition rates associated with many intervention programs, broader-gauged strategies of health promotion will be required that combine behavioral, organizational, environmental, regulatory, and political initiatives to alleviate community sources of illness and injury (Atwood et al., 1997; Montes et al., 1995; Winkleby, 1994; Winett et al., 1989). The limitations of earlier disease prevention and health promotion programs, noted previously, highlight the need for a major paradigm shift away from narrowly focused interventions aimed primarily at changing individuals' health behavior toward more comprehensive formulations that address the interdependencies among socioeconomic, cultural, political, environmental, organizational, psychological, and biological determinants of health and illness (Richmond and Kotelchuck, 1991; Schneider Jamner, this volume's introduction; Stokols, 1996; Winett et al., 1989).

Researchers in the field of public health have recognized for many years that patterns of health and illness are closely linked to a variety of sociocultural, political, and physical-environmental conditions within communities (Breslow, 1996; Cassel, 1964; Catalano, 1979; Detels and Breslow, 1997; Durkheim, 1951; McKinlay, 1975; Syme, chapter 4). The "new public health" outlined in the Ottawa Charter gave explicit emphasis to social causes of illness, above and beyond the physical-environmental health threats that exist in certain communities (Kickbush, 1989; Ottawa Charter for Health Promotion, 1986). The social ecological paradigm for health promotion extends these earlier notions by providing a set of conceptual and methodological principles, drawn largely from systems theory, for organizing comprehensive, community-based health promotion programs (Emery and Trist, 1972; Green and Ottoson, 1994; McLeroy et al., 1988; Miller, 1978; Moos, 1979).

The next section of the chapter outlines some of the developments, both in the field of public health and in society as a whole, that have led to the development of a broader, more integrative approach to wellness promotion—the *social ecological model*—which emphasizes the joint influence of behavior and environment on wellness rather than focusing exclusively on either category of health-determining factors.

SCIENTIFIC AND SOCIETAL
ORIGINS OF WELLNESS PROMOTION

We live in an era in which the dominant causes of morbidity and mortality are strongly linked to human behavior at the individual, community, and government levels (Detels et al., 1997). A crucial challenge for the 21st century is to develop programs and policies that will establish health-promotive environments at local, regional, and global levels—those that minimize individuals' exposure to health-threatening conditions and support their efforts to promote personal and collective wellness. The enormity of this task stems from the complex web of health-determining factors that impinge on individuals, organizations, and whole communities. Although these complexities make the task of promoting human wellness seem rather daunting, the "small wins" approach to social problems (Weick, 1984) suggests that as incremental health promotion and environmental protection strategies are adopted in local communities, they can exert a positive, albeit gradual, influence on population health.

Essential prerequisites for developing effective environmental design and public policy programs to create healthful surroundings are sound theoretical analyses of key concepts such as "health," "wellness," "wellness promotion," and "healthy environments." A review of the relevant research literature on topics such as health promotion, environmental stress, and environmental risk assessment, however, reveals important gaps in our understanding of these issues. For example, health is often defined in individualistic and physicalistic terms with explicit emphasis on "soundness of body or mind and freedom from disease or ailment" (*Webster's*, 1989). Analyses that define health simply as the absence of personal illness or injury, however, give little or no consideration to issues of collective well-being (e.g., social cohesion and sense of community; cf. Sarason, 1974) and optimal states of wellness (e.g., strong feelings of personal commitment to one's social and physical milieu; cf. Pelletier, 1994). The term "wellness" is used in this volume to refer to the broader conception of health, which encompasses not only the absence of illness symptoms but also very positive states of well-being.

The terms "disease prevention" and "health protection" have been used to describe various medical and public health strategies aimed at preventing the onset of physical and mental illness (e.g., inoculation against infectious diseases, enhanced community sanitation services, reduction of workplace hazards, and governmental regulation of food and drug safety). The concepts of health or wellness promotion, however, differ from the disease prevention orientation in that they place greater emphasis on the role of individuals, groups, and organizations as active agents in shaping health practices and policies to optimize both individual and collective well-being (e.g., U.S. Public Health Service, 1979, 1991; Williams, 1982; Winett et al., 1989; World Health Organization, 1984).

The majority of health promotion programs implemented in corporate and community settings have focused on changing individuals rather than their environments, organizations, or institutions. That is, they have been designed to modify individuals' health habits and lifestyles (e.g., exercise and dietary regimens) rather than to provide environmental resources and interventions that promote enhanced well-being (e.g., installation of improved ventilation systems within buildings to enhance indoor air quality, design of safe stairways to reduce falls and injuries, modification of agricultural machinery to reduce occupational injuries, and provision of insurance coverage for preventive risk-factor screenings among the elderly). Much recent research, however, suggests the potential value of environmental and institutional interventions as an adjunct to behaviorally oriented health promotion programs (e.g., Archea, 1985; Archea and Connell, 1986; Beck, chapter 16; Green and Kreuter, 1990;

Greenberg, 1986; Hedge, 1989; Karasek and Theorell, 1990; Lawrence, 1990; Mendell and Smith, 1990; Robertson, 1986; Schenker, chapter 21; Syme, 1990; Williams, 1982; Winett et al., 1989).

CONCEPTUAL ORIENTATION AND SCOPE

The chapters in this volume reflect recent efforts to develop broader and more comprehensive strategies for promoting human wellness. These strategies recognize the multiplicity of factors that influence personal and collective well-being and emphasize the multidisciplinary foundations of scientific research, professional practice, and health policy analysis in the field of wellness promotion. Taken together, these chapters reflect several themes that are intrinsic to the social ecological paradigm as a basis for understanding the community and environmental origins of public health problems and for organizing disease prevention and wellness promotion programs that can effectively ameliorate those problems. Specifically, the chapters in this volume highlight the following:

1.   The advantages of implementing disease prevention and wellness promotion programs that target multiple health risks and illnesses (e.g., cancer, cardiovascular disease, AIDS and HIV, unintentional injuries, and community violence) rather than focusing narrowly on singular disease categories

2.   The strategic value of identifying and reducing threats to public health at several community levels and in the context of multiple settings (e.g., residential settings, schools, workplaces, and health care facilities)

3.   The well-documented links among poverty, minority status, and susceptibility to disease and the importance of targeting vulnerable groups in the population for preventive services and wellness programs

4.   The advantages of combining multiple strategies of disease prevention and wellness promotion (e.g., lifestyle change, health education, medical practice, environmental enhancement, media campaigns, and regulatory initiatives) within comprehensive health promotion programs

5.   The challenge of rigorously evaluating the health benefits, cost-effectiveness, and sustainability of alternative disease prevention and wellness promotion programs

A major goal of this chapter is to delineate the core theoretical and programmatic assumptions that underlie the social ecological approach to wellness promotion and the ways in which these assumptions are relevant to the research and intervention programs described in several chapters of this volume.

THE SOCIAL ECOLOGY OF HEALTH PROMOTION: CORE ASSUMPTIONS

The term "ecology" pertains broadly to the interrelations between organisms and their environments (Hawley, 1950). From its early roots in biology, the ecological paradigm has evolved within several disciplines (e.g., sociology, psychology, economics, and public health) to provide a general framework for understanding the nature of people's transactions with their physical and sociocultural surroundings (e.g., Barker, 1968; Cassel, 1964; Catalano, 1979; Park and Burgess, 1925; Rogers-Warren and Warren, 1977). The field of social ecology gives greater attention to the social, institutional, and cultural contexts of people-environment relations than did earlier versions of human ecology, which were more closely oriented to biological processes and the geographic environment (e.g., Alihan, 1964; Binder et al., 1975; Michelson, 1970). The social ecological perspective encompasses certain core assumptions about the dynamics of human health and the development of effective strategies to promote personal and collective well-being. These assumptions are outlined here.

First, the healthfulness of a situation and the well-being of its participants are assumed to be influenced by multiple facets of both the physical environment (e.g., geography, architecture, and technology) and the social environment (e.g., culture, economics, and politics). Moreover, the health status of individuals and groups is influenced not only by environmental factors but also by a variety of personal attributes, including genetic heritage, psychological dispositions, and behavioral patterns. Thus, efforts to promote human well-being should be based on an understanding of the dynamic interplay among diverse environmental and personal factors rather than on analyses that focus exclusively on environmental, biological, or behavioral factors (cf. Moos, 1979; Stokols, 1996). For example, chapter 5 by Strohman highlights the joint influence of individuals' genetic heritage and the social environment on their susceptibility to various illnesses. Also, Minkler's research demonstrates the value of community organizing techniques aimed at ameliorating health-threatening conditions in a residential area (e.g., the threat of street crime and violence) as a basis for enhancing the health-promotive behavior of elderly neighborhood members. And Margen and Lashof emphasize the ways in which poverty, inequality of income distribution, and minority status jointly undermine the health of individuals and vulnerable subgroups in the population.

Second, analyses of health and health promotion should address the multidimensional and complex nature of human environments. As noted previously, environments can be described in terms of their physical and social components, but they also can be characterized in terms of their objective (actual) or subjective (perceived) qualities and their scale or immediacy to individuals and groups (proximal vs. distal). Furthermore, environments can be described as an array of independent attributes (e.g., lighting, temperature, noise, space arrangement, and group size) or in terms of the composite relationships among several features, as exemplified by constructs such as behavior settings, person-environment fit, and social climate (Stokols, 1987). The highly variegated nature of human environments has direct implications for the design and evaluation of health promotion programs, as illustrated by several of the chapters in this volume. For example, chapter 9 by Guendelman highlights the diversity of environmental factors that affect pregnancy outcomes in immigrant and nonimmigrant populations, including the level of social support available to individuals, the nutritional content of their diet, and the quality and availability of prenatal care. Schenker's chapter similarly illustrates the multiple environmental factors that influence agricultural workers' health, including their levels of exposure to sunlight, pesticides, and unsafe equipment. And the chapters by Stanton, Danoff-Burg, and Gallant; Roach; and Villablanca reveal the subtle ways in which societal and cultural values influence the direction and funding of health research programs and sometimes lead to racially, culturally, and gender-biased interpretations of research findings.

Third, just as environments can be described in terms of their relative scale and complexity, the participants in those environments can be studied at varying levels ranging from individuals, small groups, and organizations to larger communities and populations. Rather than focusing solely on individuals or aggregates, the social ecological perspective incorporates multiple levels of analysis and diverse methodologies (e.g., medical exams, questionnaires, behavioral observations, environmental recordings, and epidemiologic analyses) for assessing the healthfulness of settings and the well-being of individuals and groups. For example, chapter 7 by Birckmayer and Weiss shows that the evaluation of well-ness promotion programs can employ many types of measures at different levels of intervention, from indices of individual attitude and behavior change to measures of the health impacts of organizational policy changes. The chapters by Syme and Schneider Jamner also note that evaluations of community-based wellness promotion programs, ideally, should incorporate qualitative as well as quantitative measures to provide a more complete assessment of intervention outcomes.

Moreover, the social ecological perspective assumes that the effectiveness of health promotion programs can be enhanced through the coordination of individuals and groups acting at different levels, for example, family members who make efforts to improve their health practices, corporate managers who shape organizational health policies, and public health officials who supervise community health services (e.g., Green and Kreuter, 1990; Pelletier, 1984; Winett et al., 1989). Accordingly, chapter 24 by Waldo and Coates suggests that HIV and AIDS prevention efforts should engage multiple social units to promote health-enhancing behavioral changes, including individuals, small groups, organizations, and community decision-making groups. The chapter by East highlights the influential role of childbearing teens in shaping the sexual practices and likelihood of unwanted pregnancy among their younger sisters, and that by Nader underscores the value of collaborative partnerships linking universities with other community groups as a basis for promoting wellness among children and their families.

Fourth, the social ecological perspective incorporates a variety of concepts derived from systems theory (e.g., interdependence, homeostasis, negative feedback, and deviation amplification; see Cannon, 1932; Emery and Trist, 1972; Katz and Kahn, 1966; Maruyama, 1963) to understand the dynamic interrelations between people and their environments. Thus, people-environment transactions are characterized by cycles of mutual influence whereby the physical and social features of settings directly influence their occupants' health, and, concurrently, the participants in settings modify the healthfulness of their surroundings through their individual and collective actions. These cycles of mutual influence between individuals and their environments are evident in chapter 11 by Sanders-Phillips, showing that individuals' routine exposure to community violence leads to feelings of disempowerment, helplessness, and depression, which in turn preclude their efforts to adopt health promotive practices related to dietary improvement and physical activity. Similarly,

Duxbury's chapter shows that wellness among the elderly depends on the degree of fit between individuals' functional abilities on the one hand and environmental constraints on their daily activities on the other. Either or both of these elements can be modified to promote higher levels of person-environment fit (cf. Lawton, 1999).

Moreover, the social ecological model views human environments as complex systems in which local settings and organizations are nested within more complex and remote regions. Accordingly, efforts to promote human well-being must take into account the interdependencies that exist among immediate and more distant environments. For example, the occupational health and safety of community work settings are directly influenced by state and national ordinances aimed at protecting environmental quality and public health (cf. Schenker, chapter 21). Similarly, research conducted as part of the Violence Prevention Initiative in California (Wallack, chapter 19; Wintemute, 1992) demonstrates the substantial impact of public policies (especially those regulating the production and sale of firearms) in lowering rates of community violence, injury, and homicide. Additionally, Hofmann (chapter 20) contends that managed care policy reforms guaranteeing age-appropriate health care to teenagers would be one of the most effective strategies for reducing unwanted teen pregnancies and abortions.

Finally, owing to the complexity of human environments and an explicit emphasis on multilevel and multimethod analyses of behavior, the social ecological perspective is inherently interdisciplinary in its approach to health research and the development of health promotion programs. The ecological perspective draws on the fields of medicine and public health, as well as the behavioral and social sciences, in the study and promotion of human well-being. The chapter authors represented in this volume, for example, bring a wide range of disciplinary training and perspectives to the field of wellness promotion, including molecular genetics, medicine, epidemiology, psychology, sociology, anthropology, and economics. Moreover, social ecological approaches to wellness promotion link the community-wide, preventive strategies and epidemiologic orientation of public health with the individual-level, therapeutic and curative strategies of medicine. For example, the California Smokers' Helpline described in chapter 14 by Zhu and Anderson epitomizes a health-promotive intervention that combines the broad scope and "reach" of a statewide public health program with the intensity of a more personalized clinical intervention. Similarly, the medical education programs described in chapter 17 by Slavin and Wilkes introduce physicians to a variety of public health and behavioral medicine concepts and train them to be more effective change agents for promoting wellness among their patients.

The social ecological perspective also incorporates the behavioral and social science emphases on (1) the active role played by individuals and groups in modifying their own health behavior and well-being, (2) the development and testing of theoretical models describing people-environment transactions, and (3) the importance of conducting evaluative studies to assess the cost-effectiveness and social impact of wellness promotion programs (e.g., Cassel, 1964; Engel, 1976; Evans, 1988; Ganiats and Sieber, chapter 12; Henderson and Scutchfield, 1989; Kaplan, chapter 3; Schwartz, 1982; Williams, 1982; Winett et al., 1989). For example, the statewide *Wellness Guide* described in chapter 4 by Syme exemplifies a community-level intervention whose development and evaluation were guided by psychological and sociological theories of the links between personal and community empowerment on the one hand and the likelihood and efficacy of individuals' health-promotive behavior on the other.

The core assumptions and themes inherent in ecological approaches to wellness promotion are elaborated on in subsequent chapters of the volume. For example, the multiple dimensions of environments and the ways in which they are related to individual and collective well-being are examined in the chapter by Stokols in part 1. The interactions among several categories of environmental and personal determinants of health also are discussed in that chapter. Moreover, social ecological perspectives on health suggest that the effectiveness of wellness promotion efforts can be enhanced through multilevel intervention "packages" (Geller, 1987; Weiss, 1991; Williams, 1982; Winett et al., 1989) combining both behavioral and environmental modification strategies. Thus, chapter 16 by Beck describes a multifaceted intervention for promoting wellness among the elderly that includes a social, medical, and environmental assessment, followed by the provision of specific recommendations for individual behavior change and environmental modifications (e.g., installation of handrails in bathrooms to prevent falls).

Taken together, the chapters in this volume highlight the growing importance of developing more integrative and broader-gauged strategies for promoting human wellness. The principles of social ecology outlined here and elaborated on in subsequent chapters provide a valuable foundation for establishing more integrative and effective approaches to wellness promotion research, practice, and policy during the 21st century.

NOTES

The author thanks Dr. Margaret Schneider Jamner for her helpful comments on an earlier version of the chapter.

REFERENCES

Adler, N. E., Boyce, T., Chesney, M. A., et al. (1994). Socioeconomic status and health: The challenge of the gradient. *American Psychologist* 49, 15–24.

Alihan, M. A. (1964). Social ecology: A critical analysis. New York: Cooper Square Publishers.

Allen, J., and Allen, R. F. (1986). Achieving health promotion objectives through cultural change systems. *American Journal of Health Promotion* 1, 42–49.

Archea, J. C. (1985). Environmental factors associated with stair accidents by the elderly. *Clinics in Geriatric Medicine* 1, 555–569.

Archea, J., and Connell, B. R. (1986). Architecture as an instrument of public health: Mandating practice prior to the conduct of systematic inquiry. In H. Wineman, R. Barnes, and C. Zimring, eds., *Proceedings of the seventeenth annual conference of the Environmental Design Research Association*. Pp. 305–309. Washington, D.C.: Environmental Design Research Association.

Atwood, K., Colditz, G. A., and Kawachi, I. (1997). From public health science to prevention policy: Placing science in its social and political contexts. *American Journal of Public Health* 87, 1603–1606.

Barker, R. G. (1968). *Ecological psychology: Concepts and methods for studying the environment of human behavior.* Stanford, Calif.: Stanford University Press.

Bellingham, R. (1990). Debunking the myth of individual health promotion. In M. E. Scofield, ed., *Occupational medicine: Worksite health promotion.* Pp. 665–675. Philadelphia: Hanley and Belfus.

Binder, A., Stokols, D., and Catalano, R. (1975). Social ecology: An emerging multidiscipline. *Journal of Environmental Education* 7, 32–43.

Brennan, A. J. (1982). Health promotion: What's in it for business and industry? *Health Education Quarterly* 9, 9–19.

Breslow, L. (1996). Social ecological strategies for promoting healthy lifestyles. *American Journal of Health Promotion* 10, 253–257.

Breslow, L., and Johnsen, M. (1993). California's Proposition 99 on tobacco and its impact. *Annual Review of Public Health* 14, 585–604.

Cannon, W. B. (1932). *The wisdom of the body.* New York: W. W. Norton.

Cassel, J. (1964). Social science theory as a source of hypotheses in epidemiological research. *American Journal of Public Health* 54, 1482–1487.

Catalano, R. (1979). *Health, behavior, and the community: An ecological perspective.* Elmsford, N.Y.: Pergamon Press.

DeJoy, D. M., and Wilson, M. G., eds. (1995). *Critical issues in worksite health promotion.* Boston: Allyn and Bacon.

Detels, R., Holland, W. W., McEwen, J., and Omenn, G. S., eds. (1997). *Oxford textbook of public health: Volumes 1, 2, 3.* 3rd ed. New York: Oxford University Press.

Detels, R., and Breslow, L. (1997). Current scope and concerns in public health. In R. Detels, W. W. Holland, J. McEwen, and G. Omenn, eds., *Oxford textbook of public health, Volume 1: The scope of public health.* 3rd ed. Pp. 3–17. New York: Oxford University Press.

Durkheim, E. (1951). *Suicide: A study in sociology.* New York: The Free Press.

Eisenberg, D. M., Kessler, R. C., Foster, C., et al. (1993). Unconventional medicine in the United States. *New England Journal of Medicine* 328, 246–252.

Emery, F. E., and Trist, E. L. (1972). *Towards a social ecology: Contextual appreciations of the future in the present.* London: Plenum Press.

Engel, G. L. (1976). The need for a new medical model. *Science* 196, 129–136.

Erfurt, J. C., Foote, A., and Heirich, M. A. (1991). The cost-effectiveness of worksite wellness programs for hypertension control, weight loss, and smoking cessation. *Journal of Occupational Medicine* 33, 962–970.

Evans, R. I. (1988). Health promotion—Science or ideology? *Health Psychology* 7, 203–219.

Fielding, J. E., and Halfon, N. (1994). Where is the health in health system reform? *Journal of the American Medical Association* 271, 1292–1296.

Fielding J. E., and Piserchia, P. V. (1989). Frequency of worksite health promotion activities. *American Journal of Public Health* 73, 538–542.

Fisher, E. B., Jr. (1995). Editorial: The results of the COMMIT Trial. *American Journal of Public Health* 85, 159–169.

Fontanarosa, P. (1995). The unrelenting epidemic of violence in America: Truths and consequences. *Journal of the American Medical Association* 273, 1792–1793.

Fries, J. F., Harrington, H., Edwards, R., et al. (1994). Randomized controlled trial of cost reductions from a health education program: The California Public Employees' Retirement System (PERS) Study. *American Journal of Health Promotion* 8, 216–223.

Fries, J. F., Koop, C. E., Beadle, C. E., et al. (1993). Reducing health care costs by reducing the need and demand for medical services. *New England Journal of Medicine* 329, 321–325.

Geller, E. S. (1987). Applied behavior analysis and environmental psychology: From strange bedfellows to a productive marriage. In D. Stokols and I. Altman, eds., *Handbook of environmental psychology: Volume 1.* New York: John Wiley and Sons, 361–388.

Green, L. W., and Kreuter, M. W. (1990). Health promotion as a public health strategy for the 1990s. *Annual Review of Public Health* 11, 319–334.

Green, L. W., and Ottoson, J. M. (1994). *Community health.* 7th ed. St. Louis: Mosby.

Greenberg, M. R. (1986). Indoor air quality: Protecting public health through design, planning, and research. *Journal of Architectural and Planning Research* 3, 253–261.

Hawley, A. H. (1950). *Human ecology: A theory of community structure.* New York: Ronald Press.

Hedge, A. (1989). Environmental conditions and health in offices. *International Review of Ergonomics* 2, 87–110.

Henderson, D. A., and Scutchfield, F. D. (1989). Point-counterpoint: The public health versus medical model of prevention. *American Journal of Preventive Medicine* 5, 113–119.

Karasek, R., and Theorell, T., eds. (1990). *Healthy work: Stress, productivity, and the reconstruction of working life.* New York: Basic Books.

Katz, D., and Kahn, R. L. (1966). *The social psychology of organizations.* New York: John Wiley and Sons.

Kickbush, I. (1989). Approaches to an ecological base for public health. *Health Promotion* 4, 265–268.

Lawrence, R. J., ed. (1990). Housing, health, and well-being. Special issue of the *Journal of Sociology and Social Welfare* 17.

Lawton, M. P. (1999). Environmental taxonomy: Generalizations from research with older adults. In S. L. Friedman and T. D. Wachs, eds., *Measuring environment across the lifespan.* Pp. 91–124. Washington, D.C.: American Psychological Association.

Marlatt, G. A., and Gordon, J. R. (1985). *Relapse prevention: A self-control strategy for the maintenance of behavior change.* New York: Guilford Press.

Maruyama, M. (1963). The second cybernetics: Deviation-amplifying mutual causal processes. *American Scientist* 51, 164–179.

McGinnis, J. M., and Lee, P. R. (1995). Healthy People 2000 at mid decade. *Journal of the American Medical Association* 273, 1123–1129.

McKinlay, J. B. (1975). A case for refocusing upstream: The political economy of illness. In A. J. Enelow and J. B. Henderson, eds., *Applying behavioral science to cardiovascular risk.* Washington, D.C.: American Heart Association.

McLeroy, K. R., Bibeau, D., Steckler, A., and Glanz, K. (1988). An ecological perspective on health promotion programs. *Health Education Quarterly* 15, 351–378.

Mendell, M. J., and Smith, A. H. (1990). Consistent pattern of elevated symptoms in air-conditioned office buildings: A reanalysis of epidemiologic studies. *American Journal of Public Health* 80, 1193–1199.

Michelson, W. H. (1970). *Man and his urban environment: A sociological approach.* Reading, Mass.: Addison-Wesley.

Miller, J. G. (1978). *The theory of living systems.* New York: McGraw-Hill.

Montes, J. H., Eng, E., and Braithwaite, R. L. (1995). A commentary on minority health as a paradigm shift in the United States. *American Journal of Health Promotion* 9, 247–250.

Moos, R. H. (1979). Social ecological perspectives on health. In G. C. Stone, F. Cohen, and N. E. Adler, eds., *Health psychology: A handbook.* Pp. 523–547. San Francisco: Jossey-Bass.

Newsweek. (1998). Making tobacco say "Aaaaah." March 16, 33.

O'Donnell, M. P., and Harris, J. S., eds. (1994). *Health promotion in the workplace.* 2nd ed. Albany, N.Y.: Delmar Publishers.

Ottawa Charter for Health Promotion. (1986). *Health Promotion,* 1, iii–iv.

Park, R., and Burgess, E., eds. (1925). *The city.* Chicago: University of Chicago Press.

Pelletier, K. R. (1984). *Healthy people in unhealthy places: Stress and fitness at work.* New York: Dell Publishing.

———. (1994). *Sound mind, sound body: A new model for lifelong health.* New York: Simon and Schuster.

———. (1996). A review and analysis of the health and cost-effective outcome studies of comprehensive health promotion and disease prevention programs at the worksite: 1993–1995 update. *American Journal of Health Promotion* 10, 380–388.

Pertschuk, M., and Shopland, D. (1989, September). *Major local smoking ordinances in the United States.* National Institutes of Health Publication 90-479. Washington, D.C.: U.S. Government Printing Office.

Prochaska, J. O., DiClemente, C. C., and Norcross, J. C. (1992). In search of how people change: Applications to addictive behaviors. *American Psychologist* 47, 1102–1114.

Richmond, J. B., and Kotelchuck, M. (1991). Coordination and development of strategies and policy for public health promotion in the United States. In W. W. Holland, R. Detels, and G. Knox, eds., *Oxford textbook of public health.* Pp. 441–454. Oxford: Oxford Medical Publications.

Robertson, L. S. (1986). Behavioral and environmental interventions for reducing motor vehicle trauma. In L. Breslow, J. E. Fielding, and L. B. Lave, eds., *Annual Review of Public Health* 7, 13–34. Palo Alto, Calif.: Annual Reviews Inc.

Rogers-Warren, A., and Warren, S. F., eds.. (1977). *Ecological perspectives in behavior analysis.* Baltimore: University Park Press.

Rosenstock, L., Olenac, C., and Wagner, G. R. (1998). The National Occupational Research Agenda: A model of broad stakeholder input into priority setting. *American Journal of Public Health* 88, 353–356.

Sarason, S. B. (1974). *The psychological sense of community.* San Francisco: Jossey-Bass.

Satcher, D., and Hull, F. (1995). The weight of an ounce. *Journal of the American Medical Association* 273, 1149–1150.

Schauffler, H. H. (1993). *Health promotion and disease prevention in health care reform.* Contract report to The California Wellness Foundation. Berkeley: School of Public Health, University of California.

Schwartz, G. E. (1982). Testing the biopsychosocial model: The ultimate challenge facing behavioral medicine. *Journal of Consulting and Clinical Psychology* 50, 1041–1053.

Stokols, D. (1987). Conceptual strategies of environmental psychology. In D. Stokols and I. Altman, eds., *Handbook of environmental psychology, Volume 1.* New York: John Wiley and Sons, 41–70.

———. (1996). Translating social ecological theory into guidelines for community health promotion. *American Journal of Health Promotion* 10, 282–298.

Stokols, D., Pelletier, K. R., and Fielding, J. E. (1995). Integration of medical care and worksite health promotion. *Journal of the American Medical Association* 273, 1136–1142.

Syme, S. L. (1990). Health promotion: Old approaches, new choices, future imperatives. Presented at the Conference on "The New Public Health: 1990," Los Angeles, April.

Thompson, R. S., Taplin, S. H., McAfee, T. A., et al. (1995). Primary and secondary prevention services in clinical practice: Twenty years' experience in development, implementation, and evaluation. *Journal of the American Medical Association* 273, 1130–1135.

U.S. Department of Health and Human Services. (1992). 1992 National Survey of Worksite Health Promotion Activities. Final Report PB93-500023. Washington, D.C.: U.S. Government Printing Office.

U.S. Food and Drug Administration. (1996). Executive summary: The regulations restricting the sale and distribution of cigarettes and smokeless tobacco to protect children and adolescents. http://www.fda.gov/opacom/campaigns/tobacco/execrule.html.

U.S. Preventive Service Task Force. (1989). *Guide to clinical preventive services: An assessment of the effectiveness of 169 interventions.* Baltimore: Williams and Wilkins.

U.S. Public Health Service. (1964). *Smoking and health: Report of the Advisory Committee to the Surgeon General of the Public Health Service.* PHS Publication 1103. Washington, D.C.: U.S. Government Printing Office.

———. (1967). *The health consequences of smoking: A Public Health Service review.* PHS Publication 1696. Washington, D.C.: U.S. Government Printing Office.

———. (1979). *Healthy people: The Surgeon General's report on health promotion and disease prevention.* DHEW Publication (PHS) 79-55071. Washington, D.C.: U.S. Government Printing Office.

———. (1991). *Healthy People 2000: National health promotion and disease prevention objectives.* PHHS Publication (PHS) 91-50212. Washington, D.C.: U.S. Government Printing Office.

———. (1992). *Business responds to AIDS.* Washington, D.C.: U.S. Government Printing Office.

Webster's Encyclopedic Unabridged Dictionary of the English Language. (1989). New York: Portland House.

Weick, K. E. (1984). Small wins: Redefining the scale of social problems. *American Psychologist* 39, 40–49.

Weiss, S. M. (1991). Health at work. In S. M. Weiss, J. E. Fielding, and A. Baum, eds., *Perspectives in behavioral medicine: Health at work.* Pp. 1–10. Hillsdale, N.J.: Lawrence Erlbaum Associates.

Wells M., Stokols D., McMahan S., and Clitheroe, C. (1997). Evaluation of a worksite injury and illness prevention program: Do the effects of the REACH OUT Training Program reach the employees? *Journal of Occupational Health Psychology* 2, 25–34.

Williams, A. F. (1982). Passive and active measures for controlling disease and injury: The role of health psychologists. *Health Psychology* 1, 399–409.

Williams, A. F., Karpf, R. S., and Zador, P. F. (1983). Variations in minimum licensing age and fatal motor vehicle crashes. *American Journal of Public Health* 73, 1401–1403.

Winett, R. A., King, A. C., and Altman, D. G. (1989). *Health psychology and public health: An integrative approach.* New York: Pergamon Press.

Winkleby, M. A. (1994). The future of community-based cardiovascular disease intervention studies. *American Journal of Public Health* 84, 1369–1372.

Wintemute, G. J. (1992). From research to public policy: The prevention of motor vehicle injuries, childhood drownings, and firearm violence. *American Journal of Health Promotion* 6, 451–464.

World Health Organization. (1984). Health promotion: A discussion document on the concept and principles. *Health Promotion* 1, 73–76.

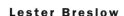

2

Lester Breslow

THE SOCIETAL CONTEXT OF DISEASE
PREVENTION AND WELLNESS PROMOTION

From time immemorial, people have been concerned, collectively as well as individually, about avoiding health impairment and prolonging life. In society they have developed two increasingly specialized arms for advancing their health interests: (1) sets of healers, now long dominated by physicians, for dealing with individuals' problems, and (2) community health protection, to which public health personnel are devoted. The first set focuses on people one at a time and the second on the population as a whole. Physicians have tended to emphasize cures, whereas public health has focused attention on prevention, though considerable overlap in these emphases has occurred. Both are supported by society to varying degrees in different times and situations, generally corresponding to the value that society places on them for safeguarding health.

COMMUNICABLE DISEASES

Most health problems arise in a societal context. Thus, tuberculosis, influenza, pneumonia, and other respiratory-borne and acute intestinal diseases dominated the health scene during the early days of the industrial revolution and even into the 20th century. Exhausting factory work, crowded housing and work space, polluted water, and inadequate nutrition largely determined that disease pattern. The latter has steadily been yielding both to social reform of poor living conditions and to social implementation of scientific-technical advances in microbiology and immunity.

THE CHRONIC DISEASE EPIDEMIC

Progress against the communicable diseases has led to longer lives. Steady improvement in technology and living conditions, however, created opportunity for increasing segments of the population—at first for the more affluent and subsequently most other people—to luxuriate in ways that induced other kinds of health damage. Physical inactivity; excessive calorie consumption, especially in the form of fats and sweets; and access to new forms of tobacco eventuated in the 20th-century epidemics of cardiovascular disease, lung cancer, diabetes, and other chronic diseases.

In the struggle against this new set of health problems, treatment dominated in the beginning, but prevention is now emerging as the major approach. The 1957 report of the Commission on Chronic Illness, which brought together the American Medical Association, American Public Health Association, American Hospital Association and American Public Welfare Association, introduced and delineated the key concepts for chronic disease prevention: primary and secondary prevention.[1] The former was defined as "averting the occurrence of disease" and the second as "halting the progression of disease from its early unrecognized stage to a more severe one and preventing complications or sequelae of disease."[2] Continued development of knowledge concerning the causation of chronic disease, especially behavioral risk factors, has enhanced prospects for primary prevention. Similarly, continuing technological advances in screening for early signs of disease have led to improvements in secondary prevention. As the 20th century comes to a close, social support for primary and secondary prevention of chronic disease is growing rapidly.

A NEW CONCEPT OF HEALTH

Meanwhile, something beyond prevention of disease as a health goal is gaining recognition. The World Health Organization (WHO) has defined health as "a state of complete physical, mental and social well-being, not merely the absence of disease and infirmity."[3] Though denigrated for years as wooly-headed and not useful in scientific work, the concept recently appears to be achieving greater credibility. Documents such as the Lalonde Report[4] and the Ottawa Charter for Health Promotion,[5] as well as the growing use of the term "health promotion" (often in connection with disease prevention), indicate a fundamental change in thinking about health.[4,5] That change reflects socially determined progress against disease to the point that it is possible to envisage a higher state of health than the absence of disease.

Gradual acceptance of that idea appears due to continuing advances not only against the communicable diseases but also against the noncommunicable chronic diseases. The prescience of the first WHO leaders is shown in the fact that mortality from major forms of chronic disease such as heart disease and cancer was still rising at the midcentury point; since then, however, both have passed their epidemic peaks and are declining, thus opening the path to a new view of health.

Overcoming the chronic diseases is resulting both from their declining incidence and from lowering their fatality. Social support of primary and secondary prevention has played a substantial role in that development.

IMPAIRMENT AS THE ISSUE

An important consequence of delaying mortality among those afflicted with chronic disease has been the extension of life expectancy within the population as a whole. Aging of the population, with its accompanying accumulation of multiple pathologies from life's stresses, is stimulating concern about functional impairment, with its social as well as individual implications.

One sign of that concern may be seen in efforts to measure health impairments. One of the first to emerge was the set of activities of daily living (ADLs) proposed by Katz, Downs, Cash, and Grotz in 1970.[6] They listed six activities necessary for living, such as eating and toileting, and began measuring the extent to which individuals could perform these functions without aid from others. This process permitted delineating the need for care, with treatment as the primary aim. Since the ADLs earmarked only those persons requiring extensive care, a next step was to define instrumental activities of daily living (IADLs).[7] These included such items as ability to perform household chores or to go shopping. Subsequently, advanced activities of daily living (AADLs) have been proposed[8] and include such behaviors as participation in regular exercise.

Noteworthy in this evolution of ADLs, IADLs, and AADLs has been the shift in focus from disease to impairments. That shift reflects a growing social concern in the health arena with loss of capacities for living, not merely with the traditional "causes" of disease and death. The focus on these functional criteria for health status also reflects the greater numbers of people living with chronic disease and their associated disabilities due to life-extending treatments and medications.

WELLNESS AS A CONCEPT

Wellness as a health goal is still a relatively crude concept. It has not yet become sufficiently explicit and standardized to permit clear delineation in a person or measurement in a population. In dealing with health, we are still strongly inclined to diagnose and count diseases and to determine the number of ADLs, IADLs, and AADLs that people can perform.

The term "wellness promotion" implies a step beyond prevention of disease and impairment. All the items that might be listed under the rubric of wellness apply to relative states of health rather than to gradations of disease or impairment. Promotion of wellness may similarly be viewed as actions to achieve higher levels of health above and beyond the reduction of impairment.

Disease and impairment have been quite well delineated; wellness has not. It is therefore necessary to make wellness as a state of health more explicit in order to advance understanding of how to promote it. This constitutes an important, current challenge to health science.[9]

SOCIAL ASPECTS OF DISEASE
PREVENTION/WELLNESS PROMOTION STRATEGY

Despite the elementary state of the wellness concept, it already appears that many of the same things that must be attacked in order to prevent disease also need attention in achieving wellness. For example, avoiding smoking both prevents lung disease and enhances pulmonary function; physical exercise both prevents cardiac disease and strengthens musculoskeletal function. Thus, in many respects disease prevention and wellness promotion constitute the two aspects of a positive health strategy.

Several levels of action are desirable in this strategy: individual, interpersonal, and social. In behavior affecting one's own health (and that is an increasingly important factor), the individual makes the final decision; he/she ultimately determines what and how much to eat, how much alcohol to drink, and the like. Because health determinants nowadays consist largely of *access* rather than *exposure* to risk factors, opportunity and inducements for individual health-related choice must be the intervention end target. One does not exercise such choice in a vacuum. Rather, that is done in the context of family, friends, peers, professional advisers, and the whole social milieu. Therefore, simple appeals to individuals may not be very effective since they constitute only one influence on the choice to be made; also, they may easily take the form of "blaming the victim." Interpersonal intervention, on the other hand—for example, by peers or physicians—may carry considerable weight with the individual because of the substantial tendency to follow such leads.

The third, and probably most effective, level of intervention for behavior that protects health is the social environment. Since behavior adverse to health arises so largely from societal influences—for example, inducing youngsters to smoke cigarettes, tolerating excessive use of alcoholic beverages, and failing to provide adequate opportunity for physical exercise in the inner city—such influences must be dealt with on the social level. In an earlier day, health advance necessitated creating a social milieu that favored hand washing and not spitting; now it has become necessary to establish new social hygiene standards: not smoking, drinking modestly if at all, exercising, and eating sensibly.

Exemplifying the societal approach to disease prevention and wellness promotion, and the struggles involved, is the California tobacco control program.[10] Activists against the number one cause of death in the United States—in major voluntary health agencies, public health and medicine, and elsewhere—had not prevailed in the legislature over tobacco industry interests. Therefore, taking advantage of the state's legislative initiative process, they succeeded in getting Proposition 99 passed in a general election. The latter increased the tax on cigarettes 25 cents a pack and allocated 20 percent of the funds to prevention efforts, the rest to medical, hospital, research and other purposes. The broad-scale program implemented with the prevention funds by the California Department of Health Services stimulates tobacco control activity in local health departments, schools, and a wide variety of community agencies throughout the state. These local efforts, and subsequent state action, stopped smoking in public buildings, workplaces, and restaurants; stepped up enforcement of laws forbidding tobacco sales to minors; removed vending machines from many places; and otherwise severely discouraged smoking. Vigorous communication via television, radio, and other media did likewise. Schools introduced materials and in other ways encouraged students to combat pro-smoking influences. The social milieu in the whole country was, of course, tilting strongly against smoking. The program's specific effectiveness, however, is indicated by the fact that the rate of smoking decline in California doubled through the next six years, bringing the prevalence down below all other states except Utah.

The tobacco industry fought back intensively with political contributions and lobbying, formation of phony "public" organizations to oppose local control activities, and heavy promotion of products. The governor and the legislature then joined in substantially disrupting the program by diverting prevention monies to medical services, until the antitobacco forces obtained court action to stop such diversion of funds. Now efforts are under way to restore the program.

The California tobacco control experience has indicated how sharply social trends and conflicts can affect health-related behavior and thus disease prevention and wellness promotion. Other elements of such efforts are likewise embedded in social context, which must be considered in order to achieve effective action.

REFERENCES

1. Commission on Chronic Illness. 1957. *Chronic Illness in the United States.* Cambridge, Mass.: Harvard University Press.
2. Commission on Chronic Illness. 1957. *Chronic Illness in the United States. Volume I: Prevention of Chronic Illness.* Cambridge, Mass.: Harvard University Press.
3. World Health Organization. 1984. Health promotion: A discussion document on the concept and principles. *Health Promotion 1,* 73–76.
4. Government of Canada. 1974. A new perspective on the health of Canadians (Lalonde Report). Department of National Health and Welfare, Ottawa.
5. Ottawa Charter for Health Promotion. 1986. *Canadian Journal of Health Promotion 77,* 425–436.
6. Katz, S., Downs, T. D., Cash, H. R., and Grotz, R. C. 1970. Progress in development of the index of ADL. *Gerontologist 10,* 20–30.
7. Avlund, K., Schultz-Larsen, K., and Kreiber, S. 1993. The measurement of instrumental ADL: Content validity and construct validity. *Aging 5,* 371–383.
8. Reuben, D. B., Laliberte, L., Hiris, J., and Mor, V. 1990. A hierarchical exercise scale to measure function at the Advanced Activities of Daily Living (AADL) level. *Journal of the American Geriatrics Society 38,* 855–861.
9. Breslow, L. 1999. From disease prevention to health promotion. *Journal of the American Medical Association 281,* 1030–1033.
10. Breslow, L., and Johnsen, M. 1993. California's Proposition 99 on tobacco and its impact. *Annual Review of Public Health 14,* 585–604.

3

Robert M. Kaplan

PROMOTING WELLNESS

Biomedical versus Outcomes Models

This chapter grew out of my experience of being named as the Wellness Lecturer at the University of California, San Diego, in 1991. It is remarkable to consider what changes have occurred over these last few years. Yet, it is also remarkable that we still face many of the same problems. In 1991, managed care had captured only a small percentage of the health care market in the United States. Today, managed care is a dominant force in most areas of the country. In 1991, few observers challenged the autonomy of physicians as sole decision makers. Today, practice guidelines for the individual health care providers are an accepted part of practice. Finally, the use of public health and preventive health care approaches, although recognized as important in 1991, were not common parts of practice. Today, the reorganization of health care has provided new opportunities for incorporation of prevention paradigms. These changes have stimulated rethinking of the basic foundations of health care organization and delivery, and this chapter addresses some of the related issues. We will begin by considering the framework proposed in 1991.

WHAT ARE THE PROBLEMS?

The major problems in the American health care system might be described as the three A's: affordability, access, and accountability (Kaplan, 1993). Similar problems were identified by Relman (1989).

Affordability

The affordability problem results from our inability to pay for all the health care that is desired. Health care costs in the United States grew remarkably between 1940 and the mid-1990s. In 1940, approximately four billion dollars per year were spent on health care in the United States. That amount tripled by 1950 and continued to escalate at an exponential rate through the early 1990s. Health expenditures were over a trillion dollars in 1996. It now takes just over a day to match the yearly expenditure from 1940.

The high costs of American health care cause very serious problems for U.S. products in the world marketplace. This is because the costs of health care are represented in every product that the United States exports. Since our per capita expenditures on health care are twice what they are in countries such as Great Britain or Japan, health care costs contribute proportionally more to the expense of American exports. We pay for expensive health care in many different ways. In some cases patients pay more for services. However, we also pay for high health care costs when we purchase consumer products. Part of the price of each product is the health insurance paid on behalf of the workers. More important, workers are doubly affected by increased health care costs. When their employers pay more for health insurance, workers get lower wages and retirement benefits (Center for Health Economics Research, 1994). If spending on health benefits rises, other aspects of compensation may be held constant or may decline.

Access

The United States remains the only industrialized country that does not provide universal access to health care. Part of the problem is that health care is usually unaffordable without insurance. The exact number of uninsured people is difficult to determine. Current estimates suggest that over 40 million Americans have no regular source of health care. The only group that has universal coverage is the elderly since virtually all Americans older than age 65 are covered by the Medicare program. The uninsured are not necessarily the unemployed. In fact, the majority of those without health insurance are working or dependents of workers. However, many employers provide either no health insurance or inadequate coverage.

Accountability

Health care may be the only major American industry that is not held accountable for what it produces. Although we produce more health care services per capita than any country in the world, it is not clear that Americans are in any way healthier than residents of other developed countries, where considerably less is spent on health care. Patient satisfaction surveys suggest that consumers are significantly more satisfied with health care services in countries that spend considerably less. One analysis compared satisfaction and expenditures in 10 countries (the United States, Canada, France, Germany, Sweden, Australia, the Netherlands, Italy, Japan, and the United Kingdom). Among these countries, the United States spends more per capita and is significantly lower in the percentage of consumers satisfied with the services they receive (Blendon et al., 1990).

In summary, the U.S. health care system is in serious trouble. Solutions to these problems require that we consider all three dimensions. In addition, we must challenge some of the most basic models of health care. The accountability piece of the puzzle is perhaps the most challenging. In order to address accountability, we must address central ideas about the purpose of health care. Most of this chapter reviews methods for accounting for health care benefits.

BIOMEDICAL AND OUTCOMES MODELS

Health care has been dominated by a traditional biomedical model. According to this model, human pain and suffering are caused by disease processes. Disease activity is measured by judgments of trained physicians and by physiological measures, including blood chemistry or radiographic evidence of pathology. The traditional medical model recognizes behavioral factors as predictors of these outcomes. Behavioral risk factors might be cigarette smoking, high-risk behaviors, or the consumption of a high-fat diet (Kaplan, 1984). In addition, the traditional biomedical model suggests that disease process is determined by genetic predispositions, environmental exposures, and the aging process itself. The disease process is also affected by medical care and the use of regular medical tests (Wilson and Cleary, 1995).

According to the traditional biomedical model, the purpose of medicine is to find disease pathology and to fix it. We sometimes refer to this as "find it–fix it medicine." For problems such as high blood pressure, for example, the physician's task is to diagnose the problem and to administer a medicine that will make blood pressure normal. The measure of success is a blood pressure reading that falls within a defined range of normality. Unfortunately, many medical procedures may affect biological processes, but may not affect life expectancy or life quality. It has been estimated that 30% to 50% of all medical procedures have little effect on long-term outcomes (Brook and Lohr, 1987). Further, some procedures may have a negative effect on survival and quality of life.

An alternative model for health care, known as the outcomes model, is similar to the traditional biomedical model. However, the ultimate outcome is not a measure of disease process. The goals of health care are to extend the duration of life and/or to improve the quality of life. Disease processes are of interest because pathology may either shorten life expectancy or make life less desirable. The same variables that predict disease process may also predict life expectancy or quality of life. However, in contrast to the traditional biomedical model, behaviors or biological events may affect life expectancy independently of disease process. Further, the measures of success in the outcomes model are different than those in the traditional biomedical model. The outcomes model emphasizes quality of life and life duration instead of clinical measures of disease process. As similar as these two models appear, they lead to substantially different approaches to organizing, financing, and delivering health care (Kaplan, 1990). These distinctions are addressed in the following sections.

Valuing Health Services

The traditional biomedical model uses procedures to fix biological problems. The greater use of procedures in the United States than in other countries resulted in the American system becoming more expensive than the systems in other countries. By 1990, it was clear that cost control would dominate the health policy agenda throughout the decade. Often, cost reduction is considered the major objective of health care reform. Pauly (1995), for example, argues that cost should be the central consideration in policy analysis. However, too much attention to cost may neglect the primary mission of health care. For example, if cost is the only criterion, the development of guidelines for appropriate care may exclude expensive services. In order to choose between alternative health programs, it is best to evaluate not only the costs but also the benefits (Sturm and Wells, 1995). Such an evaluation recognizes all financial and health outcomes as either a cost or a benefit. Financial outcomes are easily understood, but clinical outcome measures are often poorly understood, especially from a patient perspective. For example, a change in an arterial blood gas value is not an ideal health outcome measure because it may not mean much to a patient or to a public policy maker. On the other hand, restoration or preservation of the ability to perform activities of daily living is the goal of many therapies. Because patient-centered outcomes are measurable and meaningful, a paradigm shift in medicine is beginning to embrace patient-centered reports.

Despite the improvements in measuring patient outcomes, determining the value of health services has been particularly difficult. In contrast to cost-benefit analysis, which focuses on the dollar returns for investing in particular programs, or consumer willingness to pay for service, cost-utility analysis used in some health services evaluations considers the health outcomes of a program, weighted by patient preferences for outcomes, in relation to the financial costs of the program. In economics, the value of a product is related to the willingness of consumers to pay for it. For example, the value of a Mercedes-Benz automobile is set by the price that consumers are willing to pay for the car. If the price is too high, few cars are sold. Health services are difficult to value in this manner because consumers rarely pay for them directly. Instead, the charges are paid by third parties. Third-party payment leaves consumers out of the loop and makes it difficult to establish whether the services are valuable to patients.

A GENERAL HEALTH POLICY MODEL

In order to understand health outcomes, it is necessary to build a comprehensive theoretical model of health status. The major aspects of the model include mortality (death) and morbidity (health-related quality of life). In several papers, we have suggested that diseases and disabilities are important for two reasons. First, illness may cause the life expectancy to be shortened. Second, illness may make life less desirable at times prior to death (diminished health-related quality of life) (Kaplan and Anderson, 1988; Kaplan et al., 1993).

Over the last two decades, a group of investigators at the University of California, San Diego, has developed the General Health Policy Model (GHPM). Central to the model is a general conceptualization of quality of life. The model separates aspects of health status and life quality into distinct components. These are life expectancy (mortality), functioning and symptoms (morbidity), preference for observed health states (utility), and duration of stay in health states (prognosis). Each component is described here in more detail.

Mortality. A model of health outcomes necessarily includes a component for mortality. Indeed, many public health statistics focus exclusively on mortality through estimations of crude mortality rates, age-adjusted mortality rates, and infant mortality rates.

Morbidity. Health-related quality of life is also an important outcome. Most public health indicators are relatively insensitive to variations toward the well end of the death-wellness continuum. Measures of mortality, to give an extreme example, ignore all variations of morbidity: a person in a coma is considered equivalent to an asymptomatic person at full function. Both, after all, are alive. In addition, disability measures often ignore those who are relatively healthy. For example, the RAND Health Insurance Study reported that about 80% of the general population have no dysfunction. Thus, they would estimate that 80% of the population is well. But in studies that assess symptoms and function, only about 12% of the general population report no symptoms on a particular day (Kaplan et al., 1976). In other words, health symptoms or problems are a very common aspect of the human experience. Some might argue that symptoms are unimportant because they are subjective and unobservable. However, symptoms are highly correlated with the demand for medical services, expenditures on health care, and motivations to alter lifestyles. Further symptoms lower quality of life even if a disease cannot be detected. Thus, we feel that the quantification of symptoms is very important when assessing morbidity. The GHPM, using the Quality of Well-Being (QWB) scale described later, considers functioning in three areas (mobility, physical activity, and social activity) and symptoms.

Utility (Relative Importance). Not all outcomes are equally important. For example, a treatment that prevents nausea is not equivalent to one that prevents death. Given that mortality and the various components of morbidity can be tabulated, it is important to consider their relative importance. A key component of the GHPM attempts to scale the various health outcomes according to their relative importance. This exercise adds the "quality" dimensions to health status. In the preceding example, the relative importance of dying would be weighted more than developing nausea. The weighting is accomplished by rating all states on a quality continuum ranging from 0 (for dead) to 1.0 (for optimum, asymptomatic functioning). These ratings are typically provided by independent judges who are representative of the general population. Using this system it is possible to express the relative importance of states in relation to the life-death continuum. A point halfway on the scale (0.5) is regarded as halfway between optimum function and death. The quality-of-life weighting system for the QWB has been described in several different publications (Kaplan et al., 1976, 1978, 1979).

Prognosis. In the GHPM, the term "prognosis" refers to the probability of transition among health states over the course of time and includes consideration of duration of problems. A headache that lasts one hour is not equivalent to a headache that lasts one month. A cough that lasts three days is not equivalent to a cough that lasts three years. In considering the severity of illness, duration of the problem is central. As basic as this concept is, most contemporary models of health outcome measurement completely disregard the duration component. The GHPM considers the point at which the problem begins. A person may have no symptoms or dysfunctions currently but may have a high probability of health problems in the future. The prognosis component of the model takes these transitions into consideration. A discount rate is used for future outcomes if the utility of a future outcome is not the same as that of a present outcome. For example, a daylong headache that will begin a year from now may be less of a concern than a daylong headache that will start immediately.

The components of the model can be integrated to express outcomes in terms of quality-adjusted life years (QALYs). A QALY is defined as the equivalent of a completely well year of life, or a year of life free of any symptoms, problems, or health-related disabilities. A principal advantage of the QALY is that it provides a common metric that allows different programs to be directly compared. The quality-adjusted life expectancy is the current life expectancy adjusted for diminished quality of life associated with dysfunctional states and the duration of stay in each state.

Consider, for example, a person with a rare lung disease and in a state of functioning and symptoms that is rated by community peers as 0.5 on the 0-to-1.0 utility scale described previously. If the person remains in that state for one year, he or she would have lost the equivalent of one-half of one year of life. However, a person who has the flu may also be rated as 0.50. In this case, the illness might last only three days, and the total loss in QALYs might be $3/365 \times 0.50$, which is equal to 0.004 QALYs. By itself, it is clear that the flu does not produce as significant a health outcome as the lung disease. But suppose that 5,000 people in a community get the flu. The QALYs lost would then be $5,000 \times 0.004$, which is equal to 20 years, or greater than the one person with the rare lung disease. This indicates that the flu may be a greater health policy problem than the rare disease.

Now suppose that a vaccination becomes available and that the threat of the flu can be eliminated by vaccinating the 35,000 people in the community. The cost of the vaccine is $5 per person, or $175,000. The average cost/utility of the program would be as follows:

$$\frac{net\ cost}{net\ utility} = \frac{\$175K}{20\ QALYs} = \$8,750/QALY$$

Using the concept of the QALY, the net cost/utility ratio of two alternative programs can be calculated as follows:

$$\frac{net - incremental\ cost}{net - incremental\ QALY} = \frac{net\ cost\ of\ treatment_2 - net\ cost\ of\ treatment_1}{[QALY_2 - QALY_1]}$$

It is important to consider the *marginal,* or incremental, cost/utility of programs. Although we could compare the simple costs and effects of different programs, we most often have to decide how much we are willing to pay in order to add an additional benefit. For example, behavior modification has been shown to be valuable for helping people kick the smoking habit. However, the benefits might be enhanced if nicotine replacement therapy is added to behavior modification. Analysis might show that both behavior modification and behavior modification plus nicotine replacement reduce tobacco use. However, we must decide if we are willing to pay the extra expense for adding nicotine replacement. Usually, we must choose between several programs.

Another way to evaluate outcomes is within "policy space." Various approaches to cost/benefit and cost/utility analysis occasionally produce different results. The output for cost/benefit analysis is in monetary terms—a program that produces cost savings. Cost/utility analysis

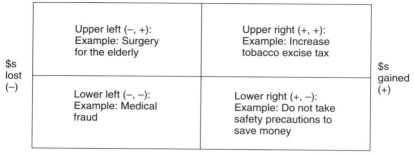

QALYs gained

Upper left (−, +): Example: Surgery for the elderly	Upper right (+, +): Example: Increase tobacco excise tax
Lower left (−, −): Example: Medical fraud	Lower right (+, −): Example: Do not take safety precautions to save money

$s lost (−) $s gained (+)

QALYs lost

Figure 3.1. Two-dimensional policy space from Anderson et al. (1986). Tobacco excise tax may be one of the few policy examples that is in the upper-right quadrant.

focuses on the cost to produce a QALY. Anderson et al. (1986) integrated the concepts of QALYs and net dollars returned within a common framework. This was accomplished by creating a two-dimensional policy space as illustrated in Figure 3.1. The *x*-axis in the figure represents net dollars returned per person. Returns are defined as benefits minus costs in dollar units. The *y*-axis displays well years lost or gained through a particular treatment program, clinical intervention, or policy change.

The right half of the plane would be used to represent programs in which benefits exceed costs, while the left half would display situations in which costs exceed benefits. The upper half of the figure displays outcomes that have positive health effects in terms of QALYs. Those in the bottom half of the figure would be used to represent negative health outcomes in well-year units.

The two-dimensional space yields four quadrants. One quadrant, the lower left, represents unsuitable alternatives. In these cases, dollars are being spent, and negative health consequences occur. Administration of a uniformly toxic treatment might be represented by this quadrant. The upper-right quadrant represents the most attractive alternatives. Here, QALY health benefits are gained, and there are also economic benefits. Increasing tobacco excise tax may be one of the few true examples of such a program. The upper-left quadrant shows QALY gains, but with more significant costs associated with these improvements. Transplantation surgery for the elderly might be described by this quadrant. Here there are significant health benefits, but the recipients may not return to the productive economic sector.

The lower-right quadrant represents another level of economic trade-off. Here, society may be willing to sacrifice some health benefits in exchange for cost savings. Anderson and colleagues suggested that these trade-offs may be common in studies involving nuclear power; pollution control; occupational, environmental, and consumer product safety; highway speed limits; and so on.

DECISIONS: OUTCOMES VERSUS TRADITIONAL BIOMEDICAL MODELS

Although the traditional biomedical model and the outcomes model are similar in many ways, they lead to different decisions about the use of resources for prevention. In the following sections, several examples are reviewed.

Diagnosis versus Outcomes

The traditional biomedical model is centered on medical diagnoses. Diagnosis defines the problems that have been found and gives direction about what needs to be fixed. The traditional system pays providers for using diagnostic tests to find problems and for using therapeutic interventions to fix the problems. Despite the importance of diagnosis, it often obscures or confuses the importance of some health problems. There are at least three reasons why focusing on diagnosis may have led us in some wrong directions. First, diagnoses do not always lead to better health outcomes. Often, people are placed in categories, but identification of a condition does not necessarily mean that an effective treatment can be applied. Second, diagnoses are not always correct, and in some cases, individuals will be treated for conditions they do not have or will fail to be effectively treated because the correct diagnosis was overlooked. Third, in many cases, poor health outcomes result from risky behavior or from exposure to risk factors. Community health outcomes can be enhanced by removing the risk factor or by modifying behavior. The identification of a disease on the pathway between the risk factor and the outcome is interesting but not essential.

There are approximately 2,150,000 deaths in the United States each year. Deaths are tallied according to major and underlying cause. The traditional biomedical model emphasized disease-specific causes of death, and therefore pathways to prevention typically considered risk factors for particular diseases. For example, cigarette smoking is associated with deaths from cancer of the lung. Thus, efforts to reduce lung cancer concentrate on smoking cessation. However, most of the major causes of death are associated with a variety of different risk factors. Further, many risk factors are associated with death from a variety of different causes. For example, tobacco use causes not only lung cancer but also a wide variety of other malignancies, heart disease, stroke, and birth complications (Kaplan et al., 1995). By concentrating on diagnoses, the traditional model often misses the relationship between behaviors and outcomes.

Major nongenetic contributors to mortality were examined in an important analysis by McGinnis and Foege (1993). When these external factors are considered independent of the disease model, clear priorities for prevention emerge. A summary of the estimates for actual causes of death in the United States is presented in Table 3.1. Tobacco use is associated with more than 400,000 deaths each year, while diet and activity patterns account for an additional 300,000. These dwarf the number of deaths associated with problems that the public is generally concerned about, such as illicit drug use. The McGinnis and Foege analysis challenged us to think differently about the way we track health indicators in the United States. Only a small fraction of the trillion dollars the United States spends annually on health care is devoted to the control of the major factors that cause premature mortality in the United States. Estimates suggest that less than 5% of the total annual health care budget is devoted to prevention efforts (Rothenberg et al., 1987). If the focus of attention shifts from finding and fixing diseases to producing QALYs, it becomes clear that preventive efforts to reduce tobacco, drug, and alcohol use and to promote exercise deserve greater attention.

It is commonly argued that traditional fee-for-service medicine provides few incentives to offer preventive services. Indeed, the higher the rates of service utilization, the greater the revenue. One attractive feature of managed care is that there are substantial incentives to prevent illness and to reduce health care utilization. From a public health perspective, managed care organizations have responsibility for a defined population. If they can keep this population healthy by investing in prevention, they may ultimately profit by having reduced costs and higher consumer satisfaction.

TABLE 3.1   ACTUAL CAUSES
OF DEATH—UNITED STATES, 1990

Factor	Deaths	Percentage
Tobacco	400,000	19
Diet-activity patterns	300,000	14
Alcohol	100,000	5
Microbial agents	90,000	4
Toxic agents	60,000	3
Firearms	35,000	<2
Sexual behavior	30,000	1
Motor vehicles	25,000	1
Illicit use of drugs	20,000	<1
Total	1,060,000	50

SOURCE: McGinnis and Foege (1993).

The traditional biomedical model has dominated thinking about prevention. Most of the 3% to 5% of the health care dollar used for prevention is devoted to clinical preventive services offered by physicians. For example, the great majority of expenditures on prevention relate to screening for diseases, such as breast cancer, cervical cancer, and prostate cancer. The purpose of the prevention service is to detect a disease that already exists and intervene medically so that progression is retarded. The screening tests have become profitable for the providers who offer them, and there is growing concern about abuses or profiteering by those who administer tests to people who do not need them.

Guidelines for preventive services might limit reimbursement to those services recommended in the Guide to Clinical Preventive Services. The U.S. Preventive Services Taskforce has prepared this excellent document that describes the appropriate use of a wide variety of medical preventive services. The strong emphasis in the Guide is on the appropriate use of medical screening tests by physicians. The latest version of the guide includes 70 chapters. There are 11 chapters devoted specifically to counseling (tobacco, physical activity, diet, motor vehicle injuries, household and recreational injuries, youth violence, low-back pain, dental/periodontal disease, HIV and STD, unintended pregnancy, and gynecological cancers). However, most of the guidelines advise physicians on testing and the medical implications for those who have been found to have a disease. For example, 47 of the 60 sets of guidelines in the first edition of the Guide concern the application of medical screening tests. Another five consider immunizations and chemoprophylaxis. The remaining eight guidelines are on counseling.

The guidelines for preventive services arise from the traditional find it–fix it model. The emphasis is on using medical screening tests that identify diseases that already exist. These are the services that have traditionally generated fees for providers. The limited yield from this approach is reviewed in the next section. The current environment favors an outcomes-oriented approach. According to the outcomes model, diagnosis and treatment are important only if they make life longer and/or better.

Medical Geography

The traditional biomedical model of health care rests on several important assumptions. One assumption is that medical technology enhances health outcomes and that there is a pool of untreated disease on which these technologies might be successfully deployed. If this is true, then more applications of medical technologies should result in better health outcomes. A second assumption is that any well-trained doctor presented with the same problem will come to the same diagnosis. However, it has been known for some time that there is substantial variation in the rate at which problems are diagnosed and treated in different communities. Thus, even though the distribution of a disease may be the same in different communities, the rate at which diseases are diagnosed varies substantially. Wennberg and colleagues have devoted the past quarter of a century to a description of this problem (Wennberg, 1996).

Wennberg argues that a major factor in the use of medical services is "supplier-induced demand." This implies that providers create demand for services by diagnosing illness. Most surgical subspecialists would agree there is a need to perform surgery on some well-defined cases. These might include amputation of a toe with gangrene, removal of some well-defined tumors, or intervention to repair a compound fracture. However, there is also substantial discretion in the use of some medical and surgical procedures. This is well illustrated by the comparison of procedures in two communities: Boston, Massachusetts, and New Haven, Connecticut.

Boston and New Haven are similar in a variety of ways. Both are traditional New England cities that have multiethnic populations. The two cities have approximately the same climate, and both cities are home to prestigious Ivy League universities. Since the cities are near each other, we would expect that the costs of medical care should be approximately the same. Using data from the mid-1970s, Wennberg and colleagues (1990) demonstrated that, in fact, medical care costs in Boston were nearly twice as high as they were in New Haven.

Figure 3.2 shows the distribution of costs in Connecticut service areas and in Massachusetts services areas in the 1970s. In 1975, Medicare was paying $324 per recipient per month in Boston and only $155 per month for residents of New Haven. The situation has not changed much. In 1989, per capita hospital expenditures for acute care were $1,524 for residents of Boston and $777 for those living in New Haven.

Further study by Wennberg and his colleagues showed that Boston has more hospital capacity than does New Haven. In Boston, there are 4.3 hospital beds for every 1,000 residents, while in New Haven, there are fewer than 2.3 beds per 1,000 residents. Residents of Boston are more likely to be hospitalized for a wide variety of acute medical conditions than are residents of New Haven. For many different medical conditions, such as pneumonia or congestive heart failure, Bostonians are more likely to be cared for as hospital inpatients, while residents of New Haven are treated outside the hospital.

Some of the differences between Boston and New Haven might be attributed to the greater development of hospital facilities. New Haven has only one major medical school (Yale), while Boston has three medical schools. The Harvard Medical School is associated with several different teaching hospitals. Further, Boston has four hospitals associated with different religious establishments, while there is only one religious-affiliated hospital in New Haven.

The Boston–New Haven comparison is particularly interesting from a public policy perspective. Medicare is a federal program that hopes to provide equal benefit to all its recipients. Yet, on average, Medicare spends twice as much per capita in Boston as it does in New Haven (Wennberg et al., 1996) for the same care. Are New Haven residents getting a bad deal? Since the government is spending less on New Haven residents, it might be argued that their health should suffer. However, outcomes evidence does not show that residents of Boston are any healthier than residents of New Haven. In fact, some evidence implies that Boston residents may be worse off. For example, people in Boston are more likely to be rehospitalized for the same condition than are people in New Haven. Residents of Boston appear to have more complications from medical treatment. More may not necessarily be better. Indeed, there is some evidence that more may be worse (Fisher et al., 1994). In the next section, we consider this question. Under a traditional model that focuses on diagnosis, more facilities will lead to more diagnoses.

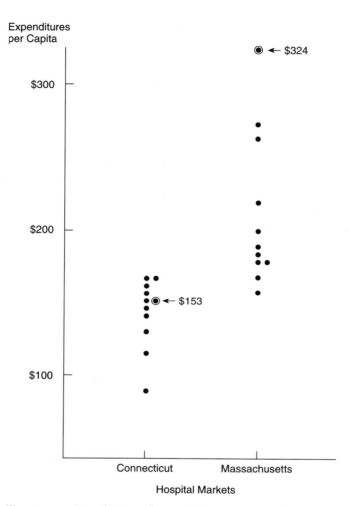

Figure 3.2. Distribution of costs in Connecticut service areas and in Massachusetts service areas in the 1970s. Each dot represents one of the 11 most populated market areas in Connecticut or Massachusetts. Per capita expenditures for hospitals are generally lower in Connecticut, but there is a twofold range of variation. The circled dots represent the New Haven and Boston markets, where the majority of hospitalizations occur in teaching hospitals. Adapted from Wennberg (1990).

The outcomes model regards diagnosis as important only if it leads to patient betterment.

A War on Cancer

Numerous studies raise questions about the association between volume of medical care and community health status. Two recent examples come from studies on the treatment of cancer and the treatment of cardiovascular disease. In 1971 Congress passed the National Cancer Act, which was also described as President Nixon's War on Cancer (National Cancer Act, PL 99-158, 1971). The purpose of the National Cancer Act was to deploy significant resources toward the eradication of cancer. Most of those resources have been directed toward treatment, with relatively few resources devoted to cancer cause and prevention. Progress in the War on Cancer was recently evaluated by Bailar and Gornik (1997). Figure 3.3 summarizes recent trends in cancer mortality in the United States between 1996 and 1994. Mortality from cancer appeared to peak in about 1991 and has gone down slightly since then. Overall, there have been slight increases in cancer mortality since the War on Cancer began in 1971. However, changes in cancer death rates have been relatively modest. The American Cancer Society provides data on cancer mortality trends over the past 60 years for men (Figure 3.4) and women (Figure 3.5). For both men and women, there have been significant declines in cancers of the stomach and significant increases in cancers of the lung. For women, there have also been significant declines in cancers of the uterus and small declines in cancers of the colon and rectum. However, for most sites, the proportions of people dying of cancers have been relatively unaffected by major changes in medical care. The rapid increase in deaths from cancers of the lung can be attributed almost exclusively to the use of cigarettes. It is encouraging that deaths from lung cancer appear to have peaked for males by 1990 and are now declining as cigarette use has decreased. Rates of lung cancer for women, however, are continuing to increase.

One example of the differences between the traditional biomedical and the outcomes models concerns screening and treatment for prostate cancer. The War on Cancer followed a traditional find it–fix it biomedical model. The identification of cancer dictates treatment, which in turn is evaluated by changes in biological process or disease activity. In the case of prostate cancer, a digital rectal exam may identify an asymmetric prostate, leading to a biopsy and the identification of prostate

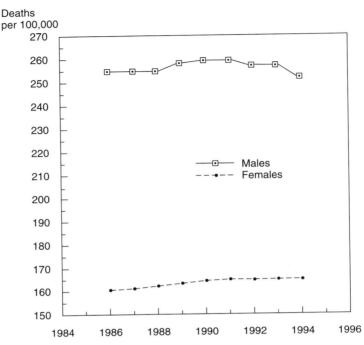

Figure 3.3. Trends in cancer mortality in the United States, 1986 and 1994. Data from Bailar and Gornik (1997).

cancer. Diagnosis of cancer often leads to a radical prostectomy (surgical removal of the prostate gland). The success of the surgery would be confirmed by eradication of the tumor, reduced prostate-specific antigen (PSA), and patient survival.

In contrast to the traditional biomedical model, an outcomes perspective embraces public health notions of benefit. Instead of focusing on disease process, benefit is defined in terms of life duration and quality of life. Studies have demonstrated that serum PSA is elevated in men with clinically diagnosed prostate cancer (Hudson et al., 1989) and that PSA levels above 4.0 ng/mL have positive predictive value for prostate cancer. Despite the promise of PSA screening, there are also significant controversies. Prostate cancer is common for men age 70 years and older (Lu-Yao et al., 1994). Averaging data across eight autopsy studies, Coley et al. (1997) estimated the prevalence of prostate cancer to be 39% in 70- to 79-year-old men. The treatment of this disease varies dramatically from country to country and within regions of the United States. For example,

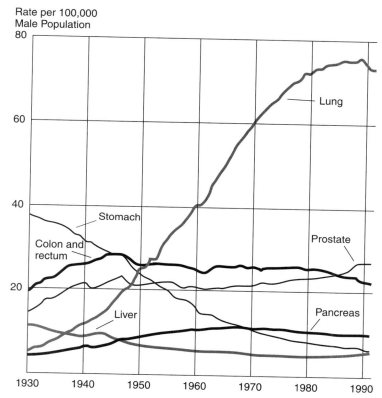

Figure 3.4. Trends in cancer mortality by site for men. Source: American Cancer Society (1997).

radical prostectomy is done nearly twice as often in the Pacific Northwest as it is in New England, yet survival rates and deaths from prostate cancer are no different in the two regions (Fleming et al., 1993). PSA screening finds many cases. However, in the great majority of cases, the men would have died of another cause long before developing their first symptom of prostate cancer. When the disease is found, it is often "fixed" with surgical treatment. However, the fix has consequences, often leaving the man incontinent and/or impotent. The outcome model considers the benefits of screening and treatment from the patient's perspective. Often, using information provided by patients, it is concluded that quality-adjusted life expectancy is optimized without screening and treatment (Kaplan, 1997).

In considering changes in mortalities since 1970, Bailar and Gornik

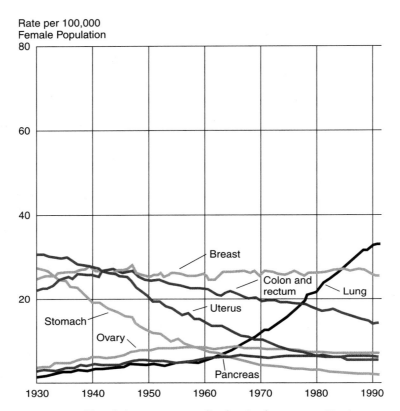

Figure 3.5. Trends in cancer mortality by site for women. Uterine cancer death rates are for cervix and corpus combined. Source: American Cancer Society (1997).

(1997) concluded that cancer has not been defeated. The find it–fix it model has found and treated significantly more cancer, but the increased treatment has not produced clear public health benefits. In fact, they argue that it is time to reevaluate the dominant strategy of the past 40 years, which placed most emphasis on improving treatments and little emphasis on prevention. The major increases in cancer have been associated with cigarette smoking, yet few of the resources have been devoted to the eradication of tobacco use. The outcomes model clearly leads toward an emphasis on factors that alter health outcomes. Bailar and Gornik concluded, "A national commitment to prevention of cancer, largely replacing reliance on hopes for universal cures, is now the way to go" (1997, p. 1574).

Looking into Arteries

Other examples come from the treatment of cardiovascular disease. Acute myocardial infarction is the most common cause of morbidity and mortality in both the United States and Canada. However, the two countries approach the treatment of cardiovascular disease differently. Invasive cardiac procedures, such as coronary angiography, are performed considerably more often in the United States than in Canada. Some years ago, we noted that about eight of every ten well-insured patients in San Diego received angiography following a heart attack, if they were treated in private hospitals (Nicod et al., 1991). However, only 40% patients at the San Diego Veterans Affairs Health Center received the procedure following a heart attack. In Vancouver, only 20% of post–myocardial infarction patients got angiography, and only 10% of patients in Sweden received the procedure. This variation would be acceptable if we knew that more care led to better health. However, there was little evidence that more aggressive care produced better results. Controlling for the seriousness of the heart attack (measured by the ejection fraction), the probability of surviving a heart attack in San Diego, Vancouver, and Sweden was comparable.

More recently, the use of invasive cardiac procedures in the United States and Canada was evaluated for 224,258 elderly Medicare recipients in the United States and 9,444 older patients in Ontario, Canada. Each of these patients had been the victim of heart attack after 1991. Among American patients, 34.9% underwent coronary angiography, while only 6.7% of the Canadian patients received this procedure. Having coronary angiography increases the likelihood that other invasive procedures will be performed. Among the American patients, 11.7% underwent transluminal coronary angioplasty in comparison to 1.5% of the Canadian patients. Further, 10.6% of the American patients versus only 1.4% of the Canadian patients underwent coronary artery bypass surgery. Figure 3.6 summarizes both the procedure rates and the mortality rates for these patients. It might be presumed that American patients are better off because they are more likely to obtain the latest procedures. However, mortality rates 30 days following the attack were comparable in the two countries (21.4% vs. 22.3%). Further, the mortality rates one year later were virtually identical (34.3% in the United States vs. 34.4% in Canada). These data suggest that the use of high-technology medical procedures is much more likely in the American system than in

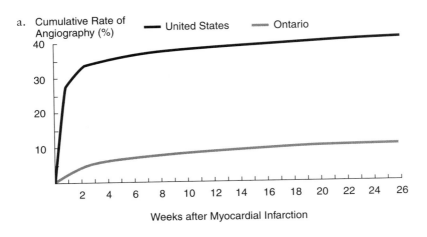

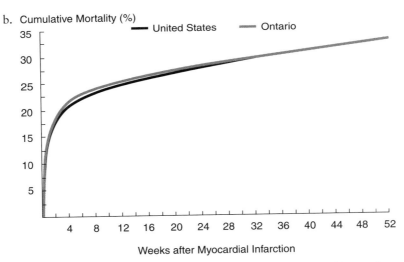

Figure 3.6.   Rates of coronary angiography (section a), cardiovascular procedures (section b), and heart disease mortality (section c) in the United States and Canada. Adapted from Tu et al. (1997).

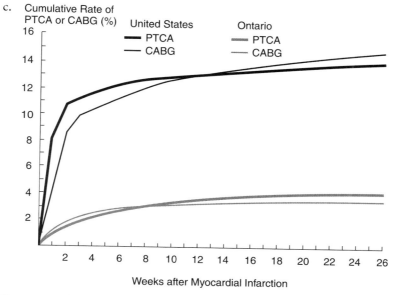

c. Cumulative Rate of PTCA or CABG (%)

Weeks after Myocardial Infarction

Figure 3.6. (*continued*)

the Canadian health care system. However, there is no clear evidence that patients benefit, at least in terms of survival (Tu et al., 1997).

These findings suggest that the find it–fix it approach to established coronary heart disease may have limited benefits. The procedures are expensive but may not extend life. An alternative might be to invest in programs that attempt to enhance outcomes by promoting health in entire communities. For heart disease, this might be accomplished by changing behaviors to reduce cholesterol. Programs to lower cholesterol might have only a small benefit for individuals but might have a substantial benefit for communities. As many as 40% of men and 20% of women have serum cholesterol levels less than 240 mg/dl. One analysis considered the benefits of population-wide heart disease prevention programs in California and Finland. Some of these programs have been criticized because they reduce serum cholesterol by only 1% to 4%. However, these slight reductions in average serum cholesterol may have contributed to as much as one-third in the decline in coronary heart disease in the United States since the mid-1960s. The education programs in Finland and California use media campaigns and face-to-face instruction. The programs cost about $4.95 per person per year and, on average, produce a reduction of about 2% in serum cholesterol. The programs produce a quality-adjusted year of life at about $3,200 for individuals at risk for coronary heart disease. A more intensive program that reduces serum cholesterol by about 3% might cost $16.55 for the first year and $8.28 per year thereafter and could produce a year of life at about $6,100. Even though advances in medical care have cut mortality from coronary heart disease (Hunink et al., 1997), the evidence suggests that population-based efforts to reduce serum cholesterol should become part of U.S. health policy (Tosteson et al., 1997).

THE OREGON EXPERIMENT

There have been a few attempts to apply outcomes thinking to health policy. One heroic attempt to apply an outcomes model to public policy was considered by the State of Oregon. In the late 1980s, Oregon was faced with the fact that costs of health care were expanding much more rapidly than the budgets for Medicaid. Collectively, Oregon citizens spent approximately $6 billion on health care in 1989, which is about three times what they spent in state income taxes. Oregon also recognized that American health care is not a two-tiered system but rather a three-tiered system. The three-tiered system includes people who have regular insurance and can pay for their care, people enrolled in Medicaid, and a growing third tier of people who had no health insurance at all. By 1993, this third tier represented about 450,000 citizens, or about one-fifth the population of the state. In addition, another 230,000 were underinsured, and the trend indicated that the number of uninsured and underinsured was steadily increasing. In order to address the growing crisis of funding for health care, the only alternatives were to (1) change eligibility criteria and remove some individuals from the Medicaid rolls, (2) continue to provide care to a large number of people but limit the care they receive, or (3) increase revenues (taxes) to pay for the current system.

Led by a grassroots citizens group known as Oregon Health Decisions, it was argued that Oregon, like other states and countries, was already rationing health care. The problem was that rationing was implicit and not open to public scrutiny. In fact, people were being rationed rather than services. In other words, many individuals in need of care received none because they were in the wrong category. Pregnant women, for example, were covered. A young woman employed as an hourly worker may be ineligible for health care, but an unemployed woman would be eligible if she were to become pregnant. Thus, the system created incentives to become pregnant in order to have a regular source of health care. The system allowed health care under Medicaid for poor families with young children but disallowed coverage for poor families with older children. Oregon, like many other states, defined Medicaid eligibility for the Aid for Families with Dependent Children (AFDC) as 50% of the poverty line. That policy set the criterion income at about $5,700 per year for a family of three. A hard-working independent carpenter earning $11,000 annually might be completely excluded by the system even though he was at high risk for injury.

These arguments caught the attention of John Kitzhaber, M.D., the president of the state senate and now the governor of Oregon. Under Kitzhaber's leadership, Oregon passed three pieces of legislation to attack this problem (Kitzhaber, 1990). In this chapter we focus most specifically on Senate Bill 27, which mandated that health services be prioritized from most to least important. The purpose of the prioritization was to eliminate services that did not provide benefit. The process of creating the prioritized list was an extremely difficult one. The commission began by attempting to create a prioritized list of all health services. However, it soon became apparent that this was a nearly impossible task. Thus, the commissioners began searching for a combination of conditions and treatments that could be lumped together. They refer to these as condition-treatment pairs. Examples of these condition-treatment pairs are shown in Table 3.2. For example, the condition of rectal prolapse is paired with the treatment partial colectomy, while osteoporosis is paired with medical therapy.

A Health Services Commission was created in order to develop the prioritized list. This commission obtained several sources of information. First, it held public hearings to learn about preferences for medical care in the Oregon communities. These meetings helped clarify how citizens viewed medical services. Various approaches to care were rated and discussed. On the basis of 48 town meetings that were attended by more than 1,000 people, 13 community values emerged. These values included prevention, cost-effectiveness, quality of life, ability to function, length of life, and so on. The major lesson from the community meetings was that citizens wanted preventive services. Further, the people consistently stated that the state should forgo expensive heroic treatments for individuals or small groups in order to offer basic services for everyone. In order to pay for these basic services, it was necessary to reduce spending elsewhere, and it was therefore important to rank services according to their desirability as determined by studies of community values. The commission chose to evaluate services using the QWB scale and a modified GHPM.

TABLE 3.2 EXAMPLES
OF CONDITION-TREATMENT PAIRS

Condition	Treatment
Rectal prolapse	Partial colectomy
Osteoporosis	Medical therapy
Ophthalmic injury	Closure
Obesity	Nutritional and lifestyle counseling

Two factors influenced the commission's decision to modify the standard GHPM approach. First, the commission could not conduct clinical trials for each of the many condition-treatment pairs. Further, estimation of treatment benefit using the QWB cannot be left to laymen. Thus, the commission formed a medical committee that had expertise in essentially all specialty areas and nearly all the major provider groups in the state. The Oregon citizens were concerned about using weights from California in assigning priorities in their state. Thus, 1,001 Oregon citizens participated in a separate weighting experiment. The weights were obtained in a telephone survey that was conducted by Oregon State University.

Multiple Lists

The Oregon Health Services Commission created multiple versions of the prioritized list. The first list was created in 1990. This list rank-ordered 1,692 condition-treatment pairs. The Health Services Commission used rough estimates of QWB changes and cost to create this list. Although this list has been the target of extensive criticism, the Health Services Commission probably intended it to be a working document rather than a final list. While they were working on the list, they completed a first draft that was discussed at a public meeting.

The list was put together in a hasty manner. As a result, there were some obvious problems. For example, 314 different medical therapies were all valued at $98.51, and an additional 177 were all estimated to cost $2,560.65 (Tengs et al., 1996). The last 193 pairs on the 1,692-item list were ranked alphabetically according to diagnosis. In addition, there were many counterintuitive orderings on the list. For example, treatment for thumb sucking was ranked higher than treatment for AIDS. Although the 1990 list was clearly flawed, it is also important to emphasize that it was never officially released. There are many reasons why the list may not have been dependable. Perhaps most important was that the overburdened staff was required to evaluate many condition-treatment pairs in a very short period of time. In most cases, systematic data were not available to guide their evaluations.

Perhaps the most discussed list was the one released in 1991. This list included 709 items. The list was based on the QWB scale to estimate benefit and included estimates of costs. In the 1991 list, the system was reorganized according to three basic categories of care: essential, very important, and valuable to certain individuals (Table 3.3). Within these major groupings there were 17 subcategories. Nine of the 17 subcategories were classified as essential. The commission decided to place greatest emphasis on problems that were acute, fatal, and reversible. In these cases, treatment prevents death, and there is full recovery, for example, appendectomy for appendicitis and nonsurgical treatment for whooping cough. Other subcategories classified as essential included maternity care, treatment for conditions that prevent death but do not allow full recovery, and preventive care for children.

Listed as very important were treatments for nonfatal conditions that would return the individual to a previous state of health. Also included in this category were acute, nonfatal, one-time treatments that might improve quality of life. These might be hip replacements and cornea transplants. At the bottom of the list were treatments for fatal or nonfatal conditions that did not improve quality of life or extend life. These might be progressive treatments for the end stages of diseases such as cancer and AIDS or care for conditions for which the treatments were known not to be effective. In the revised approach, the commission decided to ignore cost information and to allow their own subjective judgments to influence the rankings on the list. Table 3.4 summarizes the conditions selected from the top of the list, the middle of the list, and the bottom of the list. Unfortunately, the final exercise in Oregon resulted in many deviations from the GHPM. However, the exercise demonstrates an attempt to resolve the healthcare crisis on the basis of health outcome.

One of the most important criticisms of the Oregon plan has been offered by Tengs and her associates (Tengs, 1996; Tengs et al., 1996). These investigators used rank-order correlational methods to compare the Oregon lists with cost-effectiveness analyses that have been published in the literature. They report that the 1990 list showed essentially no correlation with published cost-effectiveness analyses. The 1991 list was correlated 0.39 with published studies, while the correlation of the 1992 list was 0.25. The correlation with the 1993 list was 0.24. The Tengs analyses are important, and they have received widespread attention as criti-

TABLE 3.3   SUBCATEGORIES OF
1991 OREGON LIST

Essential

1. Acute fatal—treatment prevents death and allows full recovery: appendectomy for appendicitis; nonsurgical treatment for whooping cough; repair of deep, open wound in neck; nonsurgical treatment for infection of the heart muscle (myocarditis)

2. Maternity care, including most newborn disorders: obstetrical care for pregnancy; care of the newborn

3. Acute fatal—treatment prevents death but does not allow full recovery: nonsurgical treatment for stroke; all treatment for burns; treatment for severe head injuries

4. Preventive care for children: immunizations and well-child exams

5. Chronic fatal—treatment improves life span and quality of life: nonsurgical treatment for insulin-dependent diabetes; medical and surgical treatment for treatable cancer of the uterus; medical treatment for asthma; drug therapy for HIV disease

6. Reproductive services—excludes maternity and infertility services: birth control and sterilization

7. Comfort care: pain management and hospice care for the end stages of diseases such as cancer and AIDS

8. Preventive dental care—adults and children: exams; cleaning and fluoride treatment

9. Proven effective preventive care for adults: mammograms; blood pressure screening; Pap smears

Very Important

10. Acute nonfatal—treatment causes return to previous health: nonsurgical treatment for acute thyroiditis; medical treatment for vaginitis; fillings for cavities

11. Chronic nonfatal—one-time treatment improves quality of life: hip replacement; corneal transplants for cataracts; rheumatic fever

12. Acute nonfatal—treatment without return to previous health: relocation of dislocated elbow; repair of cut to cornea

13. Chronic nonfatal—repetitive treatment improves quality of life: nonsurgical treatment for rheumatoid arthritis; gout; migraine headaches

Valuable to Certain Individuals

14. Acute nonfatal—treatment speeds recovery: medical treatment for viral sore throat; diaper rash

15. Infertility services: medical treatment for infertility; in vitro fertilization; artificial insemination

16. Less effective preventive care for adults: routine screening for those people not otherwise at risk, such as diabetes screening if the person is under 40 years old and not pregnant

17. Fatal or nonfatal—treatment causes minimal or no improvement in quality of life: aggressive treatment for end stages of diseases such as cancer and AIDS; medical treatment for nongenital warts.

NOTE: Every person is entitled to services necessary for a diagnosis. Each health service on the list is presumed to include necessary ancillary services, such as hospital care, prescription drugs, and medical equipment and supplies necessary for successful treatment.

SOURCE: Oregon Health Services Commission.

TABLE 3.4   EXAMPLES OF CONDITION-
TREATMENT PAIRS FROM TOP, MIDDLE, AND
BOTTOM OF LIST

Top 10
1. Medical treatment for bacterial pneumonia
2. Medical treatment of tuberculosis
3. Medical or surgical treatment for peritonitis
4. Removal for foreign body from pharynx, larynx, trachea, bronchus, and esophagus
5. Appendectomy
6. Repair of ruptured intestine
7. Repair of hernia with obstruction and/or gangrene
8. Medical therapy for croup syndrome
9. Medical therapy for acute orbital cellulitis
10. Surgery for ectopic pregnancy

Middle 10
350. Repair of open wounds
351. Drainage and medical therapy for abscessed cysts of Bartholin's gland
352. Medical therapy for pilonidal cyst with abscess
353. Medical therapy for acute thyroiditis
354. Medical therapy for acute otitis media
355. Drainage tubes or tonsil–adenoidectomy for chronic otitis media
356. Surgical treatment for cholesteatoma
357. Medical therapy for sinusitis
358. Medical therapy for acute conjunctivitis
359. Medical therapy for spina bifida without hydrocephalus

Bottom 10
700. Mastopexy for gynecomastia
701. Medical and surgical therapy for cyst of the kidney
702. Medical therapy for end-stage HIV disease (comfort care excluded— it is high on list)
703. Surgery for chronic pancreatitis
704. Medical therapy for superficial wounds without infection
705. Medical therapy for constitutional aplastic anemia
706. Surgical treatment for prolapsed urethral mucosa
707. Paracentesis of aqueous for central retinal artery occlusion
708. Life support for extremely low birth weight (<500 g) and under 23-week gestation
709. Life support for anencephalous

cisms of the Oregon process and the GHPM. However, the Tengs et al. analyses did not apply the GHPM and do not consider health-related quality of life. In fact, all of the analyses used in their evaluation were studies that valued the cost per year of life saved, and studies considering cost per quality-adjusted life year were systematically eliminated. Since one of the most important aspects of medical care is to improve functioning and the quality of life, this could be a serious problem. The rationale for disregarding health-related quality of life was that too few studies have evaluated these outcomes. On the other hand, it is not clear that the correlation between rigorous cost-effectiveness analysis and the Oregon process would have been improved by inclusion of quality of life data. As Tengs (1996) notes, problems with the 1991 Oregon list included poor measures of cost, failure to discount future costs, and considering health outcomes for only the first five years after treatment.

It is of interest to note that the 1991 list, the one closest to using the GHPM, showed the strongest correlation with the published literature. The correlation of .39 is statistically significant and substantial. It is important to emphasize that the Oregon project and the previously published analyses were conducted using very different methods. Further, the Tengs's analysis makes the assumptions that the rank ordering of previously published studies is correct and that failure to replicate this rank ordering must be incorrect. It is known that there is substantial variability in the estimates of cost-effectiveness across published studies.

Perhaps the most misunderstood aspect of the Oregon experience is the belief that Oregon rationed health care on the basis of cost-effectiveness. Tengs (1996) argued that Oregon intended to allocate resources using a systematic approach. However, in response to political pressures and political realities, the state abandoned the use of systematic decision analysis. They first eliminated cost for consideration, and then they eliminated quality of life from the analysis and focused on subjective estimates of treatment effectiveness over a short time interval of five years. Not only did the system applied in Oregon differ from systematic cost-effectiveness analysis, but in fact the priorities were only weakly related to results from systematic analysis.

Update on the Oregon Plan

Despite all the criticisms of the Oregon plan, there is some evidence that the outcomes approach produced benefits. The Medicaid portion of the Oregon Health Plan enrolled 120,000 new members during its first year. This was equal to the number projected for the five-year life span of the demonstration project. The initial evaluation showed that emergency room visits declined 5.3% in 1994 and that urgent care visits declined by 1%. A 1995 evaluation suggested that emergency room visits dropped an additional 2.1% overall and 6.2% in Oregon's rural areas. One of the advantages of the program is that insuring more people reduces bad debt and the need for cost shifting. In 1994, charity care declined 18.7%, and bad debts 10.6%, in Oregon. In the Portland metropolitan area, these reductions were 23.8% and 15.7%, respectively. In 1995, charity care was reduced by over 30% relative to the 1994 levels.

One of the interesting results of the plan was that the number of Oregon families receiving AFDC declined. Since it was no longer necessary to be in AFDC in order to get health care, the incentives for being on welfare were removed (Conviser, 1997).

CONCLUSIONS

This chapter has outlined a new paradigm for thinking about alternatives in health care. In short, it is suggested that limited health care resources be used to maximize life expectancy and health-related quality of life. Services that do not achieve their objectives should not be funded, and the savings should be used to extend basic health care benefits to people currently uninsured. The proposed model is consistent with the thinking of several groups, including scholars in the United States (Office of Technology Assessment, 1979; Russell, 1986; Weinstein and Stason, 1976, 1977), the United Kingdom (Drummond et al., 1987; Maynard, 1991; Williams, 1988), Canada (Torrance, 1986, 1987), and Australia (Richardson, 1991). Although the exact methodologies proposed by these different research groups vary slightly, the theory is nearly identical. Patrick and Erickson (1993) offered a detailed account of the methodological steps required to implement the system. Methods are now available to begin guiding policy decisions. However, our information base for the implementation of the model is still incomplete.

The attractiveness of the outcomes model arises from several of its qualities. For example, it makes all choices explicit, so that anyone can evaluate the assumptions used to make decisions. The model requires a large amount of data on health outcomes, much more than what we have available for most health care programs. Little research has been completed that measures outcomes in a manner that would be useful in applying the model. This requires either that we obtain the data directly (through clinical trials or other means) or that the data be estimated. Though there is extensive experience in using estimated data (e.g., Naglie and Detsky, 1992; Weinstein and Stason, 1976), there is evidence that the methods used in this approach may be faulty (Fryback et al., 1993). A second drawback is the effort required to complete an evaluation.

Work is needed on methods to simplify the evaluation without detracting from the strengths of the model.

In conclusion, problems in health care might be characterized by the three A's: affordability, access, and accountability. These three problems are interrelated. Health care became expensive because a traditional biomedical model rewarded providers for doing procedures on the basis of diagnoses. The excessive expense of care made the costs prohibitive, and many people lost access to the system. However, the expensive system has been unable to demonstrate that it provides benefits to patients. An alternative to the biomedical model, known as the outcomes model, emphasizes that health services must be valued in terms of their impact on life expectancy and their effects on patient-reported quality of life. The outcomes model suggests that population health status might be enhanced if resources are shifted away from procedure-based reimbursement and toward primary prevention.

NOTE

Supported in part by a scholars' grant from the American Cancer Society.

REFERENCES

American Cancer Society. (1997). *Cancer Facts and Figures—1997*. Atlanta: American Cancer Society.

American College of Physicians. (1997). Screening for prostate cancer. *Annals of Internal Medicine* 126, 480–484.

Anderson, J. P., Bush, J. W., Chen, M. M., and Dolenc, D. C. (1986). Policy space areas and properties of benefit-cost/utility analysis. *Journal of the American Medical Association* 255(6), 794–795.

Bailar, J. C., and Gornik, H. L. (1997). Cancer undefeated. *New England Journal of Medicine* 336, 1569–1574.

Blendon, R. J., Leitman, R., Morrison, I., and Donelan, K. (1990). Satisfaction with health systems in ten nations. *Health Affairs* 9, 185–192.

Brook, R. H., and Lohr, K. N. (1987). Monitoring quality of care in the Medicare program: Two proposed systems. *Journal of the American Medical Association* 258, 3138–3141.

Center for Health Economics Research. (1994). *The Nation's Healthcare Bill: Who Bears the Burden?* Waltham, Mass.: Center for Health Economics Research.

Coley, C. M., Barry, M. J., Fleming, C., et al. (1997). Early detection of prostate cancer. Part II: Estimating the risks, benefits, and costs. *Annals of Internal Medicine* 126, 468–479.

Conviser, R. (1997). A brief history of the Oregon Health Plan and its features. Unpublished paper, Oregon Health Services Commission, Salem, Oregon.

Drummond, M., Stoddart, G., Labelle, R., and Cushman, R. (1987). Health economics: An introduction for clinicians. *Annals of Internal Medicine* 107, 88–92.

Fisher, E. S., Wennberg, J. E., Stukel, T. A., and Sharp, S. M. (1994). Hospital readmission rates for cohorts of Medicare beneficiaries in Boston and New Haven. *New England Journal of Medicine* 331, 989–995.

Fleming, C., Wasson, J. H., Albertsen, P. C., et al. (1993). A decision analysis of alternative treatment strategies for clinically localized prostate cancer. *Journal of the American Medical Association* 269, 2650–2658.

Fryback, D. G., Dasbach, E. J., Klein, R., et al. (1993). The Beaver Dam Health Outcomes Study: Initial catalog of health-state quality factors. *Medical Decision Making* 13(2), 89–102.

Hudson, M. A., Bahnson, R. R., and Catalona, W. J. (1989). Clinical use of prostate specific antigen in patients with prostate cancer. *Journal of Urology* 142, 1011–1017.

Hunink, M. G., Goldman, L., Tosteson, A. N., et al. (1997). The recent decline in mortality from coronary heart disease, 1980–1990: The effect of secular trends in risk factors and treatment. *Journal of the American Medical Association* 277(7), 535–542.

———. (1993b). Application of a general health policy model in the American healthcare crisis. *Journal of the Royal Society of Medicine* 86, 277–281.

———. (1997). Decisions about prostate cancer screening in managed care. *Current Opinion in Oncology* 9, 480–486.

Kaplan, R. M. (1984). The connection between clinical health promotion and health status: A critical overview. *American Psychologist* 39(7), 755–765.

———. (1990). Behavior as the central outcome in health care. *American Psychologist* 45, 1211–1220.

Kaplan, R. M., and Anderson, J. P. (1988). A general health policy model: Update and applications. *Health Services Research* 23, 203–235.

Kaplan, R. M., Anderson, J. P., and Ganiats, T. G. (1993). The quality of well-being scale: Rationale for a single quality of life index. In S. R. Walker and R. Rosser, eds., *Quality of Life Assessment and Applications.* Pp. 65–94. London: MTP Press.

Kaplan, R. M., Bush, J. W., and Berry, C. C. (1976). Health status: Types of validity and the index of well-being. *Health Services Research* 11(4), 478–507.

———. (1978). The reliability, stability, and generalizability of a health status index. *Proceedings of the Social Status Section,* American Statistical Association, 704–709.

———. (1979). Health status index: Category rating versus magnitude estimation for measuring levels of well-being. *Medical Care* 17(5), 501–525.

Kaplan, R. M., Orleans, C. T., Perkins, K. A., et al. (1995). Marshaling the evidence for greater regulation and control of tobacco products: A call for action. *Annals of Behavioral Medicine* 17, 3–14.

Kitzhaber, J. (1990). The Oregon Basic Health Services Act. Oregon State Senate, Salem, Oregon.

Lu-Yao, G. L., Baron, J. A., Barrett, J. A., and Fisher, E. S. (1994). Treatment and survival among elderly Americans with hip fractures: A population-based study. *American Journal of Public Health* 84, 1287–1291.

Maynard, A. (1991). Economic issues in HIV management. In A. Maynard, ed., *Economic Aspects of HIV Management.* Pp. 6–12. London: Colwood House Medical Publications.

McGinnis, J. M., and Foege, W. H. (1993). Actual causes of death in the United States. *Journal of the American Medical Association* 270, 2207–2212.

Naglie, I. G., and Detsky, A. S. (1992). Treatment of chronic nonvalvular atrial fibrillation in the elderly: A decision analysis. *Medical Decision Making* 12, 239–249.

Nicod, P., Gilpin, E. A., Dittrich, H., et al. (1991). Trends in use of coronary angiography in subacute phase of myocardial infarction. *Circulation* 84(3), 1004–1015.

Office of Technology Assessment, U.S. Congress. (1979). *A Review of Selected Federal Vaccine and Immunization Policies: Based on Case Studies of Pneumococcal Vaccine.* Washington, D.C.: U.S. Government Printing Office.

Patrick, D. L., and Erickson, P. (1993). *Health Status and Health Policy: Allocating Resources to Healthcare.* Cambridge, Mass.: Cambridge University Press.

———. (1995). When does curbing health costs really help the economy? *Health Affairs* (Millwood) 14, 68–82.

Relman, A. (1989). Confronting the crisis in health care. *Technology Review,* July, 31–40.

Richardson, J. (1991). Economic assessment in healthcare: Theory and practice. Melbourne, Australia: Monash University National Centre for Health Program Evaluation.

Rothenberg, R., Masca, P., Mikl, J., et al. (1987). Cancer. *American Journal of Preventive Medicine* 3(Suppl.), 30–42.

Russell, L. (1986). *Is Prevention Better Than Cure?* Washington, D.C.: The Brookings Institution.

Sturm, R., and Wells, K. B. (1995). How can care for depression become more cost-effective? *Journal of the American Medical Association* 273, 51–58.

Tengs, T. O. (1996). An evaluation of Oregon's Medicaid rationing algorithms. *Health Economics* 5(3), 171–181.

Tengs, T. O., Meyer, G., Siegel, J. E., et al. (1996). Oregon's Medicaid ranking and cost-effectiveness: Is there any relationship? *Medical Decision Making* 16, 99–107.

Torrance, G. W. (1986). Measurement of health state utilities for economic appraisal: A review. *Journal of Health Economics* 5, 1.

———. (1987). Utility approach to measuring health-related quality of life. *Journal of Chronic Diseases* 40, 593–600.

Tosteson, A. N., Weinstein, M. C., Hunink, M. G., et al. (1997). Cost-effectiveness of populationwide educational approaches to reduce serum cholesterol levels. *Circulation* 95, 24–30.

Tu, J. V., Pashos, C. L., Naylor, C. D., et al. (1997). Use of cardiac procedures and outcomes in elderly patients with myocardial infarction in the United States and Canada. *New England Journal of Medicine* 336, 1500–1505.

Weinstein, M. C., and Stason, W. B. (1976). *Hypertension: A Policy Perspective.* Cambridge, Mass.: Harvard University Press.

———. (1977). Foundations of cost-effectiveness analysis for health and medical practice. *New England Journal of Medicine* 296, 716.

Wennberg, J. E. (1990). Small area analysis and the medical care problem. In L. Sechrest, E. Perrin, and J. Bunker, eds., *Research Methodology: Strengthening Causal Interpretations of Nonexperimental Data.* Pp. 177–206. USPHS/UDHHS Publication (PHS) 90-3454. Washington, D.C.: U.S. Government Printing Office.

———. (1996). On the appropriateness of small-area analysis for cost containment. *Health Affairs* (Millwood) 15, 164–167.

Williams, A. (1988). The importance of quality of life in policy decisions. In S. Walker and R. Rosser, eds., *Quality of Life: Assessment and Application.* Pp. 279–280. London: MTP Press.

Wilson, I. B., and Cleary, P. D. (1995). Linking clinical variables with health-related quality of life: A conceptual model of patient outcomes. *Journal of the American Medical Association* 273, 59–65.

███

4

S. Leonard Syme

COMMUNITY PARTICIPATION, EMPOWERMENT, AND HEALTH

*Development of a Wellness
Guide for California*

INTRODUCTION

Interventions are the key element in public health practice. Every discipline in public health attempts, directly or indirectly, to prevent disease
or promote health through interventions. Many of these have successfully improved public health through the implementation of government
regulations for water, milk, and food quality as well as for sewage control, housing standards, highway and automobile safety, and occupational hazards. However, in comparison to such structural changes, when
interventions have required that people learn the facts and then change
their own high-risk behavior, results have not been as impressive.

We need to review this failure and think about alternative ways of at-
tacking this problem.

THE MULTIPLE RISK FACTOR INTERVENTION TRIAL

It is instructive to begin with the classic failure, that of the Multiple Risk
Factor Intervention Trial (MRFIT).[1] That trial, which began in 1971
and ended in 1981, was intended to reduce the death rate from coronary
heart disease in the United States by getting men in the top 10% risk
group to lower their risk through behavioral change. A massive screening of 361,662 men in 20 cities throughout the country identified those
at highest risk, using high serum cholesterol, cigarette smoking, and high
blood pressure as determinants. After three intensive screening exams,

6,428 men were selected and randomized to intervention in MRFIT clinics while another 6,438 men, chosen at random, were informed of their risk and sent back to their own doctors.

Prior to randomization, all these men were informed about the requirements of the trial. They had to agree ahead of time to be randomly assigned either to the clinic or to their own doctors. Those randomized to the clinic had to be willing to stop smoking, change their diet, take medication for high blood pressure, agree to come to the clinic once or twice a week during the early phases of the trial, bring family members when requested, and continue their participation for six to eight years. Participants were urged not to enter the trial if they had any doubts or reservations about these terms. In addition, some volunteers were rejected by staff psychologists because it was thought that they might not be good participants. As a result, the final group of men was carefully selected, highly motivated, and highly informed.

The MRFIT cost $180 million. It was probably the most intensive and expensive clinical trial ever developed to educate people and get them to change their behavior. The trial failed.[2] Despite the fact that each clinic in the trial had a large staff of specially trained counselors who worked very closely with each participant for the entire period, after six years 65% of the participants were still smoking, only half the men with hypertension had their blood pressure under control, and there were so few dietary changes that they are not even worth mentioning.

There are several explanations for the failure of MRFIT. One, of course, is that the men in the special intervention group did not change their behavior enough; another is that men in the control group changed *too* much.

During posttrial debriefing with the men in the control group, it was learned that when they were randomized to the control group, many simply changed behaviors on their own. This is an important phenomenon because it suggests that providing people with information about their risk is not a waste of time, and it also points out the importance of how that information is transmitted. In MRFIT, the control group members were provided with personalized and relevant information about threats to their health, but they were forced to find their own solutions. The men in the special intervention group with whom the clinics worked so intensively did not have better results than those men relegated to the control group.

The results from MRFIT were, of course, disappointing. Even more discouraging is the fact that even when people *do* successfully change high-risk behaviors, new people continue to enter the "at-risk" population to take their place. For example, every time a man in MRFIT stopped smoking, one or two children in a school yard somewhere were probably taking their first tentative puffs on a cigarette. In trials like MRFIT, nothing is done to change the distribution of disease in the population because such programs do not address the forces in society that caused the problem in the first place.

COMMUNITY INTERVENTION STRATEGIES

The MRFIT is just the most dramatic in a long list of failures we have experienced over the years in attempting to get people to change their behavior and maintain those changes over time. As a result of the MRFIT failure and others like it, some of us in public health began to explore new and different intervention alternatives. One of the most interesting of these was to develop community intervention programs rather than continuing to focus on individuals. If we could not get individuals to change their behavior, perhaps we could succeed by changing the communities in which people live.

In 1984, I began a collaboration with Enid Hunkeler of the Kaiser Health Plan Division of Research to design and execute a community-based smoking intervention program in Richmond, California. At the beginning of this project, we assessed smoking behavior, knowledge, and attitudes in a random sample of residents living in a targeted area of Richmond. At the end of five years, we did a second survey with another random sample in the area to assess changes in behavior, knowledge, and attitudes. In the interval between the two surveys, we implemented an ambitious and intensive antismoking program. We worked with business and government leaders and identified a local captain on every block of the research area. We helped local children make an antismoking video featuring their own dancers and musicians performing their own music. (This video was shown for the first time in a large auditorium to a standing-room-only audience.) Data from an extensive process evaluation study directed by Professor Troy Duster of the Institute for Social Change at the University of California, Berkeley, confirmed that the project was implemented very effectively. Unfortunately, after five years of work, the smoking cessation results in Richmond were no better than they were in our two comparison cities (San Francisco and Oakland).

It is not entirely clear why this carefully designed project failed, but we can speculate on some possible reasons. For years, Richmond has been battling unemployment, crime, drugs, severe air pollution from several nearby oil refineries, and an absence of community services. Of all the problems experienced by residents of this community, cigarette smoking is very low on their list. Our research group did not take adequate account of this, instead descending on the residents with a set of plans and priorities that reflected the assumption that *our* problems were *their* problems. The children's video, a project developed on the initiative of the residents, may have been the most successful part of the intervention; unfortunately, since our project, sponsored by the National Institutes of Health, focused on adults and not children, funds to evaluate the video project were not available.

The nationwide Community Intervention Trial for Smoking Cessation (COMMIT)[3] followed basically the same design as the Richmond project. This trial involved more than 10,000 heavy smokers in 11 intervention cities. A matched group of another 11 cities served as the control group. In the intervention cities, the goal was to create a social climate that did not support tobacco use. Efforts were made to implement smoke-free policies at work sites and elsewhere in the community, provide a newsletter and other information, and train people to become smoking counselors. At the end of this massive and ambitious nationwide trial, no difference was observed in quit rate among heavy smokers between the intervention and control communities. Approximately 18% quit in both communities. Among light to moderate smokers, 31% quit in the intervention cities while 28% quit in the control communities. It is important to note that this study was expertly done by some of the best smoking cessation interventionists in the country, and it, too, failed.

During the time of the MRFIT, Richmond, and COMMIT studies, three major community intervention programs targeting coronary heart disease were also under way. These three interventions were the Stanford Five-City Coronary Heart Disease Project,[4] the Minnesota Heart Health Program,[5] and the Pawtucket (Rhode Island) Community Heart Health Program.[6] These were long-term trials involving intensive educational campaigns focused on coronary heart disease risk factors. Each of these projects was well designed, and all were implemented with energy and enthusiasm. None have yet reported their morbidity and mortality data, but they have published their risk-factor results. No differences were found in Minnesota and Rhode Island between the communities targeted for intervention and those that served as control communities; some modest changes were seen in the Stanford study for two risk factors. Given the monumental effort involved in the studies, these results can be seen only as disappointing.

WHERE WE STAND

Notwithstanding the failures of intervention efforts that relied primarily on the dissemination of information, it is important to recognize the successes that have taken place. Death rates from coronary heart disease in the United States have plummeted since 1968 despite the failure of various clinical trials designed to do just that. A conference, sponsored by the National Heart, Lung, and Blood Institute, was organized to explain this remarkable phenomenon, but it could not account for it in terms of less fat in the American diet, better control of hypertension, reduction in cigarette smoking, increases in physical activity, new surgical techniques, or better community resuscitation programs. Although the reduction in death rates is real and something is happening to explain it, we do not know what that something is.

Cigarette smoking rates have plummeted as well. Compared to overall prevalence rates of around 45% several years ago, current rates are now in the mid-20% range. Although more than 90% of this reduction has been achieved by individuals working on their own, it does appear that this success is due, in part, to information provided to them on the dangers of smoking.[7]

More discouraging is the fact that despite our best efforts to inform people about the risks of smoking, the rate among many minority populations is unchanged, and the rate among women continues to rise. And, most troubling, the smoking rate among American high school students has risen from 27% in 1991 to 35% in 1995. Among young Black males, the rate of smoking has doubled during that time (28%), while among young White males and females, the prevalence of smoking is now 37% and 40%, respectively. Among 8th-, 10th-, and 12th-graders, daily smoking rates increased by about 50% between 1991 and 1996. One of every five 12th-graders now smokes daily.[8] This is very sad news.

More people in the United States are physically active than ever before, but this phenomenon occurs mostly among the upper-middle class.[9] In the general population, the prevalence of obesity is actually increasing, with one-third of Americans now overweight.[10] And pregnant women drank more alcohol in 1995 than they did four years earlier (3.5% of pregnant women had seven or more drinks per week, a 400% increase from 1991).[11]

Clearly, there have been successes and failures, but we do not always know why, and we have not always been able to stop the harmful things from happening. Thus, the current situation is confusing. Providing information is certainly of value, but we very often find that it is not enough.

CHANGING THE PARADIGM

The field of public health faces some difficult challenges. Suggestions have been made to improve this situation, but while they are reasonable, they are not, in my opinion, enough to solve the problem. One of these suggestions is that we develop and use more innovative and rigorous research designs. Part of that process would require us to improve our definitions as well as our measurement and assessment methods. The way in which we define disease, for example, has actually caused us much harm. We typically use a disease classification scheme that is firmly rooted in the clinical model of disease. Thus, we study such chronic problems as coronary heart disease, cancer, and arthritis as separate entities. This type of classification may be useful in the individual diagnosis and treatment of disease, but it is not helpful if our goal is prevention. It would make more sense to develop a classification scheme based on the risk factors that clinical conditions have in common.

Historically, this is the approach that was used so successfully in the study of infectious diseases. In that work, the key public health concepts were the study of diseases that were water, food, vector, and air borne. In a similar vein, in the study of diseases in the developed world today, it probably would be more useful to study smoking diseases, poverty diseases, nutritional deficiency or excess diseases, and sexually transmitted diseases. By studying only clinically defined diseases, we make it virtually impossible to see underlying commonalities, to see what forces in the community are causing problems, and to see how better to target interventions.[12] This risk-factor focus would be of great value in improving assessment and measurement methods because it would be more likely to influence researchers to measure the right things.

Another suggestion is that we use qualitative methods more frequently in our work. There is often a reluctance to utilize such methods in favor of more rigorous quantitative assessment, even when quantitative approaches may be missing important issues. For example, we all know that in studying older people, quality of life may be more important than a tabulation of illnesses, but we are not very practiced in ways to measure this. Similarly, we all know that early childhood development is important for adult health and well-being, but it is rarely studied in public health because children do not have enough disease to fit the usual epidemiologic model. Clearly, we are not well served by focusing solely on the quantitative assessment of the usual issues. In addition, we tend to rely on linear multivariate statistical methods to analyze our data when we might be better served by such alternative approaches as "grade of membership" or other nonlinear methods.

While these suggestions have merit and need to be considered, there is an even more important problem that must be addressed if we hope to deal effectively with the intervention challenge we face. We need to understand better the community and environmental forces that cause disease and that might be successfully targeted for intervention. It is, of course, not easy to select important community and environmental risk factors, but there is one factor about which there can be no argument: social class.

ONE APPROACH TO UNDERSTANDING COMMUNITY FACTORS: SOCIAL CLASS

Until recently, social class had not been widely studied in public health despite the fact that the lower people are in terms of social class—however that term is defined—the higher are the rates of virtually all diseases and conditions. Although this phenomenon is universally recognized, almost nothing is known about why it occurs. While the list of possible causes is long and well recognized—including such factors as poverty, substandard housing, unemployment, poor nutrition, inadequate medical care, and low education—the relative importance of these various factors is not clear because social class is so rarely studied as the focus of research. In fact, social class is of such overwhelming power that it is typically "held constant" in research so that *other* things can be studied. If that were not done, social class would swamp all other factors, and it would be impossible to see the role of any other issues. Consequently, virtually nothing is known about the various subcomponents associated with social class.

One might justifiably argue: Why do we *need* to study the relative importance of this or that factor associated with social class? Is it not enough to recognize that people who are lower down the social ladder have higher rates of disease and then take some kind of action on the basis of that information? Do we need to fuss about the statistical details? Unfortunately, if we simply say that people in lower social class positions are in trouble and should be helped, we often end up being criticized for trying to change the world and are told that it is too difficult, too revolutionary, and too impractical. Then we withdraw, and instead we try to help people stop smoking cigarettes. If it were possible to isolate and identify a few important issues about social class, we could at least begin to think about interventions in a more practical and concrete way.

The Study of British Civil Servants

An example of how we might study social class is provided by the work of Michael Marmot and his associates. In their study of British civil servants, these researchers showed that those at the very bottom of the civil service hierarchy had heart disease rates that were four times higher than those at the top.[13] After adjusting for blood pressure, serum cholesterol, smoking, fibrinogen, social support, and other well-known heart disease risk factors, the difference between these groups was still threefold. But Marmot's study revealed something else as well: Those civil servants one step down from the top of the hierarchy—people who were professionals and executives, such as doctors and lawyers—had heart disease rates that were twice as high as those at the very top. Those at the very top were upper-class directors of agencies, all of whom had been educated at Oxford and Cambridge and most of whose careers were destined to end in knighthood.

It is not surprising that individuals at the *bottom* had higher rates of disease than those at the top, but it *is* surprising that doctors and lawyers, one step down from the top, also had higher rates. Doctors and lawyers are not poor, they do not live in run-down houses or suffer from inadequate medical care, and they are not hampered by poor education or poor nutrition. Therefore, it is not just that those at the bottom who have the highest rates of heart disease; there is a gradient of disease from the top of the British civil service hierarchy to the bottom. At first it was thought that this phenomenon might for some reason be unique to the British civil service. It is not. A similar gradient has been found almost everywhere in the industrialized world and for virtually every disease that has been studied.[14] How can this gradient be explained?

THE CONCEPT OF CONTROL

One hypothesis that seems to make sense in explaining this phenomenon is that as one moves down the social class hierarchy, one has less opportunity to influence the events that affect one's life. If this idea about control of one's destiny turns out to be useful, there *are* things that can be done to intervene, such as providing information to people so that they can take greater control of their lives. The term *empowerment* is much used these days, and even though it has lately taken on a faddish connotation, it may nevertheless be a central and crucial concept.[15] Indeed, this idea in one form or another has been used by scholars for many years under the headings of mastery, self-efficacy, locus of control, learned helplessness, controllability, predictability, desire for control, sense of control, powerlessness, hardiness, competence, and sense of coherence.

The concept of control has recently been found to be of great value in studying job stress and health. Early efforts to study the impact of job stress by focusing exclusively on job demands failed to identify any health consequences. However, when Robert Karasek and Tores Theorell added the concepts of discretion, latitude, and control to the notion of job demands, they were able to show very important effects on health.[16] Interestingly, Marmot and his associates recently published a paper that finally solved the gradient-of-disease problem among the British civil servants: When the concept of control was added to their analysis, the gradient of disease was virtually eliminated.[17]

A Successful Intervention

One very impressive and successful community intervention began in 1971 in North Karelia, Finland. The North Karelia project was instituted as a result of demands *from the community* and began when a local newspaper reported that North Karelia had the world's highest death rate from coronary heart disease. This article caused great consternation and prompted community leaders to demand that national public health authorities do something to help them. In other words, the priorities for intervention were established by the citizens themselves, not by public health professionals. When the government team arrived, it was warmly greeted by an enthusiastic population. The intervention itself focused on structural changes rather than just information and education; for example, local meat and dairy producers agreed to lower the fat content of their foods, and, in the evenings, schools were used as community discussion centers.[18]

Between 1970 and 1997, the death rate from coronary heart disease in North Karelia dropped more than 60%. This is a faster rate of decline than was recorded elsewhere in Finland or in any other European country.[19] This decline is not simply due to improved medical care, because case-fatality rates were unchanged; the big improvement was a reduction in new and recurrent cases of coronary heart disease, a change due primarily to improved primary prevention. While declines in mortality rates and risk factors have also been observed during this same period of time in other parts of Finland, the changes in North Karelia have been by far the most impressive.[20] One major difference between the highly successful North Karelia study and the other major community-level coronary heart disease intervention projects that failed was the active involvement of community workers in initiating and facilitating the project.

THE WELLNESS GUIDE

Drawing on the concepts of social class and control of destiny and the strategies of community-initiated interventions (as in North Karelia), a group of us in the Berkeley School of Public Health have spent approximately 10 years developing *The Wellness Guide* for California. Our goal was to inform Californians about the determinants of a healthy lifestyle and to communicate that there are choices that they can make and community resources that are available to help them. The *Guide* was developed with the active and intensive involvement of more than 400 community members who selected the topics to be covered, dictated much of the content, and guided the writing. It was specifically designed to empower people in lower social class positions because these are the people who bear the largest burden of disease and possess the fewest resources for dealing with these problems.

Interestingly enough, community members were initially involved only reluctantly. The first effort consisted of an 80-page guide, written entirely by university professionals, to help people deal with life problems from conception and birth to old age and death. We thought that we had done a good job in preparing this document. However, when we pretested it among the people for whom it was intended, we got a rude shock. Most of them found our efforts amusing but not very helpful or relevant. One man said, "You folks up at the university have done it again. If you want to know what problems we face, why don't you just *ask* us?"

We spent the next full year learning from our intended audience what they saw as their major life problems and what they knew about ways to solve those problems. This was an eye opener. For example, we had not realized that one of the biggest problems faced by 8- to 12-year-old girls was "being stuck with a bad reputation." Nor were we aware that many people did not know precisely what a budget was or how to make one.

In the end, children helped with the section on children, people with mental illness helped with that section, old people worked on the aging section, and so on. We also received significant input from members of the Hispanic community in developing and adapting the *Guide* into its Spanish-language version: *La Guía del Bienestar.* Following a difficult year of listening and learning, we received major funding from The California Wellness Foundation to design, print, and distribute the *Guide* to 100,000 mothers in the Women, Infants and Children (WIC) Program, a nutrition program intended for low-income pregnant women and mothers of small children. Before distributing the *Guide,* we held 12 regional workshops throughout the state to train WIC staff in how to use the *Guide* with their clients most effectively.

Once our work was under way, The California Wellness Foundation selected and funded an independent group of researchers to evaluate our project. Three outcomes were selected for study: Did the mothers who received the *Guide,* in comparison to those who did not, (1) have more sense of control and confidence in solving life problems, (2) know more about ways to solve those problems, and (3) change their behavior?

A complex, multistage, stratified random sampling design was used to select WIC mothers for study. In the end, 1,189 mothers were chosen for the baseline survey from 36 clinics in the state. As shown in Table 4.1, 816 mothers received the *Guide* in English or Spanish, while 373 did not. Approximately four months after the baseline survey, another random sample was selected to see whether mothers who had received the *Guide* had improved regarding their attitudes, knowledge, confidence, sense of control, and behavior. This sample consisted of 1,889 mothers, 994 of whom had received the *Guide* and a random sample of 895 mothers who had not. Finally, eight months after the baseline survey, a third independent sample was chosen, this time consisting of 672 mothers. Of this group, 362 had received the *Guide,* and 310 had not. Only a few mothers ended up in more than one sample; the three samples were independent of one another.

During all three time periods, mothers who received the *Guide* were

TABLE 4.1   RECEIPT OF *THE WELLNESS GUIDE* BY WIC PROGRAM PARTICIPANTS

	Mothers Who Received the *Guide*	Mothers Who Did Not Receive the *Guide*
At baseline	816	373
4 months later	994	895
8 months later	362	310
Total mothers	2,172	1,578
	(24 WIC clinics)	(12 WIC clinics)

TABLE 4.2   USE OF *THE WELLNESS GUIDE* AMONG WIC PROGRAM PARTICIPANTS

	8 Months after Receiving the *Guide* (%)
Had read the *Guide*	86
Still had the *Guide*	74
Changed behavior	26
Called telephone numbers	16
Intended to use the *Guide* in the future	65

almost identical to those in the control group in terms of age, level of education, literacy, and breast-feeding status. The only difference was that more mothers who received the *Guide* preferred to speak and read Spanish.

The first encouraging finding that the evaluators noted in this survey was that eight months after receiving the *Guide,* 86% of the mothers had read it, and 74% still had their copies. As shown in Table 4.2, 16% had called one or more of the telephone numbers in the *Guide,* 26% had actually made behavioral changes, and 65% intended to use the *Guide* in the future.

The second encouraging finding was that mothers who received the *Guide* were more knowledgeable and confident about solving life problems, as shown in Tables 4.3 and 4.4.

The data in Tables 4.3 and 4.4 show the percentages of improvement of mothers who received the *Guide* versus those who did not in dealing with the following problems: What would you do if (1) you needed free medical care for your children, (2) a friend told you that he or she had a serious drug problem, (3) for the past few months your family had been spending more money than it made, and (4) a friend thought that he or she was being denied government benefits he or she deserved? These four problems were actually discussed in the *Guide,* but a fifth

TABLE 4.3   KNOWLEDGE ABOUT FINDING
INFORMATION TO SOLVE PROBLEMS AMONG
RECIPIENTS AND NONRECIPIENTS OF *THE
WELLNESS GUIDE* IN THE WIC PROGRAM
(PERCENTAGE IMPROVEMENT OVER BASELINE)

	Responses 4 Months after Baseline (%)		Responses 8 Months after Baseline (%)	
Problem	*Recipients*	*Non-recipients*	*Recipients*	*Non-recipients*
Getting medical care for children	14	2*	11	−10*
Helping friend with drug problem	18	9*	24	−1*
Spending too much money	31	14*	25	−3*
Helping friend who is being denied government benefits	30	−4*	29	0*
Helping friend who is owed a tax refund	19	6*	31	−1*

*Chi-square test of difference between recipients and nonrecipients, $p < .01$.

problem was not. The purpose of asking about the fifth problem was to see whether mothers who read the *Guide* would be empowered by that reading to deal more effectively with a problem that was not referred to in the *Guide*. The fifth question was, "Suppose a friend thinks the government owes her a refund on her tax return? What would you do?"

As can be seen in Table 4.3, mothers who received the *Guide* were significantly more knowledgeable about finding information to solve problems than mothers in the control group. This is true for each of these problems at four months, and these differences are even greater at eight months. In my view, the extent of improvement in the mothers who received the *Guide* is remarkable. It is also noteworthy that the mothers who did *not* receive the *Guide* actually showed a decrease in knowledge over time.

As can be seen in Table 4.4, mothers who received the *Guide* were also significantly more confident at four months and at eight months in solving problems than mothers who had not received the *Guide*. This is important because confidence is crucial in dealing with life challenges. If people know ahead of time that they will not be able to meet such challenges, little effort will be made even to try. If people lack confidence

TABLE 4.4   CONFIDENCE IN PROBLEM
SOLVING AMONG RECIPIENTS AND
NONRECIPIENTS OF *THE WELLNESS
GUIDE* IN THE WIC PROGRAM
(PERCENTAGE IMPROVEMENT OVER BASELINE)

	Responses 4 Months after Baseline (%)		Responses 8 Months after Baseline (%)	
Problem	*Recipients*	*Non-recipients*	*Recipients*	*Non-recipients*
Getting medical care for children	17	−2**	22	0**
Helping friend with drug problem	7	−3**	10	0*
Spending too much money	1	−1*	9	−1
Helping friend who is being denied government benefits	7	4	14	13
Helping friend who is owed a tax refund	5	5	11	10**

* Chi-square test of difference between recipients and nonrecipients, $p < .05$.
** Chi-square test of difference between recipients and nonrecipients, $p < .01$.

in their ability to solve problems, it is not likely that they will be able to control their destiny.

Mothers who received the *Guide* were also asked whether they had actually done anything different as a consequence of reading it. This was an open-ended question, and a content analysis of the results was carried out. We were pleased to note that 20% of mothers had made a change after four months, and a surprising 26% of them made a change after eight months. Some of the most frequent responses are shown in Table 4.5. This type of behavioral change based on a printed document may be unique in the health education literature.

One key function of the *Guide* is its role as a directory of community resources. Every page has a listing titled "For More Help." This listing refers people to the Community Services section of their local phone book. Initially we found that the major telephone directory publishers each had a different way of classifying community services, but eventually we were able to get them all to standardize their listings and adopt the taxonomy used in the *Guide*. As a result, Californians in virtually every community can use the *Guide* in conjunction with their own phone di-

TABLE 4.5   CHANGES MADE
AS A CONSEQUENCE OF
READING *THE WELLNESS GUIDE*

Found a counselor	Decided to breast-feed
Used housing assistance	Visited an employment agency
Gained a better understanding of how to talk to kids	Located Alcoholics Anonymous group for friend
Started school	Learned how to choose a pediatrician

rectory to find local services. GTE Directories has agreed to use our system nationwide; we will soon work with the other major telephone companies to encourage them to do the same. Once this is accomplished, a national version of the *Guide* can be published.

While successes like this are rare and it is tempting to be excited about these results, it is important to realize that we have not yet been able to show that these improvements in knowledge, confidence, problem-solving skills, and behavioral changes do finally result in better health. Nevertheless, the epidemiologic evidence suggests that when people have greater control over their lives, when they are better able to influence the events that impinge on them, their health is better. There is growing evidence from the field of psychoneuroimmunology that this type of psychosocial factor can have important impacts on immunologic function,[21] and so we are optimistic and will continue to pursue this work. We were gratified that the WIC Program agreed with our assessment. To date, WIC has purchased and distributed one million copies of the *Guide* to mothers around the state.

SAN FRANCISCO BUS DRIVERS

While *The Wellness Guide* was developed with extensive community input, it nonetheless is focused on individuals and not on the social, economic, organizational, or political situations that are at the root of most problems. In fact, it might seem cruel and ineffective to suggest that people simply learn to adjust to and cope with an unfair and damaging world. This is another very important challenge that we must face.

To some extent, this issue has been addressed by a group of us at the School of Public Health in a study dealing with hypertension among San Francisco bus drivers. On the basis of a review of their preemployment medical records, we determined that the blood pressure of these bus drivers was relatively normal before they began driving city buses. The longer they drove a bus, the higher their blood pressure became, even after adjusting for increasing age. After many years of research on this problem, we believe that the cause of this situation is not to be found in the individual drivers but in the job itself. An unrealistic and brutal bus schedule not only causes enormous stress in drivers but encourages poor nutrition and little opportunity for physical exercise as well. The schedule also has a damaging effect on family life because drivers, to recover from their stressful days, often go to local taverns where they drink too much and then arrive home late. Over time, many of these drivers end up suffering from severe fatigue and depression.

Proposals to the San Francisco bus company about changing the bus schedule originally met with great resistance. The company much preferred a program that taught drivers better coping skills so that they could deal with stress more effectively. The company was also willing to instruct the drivers about nutrition and exercise and encourage them to seek medical help for high blood pressure. However, once we began working with individual drivers, two important things happened. First, the bus company became aware of the fact that the drivers had high rates not only of hypertension but also of musculoskeletal problems, gastrointestinal difficulties, and respiratory complaints—all of which were causing high rates of absenteeism, accidents, and early retirement. If we were to offer individual recommendations to drivers that focused only on blood pressure, it would not help their other problems. Further, even if some current drivers were helped, the new drivers who followed them would continue to be at risk. The company began to see that the individual approach to hypertension was not going to solve the larger problem, and they began to discuss the possibility of structural and organizational changes.

The drivers also began to appreciate the limits of an intervention that focused on them as individuals. They knew that even if they succeeded in making changes in their diet, exercise, and coping patterns, the continued heavy pressure from their jobs would eventually break them. As a consequence, the drivers, through their union, began pressing for structural changes to the job itself.

INDIVIDUAL VERSUS COMMUNITY INTERVENTIONS

It is often easier to begin intervention programs with individuals because their problems are obvious and salient. It is not as easy to recognize the often subtle or indirect relevance of social, economic, organizational, and political forces. With *The Wellness Guide,* we are training people to seek help from community resources. When those resources are found to be ineffective or absent, people begin complaining and banding together for help. Several community agencies, in fact, have used these complaints as ammunition to obtain increased funding. In a sense, then, the *Guide* is serving as a community mobilization tool.

The *Guide* is also being used to teach parents and children what they can and should expect from their schools. These "health promoters" are then encouraged to recruit other parents and students to address school-wide issues such as safety and improved parent-child communication. We are hopeful that this will provide the type of community support the schools need to increase their effectiveness and resources. In fact, schools may be the most important venue for such interventions.

It might be argued that *The Wellness Guide* approach is not ultimately the best way to deal with the effects of economic inequality in our society and that such an approach distracts us from focusing on fundamental societal reforms and makes things easier for those who remain committed to the status quo. However, by insisting on *only* fundamental and revolutionary social change, we may be doomed to programs that will not take effect for generations. Moral outrage about inequality is appropriate, but if we really want to change the world, we may have to begin by avoiding this type of artificial dichotomy. It seems clear to me that empowering individuals is a crucial and necessary first step in the movement toward societal change. One cannot stand without the other.

In my view, a good beginning toward reconciling the individual-versus-community argument can be made by empowering people very early in life. A wonderful example of this type of skills training is provided by the Perry Preschool Program in Ypsilanti, Michigan, in the 1960s.[22] Poor, Black three- and four-year-old children were invited to attend a new preschool program (a model that eventually led to the development of Head Start). The sponsors of the program were overwhelmed by the number of applicants. To be fair, they accepted a group at random for admission. The children who were accepted had one or two years of this preschool experience and no further special intervention.

These children were then interviewed in a follow-up study when they were 19 years of age. The results were astonishing. Almost 100% of them were located, and their life circumstances were compared to a random group who had not had the preschool experience. In comparison to that control group, the children from the preschool had twice the rates of high school graduation and college admission and one-half the rates of arrest, unemployment, and welfare dependency; the girls had one-half the rate of teenage pregnancy. A more recent follow-up of these children at age 27 reveals similarly powerful life changes.

It is not clear which elements of this program are responsible for these results. One feature of the program is that children who enroll in the class are asked what they would like to do. If they do not know, they are assigned to work with children who *have* declared an interest. When the new children eventually indicate areas of interest, all the resources of the school are marshaled to help them. If, for example, they are interested in airplanes, they learn, with help, to make a paper airplane and fly it. When it crashes, they are helped to redesign it and fly it again. When it crashes again, they are helped a third time. And so on, all day.

This approach encourages children to develop their own interests and to learn different ways to solve problems in the face of difficulties or failure. In short, they learn how to succeed. When these children go on to kindergarten and grade school, they do better than other poor, Black children, and this improvement tends to be cumulative over time. It is this type of empowerment that changes the lives of children and their families, and it is empowered individuals that are necessary to the initiation and maintenance of effective societal change.

SOME CONCLUDING THOUGHTS

The key lesson we health professionals should learn from the mistakes of the past is to be creative and inventive enough to become experts in the role of not being an expert.[23] An excellent article titled "Sustaining Interventions in Community Systems: On the Relationship between Researchers and Communities" reveals the problem we face in its last sentence: "Those psychologists willing to apply their expertise to community health will face extraordinary challenges in translating their expertise to the needs of communities."[24] It has been suggested by Professor Meredith Minkler that this sentence should read, "Those psychologists [and others, of course] willing to acknowledge the expertise of communities will face extraordinary challenges in letting go of power so that communities can use their expertise (aided by outside resources) to build on their strengths and address what they define as the needs of their communities."

John McKnight eloquently expresses the problem this way:

> The dilemma we face is lack of familiarity with the real community. We have great professional skills in managing and working within our systems, but

our skills are much less developed once we leave the system's space and cross over the frontier into the community. Indeed, many professionals are confused and frustrated when they attempt to work in community space, which seems very complex, disordered, unstructured, and uncontrollable. And many health professionals begin to discover that their powerful tools and techniques seem weaker, less effective, and even inappropriate in the community.[25]

Most educational interventions, either individual or community based, have thus far not proven to be effective. Most people do not change high-risk behaviors, and those who do seem to do so for reasons unrelated to our special efforts. It is important to learn what we can from the successes that we have seen. In my view, the common element in these successes is that people have found ways to influence the events that impinge on them and to change behaviors that do not support a healthy lifestyle. To do this, of course, they need information that they can shape to fit their life and social circumstances. This is a major challenge to those of us in public health. We have not paid sufficient attention to this problem in our training, research, or intervention programs. We need to do better.

NOTE

Prepared for the 1997 California Wellness Foundation/University of California Wellness Lecture Series under a grant from The California Wellness Foundation.

REFERENCES

1. Multiple Risk Factor Intervention Trial Research Group. 1981. The Multiple Risk Factor Intervention Trial. *Preventive Medicine* 10, 387–553.
2. Multiple Risk Factor Intervention Trial Research Group. 1982. Multiple Risk Factor Intervention Trial: Risk factor changes and mortality results. *Journal of the American Medical Association* 248, 1465–1477.
3. Community Intervention Trial for Smoking Cessation (COMMIT): II. 1995. Changes in adult cigarette smoking prevalence. *American Journal of Public Health* 85, 193–200.
4. Farquar, J. W., Fortmann, S. P., Flora, J. A., et al. 1990. Effects of community-wide education on cardiovascular disease risk factors. *Journal of the American Medical Association* 264, 359–365.
5. Luepker, R. V., Murray, D. M., Jacobs, D. R., et al. 1994. Community education for cardiovascular disease prevention: Risk factor changes in the Minnesota Heart Health Program. *American Journal of Public Health* 84, 1383–1393.

6. Lefebvre, R. C., Lasater, T. M., Carleton, R. A., and Peterson, G. 1987. Theory and delivery of health programming in the community: The Pawtucket Heart Health Program. *Preventive Medicine* 16, 80–95.

7. Fiore, M. C., Novotny, T. E., Pierce, J. P., et al. 1990. Methods used to quit smoking in the United States: Do cessation programs help? *Journal of the American Medical Association* 263, 2760–2765.

8. Novotny, T. E. 1996. Smoking among Black and white youth: Differences that matter. *Annals of Epidemiology* 6, 474–475.

9. Caspersen, C. J., Christenson, G. M., and Pollard, R. A. 1986. Status of the 1990 physical fitness and exercise objective: Evidence from NHIS 1985. *Public Health Reports* 101, 587–592.

10. 1997. Update: Prevalence of overweight among children, adolescents, and adults—United States, 1988–1994. *Morbidity and Mortality Weekly Report* 6(9), 199–202.

11. U.S. Department of Health and Human Services. 1997. *The Ninth Special Report to the U.S. Congress on Alcohol and Health.* Washington, D.C.: U.S. Department of Health and Human Services, Public Health Service, National Institute of Alcohol and Alcohol Abuse.

12. Syme, S. L. 1996. Rethinking disease: Where do we go from here? *Annals of Epidemiology* 6, 463–468.

13. Marmot, M. G., Rose, G., Shipley, M., and Hamilton, P. J. S. 1978. Employment grade and coronary heart disease in British civil servants. *Journal of Epidemiology and Community Health* 3, 244–249.

14. Adler, N. E., Boyce, W. T., Chesney, M. A., et al. 1994. Socioeconomic status and health: The challenge of the gradient. *American Psychologist* 49, 15–24.

15. Syme, S. L. 1990. Control and health: An epidemiological perspective. In Rodin, J., Schooler, C., and Schaie, K. W., eds., *Self-Directedness: Cause and Effects throughout the Life Course.* Pp. 213–219. Hillsdale, N.J.: Lawrence Erlbaum Associates.

16. Karasek, R., and Theorell, T. 1990. *Healthy Work: Stress, Productivity, and the Reconstruction of Working Life.* New York: Basic Books.

17. Marmot, M. G., Bosma, H., Hemingway, E., et al. 1997. Contribution of job control and other risk factors to social variations in coronary heart disease incidence. *The Lancet* 350, 235–239.

18. Puska, P., Nissinen, A., Tuomilehto, J., et al. 1985. The community-based strategy to prevent coronary heart disease: Conclusions from the ten years of the North Karelia Project. *Annual Review of Public Health* 6, 147–193.

19. Salomaa, V., Miettinen, H., Kuulasma, K., et al. 1996. Decline of CHD mortality in Finland during 1983–1992: Roles of incidence, recurrence, and case-fatality. *Circulation* 94, 3130–3137.

20. Vartiainen, E., Puska, P., Jousilahti, P., et al. 1994. Twenty-year trends in coronary risk factors in North Karelia and in other areas of Finland. *International Journal of Epidemiology* 23, 495–504.

21. Ader, R., ed. 1981. *Psychoneuroimmunology.* New York: Academic Press.

22. Berrueta-Clement, J. R., Schweinhart, L. J., Barnett, W. S., et al. 1984.

Changed Lives: The Effects of the Perry Pre-School Program on Youths through Age 19. Ypsilanti, Mich.: High/Scope Press.

23. Minkler, M., ed. 1997. *Community Organizing and Community Building for Health.* New Brunswick, N.J.: Rutgers University Press.

24. Altman, D. 1995. Sustaining interventions in community systems: On the relationship between researchers and communities. *Health Psychologist* 14(6), 526–536.

25. McKnight, J. L. 1994. Two tools for well-being: Health systems and communities. *American Journal of Preventive Medicine* 10(3), 23–25.

■

5

Richard C. Strohman

GENETIC DETERMINISM AS A FAILING PARADIGM IN BIOLOGY AND MEDICINE

Implications for Health and Wellness

CRISIS: WHERE IS THE PROGRAM?

The trouble with the extended theory of the gene is that genetic elements, while critical, are only one aspect of biological regulation. They cannot, in themselves, specify details of organismal phenotype, including complex diseases like sporadic cancer and cardiovascular diseases. To be sure, there are cases in which genes may be said to "cause" attributes of an organism, but these are rare; in the realm of human diseases they account for about 2% of our total disease load.[1] For the most part, complex attributes . . . phenotypes of organisms . . . are not *caused* by genes even though genes are the ultimate agents used to create phenotypes. But if genes don't determine us, if our disease causality cannot be located in genetic agents alone, if developmental processes characterized by high fidelity adherence to species form cannot be reduced to genetic programs, if the source of evolutionary change is not traced solely to random genetic mutation, then what does determine us? Where is disease causality located, where and what is the nature of programmed growth and development in living organisms, and what is the creative source of new morphology and function acting as substrates for natural selection? In short, if the program for life is not in the genes . . . and organisms are clearly programmed . . . , then where is the program?

The short answer is that the program is in no one place; it is *distributed* at many levels of the organism, and all levels are open to environmental signals. Controls may be found distributed in gene circuits, in metabolic networks, in cytoskeletal structures, in membrane units, in extracellular matrix elements, and finally in the cell as a whole and in networks of cells at the various levels of organization above the cell. These levels of control each have their own rules, and all levels are interactive with one another and, in the case of cells and organisms, with the world around them. The major new idea here is that these levels of control are not reducibly connected; it is not possible, for example, to reduce common cancer to rules that govern DNA,[2] just as it is not possible to reduce intelligence simply to the laws governing ion fluxes in brain neurons. DNA is involved in the phenotype "cancer" or "intelligence," but the cause of both lies elsewhere at higher levels of organization, including the level of the cell as a whole and the level of cell-cell networking.

This short answer is already extremely complex compared to the idea of reducibility, that ultimate control is in the gene. Part of the current maturing of biology is the surrender of simple "storybook" explanations for how life works and the acceptance that life is beginning to appear more like a complex adaptive system than like a gene machine. It is not the purpose of this chapter to treat in detail the various levels of complexity in cells and organisms, and in any case that would be beyond the reach of the author. What is attempted here is an effort to define the deficiencies evident in genetic reductionism and the problems presented by these deficiencies to medical thinking and to concepts of wellness.

Holism and Epigenesis: Alternatives to Reductionism in Biology

Reductionism is being questioned at many levels.[3,4] We are hearing of concerns about the lack of relationship between genomic and morphological complexity of cells and organisms. We hear questions concerning whether genomic databases provide the information necessary to define function at higher levels.[5,6] We are becoming aware of theories of development that do not rely so heavily on genetic mutation as the source of new morphology and action but that instead emphasize the presence of robust *generic* processes of cells and organisms that generate new phenotypes.[7] And we are learning of theories of evolution distinctly different from standard brand neo-Darwinism.[8] These are not special creation theories but scientific theories that truly aim to incorporate developmental processes into a new and more complex theory of evolution. Finally, we are beginning to see a view of complex human disease that is not reductionist in nature and does not rely on causal explanations rooted in gene mutation but rather sees disease as a function of organismal or at least organ- and tissue-level dysfunction.[9,10] In short, we are bearing witness to the reemergence of the organism as a legitimate focus of research in biology and of the genome as an embodied, experience-contingent entity. What used to be referred to as the book of life written in the concrete of DNA is now being referred to as the *flexible genome*. Genes alone are vitally important; they are *necessary but not sufficient* to determine function or dysfunction in cells and organisms (the exceptions are the rare monogenic diseases discussed here).

If we are seeing a shift away from formal reductionism that identifies genes and genetic programs as the causes of *complex* diseases, it is also a shift toward an emphasis on higher levels of analysis and in many ways involves a turn toward physiological levels analysis informed perhaps by complex adaptive systems theory.[7,8] While this shift is just beginning to be appreciated in the basic research community, where it and the accompanying revolution will certainly take some time to complete itself, the implications for medicine and for the further evolution of our concepts of health and wellness require immediate attention.[11-13] This is so for many reasons, not the least of which is that medical research continues to be dominated by molecular/genetic analysis and by a reductionist program that resists any tendency toward hierarchical analysis in which the gene appears not as sole causal agent but merely as an important part of the overall complex biological system. Genetic analysis does contribute uniquely to rare monogenic diseases (see the following discussion) but cannot extend the notion of unique genetic cause to complex diseases (common cancer and heart diseases for example) or to regulatory levels above the gene where the issues of health and wellness and their relationship to the world are most likely to be joined. This is a major problem (discussed in the following) since the stated goal of one of our most ambitious and expensive scientific projects, the Human Genome Project (HGP), is to map all complex human diseases to "Mendelian" genes.

Biological Complexity and Concepts of Wellness

Why is it that molecular/genetic reductionism does not address issues of wellness and health? First, molecular and genetic focus is almost exclusively on the diagnosis and cure of disease symptoms. This focus provides a valuable contribution because some diseases are truly genetic in the strict sense and because the design of many drugs is seen to depend more and more on a molecular understanding. However, the strategies (causal pathways) for health and wellness are profoundly different from those of genetic diseases, as will be explained here. Second, real genetic diseases are rare and account for less than 2% of the disease load in the economically advanced sectors of the postindustrial world.[1,14] Common diseases like most cancer and cardiovascular diseases that account for over 70% of premature morbidity and mortality are not genetic in the strict Mendelian sense. Nevertheless, the vast majority of our research budget is assigned to genetic-related problems.[15] This 70% represents multifactorial diseases involving many genes whose interactions with one another and with their encoded proteins define an open network sensitive to environmental signals.[1,15] The problem here is that, while the HGP will be able to provide a detailed genetic map for complex polygenic diseases, it cannot provide the instructions for reading these maps. Therefore, insights into the vast majority of complex human diseases and into their prevention are not to be expected from the HGP as such. Third, therefore, multifactorial diseases and states of health and wellness are to be seen as emergent features of these interactive informational networks. They are not reducible solely to the actions of single or even multiple genetic agents or to the actions of their encoded proteins. Fourth, while the economics of managed care forces an emphasis on disease prevention and on the superficial aspects of wellness, there is no theoretical insight into the concepts of wellness and health from fundamental research in experimental biology centered in a reductionistic genetics. Concepts of health and wellness are characteristics of whole organisms and of processes that are time and place dependent—dynamic processes open to environmental signals and contextualized by an individual's life experience. This is simply to say that in the matter of complex disease, it is necessary to go beyond the (genetic) information given, just as in the matter of a mental process, it is necessary to go beyond information in the neural cells and structures associated with that process. In complex adaptive systems like organisms and brains, even a complete description of initial conditions (even if that were possible) cannot provide a sufficient basis for predicting the outcome of the system.[8]

For all the previously stated reasons, we now find ourselves in a most critical situation in health care. Driven by economic requirements of managed care, we are coming to recognize the importance of disease prevention combined with health promotion/maintenance, and that is a giant step forward. The direction here is to extend the period of healthy life without necessarily increasing life expectancy. That is, there is increasing evidence that populations in economically advanced countries are rapidly approaching a maximum life expectancy and that further investments in this direction will be expensive without necessarily being productive. As reviewed in this chapter, even the elimination of cancer and heart disease is expected to provide only a marginal increase in life expectancy in the population as a whole. Real improvement, both in quality of life and in lowering the cost of health care, is seen increasingly to come from the effort to bring more of our population into the realm of a maximum life expectancy now enjoyed mostly by the more affluent sectors. There is overwhelming evidence that increases in life expectancy have come in the past through holistic measures and not from applications of medical technology (see the following discussion). At the same time, the community of fundamental biological researchers, as exemplified by current directions within the National Institutes of Health (NIH) and the HGP, continue to emphasize a molecular/genetic approach to disease, an approach that theoretically could marginally extend the lives of the affluent few and of the fewer with rare monogenic diseases but that says very little about substantially extending the lives of the many who, because of socioeconomic reasons, do not possess the environments necessary for a long and relatively inexpensive-to-maintain healthy life. One of the arguments made here is that our national research portfolio needs to be balanced with a larger effort dedicated to understanding the processes by which the organism integrates its world of experience into a phenotype of health and well-being. Knowledge of this integration process at fundamental levels of cells and organisms cannot fail to support the further development of health and wellness concepts now seeking recognition and resources in our health care system.

This is not in any way meant to discredit or undermine research in gene/molecular-based biology, which continues to be essential. Indeed molecular genetic research as defined by newer epigenetic approaches is essential to our understanding of the pathways from environment *to* genome and to the changes in patterns of gene expression that take place during exposure to disease-related stress. The argument here is for balancing our national research effort with a commitment to inquiry into the more complex issues of living organisms and of their interactions with the world in which they live.

BACKGROUND

The Medical-Epidemiological Background

Substantial evidence from diverse studies now points to the possibility that most human diseases in the Western world are manageable and that we are reaching a limiting plateau in our attempts to extend life. In addition, there is mounting evidence that disease management and longer life expectancy are more related to the presence of an environment appropriate to the conserved human genome than they are to the total medical intervention effort. Life span is a species constant,[16,17] and in the United States we appear now to be rapidly approaching a maximum life expectancy of age 85.[18] Even the elimination of the most serious premature killers—cancer and cardiovascular diseases—is predicted to provide a mere two to three years of additional life for the population at large.[19,20] Increases in life expectancy coming from molecular genetic approaches are not expected since monogenic diseases remain stable at only 2% of total diseases and since the afflictions of older people are seen to be multifactorial, polygenic, and therefore ultimately beyond the reach of applied molecular genetics. That is to say, progeroid syndromes have a genetic basis fundamentally different from the simple monogenic diseases afflicting mostly younger people. In younger people, but not in the older, the power of modern molecular biology is seen as sufficient to provide, in theory, a successful genetic analysis and even therapy based on a linear (single gene → single disease) format. Attempts by gene cloners, armed with advanced statistical devices, to redefine common polygenic diseases in terms of genetic tendency[21] and attempts by behavioral scholars of various backgrounds to apply monogenic "software" to the reality of polygenic human traits[22] all appear to discount the warnings coming from cell and molecular embryological studies[23,24] that genetic approaches *alone* are not sufficient to yield a satisfactory picture of complex phenotypes. These, as well as other studies discussed later in more detail, include examples of nongenetic but nevertheless cellular responses to developmental environments in which the genotype is constrained by local circumstances.

The Biomedical Paradigm
and the Problem of Informational Redundancy

The major assumption of modern biomedical research is that unique genes have unique effects. This assumption is essential in the following areas:

Medical genetics, which seeks isomorphic mapping of human diseases to Mendelian genes[25]

Molecular biology, which seeks to identify unique, genetically based mechanisms driving cellular processes[26]

Developmental biology, which presupposes (1) the presence of genetic programs, (2) additivity of gene effects, and (3) the ability to map complex developmental stages to additive programmatic sequences in DNA[27]

These assumptions and presuppositions, now experiencing major problems, are also the major features of the HGP. The HGP has become the centerpiece of the biomedical paradigm and has distilled a simplistic guide for future research and application. This guide is summarized as follows:

1. All major noninfectious diseases are caused by defective genes.

2. Diagnosis and therapy are available through genetic analysis alone.

3. Aging and other complex human behavior is genetic, and all may be mapped to Mendelian factors.

As Brenner[28] and Wilkins[27] have pointed out, however, the uniqueness assumption of genetic determinism,

$$\text{Unique Genes} \rightarrow \text{Unique Effects,}$$

is undermined by an emerging body of evidence showing functional *informational redundancy* in cell regulation. Here the focus is on redundant genes that more than one gene may specify any given function.[29] In this case the reductionistic plan to associate genetic causality with complex phenotype is brought into question since the major research approach, saturation mutagenesis, depends completely on the uniqueness equation. *This approach to understanding disease will generate a map or network of factors that interact to provide a useful background for a complex phenotype. However, as argued here, ultimate behavior is encoded not in DNA but rather in the environmentally interactive cellular epigenetic network, which includes the genome.*

Levels of Biological Regulation

It is important here to distinguish three modes of gene activity that are operative in determining complex phenotype in organisms. The first is *monogenic,* which specifies a one gene → one trait pathway. This path-

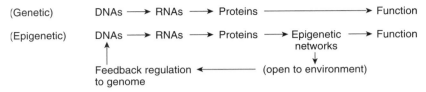

Figure 5.1.   Genetic and epigenetic regulation.

way is often influenced by environment or by other genes, but in some cases, when mutation involves a specific DNA sequence, environment is seen to be irrelevant. Diseases like sickle cell anemia and Duchenne muscular dystrophy come to mind as prime examples of monogenic diseases. The second pathway is *polygenic,* which refers to the fact that phenotype is determined by many genes acting together.

The third path is *epigenetic,* which may involve both single-gene and multigene interaction. Epigenesis implies a level of complexity beyond gene-gene interaction and extends to interaction between genes, between genes and gene products (proteins), and between all of these and environmental signals, including, of course, the individual organismal experience. But in addition, epigenetic pathways are usually thought by developmental biologists to involve progressive states of organization, each succeeding state depending on the prior state. Epigenetic pathway therefore implies great complexity of interaction as well as the production of entire states of organization arising from that interaction (see Figure 5.1). Finally, an epigenetic change in a cell, in a strict sense, is *heritable;* initial cellular responses not restricted to genomic alterations, usually called phenotypic or physiological adaptations, may persist over time and become stable so that change is transmitted to daughter cells during mitosis.

The heritable aspect of epigenetic change is an obvious aspect of differentiation where many different cell types, all with identical genomic sequences, maintain their differences over many generations. Of course, secondary changes in DNA may also contribute to the stabilization of cellular change, but these changes are not programmed by genes; they are rather programmed *into* DNA by regulatory events about which we now know quite a bit. Changes in methylation pattern, in DNA-binding proteins, or chromatin structure are examples of inherited secondary changes in DNA. These epigenetic changes result in altered transcriptional patterns and therefore in altered patterns of behavior at all levels of the organism, from cellular to integrated psychophysiological action.[30] Epigenesis has been given a modern definition as follows:

> Classical genetics has revealed the mechanisms for the transmission of genes from generation to generation, but the strategy of the genes in unfolding the developmental programme remains obscure. Epigenetics comprises the study of the mechanisms that impart temporal and spatial control on the activity of all those genes required for the development of a complex organism from the zygote to the adult.[31]

As such, the definition establishes the basis for a level of organizational control above the genome, a level that is now well established in fact, but it is a level of complexity that continues to evade decisive theoretical insight. That is, epigenetic regulation is already extending and stretching the limits of our ability to draw the limits of interactional networks that are at work in governing a major phenotype like a complex disease. For example, the mechanisms of DNA marking (e.g., methylation) may be elucidated, but what is missing is any understanding of the question, "Where and how are these mechanisms deployed in cells . . . what are the rules, the boundary conditions for such deployment?" These questions are being addressed,[10] but currently we have no consensus in biology that is necessary for a major new direction to be implemented. Courage and vision may be required on the part of our research leadership if we are to progress. Meanwhile we expect that a full description of a genetic network will come complete with a set of rules for its operation as an open system. But the rules do not come with the network diagram; they have to be discovered by human ingenuity. The differences between a genetic and an epigenetic informational system are depicted in Figure 5.1.

We have wrongly extended the theory of the gene to another area altogether; we have been lulled into reasoning that if the gene theory works at one level, from DNA to protein, it must work at all higher levels as well. We have thus extended the theory of the gene to the realm of gene management. But gene management is an entirely different process involving interactive cellular processes that display a complexity that may be described only as transcalculational, a mathematical term for "mind-boggling." This interactive complexity is *epigenetic* in nature; it involves open networks of genes, proteins, and environmental signals that may turn out to be coextensive with the cell itself. It is as if the cell has interposed between its genome and its behavior a second informational system able to integrate environmental and genetic information into its dynamical process and able to generate from this integration responses that are functional, or adaptive.

Genetic pathways specify organismal function only in rare cases, as in monogenic diseases like sickle cell anemia or muscular dystrophy, where mutation produces dysfunction in a protein of crucial importance. In these cases the cell (mostly but not always) has no compensatory mechanism, and environmental influences are nil; redundant information at either the genetic or the epigenetic level appears to be absent, and the mutant gene *becomes* the disease. But this rare event has such a powerful effect in making real the critical issues of disease and health that it has commanded our attention in other areas of our lives. Common diseases like cancer and cardiovascular problems that account for over 70% of premature morbidity and mortality are not the effects of single genes.

Epigenetic networks have been described as cellular neural networks and, given their great complexity and openness to environmental signals, most probably utilize a (nonlinear) logic and set of rules quite different from the comparatively linear rules needed for completing the genetic sequence of events. This comparison also emphasizes feedback from epigenetic networks to the genome, feedback that includes changing the patterns of gene expression. This change in pattern of gene expression is accomplished by enzymatic changes in chromosome structure and by "marking" sections of DNA chemically without changing the genetic code in any way. What is changed is the accessibility of genes to expression pathways. But the decisions to mark or not to mark are in the epigenetic and not the genetic pathway. These details of epigenetic biology, as defined by Jablonka and Holliday,[30,31] are well known and are thoroughly covered in the literature. We can see at once that failure to include epigenetic processes and their rules in predicting outcomes and basing outcome analysis only on information in DNA will lead to the anomalies that are now being seen. Thus, information for cellular integration and response is encoded not *only* in DNA, and there are no genetic programs for this process; rather integration and response come out of the dynamics of the interactive system itself. The system response includes the genome but is not reducible to it. The cell is starting to look more like a complex adaptive system rather than a factory floor of robotic gene machines, and that is well and good.

In what follows, whenever I refer to polygenic traits or diseases, I assume, along with mainstream biology, strong environmental interaction. *For my purposes, therefore, polygenic and epigenetic are synonymous.* The basic assumption is that complex disease states, at a cellular level, involve heritable changes that may include gene mutation but that also include persistent cytoplasmic changes. In addition, it must be clear what classical developmental biologists mean when they discuss complex phenotypes in terms of genotypes. What is usually meant is that all complex traits (e.g., intelligence, aggressiveness, and cancer) have some genetic basis. But this basis is so polygenic (interactive and epigenetic)— it may extend to the entire genome—that there is little in the way of practical meaning given to "genetic basis." For example, there is a genetic basis for speaking French, but the meaning of this does not go beyond the idea that there is a genetic basis for being human. In order to speak any language, we need to have something called a human genome (of which there are as many different kinds as there are humans) consisting of about 100,000 genes. But while these genes are *necessary* for speaking French, they are *not sufficient.* We also need the appropriate environment, the appropriate body, and the appropriate experience, all of which provide information not contained in the genome. Unfortunately, most behavioral and medical geneticists continue to believe that even the most complex human behavior can be reduced to genetic circuits. We now turn to examples where predictions and diagnoses based on genetic analysis alone have generated conflict and anomalous results.

CONFLICT OF THE MAJOR MEDICAL
PARADIGM WITH POPULATION GENETICS

The foundations of applied molecular genetics are twofold. The first is found in the statistical approaches designed by Fisher and Wright[32] to describe efficiency of selection in producing desired traits in agricultural populations. The second is found in the singular successful attempt in 1908 by A. Garrod to map a metabolic disease, alkaptonuria, to a Mendelian pattern of inheritance.[33] Garrod would later offer the concept of "inborn errors of metabolism" to describe a range of metabolic disorders, leading to the general emphasis on genetic disease. *The wide acceptance of the concept of genetic diseases, and the confusion of rare monogenic diseases of the Garrod type with the more common polygenic human diseases, is seen as the single most important histori-cal development underlying the widespread belief in the paradigm in question.*[34]

The tension between agricultural genetics and medical genetics has been described and analyzed most recently by Wahlsten.[35] In brief, the ar-gument is that the major statistical tool, analysis of variance (ANOVA), as developed by Fisher, is insensitive to the heredity-environment inter-action. This insensitivity is minimized in the agricultural breeding ex-periments for which ANOVA was designed because large sample size is normally the rule. In medical genetic studies (extended families) or in be-havior genetics (twin studies), the sample sizes are small, so that error is large in detecting lack of interaction between heredity and environment. As Wahlsten points out, a newer statistical approach, multiple regres-sion, is replacing ANOVA, but for the kinds of studies being discussed here, the two procedures are essentially equivalent. Experts in agri-cultural genetics generally accept significant interaction between genes and environment and are extremely cautious in applying heritability coefficients or in assigning any significant numeric value to genetic cause when dealing with complex traits. Their position is that if gene effects are interactive (not additive) with environmental effects, it is incorrect to use ANOVA for assessing genetic contribution to a par-ticular phenotype across a range of environments. Medical geneticists, however, using the same ANOVA but with significantly smaller sample size, not surprisingly do not find evidence for interaction and therefore assume that heredity and environment are additive. They then assign great significance to heritability coefficients and are confident that these numbers describe quantitatively the contribution of separate hered-ity and environment to any particular phenotype. We have a medi-cal literature, then, that asserts with great confidence, but with seri-ous theoretical reservations from sectors of population genetics, that this or that complex behavior or disease, while having an environ-mental component, also has a separate genetic component that can be discovered and utilized in pursuit of some hypothetical treatment strat-egy. It is beyond the scope of this review to enter this controversy fully. It is enough to state the minimum conclusion that medical/behavioral genetics, with a linear view of gene-disease causality, finds itself in serious debate with a significant segment of its parent science, popu-lation genetics, which sees complex traits, including disease, as highly interactive and impossible to reduce to genetic elements alone (Fig-ure 5.1).

CONFLICT OF THE MAJOR MEDICAL
PARADIGM WITH DISEASE DISTRIBUTION

Since the work of Garrod in 1908, a large number of monogenic diseases have been discovered, and there is a general misconception that all diseases are open to monogenic logic and to solution through gene therapy of some kind. In fact, the total percentage of monogenic diseases has remained constant at less than 2%. While rare monogenic diseases are legitimate targets of the new technology, most of the rest of the 98% of human diseases, including cancer and heart diseases, are not. The latter are polygenic, multifactorial diseases for which genes may be necessary but not sufficient.[1]

Diseases may be distributed according to whether they are determined before or after fertilization.[36,37] Those determined before fertilization (2%) are, of course, genetic and are mostly not preventable. Of those determined after fertilization (98%), there may be multiple causality, including early developmental effects, but in theory at least these are all preventable.

There is a second level at which the biomedical paradigm is in conflict with actual disease distribution. The problem for medical genetic theory is that the common diseases of cancer and of the circulatory system appear to be new; they were not significant causes of death and disability in the early part of the 20th century.[37] They are now the major cause of premature death and suffering in the industrial world. Clearly, this sudden shift in causality cannot be based on genetic change. Evolutionary theory and molecular biology agree completely that genetic adaptation due to mutation would take thousands of years and that change due to genetic recombination would also require much more time than the mere 50 to 100 years involved. The reasoning of medical genetics, however, is that these new diseases attack people mostly in older (post-60) age-groups. As such, the responsible genes would be beyond the reach of natural selection, which operates effectively at younger prereproductive ages. This being the case, it is argued that heart and cancer diseases are "old" entities, have always been with us (as have their genes), but show up significantly now because it is only recently that our population has aged sufficiently for them to become a problem. If this is true—so goes the argument—then these are genetic diseases, pure and simple, and may be attacked as such.

But the natural history of our complex diseases shows that, in all probability, these are not genetic diseases but are *diseases of civilization*.

Of course, they have some genetic basis, but this basis is so broad as to be trivial with regard to providing precise genetic answers. Evidence that diseases of civilization are not simply genetic includes the following. First, twin studies show extremely low concordance for most cancers and heart disease. Second, these same diseases show remarkable variation in identical populations over time and over geographic and migratory patterns. These variations disclose, for example, that diseases tend to be place (environment) specific and that when people migrate, they tend to have those diseases that are common to their host population, not those that are common to the genes they brought with them, that is, not common to their native population. These variations are reversible. Finally, these diseases are rare in populations that have not come under Western habits. Natural history studies all indicate that our major noninfectious diseases are not genetic in any straightforward causal sense; they are diseases associated with changes in environment. That is the message from the past and the present. That message, extended into the future, is that new noninfectious diseases, their prevention and therapy, will also be associated with environmental change.[36,37]

CONFLICT WITH MOLECULAR BIOLOGY OF DISEASE DIAGNOSIS

Hypertension, Myocardial Infarction, and the ACE Mutation

Restriction fragment length polymorphisms (RFLP) are being used to generate maps of genes and gene products that interact to produce a disease phenotype. The general idea here is that unique DNA sequences (mutations) can be linked to inheritance of phenotype and then mapped to specific chromosomes. Ultimately this analysis may lead to identifying mutated genes of known function and, theoretically, to gene or gene product replacement therapy. While this approach is applicable to single-gene diseases, it is highly suspect when applied to polygenic, multifactorial diseases.

The starting point for much of RFLP work was the analysis by Lander and Botstein[38] applied to the hypertensive rat.[39] This work revealed linkage of hypertension to a mutation at the ACE (angiotensin converting enzyme) locus, a gene responsible for converting angiotensin I to angiotensin II, a protein crucial to blood pressure regulation. Subsequent work, however, showed that ACE mutation was *not* linked with hypertension in humans.[40,41] More recent studies provide a strong suggestion that, even for the hypertensive rat, early developmental changes will neutralize ACE mutation and provide for near normal phenotype. Thus, if young rats are taken from genetic mothers bearing the ACE mutation and nursed by normal mothers of a related strain, the pups show decreased levels of hypertension.[42]

Myocardial infarction in humans has also been linked to ACE mutation.[41] However, in this study many individuals were identified with the identical mutation who had no heart disease. Clearly, other factors are involved. How many other genes or other factors might there be? In studies like this, the question is rarely asked. But the physiology of heart function clearly reveals that ACE-related diseases will most likely be multifactorial, polygenic entities. If so, then one expects that each of the many genes will have a small effect,[43] redundancy will be present, and any one gene or even several functionally related genes may be *necessary but not sufficient* to precipitate a heart disease. In other words, one anticipates that in this situation genetic diagnosis will not be a robust predictor of phenotype. The environment and individual natural history will be major determining factors. In the case of angiotensin-related function, it is clear that redundant epigenetic regulation will dominate a single genetic defect. Why? It is well known that in the normal or diseased human ventricle, ACE is a minor source of angiotensin II. There are many other (gene coded) serine proteases that provide for 90% of ventricular angiotensin II levels.[44]

We conclude that ACE mutation will predict neither hypertension nor myocardial infarction in humans. While an ACE mutation might have some effect, at the wider physiological–nervous system level, there will be further interactional complexity and phenotypic adaptation, including central nervous system override of renin production. These and other elements of the hypertensive control network will confound simple genetic determinism. Examples include complex cortical and medullary regulation of heart and blood pressure rhythms that are exquisitely sensitive to environmental input and personal experience.[45] While the use of ACE inhibitors may be a useful therapy for hypertension, an ACE screen for heart disease is not predicted to be efficient. Yet the biomedical community persists in calling for the use of an ACE gene screen to predict tendency for heart diseases and to emphasize genetic models of hypertension in general.[46,47] Why?

Molecular biologists are compelled to find as much detail as possible in gene-based networks like the one for hypertension, and RFLP approaches do provide the appropriate tool. In time, a gene map of extremely high density for this network will become available. But such maps, for each multifactorial trait or disease, will include perhaps hundreds of genes and interactive gene products all with input from the environment. The complexity of such a system can be described only as indeterminate since, when only six genes are involved in shaping a trait, the total number of phenotypes possible is over 4,000. There will be little of predictive value in the individual bits of genetic information defining this system. Rather, hypertension or other disease phenotype will be defined by the system as a whole and by the responses the system makes to the appropriate internal and external signaling pattern. The search for a screen that depends on a single or even a multiple number of genetic variants is an understandably oversimplified approach born of an optimism that all controls reside in genetic elements. But, as has been pointed out here, such optimism, realistic when applied to the rare monogenic diseases, is misplaced when applied to complex multifactorial systems such as hypertension.

Atherosclerosis

This is a model of multifactorial diseases. It is the major cause of death in North America and in a number of European countries.[48] Current research focus is on a hypothesis in which "response to injury" offers the most promise for understanding and perhaps control.[49] The hypothesis involves a complex etiology of atherosclerosis that includes disorders of lipid metabolism, clotting, blood pressure regulation, and carbohydrate regulation. The events proximal to the disease include lipid infiltration of blood vessel walls and loss of control of intimal cell proliferation that is postulated by some to involve, in the case of restenosis following angioplasty, tumor suppressor gene (p53) inactivation.[50,51] Thus, assuming that the hypothesis is correct, it remains highly unlikely that diagnosis or prediction of atherosclerosis will emerge from gene mutation analysis. Why? Mutation in p53 or related genes is identified as an end product in a long line of causal factors. Epidemiological studies reveal over 200 risk factors at work,[52,53] and molecular studies suggest that hundreds of genes may be involved; as many as 200 different genes are probably active in lipid metabolism alone. Using new techniques of linkage disequilibrium,[10] one may be able to detect the influences of perhaps 500 genes affecting atherosclerosis. What is the predicted benefit of measuring small effects of 500 genes? Nil. Why? Because each small effect will display strong environmental shaping, will be open to redundancy at the gene level, and will be interactive with other genes so that cooperative and compensating (epigenetic) effects can take place, all of which makes early diagnosis or prediction of final outcome based on genetic information alone extremely difficult if not impossible.

There is, however, a role for genetic analysis in the diagnosis of complex polygenic diseases like atherosclerosis. New approaches attempt to link genomic variation with specific environmental and physiological states to predict disease phenotype. They recognize that genetic and environmental signals are strongly interactive and that few signals of either kind will exert independent effects on the determination of disease susceptibility. These approaches assume "that interactive effects are translated through quantitative variation of intermediate biological and physiological agents that link discrete genome type variations and variation in risk of disease."[52] For example, Sing and his collaborators[54] have proposed a nonparametric statistical strategy for selecting combinations of genotypes, intermediate risk factor traits (physiological states), and environmental agents that can be associated with subsets of individuals showing a disease phenotype. One early result of this has been the strong association (odds ratio greater than 2) of high body mass index combined with unique apolipoprotein E genotypes with coronary artery disease. This strategy may be extended to many genomic, physiological, and environmental interactors and may reveal the role of genome type variation in nonlinear relationships with a great variety of other interactors.[55] Approaches such as this represent an upper limit of using genetic analysis coupled with other signals in a dynamic epigenetic framework to predict disease outcome. Other examples of nonlinear approaches to predict disease susceptibility rely on dynamical measures of physiological states alone and will be discussed here.

Cancer and Mutation in Regulatory Genes

The purpose of this section is, once again, to focus on an epigenetic perspective as an alternative way of thinking about disease causality. It is not the intent to dismiss mutations as an important aspect of tumor formation. However, a significant and persistent criticism of the mutational theory of cancer remains in evidence, and it behooves us to be reminded of it as a possible missing piece of our mainstream approach to cancer detection and diagnosis. This criticism should be kept in mind as we review examples here of conflicts in this area. Basically this criticism, drawn from different sources,[56-60] states the following:

1. The mutation of single genes of "major" importance, in itself, is insufficient to cause cancer at least in the early stages. Tumor suppressor genes or oncogenes are examples of major genes.

2. Early stages are often reversible and display tissuewide cellular changes inconsistent with single-gene mutation causality.

3. Early-stage changes are seen as epigenetic adaptations to environmental signals. These changes progress through intermediate states to end-stage tumors that do show many mutations that may preclude any spontaneous remission. In what follows here, discussion is restricted to polygenic cancers where there is no Mendelian segregation associated with the phenotype.

Cancer, in its multiple forms, has often been described as one of our most multifactorial and enigmatic diseases. While strong evidence exists for a genetic background, for many cancers much of this evidence is potentially confounded by congenital and familial effects; we forget that many things are inherited in addition to genes. In addition, we know that many forms of cancer have strong environmental determinants. Current research emphasis, however, is on mutation in tumor suppressor genes, which, while they will play some role in cancer, may also prove to be constrained by other factors. Here I analyze several cases and conclude that an epigenetic basis for polygenic cancer is an attractive but missing research component.

The p53 and rb Genes as Tumor Suppressors The most recent trend has been to associate unique cancers with mutation in growth control or tumor suppression genes such as p53 or retinoblastoma (rb).[61,62] These genes code for DNA-binding proteins that delay or inhibit cell replication. Mutation in both alleles would then produce defective regulation of growth and tumor formation. If one of these genes is defective at birth, then one inherits a *tendency* or *susceptibility* for cancer; the disease itself is then predicted to occur when, through somatic mutation, the second allele is also defective. But it is now clear that some form of redundancy for p53 and rb is present in cells, making it difficult or impossible to use mutational analysis alone for predicting cancer. For example, a mouse has been constructed with both p53 alleles absent (homozygous knockout).[63] In this case, it was expected that growth control in all cells would be defective with dire effects for all affected individuals. However, the affected animals were all normal at birth, and early development and growth was normal. It was only after adulthood was reached that some, but not all, of these individuals developed tumors in excess of that found in control populations. Clearly, the early phases of development that depend on stringent growth controls remain independent of p53 input or have redundant pathways around p53. The same must be said of the p53 mutant adult individuals that did not show any tumor formation. Finally, when a normal p53 gene is inserted into cancer cells, it may or may not restore normal growth regulation.[64]

More recent evidence shows that p53 protein may form heterodimers with many other cellular proteins,[65] including replication protein A, which is involved in the initial stage of DNA replication.[66] Thus, p53 regulation is a prime candidate for epigenetic control in which the final effect is modulated by a complex interaction of many bits of genetic and environmental information. Much is learned about DNA replication in p53 studies, but the emerging picture shows not single-gene control of cancer but complex interactive regulation. Epigenetic interactions of p53 protein with other gene products form a basis for explaining the varied effects observed when p53 is mutated in different genetic backgrounds[63] or when wild-type p53 fails to restore normal growth regulation to p53-defective cells.[62]

A similar story may be told for the retinoblastoma (rb) mutation (for a review, see reference 67), which arises either spontaneously or via heredity associated with a deletion in or absence of chromosome 13 in 20% to 30% of affected cases.[68,69] But 20% to 30% is not 100%, so clearly other factors are involved. Many individual rb tumors do not show mutated rb genes.[70] In addition, while expression of wild-type rb in some rb-defective cells will restore normal growth,[71] such transfection and expression fails to produce normal growth when these cells are transplanted to the eye of nude mice.[72] Homozygous rb knockout in the mouse is lethal but only late in development after lineage determination is complete and after millions of cell replications have been completed.[62] This gene, therefore, while it plays an important role in cell replication, is not essential during early development and is not sufficient to cause cancer. We must assume that epigenetic control of rb is taking place.

Finally, one of the most outstanding characteristics of neuroblastoma is spontaneous remission at 10- to 100-fold greater than that seen for any other human cancer.[73] Reversibility of tumor growth is normally thought to be inconsistent with mutation causality, especially when one eliminates from consideration the possibility of immune surveillance as the cause of remission.

A newer explanation for remission is apoptosis, but one is left with an epigenetic regulation because some aspect of cellular behavior must be presumed to signal cell death or to engage the so-called apoptosis *program*. Here again we become aware of the facile nature of molecular thinking on the issue of genetic programming and apoptosis.[74] For example, in a recent review we read, "Within a few months of birth the programme is activated: cells then *die successfully* by apoptosis and the (rb) tumor shrinks."[73] When one asks the question, "What activates the program?," the answer is usually in terms of other genes for growth factors or DNA-binding proteins. But cells reacting to stressful signals such as x-irradiation or to a loss of normal tissue environments when explanted into cell culture will display a variety of epigenetic adaptations that might easily trigger cell death.[75]

Genes for Breast Cancer Human breast cancer work is heavily invested in gene mutation causality even though a large population study tells us that less than 2.5% of breast cancer is associated with genetic determinism.[76] Many mutations are found in later stages of a variety of tumors. While it is likely that these play some role, it remains uncertain whether mutations are the cause or the effect of earlier, nongenetic lesions that, if reversed soon enough, would have deflected the tumors altogether.[56,77]

The latest focus in breast cancer has been on a familial study where linkage has been established for "cancer tendency" to a locus on chromosome 17q21.[78] The lod score (see the glossary at the end of this chapter) for linkage was 5.98, well in the range to ensure a high probability of association between the cancer and the genetic anomaly. While the technology of this linkage study may be assumed to be state of the art, we must also be aware of its problems. For example, we do not know what the frequency of this mutation might be in the general population, nor do we know the extent to which other mutations might be present in the suspect or other chromosomes of the affected women. Nor do we know the pleiotropic and epistatic effects that other genes might have in altering the penetrance of the suspected mutation. These are all questions of fundamental importance in elementary genetics.[43] We also have no knowledge of what environmental influences might be required in order for tumor formation to occur in the presence of the mutation. The mutation may be necessary but not sufficient; it may require specific environments or specific other genetic background. Finally, as mentioned at the outset of this discussion, we also know that while there is some relationship of family history to breast cancer, only 2.5% of breast tumors are genetic in origin.[76]

This breast cancer gene, BRCA1—a putative tumor suppressor gene—has now been isolated.[79] BRCA1 germ line mutations are linked to breast and ovarian cancer in a number of small families having multiple cases of these diseases. Women carrying mutant BRCA1 alleles have a significant increase of breast and ovarian cancer so this finding may prove to be extremely useful. The search for the *breast cancer gene* had been accompanied by an unnecessary hyperbolic publicity in both mass media and scientific press where an anxious expectation was developed that once the gene was found, we would be provided with important new clues for all breast cancer and perhaps for cancer in general. High expectations like this have proved mostly unfounded in the history of cancer research and serve only to frustrate public opinion and undermine confidence in research. It was sobering for many, therefore, to find that in nonfamilial breast and ovarian cancers, constituting more than 95% of the cases, BRCA1 mutations were not involved.[80] Thus, this mutation "appears to play no role in common, nonhereditary forms of breast cancer that strike about 173,000 women in the U.S. each year— a finding that undermines some long-held assumptions about how the gene works."[81]

There has also been much attention paid to another tumor suppressor gene, CDKN2, that codes for the cell cycle regulatory protein cyclin-dependent kinase-4 inhibitor (p16).[82] This (mutant) gene has been linked to a variety of tumors and has been a prime suspect for breast cancer. However, a recent report has now examined human breast carcinomas for mutations of this gene with negative results. Evidently, p16 is not involved in the formation of primary breast carcinoma.[83] In addition, it has been found that p16 mutations are found in cell lines derived from many tumors but not in primary tumors within the patients, making it clear that so-called carcinogenic mutations may be a pure artifact of cell culture.[83] The studies on p16 mutation are consistent with a hypothesis of cancer where early neoplastic change is an epigenetic one that includes mutation as an event after the fact of initiation.

OTHER CONFLICTS WITHIN BIOMEDICINE:
THE PROBLEM OF PREMATURE DIAGNOSIS

Imaging Techniques

Computed tomography and magnetic resonance imaging have become widespread and extremely expensive additions to diagnosis. The problems inherent in imaging techniques have been recently analyzed[84] and are discussed briefly here as prologue to similar problems turning up with molecular measurements that, while extremely sensitive, are also without proven meaning when applied to disease manifestation.

Imaging techniques, because they are so sensitive, often measure not disease itself but early changes in tissue that are taken as evidence that disease will develop. Early changes may, however, be extremely misleading since they often reflect reversible processes or those with extremely long lag time to any clinical manifestation. As our machines are able to detect the most incipient stages, we experience several problems.[84] First, as exemplified by thyroid cancer, is the problem of defining diseases as cellular changes that always progress to serious morbidity. In this case, clinical cancer (tumor size greater than 2 centimeters) is seen in only 0.1% of adults between the ages of 50 to 70 years. However, autopsy using increasingly thin sections of the gland could reveal at least one papillary carcinoma in 36% of adults. It was calculated that as sections became thinner, autopsy would show verifiable papillary cancer in 100% of cases. These "tumors" discovered at earliest stage represent an enormous reservoir of detectable but subclinical disease. Under these circumstances and for a variety of diseases, the patient may never experience clinical symptoms but, under aggressive medical management, may become involved in unnecessary and expensive medical procedures that are predicted to have little positive effect.[84]

The second major problem that arises has to do with the effect on reported disease frequency where frequency increases as the degree of measurement sensitivity increases. However, without any manifestation, early stage diagnosis makes it appear as if we are experiencing large increases in the disease itself. The third problem is the effect of statistical evaluations of various therapies for a disease. As the time between diagnosis and manifestation increases, it is made to appear as if various therapies are working even when nothing in the way of treatment need be involved in the statistical analysis.[84]

Antigen and Nucleic Acid Sequence Measurement

Nowhere in medical technology have we greater sensitivity of measurement than in antigen and nucleic acid chemistry. The possibility exists, however, that these measurements are often without predictive value for the diseases for which their measurement was designed. Increased levels of scrutiny can, for example, explain recent reported increased prevalence in breast, prostate, and thyroid cancer.[84] Prostate antigen testing, together with other evaluation, may prove useful. However, these tests, used alone, can provide for an enormous increase in reported prevalence and an increased *apparent* time of survival and, unless carefully applied, could lead to unnecessary treatment.

Polymerase chain reaction (PCR) is a technology used extensively to report "viral loads" in patients and has replaced measurements of actual infective units of pathogen. What PCR does is to amplify by thousands of times sequences of DNA that are present in body fluids at extremely dilute concentration. For example, it has proved to be crucial for diagnosis of HIV-related AIDS, where it is used to amplify vanishingly small amounts of *parts of* HIV sequences. But such partial sequences tell us nothing about the presence of "live" virus and could be reporting on DNA fragments resulting from a variety of sources (e.g., viral degradation). In addition, PCR is notoriously difficult to quantitate, and recent publications fail to publish standards that might show actual viral numbers. As Nobelest Kary Mullis, the inventor of PCR, himself states in a paper that was refused publication, "The vice of the PCR is that it can find the biochemical equivalent of the needle in the haystack. Viral fragments that are present only in minute quantities can be amplified and identified, but this tells us nothing about whether replicating virus is present in sufficient quantities to do harm."[85] The HIV-AIDS hypothesis remains plagued by the fact that most AIDS patients, until end-stage disease, rarely show HIV viremia (classically defined by actual virus replication), and diagnosis continues to rely on PCR and antibody measurements. In HIV and other infectious diseases, we may have abandoned, at great scientific cost, traditional rules for establishing disease causality.[86] For example, HIV, as many contend, may be caused by agents other than or in addition to HIV. But reliance on PCR tends to conceal the absence of viral units and to conceal the possibility that other causes may be involved.

CONFLICT RESOLUTION AND OTHER SPECULATION

The conflicts described here arise from attempts to apply a strict genetic-reduction analysis to the problem of complex phenotypes. Why has it been so difficult to use single-gene markers to predict polygenic cancer in individuals even when a mutation is present in an important tumor suppressor gene (rb or p53)? Why are there so many false positives and false negatives in predicting heart disease when there is a measurable defect in an important gene (ACE) involved in blood pressure regulation? Finally, why is it that the elimination (homozygous knockout) of both copies of a gene like p53—known to be important for controlled growth of cultured cells—fails to provoke any measurable defects in normal development? On the basis of a linear genetic analysis, these failed predictions should have been viewed as evidence of a failed cancer theory. However, the response from biotechnology has been to rescue the genetic theory in the face of these and many other exceptions to the rule that unique genes have predictable unique effects. Why this response should persistently come up has been treated elsewhere as part of a paradigm shift[87] in biology and medicine.[88]

The short answers, to the questions of lack of predictive power of gene analysis and of why we have thrown out the facts rather than the theory, are not too difficult. The explanation formulated here is that polygenic disease and growth regulation are not linear processes and cannot therefore be fully analyzed by a linear logic. Rather, they are representatives of complex adaptive systems that are innately unpredictable. To understand the unpredictable nature and other features of such systems, it will be necessary to develop a disease theory similar to what is found in treating nonlinear phenomena.[89]

What is needed to *supplement* genetic theory is a theory of biological complex adaptive systems.[90] If living systems were seen as complex adaptive systems, then we would not be surprised at the previously mentioned failure of prediction. In fact, they would be expected since such systems are unpredictable and actually seek out alternative pathways when perturbed by new information, either from the outside world or from within. The results of alternative pathway selection would include epigenetic change in the genome and resulting change in pattern of gene expression. In the case of mutation, however, we need to remember that it is taking place within an epigenetic framework. As explained by James Shapiro,[91] part of the adaptive response of bacterial cells to stress is the activation of a whole family of enzymes whose job is to remodel the genome, a job that will predictably increase the frequency of mutation. But in this case the mutation would not necessarily be the result of random process but part of an epigenetic response process that has become maladaptive through chronic stress. One might begin the merger of genetic reductionism and epigenetic complexity with those areas where multigenic systems are known to be coordinated by higher-order cellular responses to environmental conditions. Nobel laureate Barbara McClintock, who described mobile genetic elements long before they were discovered by molecular biology, had always been preoccupied with mechanisms that *rapidly reorganize the genome.* In one of her last reviews, she wrote of the significance of responses of the genome to challenge. She ended that article as follows: "We know about the components of genomes. . . . We know nothing, however, about how the cell senses danger and initiates responses to it that often are truly remarkable."[92]

Statements concerning cells "sensing danger" and "initiating responses" strike biologists today more as poetic meanderings than as statements with scientific value. But clearly cells and multicellular organisms display these holistic behaviors. Natural selection operates not merely at a genetic level but at all levels of biological organization,[93,94] including whole-cell and organismal behavior. Much evidence exists for the idea that cells do sense danger and respond in a manner that is not explored by reductionistic thinking. For example, when tissues are exposed to X rays, there is a tissuewide, or "field," response in the cellular population as a whole, a response that is quite separate from gene mutation but that actually induces persistent hypersensitivity to future mutation.[95] Cells exposed to the stress of removal from normal tissue constraints in vivo when explanted to cell culture adopt many morphological changes that are heritable and that, when continued over a period of time, give rise to transformation and to mutation.[96] The flip side here is the demonstrated ability of liver architecture to constrain tumor growth in an age-dependent fashion. Tumor cells explanted into young rat livers generate tumors at a much lower frequency compared to that seen when these cells are transplanted into older livers.[97] Findings like this are difficult to reconcile with singe gene mutation causality but are predicted by an epigenetic theory of cancer that locates control of single cell growth in higher (tissue and organ) levels of biological organization.

Perhaps the most important new insight into cancer is the one having to do with the source of the many (hundreds and thousands of) mutations that may be found in human tumor cells.[98] Cancer cells in culture show a hypermutation phenotype but, surprisingly, not under conditions of rapid growth. Only under conditions of nutritional stress or contact inhibition do these cells recruit an epigenetic response capable of "reorganizing the genome" through increased mutation rates. The result of this reorganization is the production of useful mutations (useful from the cancer cell point of view) allowing cancer cells to escape the various constraints that normally contain tumor expansion and metastasis. Single-gene mutation would be amply buffered by epigenetic mechanisms, including redundancy, but with stress producing 1,000- to 5,000-fold increases in mutation rates, the "cause" has to be located in the epigenetic mechanisms responsible for this extraordinarily high rate.

One may conclude that (1) higher-level epigenetic management and constraint on tumor growth delays clinical cancer and may even reverse it and that (2) epigenetic mechanisms at the intracellular level are responsible for generating increased mutation rates necessary for escape of these cells from the higher-level constraints. In other words, cancer is a cellular, epigenetic disease and not the result of single-gene mutation.

An approach to complex analysis of heart disease with multigenetic causality linked to interactive environments is the work of Sing and his group as mentioned previously (see the section "Atherosclerosis"). At these levels above the cell, for complex physiological systems, chaos theory builds on epigenetic thinking and already is providing new ways to think about complex systems.[8-10] This is particularly true for cardiac function, where sinus arrhythmia, long thought to be low-level noise or random fluctuation in heart rate, is now seen as high-order chaos.[99] Coupling of heart rate to brain function and thus to experience has long been appreciated as an observable patterned occurrence but was mostly inexplicable through standard physiological experiment.[100] Chaos theory is an old story in physiology in general[101] and is able to provide a method of revealing generic patterns in what was thought to be random variation. Recognition of these patterns allows new insights into brain-heart physiology and may even allow prediction of sudden cardiac death among patients at risk.[99]

NOTE

This chapter draws much from previously published materials by the author. See references section for the exact citations.

GLOSSARY

ALLELES. Different forms of the same gene.

ANTIGEN. A protein recognized by the immune system.

APOPTOSIS. Programmed cell death.

COMPUTED TOMOGRAPHY. A technology used to scan whole bodies for diagnostic purposes.

CONSERVED HUMAN GENOME. All genomes, including the human genome, tend to remain constant over long periods of time because of the presence in cells of formidable DNA repair systems. Mutations, for example, occur, but most are repaired.

CYTOPLASM. General term for that part of the cell surrounding the nucleus.

EPIGENETIC. Generally refers to the inheritance of factors and processes that are in addition to genes. Also refers to changes in the genome that do not involve sequence changes in DNA.

EPISTATIC. Interaction between genes.

HETEROZYGOUS. When the two alleles are different.

HOMOZYGOUS. All genes come in allelic pairs; "homozygous" refers to cases in which both alleles are the same.

HUMAN GENOME PROJECT. An international effort to identify every gene in the total of 70,000 to 100,000 genes thought to be present in all humans.

ISOMORPHIC. A linear or direct representation of one thing by another.

LOD SCORE. A technical term used to indicate linkage of a gene to a phenotype.

MENDELIAN GENE. Defined by inheritance pattern when studied in families.

METHYLATION. An epigenetic change involving addition of a chemical group (methyl group) to DNA, thus changing gene expression without changing DNA sequences within the gene.

MONOGENETIC. A phenotype (disease) said to be caused by a single gene mutation.

NUCLEIC ACID. DNA or RNA.

PCR. Polymerase chain reaction; a technique that measures extremely small samples of DNA.

PHENOTYPE. What the organism looks and behaves like; its morphology.

PLEIOTROPIC. A gene or a protein having many effects.

POLYGENIC. A phenotype shaped by many genes acting in concert.

PROGEROID. Characteristic of old age.

RETINOBLASTOMA. A disease (cancer) of the retina.

SATURATION MUTAGENESIS. An experimental procedure in which genes are randomly made mutant.

REFERENCES

1. Strohman, R. C. 1994. Epigenesis: The missing beat in biotechnology? *Bio/Technology* 12, 156–164.

2. Polanyi, M. 1968. Life's irreducible structure. *Science* 160, 1308–1312.
3. Nurse, P. 1997. The ends of understanding. *Nature* 387, 657.
4. Williams, N. 1997. Biologists cut reductionist approaches down to size. *Science* 277, 476–477.
5. Miklos, G. L. G. 1993. Emergence of organizational complexities during metazoanevolution: Perspectives from molecular biology, palaeontology and neo-Darwinism. *Memoirs of the Australasian Association of Palaeontology* 15, 7–41.
6. Miklos, G. L. G., and Rubin, G. 1996. The role of the Genome Project in determining gene function: Insights from model organisms. *Cell* 86, 521–529.
7. Goodwin, B. C. 1994. *How the Leopard Changed Its Spots: The Evolution of Complexity*. New York: Scribner's Sons.
8. Webster, G., and Goodwin, B. 1997. *Form and Transformation*. Cambridge: Cambridge University Press.
9. Golderberger, A. 1996. Non-linear dynamics for clinicians: Chaos theory, fractals, and complexity at the bedside. *The Lancet* 347, 1312–1314.
10. Schipper, H., Turley, E. A., and Baum, M. 1996. A new biological framework for cancer research. *The Lancet* 348, 1149–1151.
11. Golub, E. S. 1997. *The Limits of Medicine*. Chicago: University of Chicago Press.
12. Weiss, K. M. 1995. *Genetic Variation and Human Disease*. Cambridge: Cambridge University Press.
13. Sing, C. F., Haviland, M. B., and Reilly, S. L. 1996. Genetic architecture of common multifactorial diseases. *Ciba Foundation Symposium* 197, 211–232.
14. Weatherall, D. J. 1982. *The New Genetics and Clinical Practice*. London: Nuffield Provincial Hospitals Trust.
15. Strohman, R. C. 1993. Ancient genomes, wise bodies, unhealthy people: Limits of genetic thinking in biology and medicine. *Perspectives in Biology and Medicine* 37(1), 112–145.
16. Rose, M. R. 1991. *Evolutionary Biology of Aging*. Oxford: Oxford University Press.
17. Finch, C. E. 1990. *Longevity, Senescence, and the Genome*. Chicago: University of Chicago Press.
18. Fries, J. F., and Crapo, L. M. 1981. *Vitality and Aging: Implications of the Rectangular Curve*. New York: W. H. Freeman.
19. Tsai, S. P., Lee, E. S., and Hardy, R. J. 1978. The effect of a reduction in leading causes of death: Potential gains in life expectancy. *American Journal of Public Health* 68, 966–971.
20. Olshanky, S. J., Carnes, B. A., and Cassel, C. 1990. In search of Methuselah: Estimating the upper limits to human longevity. *Science* 250, 634–640.
21. Lander, E. S., and Schork, N. J. 1994. Genetic dissection of complex traits. *Science* 265, 2037–2048.
22. Plomin, R., Defries, J. C., and McClearn, G. E. 1990. *Behavioral Genetics*. 2d ed. New York: W. H. Freeman.
23. Goodwin, B. C. 1985. What are the causes of morphogenesis? *Bioessays* 3, 32–36.

24. Nijhout, H. F. 1990. Metaphors and the role of genes in development. *Bioessays* 12, 441–446.
25. Hood, L. 1992. In *The Code of Codes*. Edited by D. J. Kevles and L. Hood. Cambridge, Mass.: Harvard University Press.
26. Casky, T. 1992. In *The Code of Codes*. Edited by D. J. Kevles and L. Hood. Cambridge, Mass.: Harvard University Press.
27. Wilkins, A. S. 1993. *Genetic Analysis Of Animal Development*. 2nd ed. New York: Wiley-Liss.
28. Brenner, S., Dove, W., Herskowitz, I., and Thomas, R. 1990. Genes and development: Molecular and logical themes. *Genetics* 126, 479–486.
29. Tautz, D. 1992. Redundancies, development and the flow of information. *Bioessays* 14, 263–266.
30. Jablonka, E., and Lamb, M. J. 1995. *Epigenetic Inheritance and Evolution*. New York: Oxford University Press.
31. Holliday, R. 1990. *Philosophical Transactions of the Royal Society of London* B326, 329–338.
32. Provine, W. B. 1971. *The Origins of Theoretical Population Genetics*. Chicago: University of Chicago Press.
33. McKusick, V. A. 1964. *Human Genetics*. Englewood Cliffs, N.J.: Prentice Hall.
34. Yoxen, E. J. 1984. Constructing genetic diseases. In *Cultural Perspectives on Biological Knowledge,* edited by T. Duster and K. Garrett. Norwood, N.J.: Ablex.
35. Wahlsten, D. 1990. Insensitivity of the analysis of variance to heredity-environment interaction. *Behavior and Brain Science* 13, 109–161.
36. McKeown, T. 1979. *The Role of Medicine: Dream, Mirage or Nemesis?* Princeton, N.J.: Princeton University Press.
37. McKeown, T. 1988. *The Origins of Human Disease*. New York: Basil Blackwell.
38. Lander, E. S., and Botstein, D. 1989. Mapping Mendelian factors underlying quantitative traits using Rflp maps. *Genetics 121,* 185–199.
39. Jacob, H. J., Linkpaintner, K., Lincoln, S. E., et al. 1991. Genetic mapping of a gene causing hypertension in the stroke-prone spontaneous hypertensive rat. *Cell* 67, 213–224.
40. Jeunemaitre, X., Lifton, R. P., Hunt, S. C., et al. 1992. Absence of linkage between the angiotensin converting enzyme locus and human essential hypertension. *Nature Genetics* 1, 72–75.
41. Cambien, F., Poirier, O., Lecref, L., et al. 1992. Deletion polymorphism in the gene for angiotensin-converting enzyme is a potent risk factor for myocardial infarction. *Nature* 359, 641–644.
42. Myers, M. M., Brunelli, S. A., Squire, J. M., et al. 1989. Maternal behavior of shr rats and its relationship to offspring blood pressures. *Developmental Psychobiology* 22(1), 29–53.
43. Ayala, F. J., and Kiger, J. A., Jr. 1984. *Modern Genetics*. 2nd ed. Menlo Park, Calif.: Benjamin/Cummings.
44. Urata, H., Healy, B., Stewart, R. W., et al. 1990. Angiotensin: Ii-forming

pathways in normal and failing human hearts. *Circulation Research* 66, 883–890.

45. Peterson, L. H. 1972. In *Neural and Psychological Mechanisms in Cardiovascular Disease*. Milan: Casa Editrice.

46. Kurtz, T. W. 1992. The ace of hearts. *Nature* 359, 588–589.

47. Kurtz, T. W. 1992. Genetic models of hypertension. *The Lancet* 344, 167–168.

48. Higgins, M., and Higgins, R. V. 1989. Trends and determinants of coronary heart disease mortality: International comparisons. *International Journal of Epidemiology* 18, 3–12.

49. Ross, R. 1993. The pathogenesis of atherosclerosis. *Nature, 362,* 801–809.

50. Speir, E., Modali, R., Huang, E.-S., et al. 1994. Potential role of human cytomegalovirus and p53 interaction in coronary restenosis. *Science* 265, 391–394.

51. Marx, J. 1994. Cmv-p53 interaction may help explain clogged arteries. *Science* 265, 320.

52. Davignon, J., and Roy, M. 1993. Familial hypercholesterolemia in French Canadians: Taking advantage of the presence of a founder effect. *American Journal of Cardiology* 72, 6d–10d.

53. Davignon, J., Dufour, R., and Cantin, M. 1983. Atherosclerosis and hypertension. In *Hypertension,* edited by J. Genest, O. Kuchel, P. Hamet, and M. Cantin. New York: McGraw-Hill.

54. Sing, C. F., Haviland, M. B., Templeton, A. R., and Reilly, S. L. 1994. Alternative genetic strategies for predicting risk of atherosclerosis. *In Proceedings of the Xth Atherosclerosis Symposium*. Excerpta Medica International Congress Series. Amsterdam: Elsevier Science Publishers.

55. Sing, C. F., Haviland, M. B., Templeton, A. R., et al. 1992. Biological complexity and strategies for finding DNA variations responsible for interindividual variation in risk of a common chronic disease, coronary artery disease. *Annals of Medicine* 24, 539–547.

56. Prehn, R. T. 1994. Cancers beget mutations versus mutations beget cancers. *Cancer Research* 54, 5296–5300.

57. Rubin, H. 1990. On the nature of enduring modifications induced in cells and organisms. *Am. Physio. Soc.* L19–L24.

58. Farber, E., and Rubin, H. 1991. Cellular adaptation in the development of cancer. *Cancer Research* 51, 2751–2761.

59. Lijinsky, W. 1989. A view of the relation between carcinogenesis and mutagenesis. *Environmental and Molecular Mutagenesis* 14(16), 78–84.

60. Clark, W. H. 1994 What is inherited in neoplastic systems? Animal models of cutaneous malignant melanoma. *Laboratory Investigation* 71, 1–4.

61. Levine, A. J., Momand, J., and Finlay, C. A. 1991. The p53 tumour suppressor gene. *Nature* 351, 453–456.

62. Jacks, T., Faneli, A., Schmitt, E. M., et al. 1992. Effects of an rb mutation in the mouse. *Nature* 359, 295–300.

63. Donehower, L. A., Harvey, M., Slagle, B. L., et al. 1992. Mice deficient for p53 are developmentally normal but susceptible to spontaneous tumors. *Nature* 356, 215–221.

64. Baker, S. J., Markowitz, S., Fearon, E. R., et al. 1990. Suppression of human colorectal carcinoma cell growth by wild-type p53. *Science* 249, 912–915.
65. Pietenpol, J. A., and Vogelstein, B. 1993. No room at the p53 inn. *Nature* 356, 17–18.
66. Dutta, A., Ruppert, J. M., Aster, J. C., and Winchester, E. 1993. Inhibition of DNA replication factor rpa by p53. *Nature* 365, 79–82.
67. Dowdy, S. F., Hinds, P. W., Louie, K., et al. 1993. Physical interaction of the retinoblastoma protein with human D cyclins. *Cell* 73, 499–511.
68. Knudson, A. 1985. Hereditary cancer, oncogenes, and antioncogenes. *Cancer Research* 45, 1437–1443.
69. Benedict, W. F., Banetjee, A., Mark, C., and Murphee, A. 1983. Nonrandom chromosomal changes in untreated retinoblastoma. *Cancer Genetics and Cytogenetics* 10, 311–333.
70. Gardner, H. A., Gallie, B. L., Knight, L. A., and Phillips, R. A. 1982. Multiple karyotypic changes in retinoblastoma tumor cells: Presence of normal chromosome no. 13 in most tumors. *Cancer Genetics and Cyotgenetics* 6, 201–211.
71. Bookstein, R., Shew, J. Y., Chen, P. L., et al. 1990. Suppression of tumorigenicity of human prostate carcinoma cells by replacing a mutated rb gene. *Science* 247, 712–715.
72. Xu, H. J., Sumegi, J., Hu, S. X., et al. 1991. Intraocular tumor function of rb reconstituted retinoblastoma cells. *Cancer Research* 51, 4481–4485.
73. Pritchard, J., and Hickman, J. A. 1994. Why does stage 4s neuroblastoma regress spontaneously? *The Lancet* 344, 869–870.
74. Farber, E. 1994. Programmed cell death: Necrosis versus apoptosis. *Modern Pathology* 7, 605–609.
75. Rubin, H. 1994. Epigenetic nature of neoplastic transformation. In *Developmental Biology and Cancer,* edited by G. M. Hodges and C. Rowlatt. Boca Raton, Fla.: CRC Press.
76. Colditz, G. A., Willett, W. C., Hunter, D. J., et al. 1993. Family history, age, and risk of breast cancer. *Journal of the American Medical Association* 270(3), 338–343.
77. Rubin, H. 1985. Cancer as a dynamic developmental disease. *Cancer Research* 45, 2935–2942.
78. Hall, J. M., Lee, M. K., Newman, B., et al. 1990. Linkage of early-onset familial breast cancer to chromosome 17q21. *Science* 250, 1684–1689.
79. Miki, Y., Swenson, J., Shattuck-Eidens, D., et al. 1994. A strong candidate for the breast cancer and ovarian cancer susceptibility gene Brca1. *Science* 266, 66–71.
80. Futreal, P. A., Liu, Q., Shattuck-Eidens, D., et al. 1994. Brca1 mutations in primary breast and ovarian carcinomas. *Science* 266, 120–121.
81. Nowak, R. 1994. Breast cancer gene offers surprises. *Science* 265, 1796–1799.
82. Kamb, A., Nelleke, A. G., Weaver-Feldhaus, J., et al. 1994. A cell cycle regulator potentially involved in genesis of many tumor types. *Science* 264, 436–439.
83. Xu, L., Sgroi, D., Sterner, C. J., et al. 1944. Mutational analysis of Cdkn2

(Mts1/P16[ink4]) in human breast carcinomas. *Cancer Research* 54, 5262–5264.

84. Black, W. C., and Welch, H. G. 1993. Advances in diagnostic imaging and overestimation of disease prevalence and the benefits of therapy. *New England Journal of Medicine* 328(17), 1237–1243.

85. Thomas, C., Mullis, K. B., Ellison, B. J., and Johnson, P. 1993. Why there is still an HIV controversy. Unpublished manuscript.

86. Duesberg, P. H. 1992. Aids acquired by drug consumption and other non-contagious risk factors. *Pharmacology and Therapeutics* 55, 201–277.

87. Kuhn, T. 1996. *The Structure of Scientific Revolutions.* 3rd ed. Chicago: University of Chicago Press.

88. Strohman, R. C. 1997. The coming Kuhnian revolution in biology. *Nature Biotechnology* 15, 194–200.

89. Waldrop, M. M. 1994. *Complexity.* New York: Simon & Schuster.

90. Gell-Mann, M. 1994. *The Quark and the Jaguar.* New York: W. H. Freeman.

91. Shapiro, J. 1992. Natural genetic engineering in evolution. *Genetica* 86, 99–111.

92. McClintock, B. 1984. The significance of responses of the genome to challenge. *Science* 226, 792–801.

93. Gould, S. J. 1993. In *The Logic of Life,* edited by C. A. R. Boyd and D. Noble. Oxford: Oxford University Press.

94. Kaufmann, S. 1993. *The Origins of Order.* New York: Oxford University Press.

95. Frank, J. P., and Williams, J. R. 1982. X-ray induction of persistent hypersensitivity to mutation. *Science* 216, 307–308.

96. Rubin, H. 1993. Cellular epigenetics: Effects of passage history on competence of cells for "spontaneous" transformation. *Proceedings of the National Academy of Sciences USA* 90, 10715–10719.

97. McCullough, K. D., Coleman, W. B., Smith, G. J., and Grisham, J. W. 1997. Age dependent induction of hepatic tumor regression by the tissue microenvironment after transplantation of neoplastically transformed rat epithelial cells into the liver. *Cancer Research.*

98. Richards, B., Zhang, H., Phear, G., and Meuth, M. 1997. Conditional mutator phenotypes in hMSH2–deficient tumor cell lines. *Science* 277, 1523–1525.

99. Skinner, J. E., Molnar, M., Vybiral, T., and Mitra, M. 1992. Application of chaos theory to biology and medicine. *Integrative Physiological and Behavioral Science* 27, 39–53.

100. Bond, W. C., Bohs, C., Ebey, J., and Wolf, S. 1973. Rhythmic heart rate variability (sinus arrhythmia) related to stages of sleep. *Conditional Reflex* 8(2), 98–107.

101. Rossler, O. E., and Rossler, R. 1994. *Integrative Physiological and Behavioral Science* 29(3), 328–333.

PART TWO

WELLNESS PROMOTION RESEARCH: INNOVATIVE STRATEGIES AND PERSPECTIVES

P art 2 presents an array of novel approaches to human wellness promotion research and focuses attention on specific topic areas selected to exemplify how innovative methods may illuminate new solutions. Stokols (chapter 6) focuses on environmentally oriented approaches to disease prevention and health promotion. Using many examples to illustrate the potential for enhancing health by modifying the physical environment, he argues that this approach should be more consistently incorporated into wellness program planning and implementation. Sanders-Phillips (chapter 11) directs her attention to another aspect of the environment, namely, the effect of living in a community characterized by frequent violence. She points out that individuals, frequently minorities, who reside in neighborhoods where violence in both the home and the street is common face particular barriers to wellness promotion. On a more micro level, East (chapter 8) presents data that suggest that younger sisters of childbearing teens may be at high risk for becoming teenage mothers themselves. She suggests that the home environment may both directly and indirectly predispose these younger sisters to become pregnant and calls for interventions that target this at-risk population. In an interesting examination of pregnancy outcomes among immigrants, Guendelman (chapter 9) exposes the finding that despite their typically "disadvantaged" profile, certain immigrant groups actually have better pregnancy outcomes that native-born Americans. She explains this finding largely in terms of the cultural environment that these immigrants bring with them and shows how their relatively positive pregnancy outcomes tend to erode with acculturation to the typical lifestyle of native-born Americans.

In the last three chapters of part 2, the authors argue that innovative strategies of data collection and data analysis can point to important revelations in evaluating wellness promotion strategies. Roach (chapter 10) turns attention to the differences in cancer epidemiology between Whites and Blacks. He points out that preexisting societal expectations influence programs, policies, and research. These expectations frame the approach to data collection, analysis, and interpretation in such a way as to make certain conclusions more likely and may perpetuate the status quo with respect to health promotion. Similarly, Ganiats and Sieber (chapter 12) show how attachment to conventional economic analysis leads to a systematic underestimation of the value of health promotion programs. The authors provide examples of how the practice of discounting future outcomes may influence both health policy and individual behavior and call for wider incorporation of time preference as a factor in models of decision making. Finally, Birckmayer and Weiss (chapter 7) describe the use of theory-based evaluation (TBE) as a tool in wellness promotion. Compared to standard program evaluation, in which the focus is on program outcomes, TBE emphasizes the evaluation of intermediate outcomes (e.g., indicators of program implementation and mediators of behavior change) and encourages evaluators to address not only whether an intervention is effective but also why or why not. As a group, the chapters in part 2 make a case for challenging the status quo and looking beneath the surface to discover the underlying dynamics of the social and health problems that wellness professionals typically work to alleviate.

CREATING HEALTH-
PROMOTIVE ENVIRONMENTS

Implications for Theory and Research

Chapter 1 by Stokols and chapter 2 by Breslow suggest that social ecological perspectives are becoming increasingly influential as a basis
for wellness promotion research, practice, and policy. One indication of
this trend is the growing emphasis in research and intervention programs
on linking individually focused, small-group–organizational, and community environmental approaches to wellness promotion (cf. Breslow,
1996; McLeroy et al., 1988; Stokols et al., 1996; Weiss, 1991; Winett
et al., 1989). At the same time, however, the delineation of specific
environmental leverage points for wellness promotion at each level of
analysis remains an important task. This chapter gives particular attention to those sociocultural and physical-environmental qualities of organizations, institutions, and community settings that are especially health
promotive. To address these issues, a new unit of analysis for wellness promotion research, practice, and policy is proposed: the *health-
promotive* (or *wellness-promotive*) *environment*. This unit of analysis
highlights the interdependencies that exist among sociocultural, political, economic, spatial, and technological features of environmental settings, ranging from homes, neighborhoods, workplaces, and schools to
regional and global environments that influence personal and collective
well-being.

CONCEPTUALIZING HEALTH-PROMOTIVE ENVIRONMENTS

For the most part, health promotion research has focused on identifying and modifying personal behaviors that enhance physical health and reduce the risk of illness (e.g., Belloc and Breslow, 1972; Cataldo and Coates, 1986; Green, 1984; O'Donnell and Ainsworth, 1984). Examples of health-promotive behaviors are maintaining high-fiber/low-fat diets, engaging in regular aerobic exercise, using vehicle safety belts, refraining from smoking, and avoiding excessive alcohol consumption. From an ecological perspective, however, health promotion is viewed not only in terms of the specific health behaviors enacted by individuals but more broadly as a dynamic transaction between individuals, groups, and their sociophysical milieu. The social ecological approach to health promotion requires explicit analysis of the interplay between environmental resources available in an area and the particular health habits and lifestyles of the people who occupy the area (Lindheim and Syme, 1983).

As a starting point for analyzing transactions between environmental qualities, behavioral patterns, and health outcomes, it is first necessary to specify features of the environment that promote personal and collective well-being. Some suggested dimensions and criteria of health promotive environments are listed in Table 6.1, which offers a preliminary portrait of health-promotive environments and reflects certain of the previously mentioned assumptions associated with the ecological perspective on health promotion.

A basic assumption underlying the ecological perspective is that healthfulness is a multifaceted phenomenon, encompassing physical health, emotional well-being, and social cohesion. Accordingly, these different facets of healthfulness are presented in the three rows of Table 6.1, ranging from individually oriented assessments of physiological health to organizational and community-level analyses of social cohesion and health status. Explicit recognition of the multiple facets of healthfulness has important implications for ecologically oriented analyses of health promotion. For example, because environments can influence personal and collective well-being along several different "paths," the health-promotive capacity of an environment must be defined in terms of the multiple health outcomes resulting from people-environment transactions over a specified time interval. Thus, for any environmental context of behavior, it becomes important to specify key environmental resources or constraints likely to influence personal and collective well-being among members of the setting.

TABLE 6.1   SOME DIMENSIONS AND
CRITERIA OF HEALTH-PROMOTIVE ENVIRONMENTS

Environmental Resources and Behavioral Outcomes	Environmental Resources and Affordances	Behavioral, Psychological, and Physiological Outcomes
Facets of Healthfulness		
Physical Health	Injury-resistant design, ergonomically sound design, physically comfortable, nontoxic and nonpathogenic	Physiologic health, absence of illness symptoms and injury, perceived comfort, genetic and reproductive health
Mental and Emotional Well-being	Environmental controllability and predictability, environmental novelty and challenge, nondistracting, aesthetic qualities, symbolic/spiritual elements	Sense of personal competence, challenge, and fulfillment; developmental growth; minimal experience of emotional distress; strong sense of personal identity and creativity; feelings of attachment to one's physical and social milieu
Social Cohesion at Organizational and Community Levels	Availability of social support networks, participatory design and management processes, organizational flexibility and responsiveness, economic stability, low potential for intergroup conflict, health-promotive media and programming	High levels of social contact and cooperation, high levels of commitment to and satisfaction with organization and/or community, productivity and innovation at organizational and community levels, high levels of perceived quality of life, prevalence of health-promotive, injury-preventive, and environmentally protective behavior

Dimensions of Well-being

The second column in Table 6.1 lists various environmental resources that can exert a positive influence on individual and group well-being, from microlevel features of the physical environment (e.g., ergonomically sound and injury-resistant design, absence of toxic substances) to more molar or composite aspects of the sociophysical milieu (e.g., presence of pro-social environmental symbols, positive social climate, organizational programs and media to encourage health-promotive behaviors). The third column in Table 6.1 includes several behavioral, psychological, and physiological indices that can be used to assess health outcomes of people-environment transactions at different levels of analysis (e.g., absence of physiological disorders and illness symptoms; personal feelings of competence, creativity, and commitment; high levels of job satisfaction and perceived quality of work life within organizational settings).

By firmly linking the analysis of health promotion to multiple dimensions of the environment and correspondingly diverse indices of health, some important issues for future research and community intervention are raised. First, whereas scientific research on behavior change strategies and environmental protection programs generally have remained separate, the proposed ecological view of health promotion suggests the efficacy of combining these perspectives in the design and management of environmental settings (see also Geller et al., 1982, for a behavioral approach to the design of environmental protection programs). For example, automobile manufacturers can enable individuals to reduce their risk of serious injury from car crashes by installing air bags and safety belts in their vehicles. Similarly, environmental designers, facility managers, and urban planners can incorporate a variety of physical features within new or renovated settings to promote healthfulness, including the installation of physical fitness facilities on-site or adjacent to the setting to encourage health-promotive exercise regimens among occupants of the area, the specification of ergonomically sound and injury-resistant materials in the design and construction of the setting to reduce occupants' risk of injury, and the avoidance of toxic materials and potential sources of psychosocial stress (e.g., poor lighting and air conditioning systems in buildings, insufficient shielding from noise and other distractions) to minimize environmentally induced illness and discomfort.

Given the diversity of environmental conditions present in most settings, it is likely that the relationships between those conditions and multiple health indices will be quite varied and sometimes discordant. For example, the potential health benefits of a well-designed physical environment may go unrealized if the interpersonal or intergroup relationships within a setting are chronically conflicted and stressful. On the other hand, a socially supportive family or organization may enable setting members to cope more effectively with physical constraints (e.g., high spatial density, aesthetically drab surroundings, resource shortages), thereby avoiding the negative behavioral and health outcomes sometimes associated with those conditions. These examples highlight the importance of examining both physical and social dimensions of health-promotive or health-impairing environments and their joint influence on personal and collective well-being.

Similarly, several studies suggest that when environments are personally controllable and predictable, individuals' physical and emotional well-being are enhanced (e.g., Cohen et al., 1986; Gardell and Johansson, 1981; Glass and Singer, 1972; Karasek and Theorell, 1990; Sauter et al., 1989). However, to the extent that environments are too predictable and controllable, they can become so boring and unchallenging that they constrain opportunities for coping creatively with novel situations, thereby impeding developmental growth (Aldwin and Stokols, 1988; Kaplan, 1983). Thus, the same qualitative dimensions of an environment (e.g., its controllability and predictability) can be associated with contradictory health effects, depending on their magnitude (e.g., moderate vs. excessive levels of predictability) and duration (e.g., chronic vs. short-term exposure to unpredictable or excessively predictable situations).

Just as environmental conditions can vary in their magnitude and duration, health outcomes differ on these dimensions as well. For example, carcinogenic substances present in an environment may remain invisible and undetected, yet their cumulative impact on physical health can be disastrous. On the other hand, more salient short-term encounters with environmental stressors, such as uncontrollable noise or periodic crowding, may be associated with acute but nonpersisting episodes of emotional stress. Therefore, to gauge adequately the health promotive capacity of an environment, it is necessary not only to specify relevant environmental dimensions and health outcomes but also to differentiate health outcomes in terms of their severity, duration, and overall importance to members of the setting. Since many environments produce a mixture of positive and negative health outcomes, the health-promotive quality of a setting ultimately depends on its capacity to support those health outcomes most desirable and important to its members while eliminating or ameliorating those most clearly negative and detrimental to individual and social well-being.

Determining which health outcomes are of greatest importance to the occupants of a setting is not always a simple matter. Whether an individual or group places greater value on the comforts of a predictable environment or the challenges of coping with a novel one may vary in relation to their age, economic resources, and exploratory tendencies (Stokols et al., 1982). Also, residents of historically significant areas often give greater priority to the symbolic and psychological benefits of environmental preservation than to the tangible economic gains that would result from neighborhood redevelopment projects (e.g., Firey, 1945; Stokols and Jacobi, 1984). In this case, the symbolic and material benefits associated with the same environmental resources are divergent rather than compatible. Another example of voluntary trade-offs between alternative environmental arrangements and health benefits is the frequent choice of urban residents to live in a highly desirable neighborhood despite the inconveniences and strains of a long-distance commute between home and work rather than reside closer to work in a less desirable area (e.g., Campbell, 1983; Stokols and Novaco, 1981).

The environmental resources and health outcomes shown in Table 6.1 are all highly positive. This emphasis on the positive is consistent with the goals of applied environmental and health research, namely, to optimize or enhance environmental quality and human well-being (Stokols, 1978). Yet, the preceding examples of trade-offs among environmental amenities and costs serve to remind us that most situations are characterized by a mixture of positive and negative environmental circumstances and health outcomes. Thus, an important challenge for future research is to assess the overall health-promotive capacity of environments on the basis of a cumulative analysis and weighting of their positive and negative features as they affect occupants' well-being.

RELEVANCE OF ENVIRONMENTAL
SCALE AND CONTEXTUAL SCOPE
FOR HEALTH PROMOTION RESEARCH

The ecological perspective emphasizes not only the many intrasetting factors that can influence occupants' health but also the ways in which multiple situations and settings (e.g., homes, workplaces, schools, institutional environments) jointly affect the well-being of community members. The scale of environmental units relevant to individual and collective well-being ranges from specific stimuli and situations occurring within a given setting to the more complex life domains that are, themselves, clusters of multiple situations and settings. Situations are sequences of individual or group activities occurring at a particular time and place (Forgas, 1979; Pervin, 1978). Settings are geographic locations in which various personal or interpersonal situations occur on a regular basis (Barker, 1968; Stokols and Shumaker, 1981). Life domains are different spheres of a person's life, such as family, education, spiritual activities, recreation, employment, and commuting (Campbell, 1981; Stokols and Novaco, 1981). An even broader unit of contextual analysis is the individual's overall life situation (Magnusson, 1981), consisting of the major life domains in which a person is involved during a particular period of his or her life. The environmental dimensions most relevant to individual and collective well-being may vary considerably across these different levels of analysis.

The potential influence of multiple environmental settings on health outcomes raises an important question regarding the appropriate contextual scope of health promotion research. Just as environmental units can be arrayed along a continuum of scale or complexity, contextual analyses can be compared in terms of their relative scope. The contextual scope of research refers to the scale of the contextual units included in the analysis (Stokols, 1987). For example, the spatial scope of an analysis increases to the extent that it represents places, processes, and events occurring within a broad rather than a narrow region of the individual's (or group's) geographic environment. Similarly, the temporal scope of an analysis increases to the extent that it represents places, processes, and events experienced by the individual or group within an extended rather than narrow time frame. Finally, the sociocultural scope of an analysis increases to the extent that it describes behaviorally relevant dimensions of an individual's or group's sociocultural environment. It is important for health promotion researchers to be explicit about the range of settings and time periods encompassed by their analyses and the possible ways in which environmental conditions within multiple settings jointly influence individual and collective health outcomes.

Consider, for example, the challenge of preventing alcohol-related injuries. One strategy for reducing such injuries is to provide employee assistance programs at the workplace that facilitate workers' efforts to decrease their consumption of alcoholic beverages. Alternatively, a multisetting approach to this public health problem would combine employee assistance and treatment programs at the workplace with responsible beverage service programs for restaurant personnel, community-wide media campaigns to increase public awareness of alcohol-related injuries and prevention opportunities, legislative initiatives to raise the minimum age of purchase, and enforcement programs to reduce the illegal sale of alcohol to minors (Geller, 1990; Russ and Geller, 1987). The latter approach is based on a spatially broader analysis of injury prevention than the one focusing exclusively on the workplace, as it incorporates several different intervention programs implemented in multiple community settings within an extended geographic area.

Wellness promotion analyses and interventions also can be characterized in terms of their temporal scope. For example, work-site health strategies typically emphasize the provision of employee assistance and lifestyle modification programs oriented toward individual workers. They often ignore, however, the design and equipment purchasing decisions made during the construction of the work site. Yet, the physical design and furnishings of the workplace can have long-term and substantial impacts on employees' health once the facility is occupied. For example, the use of formaldehyde-laden construction materials, the installation of ineffective air conditioning and ventilation systems, poorly designed stairwells, nonadjustable seating and work surfaces, and space plans that expose workers to excessive crowding and noise all can have deleterious effects on employees' physical and mental well-being (e.g., Archea, 1985; Greenberg, 1986; Hedge, 1989; Makower, 1981; Mendell and Smith, 1990; Stellman and Henifin, 1983). Clearly, the environmental foundations for wellness promotion (or health impairment) begin to take shape far in advance of employees' direct involvement with the workplace and continue to influence their well-being once they have occupied that environment. By explicitly considering the design and construction phase prior to occupancy as well as the postoccupancy phase, the temporal scope of work-site wellness promotion is expanded to include a broader and more robust array of intervention strategies than those focusing exclusively on employee assistance and health education.

An emphasis on the temporal dimensions of people-environment transactions suggests the importance of defining the health-promotive capacity of a setting not only in terms of its immediate impact on occupants' well-being but also in terms of the potential existing within the setting for promoting and maintaining improved levels of health over extended time intervals. Just as assessments of individual health status must take into account current states of well-being as well as the prognosis for future illness or health (Kaplan, 1990; see also chapter 3), environmentally based health promotion programs must distinguish between the immediate and potential capacity of a particular setting, organization, or community to promote health among its members.

Finally, the dimension of sociocultural scope is directly relevant to research on environment-health relationships and the design of wellness promotion programs. The sociocultural scope of wellness promotion research and interventions is broadened to the extent that they encompass social and cultural factors within community settings that influence personal and collective well-being (e.g., socioeconomic status, gender, ethnicity, cultural norms about health and illness, supportive social relationships and organizational climate). Contextually oriented health research would involve comparative studies of organizational and community settings that vary across these important social and cultural dimensions. For example, Guendelman (chapter 9), Margen and Lashof (afterword), Roach (chapter 10), Sanders-Phillips (chapter 11), Syme (chapter 4), and Wallack (chapter 19) all suggest the importance of broadening the sociocultural scope of research and policy initiatives in the field of wellness promotion.

An important direction for future research is to identify the ways in which social-structural qualities of organizations and communities exert positive or negative effects on members' well-being. Several earlier studies indicate that supportive interpersonal relationships can enhance individuals' emotional and physical well-being and reduce the stressful consequences of negative life events (Berkman and Syme, 1979; Cohen and Syme, 1985; Sarason and Sarason, 1985). Social-structural qualities of settings also may play a key etiologic role in promoting social cohesion and physical and emotional well-being among setting members. For example, extensive efforts have been made to conceptualize and measure the social climate of organizations (Moos, 1976, 1987), and a number of studies have suggested a positive relationship between dimensions of social climate and the mental and physical health of setting members (e.g., Holahan and Moos, 1990; Moos, 1979). Moreover, certain organizations may be structured in ways that permit the smooth resolution of interpersonal conflicts, whereas others lack the capacity to resolve such tensions when they arise. In the former settings, shared goals among members provide a structural basis for cooperation, even when occasional conflicts develop. Also, such settings are likely to incorporate both informal and formal mechanisms of dispute resolution. In "conflict-prone" organizations, however, the positive interdependencies among members are weaker, and effective mechanisms of dispute resolution are unavailable (Stokols, 1992). To the extent that organizations promote chronic conflict among setting members or provide few resources to resolve such conflicts when they arise, they are more likely to impair the health of their members.

DEVELOPING INTERDISCIPLINARY
MODELS OF THE RELATIONSHIPS
AMONG ENVIRONMENTAL AND
BEHAVIORAL FACTORS IN HEALTH

In view of the dominant focus of earlier wellness promotion programs on modifying personal health habits and lifestyles, several theorists have called for a redirection of the field based on ecological models of research and community intervention (e.g., Geller, 1987; McLeroy et al., 1988; Winett et al., 1989). Green (1984), for example, noted a "psychological bias" in the health promotion field, in that illness-preventive interventions typically are directed at individuals in a counseling or small-group mode of delivery, with little or no theoretical input from the fields of sociology, anthropology, economics, and political science. Similarly, Syme (1990) emphasized the cost-ineffectiveness of individually oriented wellness promotion programs (e.g., the MRFIT intervention to reduce cardiovascular disease among high-risk individuals) and advocated a stronger community and environmental focus in public health research.

The conceptualization of health promotive environments offers a valuable adjunct to the individual-behavioral focus of earlier health promotion research. Yet, the social ecological approach to wellness promotion encompasses more than just the analysis of environmental factors in health and illness. The social ecological perspective requires a broader analysis of the transactions between individual and collective behavior and the various constraints and resources for health that exist within specific sociophysical environments. Thus, it is important at this point in the chapter to extend our analysis of healthy environments toward a more interactive analysis of the relationships among behavioral and environmental factors in wellness and wellness promotion.

ENVIROGENIC PROCESSES IN HEALTH
AND THEIR LINKAGES WITH BIOLOGICAL,
PSYCHOLOGICAL, AND BEHAVIORAL FACTORS

The term "salutogenesis" has been used by Antonovsky (1979) to refer to etiologic processes that enhance emotional and physical well-being. The salutogenic orientation is distinctive in its focus on the etiology of health, as compared to more traditional pathogenic models that emphasize the development of illness. Antonovsky's research has focused primarily on psychogenic factors in health, especially individuals' "sense of coherence," which enables them to resist the potentially negative health consequences of stressful life events. Construed more broadly, however, the salutogenic perspective encompasses not only psychological resistance resources but also a wide array of biological, behavioral, and environmental processes that reduce vulnerability to illness and promote enhanced levels of well-being.

Several categories of personal and environmental factors that play either an etiologic or a moderating role in human health are shown in Table 6.2. The personal factors include a variety of biogenetic, psychological, and behavioral processes that promote or undermine well-being. The environmental factors include several facets of the sociophysical environment, such as geographic, architectural/technological, and sociocultural processes that influence health. Thus, both natural and human-made features of the physical environment are included, as are multiple dimensions of the sociocultural milieu (e.g., social-structural, cultural, economic, legal, and political processes).

Much research in the field of health psychology has focused on the direct links between specific dispositional factors and personal health. For example, several studies indicate the close relationship between personal orientations, such as hostility, optimism, sense of coherence, personal hardiness, and coping efficacy, and individual well-being (e.g., Antonovsky, 1979; Barefoot et al., 1983; Friedman, 1990; Kobasa et al., 1982; Scheier and Carver, 1985; Taylor and Brown, 1988; Watson and Pennebaker, 1989). Other researchers, working from a "biopsychosocial" model of health (e.g., Engel, 1976; Schwartz, 1982), have examined the interplay between psychological dispositions, interpersonal behavior, and physiological processes underlying health and illness. Examples of this research include recent studies of the psychophysiological underpinnings of the coronary-prone and cancer-prone behavior patterns (e.g., Krantz et al., 1987; Temoshok, 1985) and the links between personal dispositions, social behavior, and susceptibility to infectious disease (e.g., Cohen and Williamson, 1991).

What have been omitted from much earlier research on psychological and behavioral factors in health are structural features of the sociophysical environment that affect individual and collective well-being, either directly or interactively in conjunction with biopsychobehavioral

TABLE 6.2   PERSONAL AND ENVIRONMENTAL
FACTORS IN HEALTH AND ILLNESS
Biopsychobehavioral Factors

Biogenetic	Psychological	Behavioral
Genetic constitution and biological resources or challenges: family history of illness, exposure to infectious pathogens (e.g., viruses, bacteria), immunologic competence, inoculation and medication history, congenital disability, disabling injuries, cardiovascular reactivity, chronological age, development stage, gender	Personal dispositions: sense of coherence, psychological hardiness, self-esteem, creativity, optimism, pessimistic explanatory style, health locus of control, interpersonal skills, extroversion, coronary-prone (Type A) orientation, cancer-prone (Type C) orientation, depression/anxiety, hostility/suspiciousness	Dietary regimens, alcohol consumption, smoking, exercise patterns, sleep patterns, safety practices (e.g., use of vehicular safety belts, bicycle helmets, safe sexual and prenatal behaviors), participation in health promotion programs, compliance with prescribed medical regimens, use of community health resources, health-relevant decisions and actions made on behalf of others

factors. These envirogenic processes in health and illness subsume geographic, architectural, and technological features of the physical environment as well as sociogenic qualities of the social and cultural environment that influence the etiology of health and illness.

An important direction for future wellness promotion research is to identify the specific mechanisms by which geographic, architectural/technological, and sociocultural factors influence health and illness. For example, five health-related functions of the sociophysical environment are outlined in Table 6.3. First, both the physical and the social environment can function as *media for disease transmission,* as exemplified by the occurrence of waterborne and airborne diseases, illnesses resulting from food contamination, and the spread of contagious disease through interpersonal contact. Second, the environment can operate as a *stressor,* evidenced by the emotional stress and physical debilitation resulting from chronic exposure to uncontrollable environmental demands, such as noise, abrupt economic change, or interpersonal conflict (e.g., Cohen et al., 1986; Dooley and Catalano, 1984; Evans, 1982;

TABLE 6.2 *(continued)*

Sociophysical Environmental Factors

Geographic	*Architectural and Technological*	*Sociocultural*
Climatic and geologic risks (e.g., earthquakes, floods, hurricanes, tornados, drought, temperature extremes), groundwater contamination, radon contamination of soil, environmental sources of radioactivity, ultraviolet radiation, atmospheric ozone depletion, global warming, health consequences of reduced biodiversity, restorative potential of wilderness and other natural environments	Injury-resistant architecture, nontoxic construction materials in buildings, ergonomic design of work areas and other environmental settings, environmental aesthetics, indoor and outdoor air pollution (e.g., "sick building syndrome"), effective design of health care facilities, vehicular and passenger safety, noise pollution, electromagnetic radiation, water quality and treatment systems, solid waste treatment and sanitation systems	Socioeconomic status of individuals and groups; social support versus isolation or social conflict, bereavement; social climate in families, organizations, and institutions; modeling and conformity processes; cultural and religious beliefs and practices; organizational or political stability; economic changes (job loss and related stressful life events); health communications and media; health promotion programs in organizations and communities (e.g., health education); health-promotive legislation and building codes; environmentally protective regulations; availability of health insurance and community health services

Rook, 1984). On the other hand, exposure to certain environmental conditions, such as natural, aesthetic, and symbolic amenities, can alleviate stress and promote physical and emotional well-being (e.g., Hartig et al., 1991; Kaplan and Kaplan, 1989; Stokols, 1990). Third, the environment functions as a *source of safety or danger,* as reflected in the health consequences of natural and technological disasters, air and water pollution, occupational hazards, interpersonal violence, and crime (e.g., Baum et al., 1983; Edelstein, 1988; Fielding and Phenow, 1988; Greenberg, 1987; Makower, 1981; Mendell and Smith, 1990). Fourth, the environment can be viewed as an *enabler of health behavior,* exemplified by the installation of safety devices in buildings and vehicles, geographic proximity to health care facilities, and exposure to interpersonal modeling or cultural practices that foster health-promotive behavior. Fifth, the environment serves as a *provider of health resources,* such as high-quality community sanitation systems, organizational and community health services, and legislation protecting the quality of physical environments and ensuring citizens' access to health insurance and community-based health care. These health-relevant functions of the environment are closely intertwined and can operate concurrently in specific environmental contexts (e.g., high rates of crime may generate increased perceptions of physical danger, physiological symptoms of chronic stress, reduced use of community health services among neighborhood residents; cf. Taylor, 1987).

Another important challenge for future research is to develop integrative models that address the joint influence of personal and environmental factors in wellness promotion and disease etiology. Some specific issues for future study suggested by the categories of variables shown in Table 6.2 are the following: (1) the prevalence of negative health effects among low socioeconomic-status groups resulting from their disproportionate exposure to geographic, architectural, and technological hazards (e.g., Bullard, 1990; Lindheim and Syme, 1983; Syme and Berkman, 1976; U.S. Public Health Service, 1991; Vaughan, 1993); (2) the relationship between individuals' age, gender, developmental stage, and their increased vulnerability to certain categories of environmental health threats, such as lead poisoning (Florini et al., 1990; Needleman et al., 1990), fatalities resulting from exposure to community violence, injuries from motor vehicle crashes and alcohol abuse among adolescents and young adults, and fatalities from the complications of falls among older adults (Sanders-Phillips, chapter 11; U.S. Public Health Service, 1991; Wallack, chapter 19); (3) the psychosocial underpinnings of high-risk behaviors (e.g., smoking, unsafe sexual practices, overexposure to ultraviolet radiation, failure to use vehicular safety belts) that predispose certain groups in the population to higher rates of illness, injury, or unwanted pregnancy (e.g., Christopherson, 1989; East, chapter 8; Hofmann, chapter 20; Jeffery, 1989; Keesling and Friedman, 1987; Robertson, 1987; Weinstein, 1987); (4) the ways in which environmental factors (e.g., geographic, architectural, and sociocultural conditions) contribute to the development, modification, and mainte-

TABLE 6.3   ENVIROGENIC PROCESSES
IN HEALTH AND ILLNESS

Environmental Dimensions	Dimensions of the Environment	
	Physical Environment	*Social Environment*
Environmental Function		
Environment as Medium of Disease	Waterborne and airborne disease, microbial contamination of food	Spread of contagious disease through interpersonal contact
Environment as Stressor	Negative affective states resulting from exposure to physical stressors such as uncontrollable noise and technological risks, negative health consequences of residential relocation	Vulnerability to health problems resulting from chronic social conflict, isolation, organizational instability, and/or abrupt economic change
Environment as Source of Safety or Danger	Exposure to climatic and geologic risks, injury-resistant environmental design, mutagenic effects of toxic environments, occupational hazards	Risk of personal injury resulting from intergroup conflict, violence, and crime
Environment as Enabler of Health Behavior	Geographic accessibility of health care facilities in the community, installation of health behavioral supports in buildings and vehicles (e.g., smoke detectors, seat belts)	Interpersonal modeling of health-promotive behavior and safety practices, health-promotive cultural and religious practices
Environment as Provider of Health Resources	Healthful lighting and air quality in buildings, community sanitation systems	Legislation pertaining to public health and safety, availability of organizational and community health services

Health-Related Functions of the Sociophysical Environment

nance of health-promotive behavior (e.g., Centers for Disease Control and Prevention, 1998; Sallis and Hovell, 1990; Winett et al., 1989); and (5) the processes by which psychological dispositions and sociophysical stressors jointly influence emotional and physical well-being (cf. Cottington and House, 1987).

The social ecological view of health promotion has important implications not only for theory development and basic research but also for public policy, community intervention, and program evaluation. We turn now to a consideration of these policy-related concerns.

COMMUNITY INTERVENTIONS TO PROMOTE
PUBLIC HEALTH: A MULTILEVEL APPROACH

The environmental and personal factors in health and illness, summarized previously, offer several leverage points for health-promotive policies and community interventions at municipal, regional, national, and international levels. Examples of these environmental design and public policy options for health promotion are summarized in Table 6.4 in relation to various categories of etiologic factors (i.e., biopsychobehavioral factors and sociophysical features of the environment). The social ecological approach to wellness promotion emphasizes the integration of person-focused and environment-focused strategies to enhance well-being.

Policies and interventions to promote wellness can be arrayed along a continuum ranging from microenvironmental settings (e.g., corporate or institutional facilities) to more molar environmental contexts (e.g., metropolitan and international regions). Each level of analysis poses opportunities for integrating person-focused and environment-focused interventions for health enhancement. For example, the advantages of combining health-promotive environmental design and management policies at the work site with behaviorally oriented programs to modify employees' health practices were noted earlier. At the community level, health promotive urban design and planning strategies (e.g., ensuring geographic accessibility of health care settings and appropriate siting of buildings away from toxic or seismic hazards) can be implemented in conjunction with effective sanitation systems and other health services (e.g., public education and risk-screening programs) to enhance the healthfulness of urban environments.

Because local and more distant environments are linked (both spatially and organizationally) within nested hierarchical systems (e.g., specific behavior settings exist as components of broader institutional, urban, and regional contexts) and are becoming increasingly interdependent because of global technological and social changes, opportunities for designing health-promotive environments at local levels will be more and more influenced by the regulatory and economic policies implemented within municipal, regional, and international contexts. Thus, an architect or facility planner working on the design of a cor-

TABLE 6.4   POLICY OPTIONS FOR HEALTH
PROMOTION AND ILLNESS PREVENTION

Focus of Health-Promotive Interventions	Examples of Health-Promotive Policies and Programs
Person Focused	
Biogenetic Factors	Preventive public health programs for risk screening, genetic counseling, inoculation; medical treatment regimens (e.g., medication, surgery)
Psychological Factors	Individual counseling and psychotherapeutic interventions
Behavioral Factors	Health behavior modification (lifestyle appraisal and modification pertaining to diet, exercise, smoking, safety practices)
Environment Focused	
Geographic Factors	Health and safety-oriented urban planning (e.g., site planning to reduce toxic or seismic hazards); land use policy and environmental law at municipal, regional, and international levels (e.g., NEPA, CEQA); strategic siting of health care facilities in the community
Architectural/ Technological Factors	Ergonomic and safety-oriented environmental design and facilities management, design of safe and health-promotive products (e.g., passenger constraints in automobiles), community sanitation systems (water treatment, air filtration)
Sociocultural Factors	Organizational development and conflict resolution, corporate health promotion programs, community health education and media programming, health-promotive legislation (e.g., regulation of health-damaging industries, health insurance and delivery of health services) and building codes

porate facility, neighborhood playground, apartment complex, hospital, or residential facility for the elderly will need to have knowledge of several disciplines, including environmental law (e.g., the regulations intended to mitigate negative impacts of proposed environmental developments), life-span human development (e.g., the specialized health and safety needs of different age-groups), and ergonomics and public health (e.g., the potential health consequences of poorly designed, toxic, or injury-prone environments). In response to the complex health challenges of the 21st century, there will be a growing need to develop broad-based, interdisciplinary graduate training programs for aspiring environmental designers, facility managers, urban planners, and public health professionals.

Among the topics likely to become more prominent in training programs for environmental planners and public health researchers are the legislative and economic strategies that have been initiated in recent years to protect environmental quality and public health. Commenting on the powerful impact of legislative interventions to enhance public health, McKinlay (1975) noted,

> One stroke of effective health legislation is equal to many separate health intervention endeavors and the cumulative efforts of innumerable health workers over long periods of time. . . . Greater changes will result from the continued politicization of illness than from the modification of specific individual behaviors. There are many opportunities for a reduction of at-riskness, and we ought to seize them. (p. 13)

The following sections of the chapter examine legislative initiatives and other community interventions that either have been implemented or could be adopted at local, state, national, and international levels to enhance environmental quality and public health.

Municipal, state, and national contexts of health promotion. In an effort to reduce the devastating personal and public health consequences of smoking (e.g., Eriksen et al., 1988; Fielding and Phenow, 1988; U.S. Public Health Service, 1979), several local governments have enacted legislation to ban smoking in public places. In California alone, 172 municipalities and counties had passed ordinances restricting smoking in workplaces and commercial settings, and nearly 400 such ordinances had been enacted nationwide by September 1989 (Pertschuk and Shopland, 1989; see also Bureau of National Affairs, 1986). In addition to protecting nonsmokers from passive smoke exposure, these actions have made smoking less socially acceptable, thereby prompting more smokers to attempt quitting. Other nonlegislated interventions to promote wellness in local communities include media campaigns to encourage heart-healthy behaviors (e.g., Farquhar et al., 1985; Maccoby and Alexander, 1980), elementary school education programs to promote bicycle helmet use among children (DiGuiseppi et al., 1989), and corporate-based programs to increase vehicle safety belt use (Geller, 1984).

At state levels, several legislative actions have been found to reduce injury and fatality rates associated with automobile crashes. These include laws mandating the use of child safety seats in automobiles (e.g., Fawcett et al., 1987; Insurance Institute for Highway Safety, 1987), laws requiring servers of alcoholic beverages to have intervention training to reduce customers' risk of alcohol-impaired driving (Geller, 1990; Russ and Geller, 1987), and laws raising the legal minimum drinking age

(Williams et al., 1983b) or the drivers' licensing age (Williams et al., 1983a). At the national level, lowering the maximum speed limit from 70 to 55 miles per hour in 1973 was associated with a substantial decrease in automobile accident injuries and fatalities throughout the United States (National Safety Council, 1987).

A notable strength of several of the local, state, and national interventions cited here is that their actual influence on public health and safety has been documented through carefully designed quasi-experimental studies. Rigorous evaluations of health promotive legislation and community interventions are essential for estimating the scientific validity and practical utility of both existing and proposed programs (e.g., Campbell, 1969; Evans, 1988; Geller, 1990; Syme, chapter 4; Wallack, chapter 19; Birckmayer and Weiss, chapter 7).

Another health-promotive strategy that has been widely used at national, state, and local levels is the enactment of legislation designed to protect natural resources and the quality of public environments. Examples of environmentally protective legislation undertaken at national levels include the 1969 National Environmental Policy Act (NEPA), the 1970 Clean Air Act, the 1972 Clean Water Act, and the 1976 Toxic Substances Control Act in the United States and the 1971 Town and Country Planning Act in Great Britain. NEPA, instituted by the U.S. Congress, requires all federal agencies to prepare detailed written statements about the potentially negative impacts that could result from any of their actions relating to the environment and proposed strategies for avoiding or mitigating those outcomes. The California Environmental Quality Act (CEQA) is one of several state analogues of NEPA that has been implemented in the United States over the past 20 years. CEQA requires that municipal and state agencies not approve a proposed environmental project unless the potentially adverse effects of the development are identified in an environmental impact report (EIR) and all feasible alternatives or mitigation measures to reduce those impacts have been incorporated into the project plans. Today, about half the states in the United States have emulated the NEPA process, and environmental impact assessment is now an established legal process in several nations (e.g., Australia, Canada, the European Community, and Great Britain; CEQA, 1986; Robinson, 1990).

International efforts to protect environmental quality and to promote public health. International efforts directed toward environmental protection and health promotion also have increased substantially in recent years. Growing public concern over global environmental problems has stimulated greater international collaboration in economic and legal matters (Silver and DeFries, 1990; Wilson and Peter, 1988; World Commission on Environment and Development, 1987). A recent example of intercity and cross-national cooperation in health promotion is the World Health Organization's Healthy Cities Project (e.g., Ashton et al., 1986; Hancock and Duhl, 1985; World Health Organization, 1984). As part of the Healthy Cities Project, public health professionals from several different countries have worked together in developing and implementing intersectoral city health plans. In support of these collaborative efforts, WHO staff provide technical assistance and resource materials to the participating cities. One product of this collaboration is a European television series on the healthy city.

An important defining attribute of healthy cities is that they continually create and improve physical and social environments conducive to the health of their residents (Duhl, 1996; Hancock and Duhl, 1985). At least 14 criteria for assessing the healthfulness of a city have been proposed, including epidemiologic indices of illness and mortality, levels of public safety, quality of the physical and social environment, quality of public health services, the degree of intersectoral collaboration in developing health policies, and the state of the local economy including unemployment levels. These criteria provide a broad framework for establishing coordinated public health plans and objectives among the participating cities.

A central concept that will guide future environmental and health promotive legislation is the notion of sustainable development. According to Robinson (1990), sustainable development is "the emerging cluster of policies by which we manage the use of the Earth's environment and natural resources to ensure the optimal level of sustainable benefits for present and succeeding generations" (p. 16). Growing concern about the sustainability of global resources highlights the crucial importance of public health forecasting, environmental simulation strategies, and the temporal dimensions of health promotion (see Table 6.2). Now more than ever, individually focused and environmentally focused efforts to enhance human health must anticipate the cumulative consequences of seemingly remote processes and distant events, for example, (1) the potential exacerbation of health problems among the elderly by elevated temperatures associated with global warming, (2) increased prevalence of cutaneous melanoma and other diseases resulting from global ozone depletion and heightened exposure to ultraviolet radiation, (3) the biogenetic consequences of exposure to toxic by-products of modern technologies, (4) the implications of reduced ecosystem biodiversity for human health and medical treatment and research programs, and (5) the ever-present threat of global nuclear war and the health consequences of nuclear weapons testing.

Amidst these somber projections of public health problems and challenges for the 21st century, the previously cited examples of municipal and international cooperation toward health promotion and environmental protection are impressive in their scope and offer a basis for optimism about the willingness of governments to work collaboratively to promote world health. Collaborative international efforts to protect the global environment and promote the well-being of the world's population give new meaning to the concept of "health behavior." Future health promotion programs must influence not only the behaviors of individuals that enhance or undermine their own well-being but also the decisions they make and the actions they take on behalf of others—ranging from small groups to urban populations—in their roles as voters, environmental planners, corporate executives, and community leaders. This distinction between *personal* and *other-directed* health behavior has important implications for the design of effective wellness promotion programs (cf. Stokols, 1996).

SUMMARY

The challenge of creating and maintaining healthy environments raises several complex theoretical, methodological, and public policy questions. For example, how shall we conceptualize healthy environments, and by what observable criteria can we determine the extent to which an environment is health promotive? Is the healthfulness of an environment defined primarily by its physical quality, or is it defined in terms of the joint influence of its material and symbolic features on the emotional and physical well-being of its occupants? Does the concept of environmental health refer to the present condition of the environment and its occupants, or does it refer to the potential that exists within a setting for promoting and maintaining improved levels of well-being over an extended period?

To address these issues, a social ecological model of health promotive environments was proposed, emphasizing the interactions among physical-material and social-symbolic features of environments as they affect the emotional, physical, and social well-being of individuals and groups. Health status was analyzed along a continuum ranging from individuals to larger aggregates and populations and in relation to microlevel, local settings (e.g., homes, offices, neighborhoods) as well as larger-scale and more distant environments (e.g., geographically and politically bounded regions). The temporal dimensions of environmental health were examined with particular emphasis on the stability or instability of healthful conditions within a setting or region and the factors that influence the healthfulness of an environment over extended periods. Finally, several directions for both basic research and the evaluation of policy initiatives to protect environmental quality and promote public health were examined at organizational, municipal, and international levels.

NOTE

Portions of this chapter were presented as part of the University of California Wellness Lectures Program in 1991 and are adapted from a subsequent article: D. Stokols (1992), Establishing and maintaining healthy environments: Toward a social ecology of health promotion, *American Psychologist, 47,* 6–22. The author thanks Dr. Margaret Schneider Jamner for her helpful comments on an earlier version of the chapter.

REFERENCES

Aldwin, C., and Stokols, D. (1988). The effects of environmental change on individuals and groups: Some neglected issues in stress research. *Journal of Environmental Psychology, 8,* 57–75.

Antonovsky, A. (1979). *Health, stress, and coping.* San Francisco: Jossey-Bass.

Archea, J. C. (1985). Environmental factors associated with stair accidents by the elderly. *Clinics in Geriatric Medicine, 1,* 555–569.

Ashton, J., Grey, P., and Barnard, K. (1986). Healthy cities: WHO's New Public Health Initiative. *Health Promotion, 1,* 319–324.

Barefoot, J. C., Dahlstrom, W. G., and Williams, R. B. (1983). Hostility, CHD incidence, and total mortality: A 25-year follow-up study 255 physicians. *Psychosomatic Medicine, 45,* 59–63.

Barker, R. G. (1968). *Ecological psychology: Concepts and methods for studying the environment of human behavior.* Stanford, Calif.: Stanford University Press.

Baum, A., Fleming, R., and Davidson, L. M. (1983). Natural disaster and technological catastrophe. *Environment and Behavior, 15,* 333–354.

Belloc, N., and Breslow, L. (1972). Relationship of physical health status and health practices. *Preventive Medicine, 1,* 409–421.

Berkman, L. F., and Syme, S. L. (1979). Social networks, host resistance, and mortality: A nine-year follow-up study of Alameda County residents. *American Journal of Epidemiology, 109,* 186–204.

Breslow, L. (1996). Social ecological strategies for promoting healthy lifestyles. *American Journal of Health Promotion, 10,* 253–257.

Bullard, R. D. (1990). *Dumping in Dixie: Race, class, and environmental quality.* Boulder, Colo.: Westview Press.

Bureau of National Affairs. (1986). *Where there's smoke: Problems and policies concerning smoking in the workplace.* Washington, DC: Author.

Campbell, A. (1981). *The sense of well-being in America.* New York: McGraw-Hill.

Campbell, D. T. (1969). Reforms as experiments. *American Psychologist, 24,* 209–219.

Campbell, J. M. (1983). Ambient stressors. *Environment and Behavior, 15,* 355–380.

Cataldo, M. F., and Coates, T. J., eds. (1986). *Health and industry: A behavioral medicine perspective.* New York: John Wiley and Sons.

Centers for Disease Control and Prevention. (1998). Panel discussion on policy and environmental actions to promote physical activity. Atlanta: Physical Activity and Health Branch, Centers for Disease Control and Prevention.

CEQA—The California Environmental Quality Act (1986). Sacramento: Governor's Office of Planning and Research, State of California.

Christophersen, E. R. (1989). Injury control. *American Psychologist, 44,* 237–241.

Cohen, S., Evans, G. W., Stokols, D., and Krantz, D. S. (1986). *Behavior, health and environmental stress.* New York: Plenum.

Cohen, S., and Syme, S. L., eds. (1985). *Social support and health.* Orlando: Academic Press.

Cohen, S., and Williamson, G. M. (1991). Stress and infectious disease in humans. *Psychological Bulletin, 109,* 5–24.

Cottington, E., and House, J. S. (1987). Occupational stress and health: A multivariate relationship. In A. Baum and J. E. Singer, eds., *Handbook of psychology and health: Volume 5.* Pp. 41–62. Hillsdale, N.J.: Lawrence Erlbaum Associates.

DiGuiseppi, C. G., Rivara, F. P., Koepsell, T. D., and Polissar, L. (1989). Bicycle helmet use by children: Evaluation of a community-wide helmet campaign. *Journal of the American Medical Association, 262,* 2256–2261.

Dooley, D., and Catalano, R. (1984). The epidemiology of economic stress. *American Journal of Community Psychology, 12,* 387–409.

Duhl, L. (1996). An ecohistory of health: The role of "healthy cities." *American Journal of Health Promotion, 10,* 258–261.

Edelstein, M. R. (1988). *Contaminated communities: The social and psychological impacts of residential toxic exposure.* Boulder, Colo.: Westview Press.

Engel, G. L. (1976). The need for a new medical model. *Science, 196,* 129–136.

Eriksen, M. P., LeMaistre, C. A., and Newell, G. R. (1988). Health hazards of passive smoking. In L. Breslow, J. E. Fielding, and L. B. Lave, eds., *Annual Review of Public Health, 9,* 47–70. Palo Alto, Calif.: Annual Reviews, Inc.

Evans, G. W., ed. (1982). *Environmental stress.* New York: Cambridge University Press.

Evans, R. I. (1988). Health promotion—Science or ideology? *Health Psychology, 7,* 203–219.

Farquhar, J. W., Fortman, S. P., Maccoby, N., et al. (1985). The Stanford Five City Project: Design and methods. *American Journal of Epidemiology, 63,* 171–182.

Fawcett, S. B., Seekins, T., and Jason, L. A. (1987). Policy research and child passenger safety legislation: A case study and experimental evaluation. *Journal of Social Issues, 43,* 133–148.

Fielding, J. E., and Phenow, K. J. (1988). Health effects of involuntary smoking. *New England Journal of Medicine, 319,* 1452–1460.

Firey, W. (1945). Sentiment and symbolism as ecological variables. *American Sociological Review, 10,* 410–418.

Florini, K. L., Krumbhaar, G. D., and Silbergeld, E. K. (1990, March). *Legacy of lead: America's continuing epidemic of childhood lead poisoning: A report and proposal for legislative action.* Washington, D.C.: Environmental Defense Fund.

Forgas, J. P. (1979). *Social episodes: The study of interaction routines.* New York: Academic.

Friedman, H. S., ed. (1990). *Personality and disease.* New York: John Wiley and Sons.

Gardell, B., and Johansson, G., eds. (1981). *Working life: A social science contribution to work reform.* New York: John Wiley and Sons.

Geller, E. S. (1984). Motivating safety belt use with incentives: A critical review of the past and a look to the future. SAE Technical Paper Series 840326. Warrendale, Pa.: Society of Automotive Engineers.

Geller, E. S. (1987). Applied behavior analysis and environmental psychology: From strange bedfellows to a productive marriage. In D. Stokols and I. Altman, eds., *Handbook of environmental psychology: Volume 1.* Pp. 361–388. New York: John Wiley and Sons.

———. (1990). Preventing injuries and deaths from vehicle crashes: Encouraging belts and discouraging booze. In J. Edwards, R. S. Tindale, L. Heath, and E. J. Posavac eds., *Social influence processes and prevention.* Pp. 249–277. New York: Plenum.

Geller, E. S., Winett, R. A., and Everett, P. B. (1982). *Preserving the environment: New strategies for behavior change.* New York: Pergamon.

Glass, D. C., and Singer, J. E. (1972). *Urban stress.* New York: Academic.

Green, L. W. (1984). Modifying and developing health behavior. *Annual Review of Public Health, 5,* 215–236.

Greenberg, M. R. (1986). Indoor air quality: Protecting public health through design, planning, and research. *Journal of Architectural and Planning Research, 3,* 253–261.

———. (1987). *Public health and the environment: The United States experience.* New York: Guilford.

Hancock, T., and Duhl, L. (1985). Healthy cities: Promoting health in the urban context. A background working paper for the Healthy Cities symposium. Lisbon, 1986. Copenhagen: WHO.

Hartig, T., Mang, M., and Evans, G. W. (1991). Restorative effects of natural environment experiences. *Environment and Behavior, 23,* 3–26.

Hedge, A. (1989). Environmental conditions and health in offices. *International Review of Ergonomics, 2,* 87–110.

Holahan, C. J., and Moos, R. H. (1990). Life stressors, resistance factors, and improved psychological functioning. An extension of the stress-resistance paradigm. *Journal of Personality and Social Psychology, 58,* 909–917.

Insurance Institute for Highway Safety (1987). Status Report, December, 1987. Washington, D.C.: Author.

Jeffery, R. W. (1989). Risk behaviors and health: Contrasting individual and population perspectives. *American Psychologist, 44,* 1194–1202.

Kaplan, R. M. (1990). Behavior as the central outcome in health care. *American Psychologist, 45,* 1211–1220.

Kaplan, S. (1983). A model of person-environment compatibility. *Environment and Behavior, 15,* 331–332.

Kaplan, R., and Kaplan, S. (1989). *The experience of nature: A psychological perspective.* New York: Cambridge University Press.

Karasek, R., and Theorell, T., eds. (1990). *Healthy work: Stress, productivity, and the reconstruction of working life.* New York: Basic Books.

Keesling, B., and Friedman, H. S. (1987). Psychosocial factors in sunbathing and sunscreen use. *Health Psychology, 6,* 477–493.

Kobasa, S. C., Maddi, S. R., and Kahn, S. (1982). Hardiness and health: A prospective study. *Journal of Personality and Social Psychology, 42,* 168–177.

Krantz, D. S., Lundberg, U., and Frankenhaeuser, M. (1987). Stress and Type-A behavior: Environmental and biological factors. In A. Baum and J. E. Singer, eds., *Handbook of psychology and health: Volume V.* Pp. 203–228. Hillsdale, N.J.: Lawrence Erlbaum Associates.

Lindheim, R., and Syme, S. L. (1983). Environments, people, and health. *Annual Review of Public Health, 4,* 335–354.

Maccoby, N., and Alexander, J. (1980). Use of media in lifestyle programs. In P. O. Davidson and S. M. Davidson, eds., *Behavioral medicine: Changing health lifestyles.* Pp. 351–370. New York: Brunner/Mazel.

Magnusson, D. (1981). A psychology of situations. In D. Magnusson, ed., *Toward a psychology of situations: An interactional perspective.* Pp. 9–32. Hillsdale, N.J.: Lawrence Erlbaum Associates.

Makower, J. (1981). *Office hazards: How your job can make you sick.* Washington, D.C.: Tilden Press.

McKinlay, J. B. (1975). A case for refocusing upstream: The political economy of illness. In A. J. Enelow and J. B. Henderson, eds., *Applying behavioral science to cardiovascular risk.* Washington, D.C.: American Heart Association.

McLeroy, K. R., Bibeau, D., Steckler, A., and Glanz, K. (1988). An ecological perspective on health promotion programs. *Health Education Quarterly, 15,* 351–378.

Mendell, M. J., and Smith, A. H. (1990). Consistent pattern of elevated symptoms in air-conditioned office buildings: A reanalysis of epidemiologic studies. *American Journal of Public Health, 80,* 1193–1199.

Moos, R. H. (1976). *The human context.* New York: John Wiley and Sons.
————. (1979). Social ecological perspectives on health. In G. C. Stone, F. Cohen, and N. E. Adler, eds., *Health psychology: A handbook.* Pp. 523–547. San Francisco: Jossey-Bass.
————. (1987). *The social climate scales: A user's guide.* Palo Alto, Calif.: Consulting Psychologists Press.
National Safety Council. (1987). *Accident facts.* Chicago: Author.
Needleman, H. L., Schell, A., Bellinger, D., Leviton, A., and Allred, E. N. (1990). The long-term effects of exposure to low doses of lead in childhood. *New England Journal of Medicine, 322,* 83–88.
O'Donnell, M. P., and Ainsworth, T., eds. (1984). *Health promotion in the workplace.* New York: John Wiley and Sons.
Pertschuk, M., and Shopland, D. (1989, September). *Major local smoking ordinances in the United States.* National Institutes of Health Publication 90-479. Washington, D.C.: U.S. Government Printing Office.
Pervin, L. A. (1978). Definitions, measurements, and classifications of stimuli, situations, and environments. *Human Ecology, 6,* 71–105.
Robertson, L. S. (1987). Injury prevention: Limits to self-protective behavior. In N. D. Weinstein, ed., *Taking care: Understanding and encouraging self-protective behavior.* Pp. 280–297. New York: Cambridge University Press.
Robinson, N. (1990). Sustainable development: An introduction to the concept. In J. O. Saunders, ed., *The legal challenge of sustainable development.* Pp. 15–34. Calgary: Canadian Institute of Resources Law.
Rook, K. S. (1984). The negative side of social interaction: Impact on psychological well-being. *Journal of Personality and Social Psychology, 46,* 1097–1108.
Russ, N. W., and Geller, E. S. (1987). Training bar personnel to prevent drunken driving: A field evaluation. *American Journal of Public Health, 77,* 952–954.
Sallis, J. F., and Hovell, M. F. (1990). Determinants of exercise behavior. In J. O. Holloszy and K. B. Pandolf, eds., *Exercise and sport sciences reviews, 18.* Pp. 307–330. Baltimore: Williams and Wilkins.
Sarason, I. G., and Sarason, B. R., eds. (1985). *Social support: Theory, research, and applications.* Dordrecht: Martinus Nijhoff.
Sauter, S. L., Hurrell, J. J., and Cooper, C. L., eds. (1989). *Job control and worker health.* Chichester: John Wiley and Sons.
Scheier, M. F., and Carver, C. S. (1985). Optimism, coping, and health: Assessment and implications of generalized outcome expectancies. *Health Psychology, 4,* 219–247.
Schwartz, G. E. (1982). Testing the biopsychosocial model: The ultimate challenge facing behavioral medicine. *Journal of Consulting and Clinical Psychology, 50,* 1041–1053.
Silver, C., and DeFries, R. (1990). *One earth, one future: Our changing global environment.* Washington, D.C.: National Academy of Sciences.
Stellman, J., and Henifin, M. S. (1983). *Office work can be dangerous to your health: A handbook of office health and safety hazards and what you can do about them.* New York: Fawcett Crest.
Stokols, D. (1978). Environmental psychology. In M. R. Rosenzweig and L. W.

Porter, eds., *Annual Review of Psychology, 29,* 253–295. Palo Alto, Calif.: Annual Reviews, Inc.

———. (1987). Conceptual strategies of environmental psychology. In D. Stokols and I. Altman, eds., *Handbook of environmental psychology, Volume 1.* Pp. 41–70. New York: John Wiley and Sons.

———. (1990). Instrumental and spiritual views of people-environment relations. *American Psychologist, 45,* 641–646.

———. (1992). Conflict-prone and conflict-resistant organizations. In H. Friedman, ed., *Hostility, coping, and health.* Pp. 65–76. Washington, D.C.: American Psychological Association.

———. (1996). Translating social ecological theory into guidelines for community health promotion. *American Journal of Health Promotion, 10,* 282–298.

Stokols, D., Allen, J., and Bellingham, R. L. (1996). The social ecology of health promotion: Implications for research and practice. *American Journal of Health Promotion, 10,* 247–251.

Stokols, D., and Jacobi, M. (1984). Traditional, present-oriented, and futuristic modes of group-environment relations. In K. Gergen and M. Gergen, eds., *Historical social psychology.* Pp. 303–324. Hillsdale, N.J.: Lawrence Erlbaum Associates.

Stokols, D., and Novaco, R. W. (1981). Transportation and well-being: An ecological perspective. In J. Wohlwill, P. Everett, and I. Altman, eds., *Human behavior and environment: Advances in theory and research, Volume 5: Transportation environments.* Pp. 85–130. New York: Plenum.

Stokols, D., and Shumaker, S. (1981). People in places: A transactional view of settings. In J. Harvey, ed., *Cognition, social behavior and the environment.* Pp. 441–488. Hillsdale, N.J.: Lawrence Erlbaum Associates.

Stokols, D., Shumaker, S., and Martinez, J. (1983). Residential mobility and personal well-being. *Journal of Environmental Psychology, 3,* 5–19.

Syme, S. L. (1990). Health promotion: Old approaches, new choices, future imperatives. Presented at Conference on "The New Public Health: 1990," Los Angeles, April.

Syme, S. L., and Berkman, L. F. (1976). Social class, susceptibility and sickness. *American Journal of Epidemiology, 104,* 1–8.

Taylor, R. B. (1987). Toward an environmental psychology of disorder: Delinquency, crime, and fear of crime. In D. Stokols and I. Altman, eds., *Handbook of environmental psychology.* Pp. 951–986. New York: John Wiley and Sons.

Taylor, S. E., and Brown, J. D. (1988). Illusion and well-being: A social psychological perspective on mental health. *Psychological Bulletin, 103,* 193–210.

Temoshok, L. (1985). Biopsychosocial studies on cutaneous malignant melanoma: Psychosocial factors associated with prognostic indicators, progression, psychophysiology, and tumor-host response. *Social Science and Medicine, 20,* 833–840.

U.S. Public Health Service (1979). *Healthy people: The Surgeon General's report on health promotion and disease prevention.* DHEW Publication (PHS) 79-55071. Washington, D.C.: U.S. Government Printing Office.

————. (1991). *Healthy People 2000: National health promotion and disease prevention objectives.* PHHS Publication (PHS) 91-50212. Washington, D.C.: U.S. Government Printing Office.

Vaughan, E. (1993). Individual and cultural differences in adaptation to environmental risks. *American Psychologist, 48,* 673–680.

Watson, D., and Pennebaker, J. W. (1989). Health complaints, stress, and distress: Exploring the central role of negative affectivity. *Psychological Review, 96,* 234–254.

Weinstein, N. D., ed. (1987). *Taking care: Understanding and encouraging self-protective behavior.* New York: Cambridge University Press.

Weiss, S. M. (1991). Health at work. In S. M. Weiss, J. E. Fielding, and A. Baum, eds., *Perspectives in behavioral medicine: Health at work.* Pp. 1–10. Hillsdale, N.J.: Lawrence Erlbaum Associates.

Williams, A. F., Karpf, R. S., and Zador, P. F. (1983a). Variations in minimum licensing age and fatal motor vehicle crashes. *American Journal of Public Health, 73,* 1401–1403.

Williams, A. F., Zador, P. L., Harris, S. S., and Karpf, R. S. (1983b). The effect of raising the legal minimum drinking age on fatal crash involvement. *Journal of Legal Studies, 12,* 169–179.

Wilson, E. O., and Peter, F. M., eds. (1988). *Biodiversity.* Washington, D.C.: National Academy Press.

Winett, R. A., King, A. C., and Altman, D. G. (1989). *Health psychology and public health: An integrative approach.* New York: Pergamon.

World Commission on Environment and Development. (1987). *Our common future.* New York: Oxford University Press.

World Health Organization. (1984). Health promotion: A discussion document on the concept and principles. *Health Promotion, 1,* 73–76.

7

**Johanna Birckmayer
and Carol Hirschon Weiss**

THEORY-BASED EVALUATION

Investigating the How and Why of Wellness Promotion Programs

Agencies and their sponsors undertake evaluation to find out how effectively a program achieves the goals set by its various publics. The emphasis has traditionally been on outcomes: How well does the program accomplish desired ends? Attention is sometimes paid to unanticipated consequences, too: What unintended outcomes appear that either negate or amplify desired outcomes?

Evaluation studies use a variety of research designs to address these questions. When some potential participants are randomly assigned to the program and others to a control group who do not receive the program, program recipients can be compared with the control group after the program is over. Since the randomization process results in equivalent groups at the start, differences between the two groups at the end can be confidently attributed to the program. The evaluator can draw conclusions with considerable confidence about how much change the program "caused." Other designs, which do not lead to such firm causal attributions, are nevertheless appropriate under certain circumstances, for example, when the evaluator has little control over assignment or when questions of causality are not salient.

In recent years, evaluators have paid increasing attention to examining program process as well, that is, how activities are implemented. The reasons for studying program process are to find out such things as the extent to which implementation follows the prescribed course or is modified to suit local circumstances, the "quality" of the implementation (at least in terms of frequency and "dosage" of service provided), characteristics of staff who deliver the program and clients who receive it, and obstacles that arise during the course of implementation that interfere with planned activities. Quantitative or qualitative data on questions of this sort provide important understanding about how the program is actually carried out.

A combination of outcome evaluation and process evaluation can produce even greater learning. Evaluations that include both kinds of data show how programs are conducted and what kinds of outcomes they generate. When outcomes are analyzed in terms of the activities and experiences offered by the program, the evaluation indicates which features of the program (and its participants) are associated with better outcomes. Thus, it may emerge that weight-loss activities offered in nonformal settings are associated with better outcomes than those offered in regular school classes.

Such evaluations have made vital contributions to the understanding of program interventions. But for all their contributions, they have not often been able to say *how and why* the program produced the outcomes observed. They can say such things as, "activities with more experienced staff tend to have better outcomes" or "participants who receive service on a face-to-face basis do better than those who receive service through telephone contact." But the reader has to speculate about how staff experience translates into more effective service or why face-to-face service works better than other forms of communication.

In many cases, the information gained is sufficient for practical purposes. A program faced with the findings in the previous paragraph can seek to employ staff with more years of experience and design activities that work in in-person modes.

But a later study may find that experienced staff do not have an edge in terms of outcomes or that telephone service that is responsive to the immediate needs of the client is actually more effective the next time around. It was not necessarily the years of experience that made staff more effective but something they did that novices did not do—something that not all staff with long experience do as a matter of course. And face-to-face service may be advantageous under some circumstances, for example, when the client has to be convinced of the service provider's expertise or good faith, but not necessarily under different circumstances.

What to do? One approach is to take a "theory-based" approach to evaluation. This chapter discusses theory-based evaluation (TBE)—what it is, what it does, and what it is assumed to contribute to more traditional evaluation fare. It is particularly fitting that we discuss TBE in wellness promotion programs because it is the field that has seen the most extensive use of TBE. Next we review six evaluation studies that have taken a theory-based approach. We look briefly at the programs, how the evaluators conducted the evaluations, and the findings that emerged. Finally, we seek to derive some lessons for the next round of TBE in wellness promotion.

WHAT THEORY-BASED EVALUATION IS

Theory-based evaluation (TBE) is a mode of evaluation that is built around the explicit or implicit assumptions on which the program is based (Suchman, 1967; Weiss, 1972, 1995, 1997, 1998; Chen and Rossi, 1987, 1992; Costner, 1989; Finney and Moos, 1989; Lipsey and Pollard, 1989; Bickman, 1990; Chen, 1990; Lipsey, 1993). The evaluator focuses on the mechanisms by which the program expects to achieve its effects. For example, a smoking prevention program offers activities that stress the perils of smoking (e.g., the known elevated risks of cancer and emphysema). The mechanism by which the program expects to keep young people from smoking is not the activities per se; it is how the participants react to the activities. Thus, one assumption is that participants gain knowledge about possible negative health effects and that the knowledge engenders fear or distaste. If this is the case, the mechanism that intervenes between program activities and refraining from smoking is assumed to be participants' increased knowledge and increased fear.

The evaluation then investigates the extent to which participants do in fact gain knowledge about the negative effects of smoking and the extent to which those with more knowledge become worried or concerned. (For further examples of TBE, see Feindler et al., 1984; Pentz et al., 1989; Donaldson et al., 1994; Goodman and Wandersman, 1994).

In sum, process evaluation collects quantitative or qualitative data on the way in which activities were carried out. Outcome evaluation collects data on the extent to which desired outcomes, in this case abstaining from smoking, were reached. The theory-based part of the evaluation focuses on the mechanisms that link process to outcome.

POSITED BENEFITS OF TBE

The benefits that advocates of TBE claim for this approach are of three kinds: advantages to program planning and improvement, advantages for the growth of knowledge about human behavior and behavior change, and advantages for the planning and conduct of the evaluation of the specific program.

Advantages for Program
Planning and Program Improvement

Theory-based evaluation provides information about the mechanisms that intervene between program activities and the achievement (or non-achievement) of expected results. When the theory on which the evaluation is based is fine grained, the evaluation can track each link in the chains of assumptions. The results of such an evaluation will show which chains of assumptions are well supported by the data collected, which chains of assumptions break down, and where in the chain they break down. For example, a program theory may be that the program increases participants' knowledge, that knowledge leads them to change their attitudes toward the risk behavior, and that attitude change leads to behavior change. Evaluation data may show, as it often does, that the program does increase knowledge and that knowledge often is associated with a change in attitude but that attitude change is not associated with change in the risk behavior. Program developers and redevelopers will then have to understand the obstacles that interfere with behavior change, that is, why people who now agree that they should not engage in a risk behavior nevertheless do so. If they find, for example, that the new attitudes tend to lapse over a short period of time, they may have to build into the program a set of ancillary activities to sustain the changed attitudes.

Advantages for Knowledge Development

Advocates of TBE hope that better knowledge about the mechanisms of change will benefit not only the specific program (or type of program) studied. The hope is that the knowledge will generalize to a wider array of change efforts. For example, if change in knowledge is not sufficient for behavior change in smoking prevention or dietary interventions, expectations for knowledge-based change may not make sense in other kinds of programming as well. Even though each evaluation study is prisoner of the unique characteristics of its setting (e.g., time, place, staff, and participants), repeated evaluations over time may be able to build a corpus of knowledge about which mechanisms work well and which work poorly. When the same kinds of theories are explored for different kinds of programs in different kinds of contexts, the findings may expand our knowledge about effective means for promoting wellness in different populations.

Such hopes are no doubt optimistic. As social science research has demonstrated over the decades, findings do not always generalize well from one setting or population to another. Furthermore, findings tend to become outmoded as times change.

But human behavior, while complex, is not random. Themes, relationships in the data, and "stories" can often be identified and, over time, may be codified into social science theories. When evaluation can test the relationships between program processes and program outcomes and the mechanisms that link the two, it can yield findings with greater relevance and staying power.

Advantages for Planning the Evaluation Study

Most immediately, a theory-based approach highlights the elements of program activity that deserve attention in the evaluation. The evaluator uses the program's assumptions as the scaffolding for the study. The evaluator can choose to collect data on the linkage mechanisms assumed to be operative in one theory or in several theories, or she can select one set of particularly central (or problematic) assumptions and direct the evaluation toward investigating that specific link in the theory chain. For example, one of the program planners' key assumptions may be that a program must be offered on a community-wide basis rather than on an individual basis, so that it changes what the relevant community regards as acceptable behavior. The theory is that individuals will not accept or sustain new behaviors unless the social groups with which they interact adopt these behaviors as their norm. Program sponsors, program planners and staff, and evaluators may choose to examine this one theoretical assumption—that the program can change community norms and that the widespread acceptance of "wellness" norms will lead to changes in individuals' behavior.

EXAMPLES OF TBE

To advance the discussions of TBE, we briefly describe six evaluations of health promotion programs that use a theory-based approach. A summary of each program's design, theory, measures, and findings is presented in Table 7.1. These studies represent fairly large, well-funded

TABLE 7.1   A SUMMARY OF SIX THEORY-BASED EVALUATIONS

Author, program	Design	Theory	Measures	Findings
Murray et al. (1994), antismoking	9th-grade students in Minnesota compared to students in Wisconsin; random survey of 3,600 students in both states conducted each year from 1986 to 1990.	Increase in antismoking activities in school and media → increase in exposure to antismoking messages → change in beliefs about health risks → decrease smoking rates.	Self-reports of exposure to pro- and antitobacco messages, antitobacco beliefs (health consequences to others, passive smoking hazard, personalized health risk), and tobacco use; expired air test for carbon monoxide to confirm smoking self-reports.	90% of schools implemented activities, but implementation was short term; 95% of youth saw or heard antitobacco ad in 1989–90, on average saw 50 ads per year; Minnesota increased exposure to antitobacco messages over Wisconsin (TV programming, net change +6.9%, p = .007; radio, net change +18.8%, p < .001; newspaper and magazine ads, net change +4.6%, p = .006; billboards, net change 3.8%, p = .09); no difference in antitobacco beliefs; 2.4% decrease in tobacco use in Minnesota, not significant compared to Wisconsin (p = .32).
Flay et al. (1995), antismoking	47 schools randomly assigned to one of five conditions: social resistance curriculum (SR), TV campaign, SR and TV combined (SR/TV), information only curriculum	IOC → increase in knowledge of effects of smoking → decrease in smoking; SR, TV, and SR/TV → increase in knowledge of effects of smoking, awareness of influences to	Self-reports of smoking knowledge, awareness of social influences to smoke, knowledge of resistance skills, refusal self-efficacy, efforts to resist smoking, smoking prevalence es-	Higher smoking knowledge in IOC group at T2–T4 (p < .001); positive effect on social influences awareness and resistance skill knowledge in SR (p < .001) and TV (p < .03)

TABLE 7.1 (*continued*)

	(IOC), and no-treatment (NOT); 340 7th-grade classrooms in study; students surveyed before intervention (T1), after (T2), 1 year after (T3), and 2 years after (T4).	smoke, skills to resist, efforts/confidence to refuse to smoke, and decrease perception of smoking acceptability (norm) → decrease in behavioral intentions to smoke → decrease in smoking.	timates (as indicator of smoking norms), approval of parental smoking, intentions to smoke, and past and current smoking.	groups and SR/TV at T2–T4 compared to NOT, SR, and TV; greater effect on social influences and resistance knowledge at T2 than SR/TV, difference faded by T4; no differences across groups on refusal self-efficacy; TV/SR positive effect on efforts at T2 ($p < .009$) and T ($p < .02$), effect faded by T4; smoking prevalence estimates lowest for SR ($p < .001$) and TV ($p < .006$) at T2, effect continued for SR at T4 ($p < .007$); no difference across groups in intentions to smoke; no difference in smoking rates.
Eisen et al. (1992), sex education curriculum	Random assignment to either the Health Belief Model (HBM) curriculum or agencies' usual sex ed program; 1,444 13- to 19-year olds attending six family planning services and one school surveyed before (T1), after (T2), and 12 months after (T3) intervention.	Increase awareness of probability and negative consequences of pregnancy, benefits of delayed sexual activity or contraceptive use, and decrease perceptions of barriers to abstinence or contraceptive use → decrease sexual activity and increase contraceptive use → decrease in pregnancy.	Self-reports of sexual and contraceptive knowledge, attitudes, and behavior.	Knowledge in both HBM and comparison class increased; HBM class greater increase ($p < .05$); health perceptions in both HBM and comparison group increased ($p < .01$); no difference between groups; no difference in continued abstinence between groups. T1 female virgins in comparison group more likely to use effective con-

TABLE 7.1 *(continued)*

Author, program	Design	Theory	Measures	Findings
Eisen et al. (1992), sex education curriculum *(continued)*				traceptives at T2–T3; T1 male virgins, no difference between programs on outcomes at T2–T3; both programs increased contraceptive efficiency, T1–T3 for nonvirgins; males in HBM group greater increase in contraceptive efficiency than comparison program ($p < .05$); no difference between programs for females.
Brug et al. (1996), nutrition education	Random assignment to program or general nutrition information; 347 employees in the Netherlands Royal Shell laboratory surveyed before and three weeks after intervention.	Change in attitudes toward desired diet, perceived social influences, self-efficacy beliefs, and intentions to change diet → reduce fat intake and increase vegetable and fruit consumption.	Self-reports of attitudes, social influences, and self-efficacy expectations; dietary fat, fruit, and vegetable intake.	Program group more positive attitudes to vegetable and fruit consumption ($p < .01$); no effect on self-efficacy or social influences; program group strongest intention to change consumption in recommended direction ($p < .01$); program group lower fat scores (26.9 vs. 27.2 grams of fat, $p < .01$); greatest effect among preintervention high fat eaters (9% vs. 3% fat reduction ($p < .01$)); both groups increased vegetable but not fruit consumption.

TABLE 7.1 (*continued*)

Puska et al. (1985), heart disease prevention	Program community compared to contiguous comparison community in Finland; independent random samples of adults before (T1), 5 years (T2), and 10 years (T3) after intervention.	Change in individuals' knowledge and attitudes and providing social and environmental support for behavior change → reductions in individuals' risk factors (smoking, serum cholesterol, and blood pressure) → reduced mortality at population level.	Self-reports of knowledge, attitudes, and behavior; physical exam measuring height, weight, blood pressure, and cholesterol.	Knowledge of risk factors increased, but change was only slightly higher in program community; no major changes in health attitudes; net reduction in smoking for program community (27%, $p < .001$); net reduction in serum cholesterol for program men ($p < .01$); net reduction for blood pressure ($p < .01$); from 1974 to 1979, coronary heart disease mortality decreased (22% in program vs. 12% in control, $p. < .05$).
Holder et al. (1997), prevention of alcohol-related injuries and death	Three experimental communities compared to matched comparison communities in United States over five-year period from 1992 to 1997.	Five main program components → produce short-term effects (e.g., alcohol server training results in fewer drinks served to intoxicated patrons, alcohol law changes results in fewer sales to youth) → combined effect of activities reduce alcohol availability and consumption, youthful drinking and drunk driving, etc. → reduced alcohol-related morbidity and mortality.	Random-digit telephone surveys of adults, youth telephone and school surveys, roadside surveys, and media coding analysis measured mediating variables; emergency room surveys, records of hospital admissions, community surveys, and death certificate data measured alcohol-related trauma and death.	Results not yet available.

efforts by social scientists to evaluate programs in which the program theory is developed during the planning process and tested during the evaluation. At the end of this section, we discuss what was learned from the TBE approach. We then discuss the application of TBE in smaller, less formal programs for which program theory is not clearly defined before the program is implemented.

Murray et al. (1994)

Murray et al. (1994) used a relatively simple theory to evaluate the effects of a statewide antismoking campaign. A tax initiative passed in 1985 by the Minnesota State Legislature designated the use of tax money from tobacco products for antitobacco programs. The initiative was expected to spur local communities and schools to develop a variety of tobacco control programs targeting school-age children. Concurrently, the Department of Health was funded to implement a statewide antismoking mass media campaign. While schools and groups receiving money from the initiative were asked to develop activities using a social influences model of smoking, programs varied across the state.

The evaluators tracked whether the initiative resulted in increased antismoking activities in schools. Exposure to these activities coupled with the media campaign was expected to change beliefs about the health risks of smoking. Changes in beliefs were hypothesized to result in lower smoking rates among youth.

A process evaluation found the Department of Health implemented a mass-media campaign from 1986 to 1990. However, schools made only short-term and erratic increases in antismoking activities.

The evaluators compared Minnesota ninth-graders to Wisconsin ninth-graders in terms of exposure to school-based and mass-media programming, beliefs, and tobacco use each year from 1986 to 1990. Minnesota students reported greater increases in exposure to antismoking messages than Wisconsin students. However, there was no difference between the two states in the pattern of change in antitobacco beliefs. Ninth-graders in both states expressed strong antitobacco beliefs at the start that remained stable over time. Reports of tobacco use in Minnesota declined, but the decrease was not significantly different from that in Wisconsin.

The tax initiative increased students' exposure to antismoking messages in mass media. However, the increase in exposure did not lead to changes in beliefs or behavior. Because of the lack of full implementation of the school-based program, the authors cannot fully determine whether or how a combined school/mass-media campaign of this type can work. They did learn that a mass-media campaign, while clearly reaching children on its own, does not produce changes in attitudes associated with smoking.

Flay et al. (1995)

In a second antismoking program, Flay et al. (1995) assessed the combined effects of a school and media smoking prevention and cessation program for seventh-graders. Schools were randomly assigned to one of five conditions: a social resistance curriculum only (SR), a television campaign only (TV), a combination of the social resistance curriculum and television (SR/TV), an information-only curriculum (IOC), and a no-treatment control group.

The program theory was defined at the outset. The IOC, SR, TV, and combined SR/TV programs were expected to increase knowledge about the effects of smoking. In the IOC program, this knowledge alone was expected to lead to changes in smoking behaviors. The SR, TV, and combined SR/TV programs included, in addition, activities designed to increase youths' awareness of factors that influence smoking and to increase youths' skills to resist smoking. In turn, students' efforts and confidence in their ability to refuse to smoke were expected to increase. Further, the program sought to change smoking norms. The combined effect of changes in these factors was expected to increase behavioral intentions to reduce, quit, or not start smoking, which in turn were hypothesized to lead to reduced smoking.

Questionnaires were used to measure all mediating and outcome measures before the intervention, immediately after, and one and two years after. For the SR, TV, and combined SR/TV programs, the evaluators found significant positive effects on health and resistance skills knowledge, estimates of the prevalence of smoking (which was assumed to reflect community norms), and efforts to quit. The knowledge and prevalence estimates effects decayed partially but remained significant at the two-year follow-up. The effect of the programs on efforts to quit did not persist at the one- and two-year follow-ups. The programs had no effect on confidence to quit or smoking intentions. None of the programs was related to actual smoking at any posttest. The only predictors of smoking at posttest were smoking at pretest and strong intentions to smoke in the future.

The authors have some difficulty interpreting the results of this study. First, they note that the group targeted, seventh-graders, have very low rates of smoking and strong antitobacco beliefs, effectively reducing the chances of finding a program effect on attitudes or behavior. They suggest that programs for this group either are not necessary or need to continue into later grades. Second, a process evaluation found variability in the curriculum delivery and poor execution of the television programming. However, because of the strong effects of the program on certain mediators, the authors are reluctant to attribute the shortcomings to implementation problems alone. They point out that the program affected knowledge about resistance skills and prevalence estimates. While these effects decayed slightly, they persisted over time. Effects on skills were smaller and decayed more quickly. On the basis of these findings, they suggest that an effective preventive program will need to commit to long-term reinforcement of both knowledge and skills. They conclude, however, that given the lack of program impact on smoking rates, the field has more to learn about how programs work.

Eisen et al. (1992)

A well-known individual-level theory of health behavior, the Health Belief Model (HBM), posits that a person's behavior is influenced by perceptions of his/her own susceptibility to the effects of an action, the potential seriousness of these effects, and perceived benefits and barriers to action. Applying the HBM to the issue of adolescent pregnancy, Eisen et al. (1992) developed a school curriculum to target the mediating factors identified in the theory. The curriculum developed was intended to increase students' awareness of the probability of becoming pregnant or causing a pregnancy, the serious negative consequences of pregnancy, and the benefits of delayed sexual activity or contraceptive use. It was also designed to decrease participants' perceptions of barriers to abstinence or contraceptive use. Changes in these mediating factors were expected to lead to changes in contraceptive and sexual behavior. Past research led the authors to believe that males and females and virgins and nonvirgins would respond differently to the program.

The evaluation was designed to assess the impact of the program on sexual behavior and the importance of the mediating factors in the HBM. Six family planning services and one school were selected to participate in the project. Youth aged 13 to 19 participating in these agencies' programs were randomly assigned to receive the HBM curriculum or the agencies' usual sex education program.

The evaluation measured sexual and contraceptive knowledge, the sexuality-related beliefs identified by the HBM model, and contraceptive and sexual behavior (the targeted outcomes) before, immediately after, and 12 months after program completion. Knowledge in both the experimental and the control group increased at posttest, with the experimental group showing a greater increase. Participants' health perceptions pre- to postintervention improved in both the control and the experimental group; the experimental group showed no greater increase than the control group.

All behavioral results were presented by gender and previous sexual experience. The HBM program produced significantly greater positive changes among males who were sexually active before the program in terms of their self-reported "contraceptive efficiency" (a measure of the consistency with which teens used effective birth control methods). Females in the comparison group who became sexually active after the initial baseline survey reported significantly more effective contraceptive use than those in the program group.

Similar to the Flay et al. study, the authors cite the low rate of sexual activity among the age-group included in the study as one possible explanation for the limited postintervention differences found between the two programs (more than half the teens were still virgins at follow-up). In addition, the authors note that the number and length of sessions of the comparison and intervention program were similar and acknowledge that the two programs may have had the same potential for impact. In part because of these design problems, the authors do not reject the potential importance of the HBM beliefs. While the evaluators did not find a difference in postintervention HBM beliefs between the HBM curriculum and comparison groups, they found that those who perceived fewer barriers and greater benefits of birth control use before the intervention were more likely to be abstinent after the intervention (if they were virgins) and more effective users of contraception (if they were sexually active). This finding suggests that at least some of the HBM beliefs are important in determining sexual behavior. The authors suggest that program theory may operate differently for the specific groups in the study. They hypothesize that the HBM program may have been more effective than the comparison program for sexually active males because it focused on increasing males' awareness of the risk of pregnancy. They suggest that in contrast, females may be saturated with messages about the threat of pregnancy and so learned less from the HBM program. The authors conclude that differences in program impact by previous sexual experience and gender indicate that programs must be tailored to specific groups.

Brug et al. (1996)

A study by Brug et al. (1996) presents a theory-based approach to evaluating a nutrition education program in the Netherlands. The program aimed to reduce fat intake and increase fruit and vegetable consumption among study participants by programming computers to ask questions about participants' dietary intake and determinants of and barriers to changing their behaviors. The computer then generated messages specifically tailored to individuals' needs. The program theory posited that the tailored messages would change individuals' attitudes toward the desired diet, perceived social influences, beliefs about their ability to perform the behavior (self-efficacy), and intentions to make dietary changes. In turn, these changes would lead participants to reduce their fat intake and increase their vegetable and fruit consumption.

In the evaluation, employees in a Royal Shell laboratory were randomly assigned to receive the program or to receive general nutrition information. Questionnaires were used pre- and three weeks postintervention to assess changes in dietary fat, fruit and vegetable intake, and changes in attitudes, social influences, and self-efficacy expectations.

At posttest, the program group that had received tailored messages had more positive attitudes toward increasing consumption of vegetable, fruits, and fat than the comparison group. No effects were found for self-efficacy or social influences. Program participants expressed stronger intentions to change their consumption of fat and fruit in the recommended direction than the comparison group. At posttest, the program group had significantly lower fat scores than the comparison group. Both groups increased their reported vegetable but not their fruit consumption with no difference found between the changes in the two groups.

The authors conclude that interventions targeting psychosocial beliefs may be more effective than programs providing dietary feedback alone. They suggest that general information regarding recommended consumption of fruit and vegetables may be adequate to induce change, whereas messages tailored to the individual may be more effective for influencing the more complex issue of fat intake.

Puska et al. (1985)

The North Karelia project in Finland is a much cited study of a community-based approach to the reduction of heart disease. The project team implemented mass-media campaigns and worked with health and community groups to provide health education information to individuals and to initiate changes in the social and physical environment to motivate and maintain behavior change. The basic theory of the program was that targeting individuals' knowledge and attitudes and providing social and environmental support for behavior change would lead individuals to reduce their risk factors for cardiovascular disease. In turn, reductions in individual risk factors, specifically smoking, serum cholesterol, and blood pressure, would lead to reduced morbidity and mortality at the population level. The authors state that the theory of how the program would work was only partially developed at the outset of the program because of the paucity of theories related to community interventions. Thus, the evaluation tracked individuals' knowledge, attitudes, and behavior, the most developed part of the program theory, while documenting program-related activities in the community through a process evaluation.

Independent random samples of adults were surveyed before the intervention in 1972 and again five and 10 years later. Results for North Karelia were compared to those of a comparison community. The surveys asked questions about health knowledge, attitudes, and behavior and included an exam to measure height, weight, blood pressure, and cholesterol. Finally, mortality rates for the two communities were compared.

The evaluation showed that knowledge of risk factors increased somewhat but that the change was only slightly higher in North Karelia. The evaluators reported no major changes in health attitude measures with little difference between the two communities. A net reduction in smoking and blood pressure was found in North Karelia over the 10-year period. A net reduction in serum cholesterol was found for men in North Karelia. Coronary heart disease mortality decreased by 22% compared to 12% in the comparison community.

The lack of change in individual's knowledge and attitudes led the authors to attribute the success of the project more to its community organization aspects than to the project's efforts to target individuals. They believe that health education messages disseminated through the media and opinion leaders gradually created an environment promoting healthier lifestyles and that these environmental changes gradually influenced individual behavior.

Holder et al. (1997)

The Community Prevention Trial provides a final example of a theory-based approach to evaluation. The study has only recently concluded, and, as study results were not yet available, the authors' paper described here reviews only the evaluation plan. The project used a combination of community awareness and policy-related activities to reduce alcohol-involved injuries and deaths. The program consisted of five main components that were expected to reinforce one another: working with community groups to plan and implement prevention activities and develop public awareness of alcohol-related trauma; working with alcohol beverage servers and retailers to design and implement safer beverage service policies; developing community programs to reduce underage drinking; working with law enforcement, retail establishments, and others to reduce drinking and driving; and using municipal control policies to reduce alcohol availability.

The hypothesized program model is presented in Table 7.2. Each component of the program is hypothesized to lead to certain short-term effects. The combined effects of the components are expected to lead to changes in intervening variables, such as alcohol availability and consumption, youthful drinking, and drinking and driving. These changes in turn are expected to lead to reductions in alcohol-related morbidity and mortality.

A process evaluation monitored the extent of implementation of the different components within each community in order to assess the timing and quality of the intervention activities. Surveys and media content analysis were used to measure changes in the mediating variables in Table 7.2. Alcohol-related trauma and death were measured using hospital and community records and surveys. Results from the three experimental communities will be compared to matched comparison communities for a five-year period from 1992 to 1997.

Results of the trial are not yet available. Therefore, we cannot yet tell how well the program theory represents the actual processes that were

TABLE 7.2   THEORY OF PROGRAM
TO REDUCE ALCOHOL-RELATED MORTALITY

Component	Program Activities	Mediating "Process Variables"	Intervention Outcomes
Community knowledge, values, and mobilization	Media advocacy, community organization	Media coverage of alcohol-related issues	
Responsible beverage service	Establishment of RBS standards, server training	Changes in server behavior, reduction in DWI	Traffic-related trauma
Underage drinking	In-school programs, zero tolerance	Restricted youth access, decreased youth drinking	
Risk of drinking and driving	Increased DWI enforcement	Lowered BACs among drivers, reductions in DWI	Non-traffic-related trauma
Access to alcohol	Density restrictions, licensing requirements	Decreased density, decreased adult drinking	

implemented or how well the program theory produces the expected results. The authors make several statements relevant to the use of TBE.
First, they state that community-based approaches are complex efforts
and that little is known about how they work. They argue that a theory-
based approach is essential to build a better understanding of these processes. Second, they argue that when the processes by which an intervention work are not well understood, it is preferable to do an in-depth
study of a few communities rather than a larger, multicommunity study.

WHAT WAS LEARNED FROM
THESE THEORY-BASED EVALUATIONS?

While each of the evaluations has some modicum of theory involved, the
authors are not always explicit about what they learned from TBE over
and above what they would have learned without it. Here we draw conclusions about findings from the theory-based approach to evaluation

based on our own interpretation of the published evaluation reports. One of the incidental learnings we derive from this review is that authors do not always make explicit the relation of their data to the theory of the program. They report in traditional ways without necessarily emphasizing insights about mechanisms of change that the theory-based approach provides. At times our interpretation ranges beyond the authors' reported conclusions (with all the perils of such extrapolation) because of this omission. We offer the following interpretations in the spirit of examining the types of learning TBE can provide. We highlight particular lessons from each study (with the understanding that more than one study may illustrate the point).

The Difficulties of Going to Scale

The antismoking program evaluated by Murray et al. was an effort to take positive evaluation findings from small-scale antismoking programs and "scale up" to the state level. Minnesota appropriated tobacco tax money for the purpose. The evaluation found that a key component of the intervention was not well implemented, and thus the learnings from the theory-based approach were limited.

The study revealed that schools did not conduct strong or consistent antitobacco interventions. Although the media component reached the ninth-grade audience, this intervention alone did not change beliefs or behavior. Because schools' enthusiasm for antismoking curricula was short-lived, the full theory could not receive an adequate test at the state level.

Finding Intermediary Changes

The study by Flay et al. confronted the endemic question of the appropriate age to begin prevention activities, an issue common to smoking, sex, and drug and alcohol programs. An outcome evaluation of the smoking program evaluated by Flay would have discovered no impact on the smoking rates of seventh-graders. This finding, coupled with low rates of smoking in the study age-group, led the authors to question the utility of targeting such a young group. However, as the authors note, results from the TBE indicating a change in attitudes among the youth suggest that programs targeting this age-group may have future effects on smoking. The additional finding that skills and knowledge have differential attrition rates suggests the need to reinforce attitude changes over time. While the two findings do not conclusively answer the question of whether seventh grade is the appropriate age to begin smoking prevention efforts, they suggest that some effects do appear in seventh-graders and that perhaps program efforts need to be reinforced over time.

Raising Questions

The theory-based evaluation of the sex education course evaluated by Eisen raises many questions about how both the HBM curriculum and the comparison program work. An outcomes evaluation that broke down study results by gender and previous sexual experience would have discovered the differential impact of the programs. Given the explicitly theory-based design of the program, it would have been reasonable to assume that participants' health beliefs were differentially influenced by the program. However, the assessment of beliefs indicates that this was not the case and leads us to question the underlying mechanisms by which both programs worked. Was the HBM curriculum simply inadequate to change important HBM beliefs? If indeed the preintervention HBM beliefs found to be associated with positive outcomes in both groups were able to be changed by the program, would the program outcomes have been different? What accounts for the differences by gender and past sexual experience when little difference was found in health beliefs? What are possible alternative intervening factors that led to the changes in behaviors found?

Identifying Possibly
Unnecessary Program Components

The Brug et al. evaluation of the computer-generated nutrition program found that certain mechanisms of change identified by the theory were affected among program participants but that others were not. Nonetheless, participants made significant improvements in their consumption of fat. An outcome evaluation would have indicated only that the program was successful. The additional findings contributed by TBE suggest the need to explore whether those program elements that were not associated with the dietary improvement can be eliminated in future programs. The authors also suggest the need to study longer-term effects of tailored nutrition programs.

Contributing to a Paradigm Shift

The North Karelia study was one of the first large-scale health promotion studies to attempt to influence the health of individuals through
community change efforts. The authors state that the program theory
was only partially developed at the start of the project because of an absence of theories about community-level change. The evaluators systematically tracked one of the proposed mechanisms of change at the
individual level—and discovering little change. Although the hypothesized individual-level mechanisms were not affected, they nevertheless
discovered an overall positive impact of the program on health outcomes. The findings supported a shift from changing only individual
knowledge and attitudes to focusing on changing the social and cultural
environments in which individuals live.

Providing Clarity and Focus for Evaluation

Twenty years later, in an evaluation of a community-level health promotion effort, Holder et al. explicitly discuss the importance of laying
out a program theory for the evaluation of large-scale community-based
programs. With the results not yet in, the benefits of the TBE approach
for exploring outcomes in this study cannot be assessed. However, the
delineation of the program theory of such a complex change effort provides the evaluator with clear guidelines for data collection and analysis
and will undoubtedly assist in the clarity of interpreting results and
drawing conclusions.

IS THEORY-BASED EVALUATION
APPLICABLE IN OTHER SETTINGS?

The evaluations described here represent well-funded, primarily re-
search-oriented projects. The programs themselves were developed based
on theory, although rather rudimentary theory in some cases, and the
evaluations test the theory embedded in the program. However, most
programs are not explicitly based on theories of change, and many are
not well-defined at the planning stage. They are often small programs,
based on practitioner experience, and funded at relatively low levels. Is
TBE relevant to them? Can it be applied in these settings, and what can
be gained? It is our belief that theory-based evaluation can be applied in

these settings and that it has the potential to provide benefits that match those provided for programs with well-articulated theory. Even if the evaluators do not adopt the language of TBE, they can incorporate elements of it into their studies.

Here are some kernels of advice gleaned from this review that we believe apply to even small, atheoretical, marginally funded programs.

Consider Theory Development as a Stage in the Evaluation

An emphasis on theory development at the start of the evaluation may be, in and of itself, the most beneficial aspect of the theory-based approach.

In many fields, programs are planned on the basis of experience, professional savvy, intuition, and beliefs in fashion in the field. There is little in this melange that is easily characterized by the name of theory. But all programs have a theoretical basis no matter how weakly the assumptions are articulated. Program people make some assumptions about why the set of activities they plan will lead to desirable outcomes. When the assumptions are tacit rather than consciously expressed, the evaluator has the task of eliciting or constructing the theoretical assumptions underlying the program. The evaluator usually undertakes this theory-surfacing exercise in conjunction with program planners and program staff.

When program staff describe their assumptions about the mechanisms by which the program will bring about change, the evaluator has to see whether the theories offered are operative. She has to learn enough about program activities—real activities in action and not just espoused ideas of activities—to figure out whether practitioners' theories are being operationalized in the program. If the program claims that its prevention goals will be realized by increasing participants' sense of self-efficacy but the evaluator finds no activities dedicated to increasing self-efficacy, she will doubt that the theory is "real" for this program. She will have to seek an alternative theory that explains why the real activities are expected to lead to the intended effects. Or she may call the absence of efficacy-building activities to the attention of program staff and perhaps encourage them to alter the program to fit their theory (or alter their theory to fit the program).

Possible sources of program theories are social science theories and research, prior evaluations, planner and practitioner expectations, the evaluator's knowledge and experience with programs of similar type, and her own logical thinking. Often the evaluator will cycle through several of these sources—asking program planners and program managers, reviewing existing theories in the field, reviewing previous research and evaluations, hypothesizing a theory on the basis of this information, and then negotiating her formulation with program managers and staff to come to an agreement that accords with their thinking.

When people do not agree on their assumptions, the evaluator may incorporate several different chains of reasoning into the study. For example, staff in a pregnancy prevention program may expect the program to work because it provides information about contraception, or because it teaches young women to be more assertive in demands on their partners, or because it makes chastity more socially acceptable within the program group, or for a number of other reasons. Rather than demanding that program staff agree on a single theory, the evaluator can design the study to collect data on several different assumptions. The study can then show which of the theories, if any, is supported by the data.

Identifying poorly defined, implausible, or hotly debated links in how a program is expected to work can force practitioners and managers to define and agree on what they believe they are doing. With greater clarity about what they are trying to accomplish, and how, program people should do a better job of developing and improving programs. And with a greater understanding of how the program is expected to work, the evaluator can better structure the evaluation to answer relevant questions and interpret study results. Even if the evaluator does not have adequate resources to collect data on all the mediating variables identified in a program theory, developing the program theory as the starting point in evaluation can be of value for program development, improvement, and evaluation.

Do Not Expect Theories to Be Completely Right

Remember when conducting a theory-based evaluation that at this stage the theory is primarily a guide to the evaluation. Managers, practitioners, and evaluators of small programs who attempt retrospectively to define program theory should not expect the theories they develop of the program to be exactly right. In fact, in none of the five theory-based evaluations described here was the original theory borne out. (The Holder et al. study of alcohol-related traffic accidents is still in progress.)

Some of the programs activated the mechanisms that were assumed to trigger desired outcomes, but the desired outcomes did not appear. Some of the programs produced the desired outcomes but not through the mechanisms that were assumed to be causal; there were no significant changes in the mechanisms. Obviously, one lesson from these theory-based evaluations is that program planners have limited understanding of how and why programs work or fail to work. Much more effort is needed to understand what it takes to get people to reduce risk behaviors and adopt positive lifestyles. The processes of change are complex, dependent on many variables and on higher-order interactions among variables. Concerted research is required to unravel the many contingencies in behavioral change.

In the studies reviewed, we have come across cases where program theories were not well supported by the data but where the evaluators were reluctant to abandon the theories. No sin inheres in such caution. One single null finding should not lead to the rejection of a sensible-sounding theory; any one study may provide misleading evidence. However, if repeated evaluations show the same pattern, if a theory is disconfirmed again and again, there seems little reason to cling to it. Evaluators should join with program planners to seek more effective theories, develop programs that embody the theories, and conduct evaluations to test them.

One reason for staying with a well-known and well-respected program theory, even when the evidence is slim, is that it often seems so intuitively right. Another reason why people sometimes cling to a familiar, if ill-supported, theory is that few alternatives seem to be waiting in the wings. If programs do not lead to desired outcomes through the mechanisms of knowledge, attitude change, social support, revisions in community norms, or whatever else the theory posits, it is usually hard to figure out what mechanisms would be effective. This represents a challenge to the whole field of wellness promotion.

Include a Process Evaluation

A TBE study should include a description of program implementation, generally called a process evaluation. Some programs do not work because planned activities are not carried out regularly or not carried out well. If an evaluation fails to collect data on the *processes* of the program, it will be unable to distinguish between "program failure" (the program was not carried out well and therefore did not lead to the desired effects) and "theory failure" (the idea underlying the program was wrong and therefore expected results did not materialize) (Suchman, 1967). If the study of implementation is forgone, the evaluator loses the ability to tell whether this particular realization of the program or the basic theory is at fault.

One possible reason for the observed outcomes of the TBE studies we have reviewed is that programs work differently for different subgroups. Or outcomes may differ according to the type and frequency of activities to which participants are exposed. Again, process evaluation is essential. The evaluator is well advised to collect data on those characteristics of participants, staff, activities, settings, and time that are likely to be salient to success. In the analysis, the evaluator can examine outcomes in light of the features of people and program activities and thus come to estimates of which activities work best for which groups under which conditions.

When a program is poorly implemented, there may not be a great need to delve deeply into all the hypothesized causal links in the theory chain. Sometimes even with a poorly conducted program, some later expectations are realized. It is difficult to explain positive outcome data by assuming that they were brought about by a weak or incompetent program. Other information is needed. On the other hand, if the outcomes of a poorly conducted program are disappointing, as one might expect, the immediate lesson is to do a better job of conducting the program — and evaluate the program in its superior version.

Use the Information TBE Can Provide

While many funders of small-scale programs ask for outcome evaluations, the results of these evaluations are rarely used to make go/no-go decisions about the program's future. Rather than using evaluative information for continuing or discontinuing the program, funders and program managers usually want information about how to improve the program. The results of theory-based evaluation may prove to be more useful than evaluations of outcomes only. Knowledge of how or why a program is failing provides managers with leads to how to improve the existing program. They can use the information to discuss why programs should work and where they are breaking down. This type of information communicates easily to policy makers and may be more convincing than the results of outcome evaluations only.

Theory-based evaluation has a longer tradition among academic researchers developing and testing program approaches than among program evaluators called in after a program is in process. We noted that traditional methods of reporting results sometimes got in the way of clearly associating the evaluation results to the theory in the evaluations reviewed. As TBE becomes more widely used in practice, evaluators will need to develop effective ways to report on the findings.

CONCLUSION

How well the evaluator is able to test a program theory is likely to be a function of three factors. The first is how well the theory is defined. The evaluator may have to consult many stakeholder groups to identify and secure agreement on the definition of the theory underlying the program. Second is how well program activities reflect the assumptions embedded in the theory. Third is the grubby matter of money and time. If TBE is carried out in full detail, it is apt to be an expensive and time-consuming enterprise.

As several of the examples show, even if an evaluation is able to track a specific theory, the interpretation of results may not be straightforward. Findings that indicate that the program altered some of the hypothesized intervening factors but not others do not lead to easy interpretation. Assessing exactly where the hypothesized theory breaks down, and why, calls for more finely grained study than most evaluations have yet included. A basic limitation is the state of knowledge in the field about which factors are effectual in bringing about change and how factors interact to change human beings and human communities. Advocates of TBE hope that over time results from TBE will lead to cumulative knowledge of change processes and consequently the development of more effective wellness programs. As some of the examples show, even within its limitations TBE is contributing to a growth in knowledge in the health promotion field.

REFERENCES

Bickman, Leonard, ed.(1990). *Advances in Program Theory*. New Directions for Program Evaluation 47. San Francisco: Jossey-Bass.

Brug, J., Steenhuis, I., Van Assema, P., and H. De Vries. (1996). "The Impact of a Computer-Tailored Nutrition Intervention." *Preventive Medicine, 25,* 236–242.

Chen, Huey-tsyh. (1990). *Theory-Driven Evaluation.* Newbury Park, Calif.: Sage.

Chen, Huey-tsyh, and Rossi, P. H. (1987). "The Theory-Driven Approach to Validity." *Evaluation and Program Planning,* 10, 95–103.

Chen, Huey-tsyh, and Rossi, P. H. eds. (1992). *Using Theory to Improve Program and Policy Evaluations.* New York: Greenwood Press.

Costner, H. L. (1989). "The Validity of Conclusions in Evaluation Research." *Evaluation and Program Planning,* 12, 345–353.

Donaldson, S. I., Graham, J. W., and Hansen, W. B. (1994). "Testing the Generalizability of Intervening Mechanism Theories: Understanding the Effects of Adolescent Drug Use Prevention." *Journal of Behavioral Medicine,* 17, 195–216.

Eisen, M., Zellman, G., and McAlister, A. (1992). "A Health Belief Model–Social Learning Theory Approach to Adolescents' Fertility Control: Findings from a Controlled Field Trial." *Health Education Quarterly,* 19(2), 249–262.

Feindler, E. L., Marriott, S. A., and Iwata, M. (1984). "Group Anger Control Training for Junior High School Delinquents." *Cognitive Therapy and Research,* 8, 299–311.

Finney, J. W., and Moos, R. H. (1989). "Theory and Method in Treatment Evaluation." *Evaluation and Program Planning,* 12, 307–316.

Flay, B. R., Miller, T. Q., Hedeker, D., et al. (1995). "The Television, School and Family Smoking Prevention and Cessation Project, VIII: Student Outcomes and Mediating Variables." *Preventive Medicine,* 24, 29–40.

Goodman, R. M., and Wandersman, A. (1994). "FORECAST: A Formative Approach to Evaluating Community Coalitions and Community-Based Initiatives." *Journal of Community Psychology,* special issue, 6–25.

Holder, H. D., Saltz, R. F., Treno, A. J., et al. (1997). "Evaluation Design for a Community Prevention Trial." *Evaluation Review,* 21(2), 140–166.

Lipsey, M. W. (1993). "Theory as Method: Small Theories of Treatments." *New Directions for Program Evaluation,* no. 57, 5–38.

Lipsey, M. W., and Pollard, J. A. (1989). "Driving toward Theory in Program Evaluation: More Models to Choose From." *Evaluation and Program Planning,* 12, 317–328.

Murray, D. M., Prokhorov, A. V., and Harty, K. C. (1994). "Effects of a Statewide Antismoking Campaign on Mass Media Messages and Smoking Beliefs." *Preventive Medicine,* 3, 54–60.

Pentz, M. A., Dwyer, J. H., MacKinnon D. P., et al. (1989). "Primary Prevention of Chronic Diseases in Adolescence: Effects of the Midwestern Prevention Project on Tobacco Use." *American Journal of Epidemiology,* 130, 713–724.

Puska, P., Nissinen, A., and Tuomilehto, J. (1985). "The Community-Based Strategy to Prevent Coronary Heart Disease: Conclusions for the Ten Years of the North Karelia Projects." *Annual Review of Public Health,* 6, 147–193.

Suchman, E. A. (1967). *Evaluative Research.* New York: Russell Sage Foundation.

Weiss, C. H. (1972). *Evaluation Research: Methods for Assessing Program Effectiveness.* Englewood Cliffs, N.J.: Prentice Hall.

Weiss, C. H. (1995). "Nothing as Practical as a Good Theory: Exploring Theory-Based Evaluation for Comprehensive Community Initiatives for Children and Families." In J. P. Connell, A. C. Kubish, L. Schorr, and C. H. Weiss, eds., *New Approaches to Evaluating Community Initiatives: Concepts, Methods and Contexts.* Washington, D.C.: Aspen Institute.

Weiss, C. H. (1997). "How Can Theory-Based Evaluations Make Greater Headway?" *Evaluation Review,* 21, 501–524.

Weiss, C. H. (1998). *Evaluation: Methods for Studying Programs and Policies.* Upper Saddle River, N.J.: Prentice Hall.

━━━

8

Patricia L. East

PREGNANCY PREVENTION
OPPORTUNITIES FOCUSING ON THE
YOUNGER SISTERS OF CHILDBEARING TEENS

This chapter describes a previously unrecognized target population for adolescent pregnancy prevention: the younger sisters of childbearing teens. Data from several studies show that the younger sisters of adolescent mothers have teenage childbearing rates two to six times higher than women in the general population (Cox et al., 1993; Friede et al., 1986; Goldfarb et al., 1977). These studies involved large samples—and, in two cases, statewide samples—of Black and non-Black adolescents in both urban and rural settings, so that such findings appear to be robust (East and Felice, 1992). The younger sisters of adolescent mothers have also been shown to have higher rates of adolescent sexual activity (East et al., 1993; Hogan and Kitagawa, 1985), to be younger at first sexual intercourse and first pregnancy (Hogan and Kitagawa, 1985), and less likely to use contraception when sexually active (Hogan et al., 1985) than other girls of their race and social class.

Although these studies are useful for identifying a population at increased risk of early sexual activity and early pregnancy, they fail to address *how* or *why* the sisters of childbearing teens become vulnerable to such outcomes. This chapter describes two groups of causal factors that predispose the younger sisters of pregnant and parenting teens to early pregnancy. The first group of causal factors concerns sisters' shared background and consists of factors equally present for all siblings within a family. These shared *preexisting predispositions* include the parenting the sisters received, their ethnic identity and socioeconomic sta-

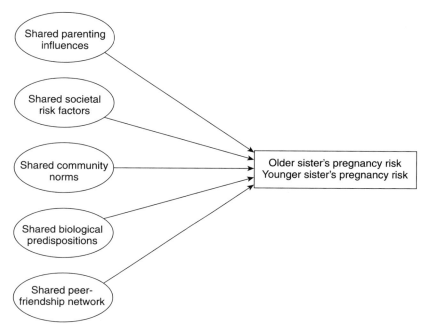

Figure 8.1.   Sisters' shared vulnerability to early childbearing.

tus, their exposure to shared community-neighborhood norms, a shared biological predisposition, and a common peer-friendship network (see Figure 8.1). The second group of causal factors that would increase a younger sister's risk for early pregnancy are factors that *result from* the older sister's pregnancy and childbearing and involve interactions between the childbearing teen and her younger sister and family during the postpartum period. These processes include social modeling of the older sister, socialization to early motherhood through child care provided to the sister's child, diminished quality of parenting by the sisters' parents, and increased family stress and family economic hardship resulting from the older sister's pregnancy.

It is further argued in this chapter that these unique effects resulting from the pregnancy of the older sister contribute to younger sisters' preexisting predispositions toward early childbearing to render younger sisters even more vulnerable to early pregnancy and early childbearing. Data are then reviewed that highlight the high level of problem and delinquent-like behavior and the relatively high rate of sexual activity among the younger sisters of childbearing teens. These behavioral proclivities are significant because they point to several transition behaviors that likely lead to teenage pregnancy and childbearing. Finally, specific considerations for intervening with this unique target population are discussed.

SISTERS' SHARED
VULNERABILITY TO EARLY CHILDBEARING
Shared Parenting Influences

One line of reasoning that can be used to explain sisters' similarity in adolescent sexual initiation and permissiveness—and, therefore, risk for adolescent pregnancy and parenthood—is that because all children within a family experience similar parenting styles and disciplinary techniques, they are equally likely to engage or not to engage in sexual activity during adolescence. It has consistently been shown that lack of parental control and discipline are related to adolescents' permissive sexual attitudes and sexual behavior (Baumrind, 1983; Ensminger, 1990; Miller, 1998; Miller et al., 1986). For example, it has been found that sexually active adolescent females have more permissive family rules about the time they are expected home on school nights (Ensminger, 1990) and have lower overall parental supervision (Miller et al., 1986) than nonsexually active girls. Most research on parents' discipline styles characterizes a parent as having a general parenting style (i.e., authoritarian, permissive, or authoritative) that is applied similarly to all children in the family (Baumrind, 1983). To the extent that parenting style *is* consistent for all children in the family—that is, that all children in the family are controlled and disciplined similarly—then all children within the family would be equally at risk for early sexual behavior and, consequently, early pregnancy and early childbearing.

Related to parents' discipline style, parent-adolescent communication has also been shown to be important for delaying adolescent sexual activity and for pregnancy prevention (Fox, 1980; Fox and Inazu, 1980; Newcomer and Udry, 1985). For example, girls who are the most effective contraceptive users prior to pregnancy are more likely than nonusers to have mothers who communicate information about how and where to obtain contraception (Moore et al., 1986a). Another study reported that daughters who talked with their mothers about sexual and contraceptive matters were more likely than others to postpone sexual activity or to employ effective contraceptive methods if they did become sexually active (Fox and Inazu, 1980). If it is the case that mothers share the same communication openness with all their daughters, then such effects would be consistent across all girls within the family. That is, all daughters of noncommunicative mothers would be equally at risk for sexual permissiveness and pregnancy, and all daughters of communicative mothers would be equally likely to postpone sexual initiation or to use effective contraception.

Another aspect of parental behavior that affects adolescent sexual activity is parents' marital status. Much research has shown that adolescents from single-parent families (i.e., in which the parent is divorced or was never married) are more likely to engage in nonmarital sexual intercourse than adolescents from two-biological-parent families (Hogan and Kitagawa, 1985; Jemmott and Jemmott, 1992; Kinnaird and Gerrard, 1986; Miller, 1998; Miller and Bingham, 1989; Newcomer and Udry, 1987). For females, the amount of time spent in a single-family household was also found to be associated with a young onset of sexual intercourse (Miller et al., 1997). Most studies examining parents' marital status as a correlate of adolescent sexual behavior conceptualize marital status not just as a family structure variable but as a proxy of parental control, family functioning, and family disruption, with adolescents in single-mother households experiencing less parental control and supervision than teens in two-parent households (Newcomer and Udry, 1987). Given that single parenthood is consistent for all children in the family, this may be another circumstance that encourages a resemblance in sibling sexual behavior during adolescence. That is, because sisters are equally exposed to the loss of parental control and the diminished parental monitoring associated with single-parent households, they would be equally at risk for permissive sexual behavior and, thus, teenage pregnancy.

Shared Societal Risks

A second conceptualization for understanding sisters' shared vulnerability to adolescent pregnancy and childbearing is that sisters within a family share a socioeconomic status, social class, and an ethnic identity that are highly correlated with early sexual initiation and early pregnancy. Key socioeconomic indicators related to adolescent pregnancy and childbearing are parental education and income, with higher maternal education correlated with later sexual initiation (Hayward et al., 1992), a greater likelihood of contraceptive use at first intercourse (Kahn et al., 1990), and a higher probability of abortion given pregnancy (Plotnick,

1992). Regarding race and ethnicity, Black and Hispanic women have teenage birth rates 2.7 times higher than White teenage women: the rates for 1994 were 108 births per 1,000 females aged 15 to 19 for both Hispanics and non-Hispanic Blacks and 40 births per 1,000 women aged 15 to 19 for non-Hispanic Whites (Moore et al., 1997). It has also been shown that teenagers from high-risk environments—characterized as low socioeconomic status, inner-city residence, and a nonintact family—have pregnancy rates as much as 8.3 times higher than girls from low-risk environments—or being of upper to middle class, residing in a suburban neighborhood, and being from an intact family (Crane, 1991; Hogan and Kitagawa, 1985). Hogan and colleagues (1985) discuss this difference as likely reflecting the lack of knowledge about and access to effective birth control in high-risk neighborhoods. Other characteristics of the neighborhood itself—such as employment opportunities, neighborhood quality, and social disorganization—also have been shown to relate to adolescent sexual activity (Brewster et al., 1993).

Several social scientists have discussed the conditions of economic uncertainty and the poor prospects for marriage and for a stable job that are endemic to poor minority youth as contributing to many teenagers' choice of early parenthood as a pathway to adulthood and adult status (Dash, 1989; Hamburg, 1986; Hayes, 1987; Luker, 1991, 1996; Moore et al., 1986b; Williams, 1991). Poverty, uncertain economic conditions, and low prospects for advancement discourage many young women from making the transition to adulthood through educational or career achievements or through parenthood after marriage. Instead, the lack of opportunity leads to frustration and the search for adult status via more accessible routes, such as through sexual activity, pregnancy, and parenting.

Sociologist Kristin Luker states that

> teen pregnancy is less about young women and their sex lives than it is about restricted horizons and the boundaries of hope. It is about race and class and how those realities limit opportunities for young people. Most centrally, however, it is typically about being young, female, poor, and non-white and about how having a child seems to be one of the few avenues of satisfaction, fulfillment, and self-esteem. (Luker, 1991, p. 83)

The disproportionate number of pregnant and parenting teenagers observed among poor, minority, inner-city residents may well reflect the absence of employment, education, or marriage options that typically mark the path from adolescence to adulthood. Such life-course experiences would be similar for all sisters in the family and thus may act to create similar early childbearing behavior among them.

Shared Community-Neighborhood Norms

Many scholars of teenage pregnancy have discussed the strong socialization pressures and multiple role models of young unmarried mothers as powerful contributors to both the acceptability of teenage pregnancy and its prevalence (Crane, 1991; East and Felice, 1992; Hogan and Kitagawa, 1985; Moore et al., 1986b). The social norm framework, derived from the family life-course perspective, states that the scheduling of life-course events associated with the transition to adulthood (e.g., moving out of one's parents' house, getting married, having a child) is relatively well defined within communities, with clear and socially recognized norms for the timing and sequencing of transitional events (Elder, 1975; Haraven, 1978; Marini, 1984; Neugarten et al., 1965). In their ethnographic studies of Black urban and rural neighborhoods, Stack and Burton (1993) discuss the community norms for early childbearing as powerful socialization pressures, with "early childbearing often considered a necessary activity" (p. 159). These expected norms, as well as community sanctions against abortion, undoubtedly reflect the high value that family and kin place on having a child of one's own. Moreover, teenage mothers within both Black and Hispanic communities are often cared for and supported by extended family to a greater extent than are White teenage mothers, with "kin-keeping" the primary means of sustenance among poor urban families (Brindis, 1992; Burton, 1990; Duany and Pittman, 1990; Ladner, 1988; Melville, 1980; Stack, 1974). Such strong family, extended-family, and community support systems work to reduce the stigma associated with nonmarital teenage childbearing and make it a more acceptable lifestyle for Black and Hispanic women.

Shared Biological Predispositions

For heuristic purposes, it is also important to consider that a shared biological predisposition may be contributing to sisters' similarity in sexual and birth timing. Numerous studies show that the timing of puberty (often measured as the age at menarche for girls) is related to the timing of first sexual intercourse, first marriage, and first birth (Presser, 1978; Udry, 1979; Udry and Cliquet, 1982). Furthermore, the timing of puberty is known to be correlated across generations, with age at menarche highly correlated for mothers and daughters and between sisters (Garn, 1980). Thus, it follows that sisters would have a similar proclivity toward early pregnancy and early sexual behavior because they share the same maturational predisposition for early puberty, a predisposition at least partly inherited from their mother. Some have argued that the intergenerational pattern of teenage childbearing may simply reflect this biological predisposition for early maturation (Kahn and Anderson, 1992), and Newcomer and Udry (1984) were able to confirm links between mothers' pubertal development, daughters' pubertal development, and daughters' sexual onset. Thus, there is reason to suspect that the increased vulnerability for early childbearing among the younger sisters of childbearing teens may have biological origins and that such influences should be carefully considered in future research.

Shared Peer-Friendship Network

Finally, it is possible that sisters have a common peer group or friendship network that is inducing *both* sisters to engage in early sex and early parenting. At least three different processes of friendship influence may be at work in creating behavioral similarity between sisters who share a common peer network. First, it is possible that the friendship network, common to both sisters, might be exerting strong and pervasive pressures for both sisters to engage in early sexual behavior (East and Shi, 1997). It is well known that friends can be powerful reference groups and socialization agents for adolescent sexual activity (East et al., 1993; Mirande, 1968). Thus, sister pairs might be similar behaviorally because both are influenced (i.e., pressured) by the shared friendship network to have sexual relationships.

Second, it is possible that the older sister actively initiates or facilitates her younger sister to join in with the older sister's friends, friends who are likely to be older and sexually active. Thus, for example, the older sister might take her younger sister to older adolescent events or parties where sexual activity will occur or where potential partners will be available. In this case, older sisters are actively accelerating the sexual experience of their younger sisters by exposing them to an older peer group. This type of facilitative process was tested specifically for White and Black older sister–younger sister pairs by Rodgers et al. (1992), who found, however, little empirical support for this type of sibling influence.

Finally, it is possible that sister pairs who share common friends have similar behavioral attributes with similar inclinations for deviance (East and Shi, 1997). In this case, the younger sister might act in ways similar to the older pregnant or childbearing sister (i.e., in problem behavior and sexual behavior) because both share similar behavioral inclinations, with the shared friendship network only a reflection of their shared behavioral dispositions. Certainly, these and other possible shared peer-friendship group influences might be at work in enhancing the behavioral similarity between sister pairs, or a combination of these processes might be operating.

The preceding discussion suggests that because sisters receive similar parenting, share societal risks, are socialized by the same community norms, have a common biological predisposition, and may share a common peer-friendship network, they are equally likely to become or not to become pregnant as teens. For the younger sister, however, there is an additional factor to consider: the *effect* of her older sister's pregnancy and childbearing on her and her family of origin. That is, the predispositions toward early pregnancy described previously *may interact with* or *contribute further to* the *effects* of an older sister's childbearing, thereby rendering younger sisters *even more vulnerable* to early sexual activity and early pregnancy (East, 1998b). These intrafamilial dynamics that occur after the older sister has had her child are described in the following.

HOW AN OLDER SISTER'S EARLY CHILDBEARING INCREASES HER YOUNGER SISTER'S RISK OF EARLY PREGNANCY

Based on theoretical considerations and drawing from various bodies of literature, Figure 8.2 presents a descriptive model of how an older sister's early childbearing affects her younger sister. Principal assumptions of the model are as follows:

1. A younger sister is prone to modeling her older sister's behavior.

2. A younger sister's child care involvement with her sister's baby socializes her for early parenting.

3. The older sister's childbearing diminishes the quality of her parents' parenting of their children and increases parental acceptance of teenage childbearing.

4. A younger sister is affected by the increased family financial hardship and increased family stress that her sister's childbearing may provoke.

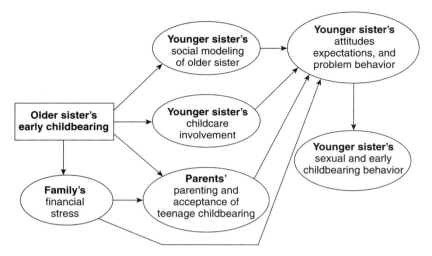

Figure 8.2.   How an older sister's early childbearing contributes to her younger sister's risk of early pregnancy.

The next section also takes up another assumption of the model: that a younger sister's attitudes, future expectations, and problem behaviors serve as important mediators to her sexual and childbearing behavior. Each of these assumptions is discussed in turn.

Younger Sisters Model Their Older Sisters' Behavior

Social learning theory (Bandura, 1977) and modeling explanations of behavior would suggest that because older siblings operate as important role models and socialization agents for younger siblings (Bryant, 1982; Cicirelli, 1982) older siblings have the capacity to shape the attitudes, values, and norms—and, ultimately, the behavior—of younger children in the family. Moreover, because large numbers of pregnant teenagers choose to keep their babies and remain at home within their family of origin (Furstenberg, 1980; Trent and Harlan, 1994), many younger siblings witness firsthand their older sister in the role of mother and, most often, of unwed mother. Furthermore, because motherhood establishes a role for the older adolescent—a role associated with status and femininity— a younger sister may become envious or jealous of her and, consequently, attempt to identify with her (East, 1996a; East and Felice, 1992). Hogan and Kitagawa (1985) discuss this socialization process whereby girls who see their sisters become teenage mothers are more likely to (1) accept adolescent parenthood as normative and (2) accept single parenthood as a way to achieve adult status. These attitudinal changes are thought to pre-cede an increased willingness to engage in early sexual activity (Plotnick and Butler, 1991). Such beliefs may be especially likely to develop among early adolescent younger sisters who are forming attitudes about school-ing, employment, marriage, and family formation (Hamburg, 1974). Thus, an older sister's early childbearing can have a profound impact on the development of her younger sisters by exposing them to a role model that appears attractive because of its associated adult status. Research on sibling influence shows that modeling is enhanced under two condi-tions: when siblings are particularly close (Rowe and Gulley, 1992; Rowe et al., 1989) and when siblings are particularly rivalrous or competitive with one another (East, 1996c). For example, East and Shi (1997) found that the extent of rivalry and competition between a pregnant or par-enting teen and her younger sister was the best predictor of whether the younger sister had engaged in delinquent-like behavior and sexual activ-ity. Rivalry was actually a better predictor of girls' behavior than the sis-ters' closeness or the conflict between them. One must also remember that sibling competition among pregnant and parenting teens and their sisters is typically occurring on a playing field of few resources and limited opportunities. Thus, where one of the few avenues to status and adulthood is *through childbearing*, it would be very understandable to see a younger sister *also* become pregnant in attempts to—consciously or subconsciously—rival the older sister.

A Younger Sister's Child Care
Involvement Socializes Her for Early Parenting

When a teenager has a baby, typically all available family resources and personnel are pooled to help parent her child (Burton, 1995, 1996a, 1996b; Burton and Bengtson, 1985; Stack, 1974, 1975). Younger siblings often participate in the care of their teenage sister's child out of social and economic necessity (Ladner, 1988). Child care assistance provided by early adolescent younger sisters may be favored over other strategies because it best utilizes available family personnel and because it fosters child care skills and parent training for girls who themselves will some-day assume parenting responsibilities for their own children.

In the author's own study on the siblings of parenting teens, it appears that many younger siblings, particularly younger sisters, help in the care of their older sister's child (East, 1996c). It also appears that younger sibling child care is a *cooperative* arrangement between the older and younger sister, with the younger sister *co-participating* in her niece's or nephew's care by performing instrumental child care tasks but clearly taking direction from the older sister. Such secondary instrumental care typically includes temporarily occupying the baby, getting a toy, getting diapers, or helping to prepare food for the baby. This pattern is similar to one observed by Weisner (1982), who noted that when mothers give older children caretaking responsibilities for their younger siblings, the mothers still retain primary control over child care.

How does helping to care for an older sister's child impact younger sisters? Many anthropologists who study caregiving by older siblings to younger ones in non-Western societies have noted that sibling caretakers gain a great deal of felt competence in their caregiving role and experience a positive sense of autonomy by carrying out their co-caregiving responsibilities (Draper, 1976; Weisner, 1982, 1986; Whiting, 1983; Whiting and Whiting, 1975). Additionally, Whiting and Whiting (1975) observed that sibling care systems involve intricate authority hierarchies and subtle patterns of rank and deference. Thus, the younger sisters, in addition to learning compliance and prosocial behavior, may learn keen positional awareness and sensitivity.

Sibling caretaking as it occurs within teenage childbearing families has been a completely neglected area of study. (Notable exceptions include Burton, 1995, and Burton, 1996b. In these works, however, Burton describes the intergenerational caregiving patterns in teenage childbearing families wherein the teen's sister provides *primary* care to her nieces and nephews, with the teen mother completely unable to cope with parenting.) In the author's preliminary work, girls who provided extensive child care assistance to their teenage sisters had more pessimistic expectations of graduating high school, had more positive intentions of an early childbearing, and exhibited more permissive sexual behavior than girls who provided little or no child care help to their teenage sisters (East and Jacobson, 2000). Thus, taking part in the care of the older sister's child may have negative ramifications for girls' development. But several questions remain. For example, what is the nature and extent of child care provided by the younger sisters of teen mothers? To what extent does such caretaking socialize younger sisters for early parenthood? Does the perceived child care competence gained by the younger sister lead her to minimize the hardships associated with early parenting or to become less diligent in pregnancy prevention? What are the effects of caretaking the older sister's baby for the younger sister's role aspirations and her attitudes about early parenting? These questions represent potentially fruitful lines for future research on how an adolescent sister's childbearing may socialize her younger sister for early pregnancy and early parenting.

Adolescent Childbearing Diminishes
the Quality of Parents' Parenting and
Increases Parents' Acceptance of Teenage Parenting

In discussing the burdens and benefits of early childbearing for the adolescent's family of origin, Furstenberg (1980) observed that the teenager's parents' own parenting likely suffers because of the increased stress and time constraints of helping to parent their daughter's child. Typically, the teenager's mother provides much hands-on child care for her grandchild (Brooks-Gunn and Chase-Lansdale, 1991; Burton, 1996a, 1996b; Stack, 1975). Because these grandparenting duties can be extensive, they can interfere with the new grandmother's ability to monitor or supervise her own children. With a new baby in the home, the grandmother may find it particularly difficult to monitor her children's out-of-home, peer-related activities. This problem is compounded by the fact that these women are usually parenting and grandparenting alone, without a co-resident adult (Burton, 1996a, 1996b; Stack, 1975). This inattentiveness or unavailability to her own children creates an opportunity for younger siblings to engage in problem or delinquent behaviors, behaviors that are likely to lead to teenage sexual activity and, consequently, teenage pregnancy (Elliot and Morse, 1989; Ensminger, 1987).

There are also several reasons to expect that the older daughter's early childbearing increases her parents' acceptance and tolerance of early nonmarital childbearing in general and of a *younger sister's* pregnancy and childbearing in particular. Having already experienced the older daughter's early childbearing, parents—as well as other family members—would likely view a teenage pregnancy by another daughter in the family with less stigma and less disgrace (East and Felice, 1994). Moreover, by the sheer fact that the older sister has had a child as a teen, she has in effect "opened the floodgates" or "broken the barrier" of what constitutes allowable and tolerated behavior for other siblings within the family.

Second, the older daughter's early childbearing may signify to her parents the lack of alternate life options available to their children, particularly their daughters. Consequently, parents may rationalize their daughter's early childbearing as a reasonable and acceptable response to the disadvantaged socioeconomic circumstances in which they live. Such tacit parental acceptance of early nonmarital parenthood has been shown to precede adolescent sexual activity and pregnancy-risk behaviors (Moore et al., 1986a; Thornton and Camburn, 1987).

To understand the consequences of adolescent pregnancy and childbearing for the family, East studied mothers in families in which only one teenager was currently pregnant and this was the first teenage pregnancy to occur within the family (East, 1999). Mothers were assessed twice, 13 months apart. Results indicated that mothers monitored and communicated less with their other children and were more accepting of teenage sex after the older daughter gave birth. These results suggest that both mothers' parenting and their attitudes may be affected by an adolescent's pregnancy and birth.

Adolescent Childbearing Increases
Family Economic Hardship and Stress

Although virtually no research has examined the economic hardship resulting from teenage childbearing on the adolescent's *family of origin,* there has been much discussion of the negative socioeconomic consequences experienced by the teenage mother herself. These studies, which take into account the socioeconomic disadvantage that *preceded* the teen's childbearing, show substantial and qualitatively important socioeconomic costs associated with teenage childbearing (Geronimus and Korenman, 1992, 1993; Hoffman et al., 1993a, 1993b). For example, Hoffman and colleagues found that, after controlling for factors associated with teenage childbearing such as race and economic disadvantage, teenage mothers were more likely to be poor and to receive welfare than were their nonteenage childbearing sisters. These socioeconomic costs were above and beyond what the teen would have experienced had she not become a mother. Given that most teens continue to live with their parents for some time after the birth (Trent and Harlan, 1994), it is likely, then, that the adolescent's family of origin also experiences *additional* and *unique* economic costs and financial strains that result directly from the teenager's childbearing.

How would such economic strain on the adolescent's family of origin affect younger sisters? There is an extensive literature that suggests that economic hardship is strongly linked with stressed intrafamilial relations (Conger et al., 1994; Elder et al., 1995), punitive and neglectful parenting (McLoyd, 1990; McLoyd et al., 1994), and adolescents' pessimistic future expectations (Galambos and Silbereisen, 1987; Lempers et al., 1989). For example, under conditions of acute economic decline, mothers tend to become physically punitive toward their adolescent children and highly critical and pessimistic about their children's future job success (McLoyd et al., 1994), and as the economic decline intensifies, the coercive, hostile parent-child exchanges increase (Conger et al., 1994). When their family experiences a significant loss of income, adolescents also reduce their own expectations about future educational and career attainments (Conger et al., 1994), and they often experience a sudden onset of delinquent-like behaviors (Galambos and Silbereisen, 1987; Lempers et al., 1989; Sampson and Laub, 1994).

The model shown in Figure 8.2 incorporates these findings about the consequences of increased family economic hardship experienced by teenage childbearing families for adverse younger sister outcomes, such as reduced future expectations and increased problem behavior. In addition, the model maps an additional pathway by which economic adversity impinges on parents' socialization of their children (e.g., through punitive parenting and stressed parent-child relations). Thus, the financial strain and hardship within the family provoked by the older sister's early parenting is believed to affect directly the expectations and behavior of younger sisters, as well as indirectly, through parents' parenting practices and expectations for their children.

Other family-related effects that might result from the older sister's childbearing include accommodating the father of baby, who may move in with the teen's family after the birth of the baby (Furstenberg, 1980). This may be more likely to occur if the father of the baby is older and able to help financially support the teen, her baby, and her family (East and Felice, 1996). The father moving in with the teen's family, however, may cause moving other family members (e.g., younger siblings) to live with kin so that there is enough room to house the father. All such household changes—as well as having a young infant in the household—would likely serve to stress all family members and strain family relations.

PREGNANCY-RISK BEHAVIORS
OF YOUNGER SISTERS OF PARENTING TEENS

Several studies have pointed to the high risk for early pregnancy among the younger sisters of pregnant and parenting teens by documenting younger sisters' relatively permissive sexual and childbearing attitudes, higher levels of problem and delinquent-like behavior (e.g., fighting, stealing, destroying property, and being picked up by the police), and higher rates of sexual activity (East, 1996a, 1996b; East et al., 1993).

These characteristics are revealing because they are considered precursors to adolescent pregnancy and childbearing (Elliot and Morse, 1989; Elster et al., 1990; Ensminger, 1987, 1990; Miller and Sneesby, 1988; Moore et al., 1995; Mott and Haurin, 1988; Plotnick and Butler, 1991; Zabin et al., 1984, 1993). Thus, once on a particular pathway, the younger sisters would become prone to engaging in other high-risk behaviors leading to teenage pregnancy, such as frequent and unprotected sexual intercourse (East, 1995). The studies on younger sisters' risk behavior are reviewed briefly in the following.

When compared to early adolescent girls with only nonchildbearing adolescent sisters, East et al. (1993) found that girls of the same age and socioeconomic status who had at least one childbearing adolescent sister had more permissive attitudes about premarital teenage sex and (among virgins only) had more positive intentions to have sexual intercourse in the near future. Results are shown in Figure 8.3. Additionally, girls with a childbearing teenage sister were almost four times more likely to have already had sex (26%) than were girls with only nonchildbearing teenage sisters (7%). This is perhaps more significant considering that girls in the study were, on average, only 13 years old.

Further study of the same sample showed that girls with a childbearing adolescent sister had significantly more permissive attitudes toward childbearing (i.e., they were more accepting of nonmarital teenage childbearing), perceived *younger* ages for typical life-course transitions (best age to first have sex, get married, have first child), and were more pessimistic about achieving school and career goals than were girls with only nonchildbearing adolescent sisters (see Figure 8.4) (East, 1996c). Moreover, the girls who had a childbearing teenage sister were more likely to have engaged in problem behaviors (with the exception of drug use), such as school truancy and smoking, and had more total problem behaviors (see Figure 8.5).

It should be noted that the differences that emerged between the two younger sister groups cannot be attributed to differences in younger sisters' age, family size, mothers' educational level, family income, or the family's current welfare status. The two sister groups were comparable with regard to all these factors, and subjects' race (which covaried with older sister's childbearing status) was statistically controlled in all analyses.

Additional findings that highlight potential prepregnancy behaviors of the younger sisters of teen mothers derive from a longitudinal study

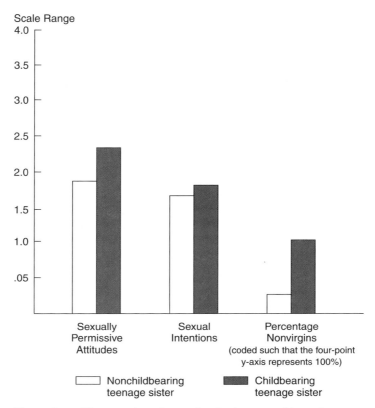

Figure 8.3. Younger sisters' sexual attitudes, sexual intentions, and sexual status by older sisters' childbearing status. Source: East et al. (1993).

conducted by East that focused on families in which only one teenager in a family was either currently pregnant or had delivered her first child no more than six months previously and in which no other sibling had ever been pregnant (East, 1996a). Thus, the current pregnancy or childbearing was the first to occur within the family. The younger sisters in such families were compared to the same-age, same-race (67% Hispanic, 33% Black) younger sisters of never-pregnant adolescents from families in which no teenage pregnancy had yet occurred.

As with the previous study, the two sets of families were carefully matched along several socioeconomic and demographic characteristics, for example, family size, family structure (e.g., two-parent or mother-only households), and parental educational levels. Nonetheless, the fam-

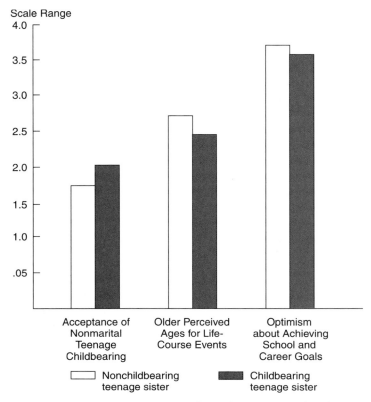

Figure 8.4. Younger sisters' attitudes and expectations by older sisters' childbearing status. Source: East 1996c.

ilies of pregnant and parenting teens had lower family incomes and were more likely to be receiving welfare at the time of the study than were the families of never-pregnant teens. Thus, these factors were statistically controlled in all analyses.

Scores for the younger sisters in each family category on several attitudinal and behavioral characteristics are shown in Table 8.1. When compared to girls with a never-pregnant older sister, girls with a pregnant older sister were significantly less optimistic about their future, were more accepting of teenage childbearing, perceived younger ages as appropriate for life-transition norms (i.e., ages for girls to first have sex, marry, and have children), and engaged in more problem behavior at school (e.g., school suspension and disruptive behavior in class) and more delinquent behavior. However, the increase in highly visible delinquent, acting-out behavior may be a short-lived phenomenon in reac-

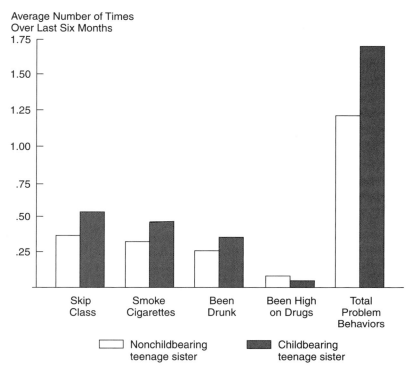

Figure 8.5. Younger sisters' problem behavior by older sisters' childbearing status. Source: East (1996c).

tion to an older sister's pregnancy since the frequency of delinquent behavior by the younger sisters of *parenting* teenagers was comparable to that for the younger sisters of never-pregnant teenagers.

Nonetheless, girls who had a parenting older sister were almost five times as likely to have already had sex (29%) as girls with a never-pregnant older sister, of whom only 6% were nonvirgins. They were also more likely to have had sexual intercourse more frequently and to have engaged in significantly more intimate sexual behaviors (ranging from kissing, to light petting, to heavy petting, to sexual intercourse).

As suggested previously, the differences between the younger sisters of never-pregnant teens and the younger sisters of pregnant or parenting teens may reflect the societal and intrafamily risk factors that may have precipitated the older sister's pregnancy. Consequently, these results need to be cautiously and judiciously interpreted, with the understanding that the differences found in younger sisters' attitudes and behavior

TABLE 8.1   MEAN SCORES OF
YOUNGER SISTERS' CHARACTERISTICS
BY OLDER SISTERS' PREGNANCY
AND CHILDBEARING STATUS

	Never Pregnant (n = 83)	Pregnant (n = 29)	Parenting (n = 51)	F(2,161)	Possible Score Range	High Scores Indicate:
Future orientation	4.43 [a,b]	4.10 [a]	4.09 [b]	3.40 * z	1–5	Optimistic expectations
Perceived maternal strictness	3.44	3.54	3.35	<1	1–5	High maternal strictness
Perceived maternal monitoring	2.99	2.98	2.94	<1	1–5	High maternal monitoring
Perceived parental approval of teenage childbearing	1.60 [b]	1.88 [c]	2.39 [b,c]	12.26 ***	1–5	High approval
Acceptance of teenage sex	2.07 [b]	2.50	2.70 [b]	3.75 *	1–5	High acceptance
Acceptance of teenage childbearing	1.84 [a,b]	2.16 [a]	2.34 [b]	3.98 *	1–5	High acceptance
Acceptance of nonmarital childbearing	2.07 [b]	2.30 [c]	2.72 [b,c]	4.12 *	1–5	High acceptance
Life-transition norms (years)— girls	21.94 [a,b]	20.92 [a]	21.08 [b]	3.07 *	—	Later ages
Life-transition norms (years)— boys	22.53 [b]	21.65	21.06 [b]	2.77	—	Later ages
Status from childbearing	1.96 [b]	2.36	2.50 [b]	5.05 **	1–5	High status
Problems of early childbearing	4.35	4.10	4.04	1.71	1–5	More problematic
Intentions of early childbearing	1.42 [b]	1.49 [c]	2.03 [b,c]	6.41 **	1–5	More definite intentions
Self-esteem	3.80	3.67	3.92	<1	1–5	High self-esteem
School problems	1.94 [a]	2.49 [a,c]	1.95 [c]	6.65 **	0–4	More frequent
Drug use	1.55	1.68 [c]	1.41 [c]	2.81	0–4	More frequent
Partying	1.26	1.36	1.34	1.51	0–4	More frequent

TABLE 8.1   (*continued*)

	Never Pregnant (n = 83)	Pregnant (n = 29)	Parenting (n = 51)	F(2,161)	Possible Score Range	High Scores Indicate:
Delinquency	1.27[a]	1.69[a,c]	1.39[c]	4.21*	0–4	More frequent
Sexual-behavior progression	3.25[b]	4.03	4.88[b]	3.31*	1–11	More intimate sexual acts
Nonvirgin status	0.06[b]	0.17	0.29[b]	6.49**	0–1	Percentage nonvirgins
Frequency of sexual intercourse among nonvirgins	0.18[b]	0.52	0.78[b]	4.51*	0–4	More frequent

NOTE: The F-statistic tests for equality of means. If the F is statistically significant (asterisked), the means are not equal. Means with the same-letter superscript in the same row are significantly different ($p < .05$). *$p < .05$. **$p < .01$. ***$p < .001$.
SOURCE: East (1996a) (adapted with permission from the Alan Guttmacher Institute).

may reflect family and societal factors instead of, or perhaps in addition to, the consequences of having a pregnant or parenting sister.

The differences between the younger sisters of *pregnant* teenagers and the younger sisters of *parenting* teenagers, however, would not be biased by selection factors. Since the intergroup social and demographic characteristics were comparable or were statistically controlled, differences between these two groups are likely to indicate how younger sisters are affected specifically by the birth of an older sister's child. Compared to girls with a pregnant older sister, girls with a parenting older sister perceived significantly greater parental approval of teenage childbearing, were more accepting of nonmarital childbearing, and had more definite intentions to have a child themselves at an early age.

Cumulatively, the results of these studies suggest that the younger sisters of childbearing teens are at greater risk for early parenthood than the younger sisters of nonchildbearing teens. Girls with adolescent childbearing sisters are more accepting of nonmarital teenage parenting, perceive younger ages for typical life-course transitions, hold more pessimistic school and career expectations, and are more likely to engage in deviant behaviors—all of which are key risk factors for early sexual behavior and early parenthood (Moore et al., 1995). However, the current findings—based on cross-sectional data—are evidence only of *associations* between an older sister's childbearing and her younger sister's attitudes and behaviors, not of causal sequences of events. Further longitudinal examination of the *changes* in younger sisters' attitudes and behaviors *as a function of an older sister's childbearing* would be necessary to show a causal relationship.

CONSIDERATIONS AND STRATEGIES
FOR INTERVENING WITH YOUNGER SISTERS

Because younger sisters of pregnant and parenting teenagers are a singularly high-risk group for early pregnancy, such adolescents are an important and strategic population to target for pregnancy prevention (East, 1996b, 1998a). The design of a prevention program for them must take into account factors related to the identification, accessibility, and participation of this population that, in turn, will likely impact the effectiveness of the intervention.

Identifying the Population

The first characteristic of younger sisters of pregnant and parenting teenagers that should be considered in designing a pregnancy prevention program is that such girls represent a relatively easily identifiable population. Virtually all protocols of teen obstetric clinics include obtaining a family history of every adolescent presenting with pregnancy. In this history, the number of younger sisters, their ages, and their living situations are often noted. In addition, the younger sisters may already be known to health care staff through the prenatal and pediatric visits of the older sister, as well as through well-child checkups of the younger sister herself. Thus, data identifying the younger sisters may be readily available to program personnel.

Involving the Family

Prevention efforts aimed at younger sisters may be optimized if family involvement is encouraged. As noted previously, adolescent childbearing has complex and multifaceted consequences for the adolescent's family of origin, affecting the family dynamics, the family's economic situation, the parents' parenting, and the younger siblings' attitudes, expectations, and behaviors. By intervening at the family level, many of the family's problems and situations can be impacted.

However, clinicians and educators designing pregnancy prevention programs must be cognizant of both the obstacles as well as the advantages of incorporating family participation in the prevention effort. For example, the active involvement of younger sisters may be facilitated by their and their mothers' motivation to learn about how to prevent a second pregnancy within the family. In addition, the prevention message may be more lasting and long-lived if the family is included in service delivery, as programs are often short term and relatively temporary. Alternately, program designers must be alert to the often strong attitudinal and behavioral influences that older sisters have on their younger sisters. Younger sisters participating in prevention programs that attempt to change their attitudes and values about early sexual involvement (e.g., abstinence-promotion programs) may feel caught in a cross-current: The messages they receive from the program about teen sex and pregnancy may compete or conflict with the messages they continue to receive at home (East and Felice, 1992). In these cases, the extent and type of parental and family involvement in the prevention effort should be carefully considered before the intervention begins. Finally, in situations of suspected abuse or incest, family or parental involvement may not be in the best interest of the younger sister, and a different approach should be sought.

Offering Disincentives to Early Childbearing

Prevention efforts should take into consideration the social reality of girls who model or mimic their older sister's early childbearing. That is, early childbearing may well seem a logical life choice for young women who perceive few alternatives. Programs that do not attempt to alter this perception are likely to fail, as they will be counteracted by messages that the girls receive at home and from peers. Thus, pregnancy prevention efforts aimed at younger sisters require a broader policy agenda that goes well beyond addressing exclusively fertility-related behaviors (e.g., contraception or abstinence). As Lizbeth Schorr (1988) has appropriately argued, at heart what is needed is a comprehensive economic agenda for providing *disincentives* to early parenting, such as job skills training, reasonable-wage job opportunities, and employment security. If young women are expected to be motivated *not* to be teen mothers, they need to have a clear vision of what they *can* do.

Promoting Alternative Role Models

Many younger sisters lack successful role models to help overcome the overwhelming odds for the inter- and intragenerational perpetuation of teenage pregnancy that has preceded them (Cox et al., 1995). The need for alternative role models is especially crucial for the younger sisters of parenting teens who remain at home with their families of origin. In these cases, the younger sister witnesses firsthand the way in which motherhood establishes a role for the older adolescent—a role associated with status, femininity, and attention—and the choice to emulate her may be particularly seductive. Thus, policy and program development strategies that incorporate caring adult role models and mentors who will inform girls that becoming a mother is not their only avenue to fulfillment and recognition seem uniquely promising for this target group.

Encouraging Group Discussion

A group discussion approach uniting younger sisters may hold many benefits. For example, participants could be asked to discuss the stresses and disruption caused by premarital parenting in general and by their sisters' parenting in particular. They could be encouraged to share their stories of how they and their families have been affected by their sisters' pregnancies and births and how they and their families are coping. As they tell their life stories in a nonthreatening, supportive environment, the younger sisters may develop a broader perspective on their own problems, and the sharing of experiences can provide a source of strength and a positive basis for pregnancy prevention.

Providing Intensive Individualized Attention

A final consideration in program design is to offer younger sisters intensive individualized attention as soon as the older sister learns that she is pregnant and begins seeking prenatal care. Service delivery could be arranged in such a way that the pregnant teen and her sister both receive care at the same site at the same time but from separate care providers, a model based on Teen-Tot Clinics or Two Generation Services (Dryfoos, 1990; Hardy and Zabin, 1991). Certainly, prevention programs that "pay attention" to younger sisters before, rather than after, they become pregnant seem particularly compelling.

Service programs for pregnant teens offer a wide variety of support services, such as individualized counseling, nutritional services, job preparation and placement, case management, special school guidance or instruction, free bus tokens, free food coupons, and sometimes monetary reimbursement or free transportation to attend prenatal clinic visits (Klerman and Horwitz, 1992). As such, it appears that a number of policies have been established that inadvertently reward young people for early childbearing. Providing personalized, concentrated care for younger sisters could serve to *counterbalance* the positive inducements that they witness their older sisters receiving as a result of their pregnancies. It will be interesting to see what impact the Federal Welfare Reform Bill—also known as the Personal Responsibility and Work Opportunity Reconciliation Act—will have on the younger siblings within teenage childbearing families. As planned, this act will impose new work requirements on individuals, cut food stamp benefits, and limit the length of time on aid to a maximum five-year lifetime limit. By removing such essential threads in teen parents' safety net, this bill will undoubtedly make it more difficult to support a child while still in school. It may also diminish the attractiveness and apparent ease of having children while one is young.

POLICY IMPLICATIONS

What are the policy implications of the research presented in this chapter? First and foremost is the need to target the siblings of pregnant and parenting teens for pregnancy prevention services. This has actually started to occur in the form of several statewide policies. For example, in 1996, the State of California—through the Department of Health Services, Maternal and Child Health Branch—legislated $3 million per year to provide Adolescent Family Life case management services specifically to the siblings of pregnant and parenting teens (California Senate Office of Research, 1997). In addition, the California Department of Education implemented a "Teenage Pregnancy Prevention Grant Program," with $10 million per year given to school programs that, among other things, "target youth who have a sibling who is a teenage parent." As a result of these initiatives, numerous programs have sprung up across the state that systematically focus prevention efforts on the siblings of pregnant and parenting teens. Although the results of these programs are not yet known, both programs are being intensely evaluated, and their results will help shed light on whether these special prevention services can reduce the teenage pregnancy rate within this population. It is also likely that these programs will serve as model programs for other states that are launching large, statewide sibling pregnancy prevention efforts.

Another trend in pregnancy prevention programs and policies is the recent emphasis on comprehensive, community-wide collaboratives aimed at reducing the teenage pregnancy rates in particularly high-risk areas and communities (Brindis, 1993). These comprehensive collaboratives are the result of several reports stating that many single-prong approaches to preventing teen pregnancy have been demonstrably unable to show sufficient scale, effectiveness, or sustainability (e.g., Kirby et al., 1997; Miller et al., 1992). For example, The California Wellness Foundation recently started "The Teenage Pregnancy Prevention Initiative," which funds broad-based, multisector community coalitions that saturate targeted areas with coordinated comprehensive services, ranging from school mentoring and life skills counseling to sexuality education and access to family planning services. These kinds of comprehensive initiatives that help create and then sustain caring communities that can effectively nurture their youth show great promise for significantly lowering California's teenage pregnancy rate—which is the highest in the nation (Henshaw, 1997)—and should be an integral component of any national pregnancy prevention policy.

CONCLUSION

The younger sisters of pregnant and parenting teens have disproportionately high rates of early childbearing and engage in teenage sexual activity at earlier ages and at higher rates than other girls of their same race, ethnicity, and social class. This chapter has highlighted several reasons why sister pairs within a family share a vulnerability to teenage childbearing, and a model was presented of how a teenager's childbearing further increases her younger sister's risk of early pregnancy. This model can be used to inform community-, school-, and hospital-based pregnancy prevention efforts in addressing the multiple factors that contribute specifically to younger sisters' vulnerability to early pregnancy. The model can also be used to better understand the mechanisms by which the younger sisters become vulnerable to such outcomes so that program developers can design and tailor more effective interventions. As researchers continue to illuminate the factors that predispose these younger sisters to early childbearing, service providers will be better able to construct effective programs to reduce within-family teenage pregnancies. A "younger sister" approach to breaking the cycle of teenage childbearing offers tremendous—and as yet untapped—potential for adolescent pregnancy prevention.

NOTE

This research was supported by grant R29-HD29472 from the National Institute of Child Health and Human Development, grant APR-000970 from the Office of Population Affairs, and a 1996 Distinguished Wellness Lecturer Award from The California Wellness Foundation and the University of California Office of Health Affairs. The author is very grateful to Erica Johnson, Lisette Lahana, Marijo Villena, and Daisy Barguiarena for their dedication and determination in recruiting and interviewing the study families whose data are presented in this chapter.

REFERENCES

Bandura, A. L. (1977). Social learning theory. Englewood Cliffs, N.J.: Prentice Hall.

Baumrind, D. (1983). Three commentaries on teenage sexuality. American Psychologist, 36, 528–531.

Brewster, K., Billy, J. O. G., and Grady, W. R. (1993). Social context and adolescent behavior: The impact of community on the transition to sexual activity. Social Forces, 71, 713–740.

Brindis, C. (1992). Adolescent pregnancy prevention for Hispanic youth: The role of schools, families, and communities. Journal of School Health, 62, 345–351.

———. (1993). Antecedents and consequences: The need for diverse strategies in adolescent pregnancy prevention. In A. Lawson and D. L. Rhode, eds., The politics of pregnancy: Adolescent sexuality and public policy. Pp. 257–283. New Haven, Conn.: Yale University Press.

Brooks-Gunn, J., and Chase-Lansdale, L. (1991). Children having children: Effects on the family system. Pediatric Annals, 20, 467–481.

Bryant, B. K. (1982). Sibling relationships in middle childhood. In M. Lamb and B. Sutton-Smith, eds., Sibling relationships: Their nature and significance. Pp. 87–121. Hillsdale, N.J.: Lawrence Erlbaum Associates.

Burton, L. M. (1990). Teenage pregnancy as an alternative life-course strategy in multigenerational Black families. Human Nature, 1, 123–143.

———. (1995). Intergenerational patterns of providing care in African American families with teenage childbearers: Emergent patterns in an ethnographic study. In V. L. Bengtson, K. W. Schaie, and L. M. Burton, eds., Adult intergenerational relations: Effects of societal change. Pp. 79–96. New York: Springer.

———. (1996a). Age norms, the timing of family role transitions, and intergenerational caregiving among aging African American women. The Gerontologist, 36, 199–208.

———. (1996b). The timing of childbearing, family structure, and the role responsibilities of aging black women. In E. M. Hetherington and E. A. Blechman, eds., Stress, coping and resiliency in children and families. Pp. 155–172. Mahwah, N.J.: Lawrence Erlbaum Associates.

Burton, L. M., and Bengtson, V. L. (1985). Black grandmothers: Issues of timing and continuity of roles. In V. Bengtson and J. Robertson, eds., *Grandparenthood: Research and policy perspectives*. Pp. 61–78. Beverly Hills, Calif.: Sage.

California Senate Office of Research. (April, 1997). *Issue brief: California strategies to address teenage pregnancy*. Sacramento, Calif.: Senate Printing Office.

Cicirelli, V. G. (1982). Sibling influence throughout the lifespan. In M. Lamb and B. Sutton-Smith, eds., *Sibling relationships: Their nature and significance*. Pp. 267–284. Hillsdale, N.J.: Lawrence Erlbaum Associates.

Conger, R. D., Ge, X., Elder, G. H., et al. (1994). Economic stress, coercive family process, and developmental problems of adolescents. *Child Development, 65,* 541–561.

Cox, J., DuRant, R. H., Emans, S. J., and Woods, E. R. (1995). Early parenthood for the sisters of adolescent mothers: A proposed conceptual model of decision making. *Adolescent and Pediatric Gynecology, 8,* 188–194.

Cox, J., Emans, S. J., and Bithoney, W. (1993). Sisters of teen mothers: Increased risk for adolescent parenthood. *Adolescent and Pediatric Gynecology, 6,* 138–142.

Crane, J. (1991). The epidemic theory of ghettos and neighborhood effects on dropping out and teenage childbearing. *American Journal of Sociology, 96,* 1226–1259.

Dash, L. (1989). *When children want children: An inside look at the crisis of teenage parenthood*. New York: Penguin.

Draper, P. (1976). Social and economic constraints on child life among the !Kung. In R. Lee and I. DeVore, eds., *Kalahari hunter-gatherers: Studies of the !Kung San and their neighbors*. Pp. 200–217. Cambridge, Mass.: Harvard University Press.

Dryfoos, J. G. (1990). *Adolescents at risk: Prevalence and prevention*. New York: Oxford University Press.

Duany, L., and Pittman, K. (1990). *Latino youths at a crossroad: Report of the Adolescent Pregnancy Prevention Clearinghouse*. Washington, D.C.: Children's Defense Fund.

East, P. L. (1995). The social contagion model and adolescent sexual behavior. *Directions in Clinical Psychology, 10,* 1–10.

———. (1996a). Do adolescent pregnancy and childbearing affect younger siblings? *Family Planning Perspectives, 28,* 148–153.

———. (1996b). Pregnancy prevention opportunities focusing on younger sisters of childbearing teens. In *1996 Wellness Lectures*. Pp. 101–127. Berkeley: University of California Regents, University of California Printing.

———. (1996c). The younger sisters of childbearing adolescents: Their attitudes, expectations, and behaviors. *Child Development, 67,* 267–282.

———. (1998a). Breaking the cycle of teenage pregnancy: Prevention opportunities focusing on the younger sisters of teen mothers. *Education and Urban Society, 30,* 157–171.

———. (1998b). Impact of adolescent childbearing on families and younger siblings: Effects that increase younger siblings' risk for early pregnancy. *Applied Developmental Science, 2,* 62–74.

————. (1999). The first teenage pregnancy in the family: Does it affect mothers' parenting, attitudes, or mother-adolescent communication? *Journal of Marriage and the Family, 61,* 306–319.

East, P. L., and Felice, M. E. (1992). Pregnancy risk among the younger sisters of pregnant and childbearing adolescents. *Journal of Developmental and Behavioral Pediatrics, 13,* 128–136.

————. (1994). The psychosocial consequences of teenage pregnancy and childbearing. In I. R. Shenker, ed., *Adolescent Medicine.* Pp. 73–92. London: Harwood Academic Publishers.

————. (1996). *Adolescent pregnancy and parenting: Findings from a racially diverse sample.* Mahwah, N.J.: Lawrence Erlbaum Associates.

East, P. L., Felice, M. E., and Morgan, M. C. (1993). Sisters' and girlfriends' sexual and childbearing behavior: Effects on early adolescent girls' sexual outcomes. *Journal of Marriage and the Family, 55,* 953–963.

East, P. L., and Jacobson, L. J. (2000). The younger siblings of teenage mothers: A follow-up of their pregnancy risk at middle adolescence. Manuscript submitted for publication.

East, P. L., and Shi, C. R. (1997). Pregnant and parenting adolescents and their younger sisters: The influence of relationship qualities for younger sister outcomes. *Journal of Developmental and Behavioral Pediatrics, 18,* 19–25.

Elder, G. H. (1975). Age differentiation and the life course. In A. Inkeles, J. Coleman, and N. Smelser, eds., *Annual Review of Sociology.* Pp. 165–190. Palo Alto, Calif.: Annual Review Company.

Elder, G. H., Eccles, J. S., Ardelt, M., and Lord, S. (1995). Inner-city parents under economic pressure: Perspectives on the strategies of parenting. *Journal of Marriage and the Family, 57,* 771–784.

Elliot, D. S., and Morse, B. J. (1989). Delinquency and drug use as risk factors in teenage sexual activity. *Youth and Society, 21,* 32–60.

Elster, A. B., Ketterlinus, R., and Lamb, M. E. (1990). Association between parenthood and problem behavior in a national sample of adolescents. *Pediatrics, 85,* 1044–1050.

Ensminger, M. E. (1987). Adolescent sexual behavior as it relates to other transition behaviors in youth. In S. L. Hofferth and C. D. Hayes, eds., *Risking the future: Adolescent sexuality, pregnancy, and childbearing.* Pp. 36–55. Washington, D.C.: National Academy Press.

Ensminger, M. E. (1990). Sexual activity and problem behaviors among black, urban adolescents. *Child Development, 61,* 2032–2046.

Fox, G. L. (1980). The mother-adolescent daughter relationship as a sexual socialization structure: A research review. *Family Relations, 29,* 21–28.

Fox, G. L., and Inazu, J. K. (1980). Patterns and outcomes of mother-daughter communication about sexuality. *Journal of Social Issues, 36,* 7–29.

Friede, A., Hogue, C., Doyle, L., et al. (1986). Do the sisters of childbearing teenagers have increased rates of childbearing? *American Journal of Public Health, 76,* 1221–1224.

Furstenberg, F. F. (1980). Burdens and benefits: The impact of early childbearing on the family. *Journal of Social Issues, 36,* 64–87.

Galambos, N. L., and Silbereisen, R. K. (1987). Influences of income change and parental acceptance of adolescent transgression proneness and peer relations. *European Journal of Psychology of Education, 1,* 17–28.

Garn, S. M. (1980). Continuities and change in maturational timing. In O. G. Brim and J. Kagan, eds., *Constancy and change in human development.* Pp. 113–162. Cambridge, Mass.: Harvard University Press.

Geronimus, A. T., and Korenman, S. (1992). The socioeconomic consequences of teen childbearing reconsidered. *Quarterly Journal of Economics, 107,* 1187–1214.

———. (1993). The socioeconomic consequences of teenage childbearing: Evidence and interpretation. *Demography, 38,* 281–290.

Goldfarb, J., Mumford, D., Schum, D., et al. (1977). An attempt to detect "pregnancy susceptibility" in indigent adolescent girls. *Journal of Youth and Adolescence, 6,* 127–144.

Hamburg, B. (1974). Early adolescence: A specific and stressful stage of the life cycle. In G. V. Coelho, D. A. Hamburg, and J. E. Adams, eds., *Coping and adaptation.* Pp. 101–124. New York: Basic Books.

———. (1986). Subsets of adolescent mothers: Developmental, biomedical and psychosocial issues. In J. Lancaster and B. Hamburg, eds., *School-age pregnancy and parenthood.* Pp. 115–145. New York: Aldine de Gruyter.

Haraven, T. K. (1978). *Transitions: The family and the life course in historical perspective.* New York: Academic Press.

Hardy, J. B., and Zabin, L. S. (1991). *Adolescent pregnancy in an urban environment: Issues, programs, and evaluation.* Baltimore: Urban and Schwarzenberg Press.

Hayes, C., ed. 1987. *Risking the future: Adolescent sexuality, pregnancy, and childbearing.* Washington, D.C.: National Academy Press.

Hayward, M. D., Grady, W. R., and Billy, J. O. G. (1992). The influence of socioeconomic status on adolescent pregnancy. *Social Science Quarterly, 73,* 750–772.

Henshaw, S. K. (1997). Teenage abortion and pregnancy statistics by state, 1992. *Family Planning Perspectives, 29,* 115–122.

Hoffman, S. D., Foster, E. M., and Furstenberg, F. F. (1993a). Re-evaluating the costs of teenage childbearing. *Demography, 30,* 1–13.

———. (1993b). Re-evaluating the costs of teenage childbearing: Response to Geronimus and Korenman. *Demography, 30,* 291–296.

Hogan, D. P., Astone, N. M., and Kitagawa, E. M. (1985). Social and environmental factors influencing contraceptive use among black adolescents. *Family Planning Perspectives, 17,* 165–169.

Hogan, D. P., and Kitagawa, E. M. (1985). The impact of social status, family structure, and neighborhood on the fertility of black adolescents. *American Journal of Sociology, 90,* 825–855.

Jemmott, L. S., and Jemmott, J. (1992). Family structure, parental strictness, and sexual behavior among inner-city black male adolescents. *Journal of Adolescent Research, 7,* 192–207.

Kahn, J. R., and Anderson, K. A. (1992). Intergenerational patterns of teenage fertility. *Demography, 29,* 39–57.

Kahn, J. R., Rindfuss, K. R., and Guilkey, D. K. (1990). Adolescent contraceptive choice. *Demography, 27,* 323–335.

Kinnaird, K. L., and Gerrard, M. (1986). Premarital sexual behavior and attitudes toward marriage and divorce among young women as a function of their mothers' marital status. *Journal of Marriage and the Family, 48,* 757–765.

Kirby, D., Korpi, M., Barth, R. P., and Cagampang, H. H. (1997). The impact of the postponing sexual involvement curriculum among youths in California. *Family Planning Perspectives, 29,* 100–108.

Klerman, L. V., and Horwitz, S. M. (1992). Reducing the adverse consequences of adolescent pregnancy and parenting: The role of service programs. *Adolescent Medicine: State of the Art Reviews, 3,* 299–316.

Ladner, J. (1988). The impact of teenage pregnancy on the black family. In H. McAdoo, ed., *Black families.* Pp. 296–305. Newbury Park, Calif.: Sage.

Lempers, J., Clark-Lempers, D., and Simons, R. (1989). Economic hardship, parenting, and distress in adolescence. *Child Development, 60,* 25–49.

Luker, K. (1991). Dubious conceptions: The controversy over teen pregnancy. *The American Prospect, 5,* 73–83.

———. (1996). *Dubious conceptions: The politics of teenage pregnancy.* Cambridge, Mass.: Harvard University Press.

Marini, M. M. (1984). Age and sequencing norms in the transition to adulthood. *Social Forces, 63,* 229–243.

McLoyd, V. C. (1990). The impact of economic hardship on black families and children: Psychological distress, parenting, and socioemotional development. *Child Development, 61,* 311–346.

McLoyd, V. C., Jayaratne, T. E., Ceballo, R., and Borquez, J. (1994). Unemployment and work interruption among African-American single mothers: Effects on parenting and adolescent socioemotional functioning. *Child Development, 65,* 562–589.

Melville, M., ed. (1980). *Twice a minority: Mexican American women.* St. Louis, Mo.: Mosby.

Miller, B. C. (1998). *Families matter: A research synthesis of family influences on adolescent pregnancy.* Washington, D.C.: National Campaign to Prevent Teen Pregnancy.

Miller, B. C., and Bingham, C. R. (1989). Family configuration in relation to the sexual behavior of female adolescents. *Journal of Marriage and the Family, 51,* 499–506.

Miller, B. C., Card, J. J., Paikoff, R. L., and Peterson, J. L. (1992). *Preventing adolescent pregnancy: Model programs and evaluations.* Newbury Park, Calif.: Sage.

Miller, B. C., McCoy, J. K., Olson, T. D., and Wallace, C. M. (1986). Parental discipline and control attempts in relation to adolescent sexual attitudes and behavior. *Journal of Marriage and the Family, 48,* 503–512.

Miller, B. C., Norton, M. C., Curtis, T., et al. (1997). The timing of sexual intercourse among adolescents: Family, peer, and other antecedents. *Youth and Society, 29,* 54–83.

Miller, B. C., and Sneesby, K. R. (1988). Educational correlates of adolescents' sexual attitudes and behavior. *Journal of Youth and Adolescence, 17,* 521–530.

Mirande, A. M. (1968). Reference group theory and adolescent sexual behavior. *Journal of Marriage and the Family, 30,* 572–577.

Moore, K. A., Miller, B. C., Glei, D., and Morrison, D. R. (1995). *Adolescent sex, contraception, and childbearing: A review of recent research.* Washington, D.C.: Child Trends, Inc.

Moore, K. A., Peterson, J. L., and Furstenberg, F. F. (1986a). Parental attitudes and the occurrence of early sexual activity. *Journal of Marriage and the Family, 48,* 777–782.

Moore, K. A., Romano, A., and Oaks, C. (1997). *Facts at a glance.* Washington, D.C.: Child Trends, Inc.

Moore, K. A., Simms, M. C., and Betsey, C. L. (1986b). *Choice and circumstance: Racial differences in adolescent sexuality and fertility.* New Brunswick, N.J.: Transaction Books.

Mott, F., and Haurin, J. R. (1988). Linkages between sexual activity and alcohol and drug use among American adolescents. *Family Planning Perspectives, 20,* 128–136.

Neugarten, C. N., Moore, J. W., and Lowe, J. C. (1965). Age norms, age constraints, and adult socialization. *American Journal of Sociology, 70,* 710–717.

Newcomer, S. F., and Udry, J. R. (1984). Mothers' influence on the sexual behavior of their teenage children. *Journal of Marriage and the Family, 46,* 477–485.

———. (1985). Parent-child communication and adolescent sexual behavior. *Family Planning Perspectives, 17,* 169–174.

———. (1987). Parental marital status effects on adolescent sexual behavior. *Journal of Marriage and the Family, 49,* 235–240.

Plotnick, R. D. (1992). The effects of attitudes on teenage premarital pregnancy and its resolution. *American Sociological Review, 57,* 800–811.

Plotnick, R. D., and Butler, S. S. (1991). Attitudes and adolescent nonmarital childbearing: Evidence from the National Longitudinal Survey of Youth. *Journal of Adolescent Research, 6,* 470–492.

Presser, H. (1978). Age at menarche, socio-sexual behavior, and fertility. *Social Biology, 25,* 94–101.

Rodgers, J. L., Rowe, D. C., and Harris, D. F. (1992). Sibling differences in adolescent sexual behavior: Inferring process models from family composition patterns. *Journal of Marriage and the Family, 54,* 142–152.

Rowe, D. C., and Gulley, B. L. (1992). Sibling effects on substance use and delinquency. *Criminology, 30,* 217–233.

Rowe, D. C., Rodgers, J. L., Meseck-Bushey, S., and St. John, C. (1989). Sexual behavior and nonsexual deviance: A sibling study of their relationship. *Developmental Psychology, 12,* 418–427.

Sampson, R. J., and Laub, J. H. (1994). Urban poverty and the family context of delinquency: A new look at structure and process in a classic study. *Child Development, 65,* 523–540.

Schorr, L. B. (1988). *Within our reach: Breaking the cycle of disadvantage.* New York: Doubleday.

Stack, C. (1974). *All our kin: Strategies for survival in a black community.* New York: Harper and Row.

―――. (1975). Who raises black children? Transactions of child givers and child receivers. In T. R. Williams, ed., *Socialization and communication in primary groups.* Pp. 183–205. New York: Hague-Mouton.

Stack, C. B., and Burton, L. M. (1993). Kinscripts. *Journal of Comparative Family Studies, 24,* 157–170.

Thornton, A., and Camburn, D. (1987). The influence of the family on premarital sexual attitudes and behavior. *Demography, 24,* 323–340.

Trent, K., and Harlan, C. (1994). Teenage mothers in nuclear and extended households. *Journal of Family Issues, 15,* 309–337.

Udry, J. R. (1979). Age at menarche, at first intercourse and at first pregnancy. *Journal of Biosocial Science, 11,* 433–441.

Udry, J. R., and Cliquet, R. L. (1982). A cross-cultural examination of the relationship between ages at menarche, marriage and first birth. *Demography, 19,* 53–63.

Weisner, T. S. (1982). Sibling interdependence and child caretaking: A cross-cultural view. In M. Lamb and B. Sutton-Smith, eds., *Sibling relationships: Their nature and significance.* Pp. 305–327. Hillsdale, N.J.: Lawrence Erlbaum Associates.

―――. (1986). Socialization for parenthood in sibling caretaking societies. In J. B. Lancaster, J. Altman, A. Rossi, and L. Sherrod, eds., *Parenting across the life span.* Pp. 237–270. New York: Aldine de Gruyter.

Whiting, B. B. (1983). The genesis of prosocial behavior. In D. Bridgemen, ed., *The nature of prosocial development.* Pp. 221–242. New York: Academic Press.

Whiting, B. B., and Whiting, J. W. (1975). *Children in six cultures: A psychocultural analysis.* Cambridge, Mass.: Harvard University Press.

Williams, C. W. (1991). *Black teenage mothers: Pregnancy and child rearing from their perspective.* Lexington, Mass.: Lexington Books.

Zabin, L. S., Astone, N. M., and Emerson, M. R. (1993). Do adolescents want babies? The relationship between attitudes and behavior. *Journal of Research on Adolescence, 3,* 67–86.

Zabin, L. S., Hirsch, M., Smith, E., and Hardy, J. B. (1984). Adolescent sexual attitudes and behavior: Are they consistent? *Family Planning Perspectives, 16,* 181–185.

9

Sylvia Guendelman

IMMIGRANTS MAY HOLD CLUES TO PROTECTING HEALTH DURING PREGNANCY

Exploring a Paradox

Poverty is a well-known determinant of health. Persons of low socio-economic status have much higher levels of morbidity and mortality than do those of higher status.[1-3] Yet recent research revealing positive pregnancy outcomes within poor immigrant groups raises the question of whether poverty is necessarily linked to adverse pregnancy outcomes. Are there protective factors that can buffer against the noxious effects of poverty during pregnancy? If so, what lessons can we learn from immigrant and refugee women about promoting healthy pregnancy outcomes?

To address these questions, this chapter attempts to identify protective factors that may be associated with favorable pregnancy outcomes among Latina and Southeast Asian women. It reports the work by Guendelman and colleagues on Latina women of reproductive age and extends previous analyses to compare Latinas and Southeast Asians. The geographic focus is predominantly on California since it is the most important immigrant-receiving state, absorbing approximately 40% of Latino and Asian newcomers. Favorable pregnancy outcomes among Southeast Asian women and Mexican immigrants have been reported in other states, suggesting that what we learn about these populations residing in California may be applicable elsewhere.

CALIFORNIA'S FERTILE GROUND

California leads the nation in rapid diversification, moving away from a White "majority" toward a predominantly Asian and Latino population. Immigration and high fertility have fueled the growth of these populations, which are increasing at a rate ten times faster than that of Whites (i.e., White non-Latinos). Newcomers from Mexico and Southeast Asia constitute more than one-third of California's immigration inflow. Immigrants to California from Vietnam, Cambodia, and Laos numbered close to 30,000 in 1993, with the majority coming from Vietnam.[4] Besides constituting the largest refugee admissions, Southeast Asians have exhibited the highest fertility rates among ethnic groups in the United States.[5] Mexico provides the largest number of Latino immigrants to California: more than 52,000 legal immigrants[4] and as many as 100,000 undocumented immigrants annually.[6] Mothers of Mexican descent—who represent the great majority of California's Latinas—also exhibit fertility rates that far surpass those of White women. Although Mexican Americans and Southeast Asians constitute 22.5% and Whites constitute 57% of the state's total population, in 1993 alone, Mexican-American and Southeast Asian women collectively gave birth to 42% (n = 243,833, out of which 228,707 were to Mexican Americans) of California's infants, compared to 37% (215,885) of infants borne by White women.[7]

Aside from their large immigration numbers and high fertility rates, it would seem that Mexican and Southeast Asian women have little in common. Indeed, these ethnic groups have very different histories in California. Mexicans have a long history in the state, while Southeast Asians are recent immigrants. Hence, whereas a large proportion of Mexican origin women of reproductive age are U.S. born, Southeast Asian women are predominantly foreign born. Whereas Mexican women most often come by choice, seeking economic opportunity for themselves or their families, Southeast Asian women have been forced to flee their war-torn native lands. Yet because Southeast Asians are admitted as refugees, they can receive resettlement funds and other assistance such as language instruction and job training. Mexican immigrants, legal or not, are ineligible for such benefits since they do not qualify for "political refugee" status. Such circumstances, which are often exacerbated by anti-immigrant attitudes, create their own set of resettlement stresses for Mexican newcomers. In addition to the differences across these populations, there are

TABLE 9.1 SOCIOECONOMIC CHARACTERISTICS OF MEXICAN-AMERICAN, SOUTHEAST ASIAN, AND NON-LATINA WHITE WOMEN IN CALIFORNIA

	Mexican-American	Cambodian	Hmong	Laotian	Vietnamese	Non-Latina White
Total California population	6,118,996	68,190	46,892	58,058	280,223	17,029,126
Total female population	2,897,838	35,203	23,041	28,666	132,467	7,800,106
Education						
Less than fifth grade (%)	17.7	47.7	58.9	44.8	12.2	0.9
High school or higher (%)	48.9	29.7	18.3	31.8	63.9	91.6
Income						
Household median ($)	27,934	17,400	15,978	16,436	32,199	39,564
Median for female > 15 years ($)	8,991	7,729	7,531	8,059	9,520	14,221
Families below poverty level (%)	19.3	46.9	59.9	50.4	25.3	5.3
Labor Force						
> 16 years in labor force	55.8	23.3	12.5	26.8	50.9	58.1

SOURCE: Census data for California, 1990.

important differences in language, culture, and social and political standing within the Mexican and Southeast Asian populations.

Despite these notable differences, similarities do exist at the population level in the general socioeconomic profiles of Mexican Americans and Southeast Asians in comparison to the majority White population of California. Both populations are characterized by low educational attainment and high incidence of poverty, especially among women. With the exception of the Vietnamese, Southeast Asian women have strikingly few years of formal schooling and high rates of unemployment and welfare dependency. They commonly lack English proficiency and transferable job skills.[5] Mexican-American women, while more active in the labor force and less likely than Southeast Asian women to have families living below the poverty level, nevertheless have very low incomes in comparison with White women (Table 9.1).

From a health perspective, Mexican-American and Southeast Asian women also share a high-risk profile. Both groups of women experience delayed entry into prenatal care, have large families with short birth-spacing intervals, and—with the exception of the Vietnamese—have high rates of teen pregnancy compared to White women (Table 9.2).

UNCOVERING THE PARADOX

These socioeconomic and health risk factors have traditionally predicted adverse pregnancy outcomes in other populations. For instance, African Americans have risk profiles that are similar to immigrants, yet on average their pregnancy outcomes are much worse.[3,8–10] Studies of White women who share similar risk factors also show increased rates of low birthweight.[3,11] Surprisingly, Mexican Americans and Southeast Asians enjoy pregnancy outcomes that are comparable to those of the overall White population despite the dramatic differences in risk profiles. In this chapter, we examine this paradox in Mexican Americans and Southeast Asians, using White women as a reference group. Space constraints preclude a consistent analysis of differences among the various Southeast Asian subgroups, but we highlight the differences between foreign-born and U.S.-born Mexican Americans.

California birth cohort files for 1990–92 indicate that infant mortality (birth to 364 days) and postneonatal mortality (28–364 days) rates among all Mexican Americans regardless of nativity states and Southeast Asians are comparable to those of Whites (Table 9.3). The infant mortal-

TABLE 9.2   REPRODUCTIVE RISK FACTORS FOR
MEXICAN-AMERICAN, SOUTHEAST ASIAN, AND
NON-LATINA WHITE WOMEN IN CALIFORNIA

	Mexican-American	All Southeast Asian	Cambodian	Laotian	Vietnamese	Non-Latina White
Late entry into prenatal care (third trimester or not at all) (%)	10.9*	6.6*	7.6*	9.6*	5.3*	3.7
Children born to women 35–44 (per 1,000 women)[a]	2.9	N.A.	3.6	3.7	2.5	1.5
Mothers < 18 years (%)	6.5*	3.6*	4.4*	8.9*	1.7*	2.5

NOTE: Estimates not available separately for Hmong in this data set.
[a] Census data for California, 1990.
*Significance compared with non-Latina Whites: p < .001.
SOURCE: Birth Cohort Files for California, 1990–92.

ity rates are comparable even with the inclusion of infants weighing less than 500 grams at birth, who are increasingly being saved with improved technology in neonatal intensive care units.

Mexican Americans do have higher neonatal (0–27 days) mortality rates (4.1 per 1,000 live births) than Whites (3.7) or Southeast Asians (3.5); however, when we restrict the comparison to births of Mexican-born women and exclude U.S.-born Mexican Americans, the neonatal mortality rates (3.9) are similar to those of Whites (Table 9.4). Since foreign-born immigrants are even poorer, less educated, and face more difficulties in access to care than native-born Mexican Americans, their more favorable pregnancy outcomes are especially puzzling.

Birthweight data provide another strong indicator of perinatal health, as infants who weigh 2,500 grams or less at birth have higher-than-average rates of morbidity, neurological impairments, and mortality during the early years of life. Among Mexican Americans in California, the rate of low birthweight is equal to that of Whites (5.1%) despite differences in socioeconomic status (Table 9.3). However, Mexican-born women have significantly lower rates than Whites (Table 9.4). The low birthweight rates among Southeast Asian women appear to be significantly higher than Whites (Table 9.3), possibly because of genetic or biological differences.[10] On average, Asian infants weigh one-half pound

TABLE 9.3 PREGNANCY OUTCOMES AMONG MEXICAN-AMERICAN,
SOUTHEAST ASIAN, AND NON-LATINA WHITE WOMEN IN CALIFORNIA

	All Mexican-Americans	Mexican-Born	All Southeast Asian	Cambodian	Laotian	Vietnamese	Non-Latina White
Infant mortality per 1,000 live births							
Including <500 g	6.6	6.1	6.2	7.4	7.3	5.4	6.4
Excluding <500 g	6.1	5.8	5.7	7.0	6.5	4.9	5.9
Neonatal mortality per 1,000 live births, including <500 g	4.1*	3.9	3.5	4.4	3.9	3.1	3.7
Postneonatal mortality per 1,000 live births	2.5	2.2	2.7	3.0	3.3	2.3	2.7
Low birthweight (%)	5.1	4.8*	6.4*	7.6*	7.7*	5.5*	5.1

NOTE: Estimates not available separately for Hmong in this data set.
  *Significance compared with non-Latina Whites: p < .001.
SOURCE: Birth Cohort Files for California, 1990–92.

TABLE 9.4   REPRODUCTIVE RISK
FACTORS AND PREGNANCY OUTCOMES
AMONG U.S.- AND MEXICAN-BORN MEXICAN-
AMERICAN AND NON-LATINA WHITE WOMEN

	U.S.-Born Mexican-American	Mexican-Born	Non-Latina White
Mean years of education[a]	11.3	7.8	12.8
Living in poverty (%)[a]	28.2	38.3	11.3
Late entry into PNC (%)	7.3*	12.3*	3.7
Mothers < 18 years (%)	11.6*	4.6*	2.5
Infant mortality per 1,000 live births			
Including <500 g	7.8*	6.2	6.4
Excluding <500 g	7.1*	5.8	5.9
Neonatal mortality per 1,000 live births	4.5*	3.9	3.7
Postneonatal mortality per 1,000 live births	3.3*	2.2	2.7
Low birth weight (%)	5.9*	4.8*	5.1

[a]Health and Nutrition Examination Surveys, 1976–80, 1982–84, NCHS.
*Significance compared with non-Latina Whites: p < .001.
SOURCE: Birth cohort files for California, 1990–92.

less than White infants.[12] Differences in birthweight distribution among Southeast Asians, however, do not appear to affect rates of infant mortality adversely.

SEEKING TO EXPLAIN THE PARADOX

Research indicates that there are no straightforward explanations for the epidemiological paradox of positive pregnancy outcomes in immigrant mothers born in Mexico and Southeast Asia. Several hypotheses have surfaced that point to deficits in these populations, such as an underreporting of infant deaths, ethnic misclassification in birth and/or death certificates, and the possibility that excess fetal deaths might eliminate weaker fetuses before birth. Other hypotheses focus on the positive or "protective" factors that may contribute to healthy outcomes. For instance, selective migration may favor healthy mothers and healthy babies, and immigrant mothers who relocate in California may bring with them certain attitudes, values, and behaviors that protect them against stresses and other adverse conditions associated with poverty and resettlement in a new society. This chapter will examine each of these issues but will emphasize a search for clues in identifying protective factors for positive pregnancy outcomes.

Underreporting / Misclassification

It has been suggested that infant mortality rates among immigrant groups may be artificially low because of underreporting of infant deaths. However, low rates of out-of-hospital births in California, coupled with the fact that the great majority of neonatal deaths occur before the first hospital discharge, make it appear that underreporting of neonatal deaths is not a significant phenomenon for Mexican Americans or Southeast Asians in this state.[13-15] Underreporting, if it does occur, is more likely to occur in the postneonatal period (28–364 days), when the child is living at home.[15]

Infant death may go unreported when a migrant family or mother returns to Mexico following birth.[16-18] Crossing the border to give birth is not an uncommon event; in fact, one study found that 10.4% of the women living in the Mexican border town of Tijuana who had given birth between 1982 and 1987 had done so in California.[19] Women gave birth across the border, by their own report, principally in order to receive adequate medical care and/or to secure U.S. citizenship for their children. The study participants then returned with the child to live in Mexico, and any postneonatal mortality that may have occurred presumably went unreported in California. A recent comparison showing Mexican-American infant mortality rates to be lower in border than in nonborder states suggests that proximity to the border might facilitate Mexican parents' return to Mexico before a child dies.[15] For obvious geographic reasons, such circumstances do not apply to the Southeast Asian populations.

Another possible source of underreporting is misclassification of ethnicity and race. Whereas inaccurate coding of race at birth and at death is low for Whites, it has not been unusual for Asians and Latinos to be misclassified—usually as Whites.[15,20,21] Although Latinos can be shown to have differing infant mortality rates in relation to Whites depending on the definitions used to code infant ethnicity,[22] researchers have, nevertheless, shown that the effect of such discrepancies is minor.[14,23] Further, the newer standard of linking birth and death certificates, which minimizes reporting inaccuracies, has raised the Mexican-American infant mortality rate only slightly.[24] In general, underreporting and misclassification should be considered in evaluating birth outcomes, but the magnitude of these effects for Latinos does not appear to be substantial. Less is known about these factors for Southeast Asian women. Available data are often aggregated into an Asian or Asian Pacific category, lacking information specific to Southeast Asians.

Underestimation of infant mortality cannot, however, explain more favorable birthweight distributions among infants of Mexico-born mothers than White mothers, unless there are selective pressures to return to Mexico when a pregnancy has complications likely to result in adverse pregnancy outcomes. Although this phenomenon has not been formally studied, evidence suggests that Mexican mothers residing in California at risk for pregnancy complications prefer health services on the U.S. side of the border because they are perceived as highly innovative and technical.[19] In addition, U.S. citizenship for the U.S.-born child of low-income immigrant parents ensures Medi-Cal insurance coverage for care after birth. The extent to which welfare reform may change these behaviors because of severe restrictions in eligibility for immigrants will require monitoring in the future.

Excess Fetal Deaths

Another conceivable deflator of the infant mortality rate might be excess fetal deaths among Latinas and/or Southeast Asians, whereby biologically weaker fetuses are eliminated and only healthy ones survive until birth.

Studies of fetal mortality are few, and they offer poor comparability because of different state reporting laws. Examination of available data in California, where the law mandates reporting of fetal deaths after 20 weeks' gestation, has not supported the hypothesis that excess late fetal deaths occur in the Latina (predominantly of Mexican birth or descent) and Southeast Asian populations. Guendelman, Chavez, and Christianson studied a large sample of low-income women enrolled in the California Comprehensive Perinatal Program and found that the fetal death rate after 20 weeks' gestation among Latinas (7.8 per 1,000 live births and fetal deaths) was actually lower than the rate among Whites (8.4).[25] These ethnic disparities persisted after controlling for sociobehavioral characteristics, such as maternal age and education, support systems, level of acculturation, tobacco use before and during pregnancy, and prenatal care.

One predictor of fetal death after 20 weeks is a history of fetal loss. By self-report, Latina women indicated having had fewer previous fetal losses than White women. Another indicator that compared favorably for Latinas was early fetal deaths. The rate of fetal death before 20 weeks' gestation for Latinas was 8.9 (per 1,000 live births and fetal deaths), whereas for Whites it was 13.4.[25] It is important to note that this study sampled a low-income clinic population motivated to seek care, and this disposition may have lowered their risk of unreported fetal death. Future research should focus on women who do not obtain prenatal care since they are at higher risk for fetal death.

Fetal death rates were also found to be lower among Southeast Asian refugees compared to the rest of the population in San Diego County.[14] Data from the 1990–92 California birth cohort files indicate comparable rates of late fetal deaths among Southeast Asian and White women (5.2 vs. 5.0 per 1,000 live births), although there are marked variations among the Southeast Asian groups (3.7 for Vietnamese, 7.0 for Cambodian, and 7.7 for Laotian women). It should be noted that a reluctance to use Western medical services, particularly among the Cambodian and Hmong, may increase lack of ascertainment.[26] In addition, the late onset of prenatal care among Southeast Asians and Mexican Americans may skew the fetal death statistics since spontaneous abortions may be occurring at home, without detection.

Clearly, more studies are needed to compare the actual rates of fetal death among our study populations and Whites. Yet the information to date offers little support for the excess fetal death hypothesis as a likely explanation of the epidemiological paradox. In fact, a large multicenter (multistate) study containing 34,350 births recently examined fetal deaths at 20 weeks' gestation or above. According to the findings, the likelihood of a fetal death for Latinos was similar (0.9 vs. 1.0) to that of Whites.[27]

Selective Migration

A cursory look at birth data from Mexico and the countries of Southeast Asia gives the impression that those who emigrate are not in the same health pool as those who stay behind. In Mexico, for example, as many as 15% of babies are born at low birthweight, and 47 infants for every 1,000 live births die in their first year.[27] Between 1980 and 1985, at the height of Southeast Asian immigration into the United States, the infant mortality rates (per 1,000 live births) for Cambodia, Laos, and Vietnam were 160, 122, and 63, respectively.[28,29]

Several studies have shown that both economic and cultural self-selection operate in voluntary migration, as from Mexico.[30-32] The unpredictability of the economic environment in the sending communities often motivates people to want to take the risks involved in relocation. Immigration is expensive; it includes monetary costs, opportunity costs, and psychic costs, which are reduced if the migrant has network connections in the host country. It is the somewhat more affluent and skilled persons rather than those in the bottom of the socioeconomic hierarchy who are most likely to go in search of higher-paying jobs and a better life.[33]

Evidence indicates that labor migration decisions are made jointly by family members within households.[35] But selection factors may vary according to gender roles and expectations. While Mexican male migrants are pushed out of their communities by lack of employment and pulled to the United States by labor and higher wages and social network ties that facilitate access to employment,[33-35] female participation in migration is more often a means of keeping the family together and providing continuity of care.[36] This being the case, health selection factors may perhaps be stronger among Mexican men, who are most often the initiators of migration, than among Mexican women, who are often the implementers of household decisions to migrate.

In the case of Southeast Asians, the rates of adverse pregnancy outcomes in refugee relocation camps, while still elevated, were much lower than in the refugees' countries of origin.[26] This indicates that perhaps sturdy women were more able and likely to leave their war-torn countries of origin behind. Moreover, health conditions including health care services were likely to be better in the refugee camps. Selection also took place through the health screenings of refugees in the refugee processing centers. These consisted of a general physical exam, a serologic test, a chest X ray, immunizations, and treatment for tuberculosis and venereal disease. Positive screens for infectious diseases resulted in quarantines in the refugee camps. On relocation, diagnostic surveillance continued, and health problems were followed up.[37] The hypothesis that migration is selective of a healthier population is further borne out by the obervation that rates of chronic disease among Southeast Asians in the United States are far lower than those observed in the countries of origin.[26]

These clues notwithstanding, the selectivity hypothesis has not been empirically tested. For instance, studies that compare the health of nonmigrants and prospective migrants who plan to emigrate from their communities of origin in Mexico with those immigrants who are residing in California are needed to assess selectivity effects.[30] Future household surveys may also want to include information from the sisters of the women interviewed in order to assess the differential effects of migration experiences.

Protective Sociocultural Factors

While the hypotheses discussed to this point offer some hints about the health paradox among immigrant mothers, perhaps most compelling from the "prevention" perspective is the idea that immigrants and refugees might be profiting from sociocultural and behavioral factors whose benefits outweigh the risks stacked against them. It appears that newcomers bring to the host society values, attitudes, and behaviors that protect them against the risks of adverse pregnancy outcomes or directly contribute to healthy outcomes.

HEALTHY HABITS

Several studies have shown that the consumption of tobacco, alcohol, and illicit drugs during pregnancy are associated with poor pregnancy outcomes. Fetal growth retardation has been associated with smoking[38,39] and with moderate to high levels of alcohol use.[40,41] Both smoking and drug use have been associated with fetal death, low birthweight, and preterm births.[10,38–43] Substance use also contributes to general pregnancy complications and congenital malformations.[3,38,42,43]

Cigarette Smoking

Cigarette smoking during pregnancy causes close to 10% of fetal and infant deaths and one-fifth of all low-birthweight births in the United States and is the single most important known cause of environmentally induced low birthweight.[10] Women who smoke are almost twice as likely to deliver a low-birthweight baby as are nonsmokers.[44] Studies

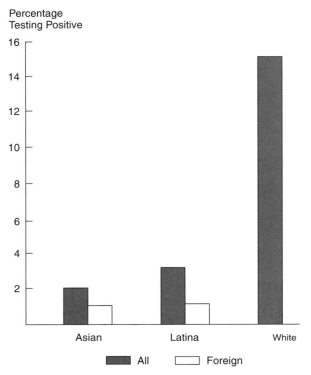

Percentage
Testing Positive

Figure 9.1. Tobacco use of Asian, Latina, and White
maternity patients. Source: Vega et al. (1993 [45]).

consistently show low prevalence rates of tobacco use among Mexican-American, including Mexico-born women, and Southeast Asian women.

Vega et al.,[45] in a study of perinatal substance use among almost 30,000 women attending 202 hospitals in California in 1992, found that Latina women, principally of Mexican birth or descent, were far less likely than White women to have reported that they smoked during pregnancy (3.3% vs. 14.8%; Figure 9.1). Foreign-born Latinas were 3.6 times less likely to smoke than native-born Latinas (1.8% vs. 6.6%). Asian women, in comparison with White and Mexican-born women, were the lowest consumers of tobacco (1.7%; Figure 9.1).

Self-reports of tobacco use in the Health and Nutrition Examination Survey (HANES) studies corroborate the finding of Vega et al. that Mexican-American women smoke less during pregnancy than do Whites. Guendelman and Abrams compared 664 Mexican-American women in the Hispanic HANES and 1,156 White women in the second HANES

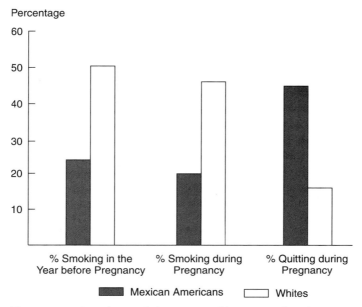

Figure 9.2.   Prevalence of cigarette smoking among low-income
Mexican-American and White women. Source: Camilli et al.
(1994 [47]).

across stages of the reproductive cycle and found that whereas 23%
of Mexican-American women smoked in the interconceptional period,
only 8.1% smoked during pregnancy. In contrast, among White women
there were nearly twice as many interconceptional smokers (43%), and
this level remained high during pregnancy (37.3%).[46]

Since Guendelman and Abrams's study used cross-sectional data, empirical evidence of quitting could not be ascertained. Yet evidence from
a recent study by Camilli, McElroy, and Reed shows that Mexican-
American smokers are more likely to quit during pregnancy than White
smokers. The authors compared 200 Mexican-American and 131 White
low-income women seeking prenatal care in a university hospital in Tuc-
son, Arizona. As shown in Figure 9.2, 24% of Mexican-American
women had smoked in the year before pregnancy, compared with 51%
of White women. Only 19% of Mexican Americans had smoked during
any part of their pregnancy, whereas 48% of their White counterparts
had done so. Furthermore, on average, Mexican Americans smoked
almost five fewer cigarettes per day than Whites (6.9 vs. 11.8). The
odds of quitting during pregnancy, as verified by urinary cotinine values,
were 4.71 times higher for Mexican Americans (95% CI 1.66–13.38).[47]

Since quitting even as late as the seventh or eighth month has a positive influence on birthweight, the health benefits to Mexican Americans are clear.[48]

Less is known about smoking before and during pregnancy among Southeast Asians. Data from 1989–91 describing women participating in the San Diego Comprehensive Perinatal Program (a state-funded program for pregnant low-income women) indicate no history of smoking for Southeast Asian women in the program.[49] In comparison, 6.7% of Mexico-born immigrants and 29.4% of White women reported having smoked previously in their lives. An earlier study of Southeast Asian women in San Diego County found that less than 2% of Southeast Asian mothers were smokers.[5] In another study, conducted in Washington State, cigarette smoking among Southeast Asian immigrants during pregnancy decreased slightly from 3% to 2.4% between 1984 and 1986.[50] These rates for Southeast Asian women are consistently lower than for Whites.

Since the bulk of evidence shows a clear and consistent association between low birthweight and infant mortality and smoking, the low rate of smoking in these immigrant populations is clearly advantageous.

Alcohol Use

Alcohol use during pregnancy has been associated with both short- and long-term negative health effects for infants, including congenital malformations and mental retardation.[48] Women who consume large amounts of alcohol during pregnancy have higher rates of low-birthweight babies than do nondrinkers.[41] While the evidence is mixed, alcohol use during pregnancy appears to be low among Mexican-American and Southeast Asian women.

Using food frequency data from two Health and Nutrition Examination Surveys (the Hispanic HANES and the second HANES), Guendelman and Abrams compared mean daily servings of beer, wine, and liquor for 664 Mexican-American women and 1,156 White women across four stages of the reproductive cycle.[46] On average, pregnant Mexican-American women consumed .02 daily servings of alcohol compared to .08 servings among pregnant White women. Interconceptional, pregnant, lactating, and postpartum Mexican Americans were far less likely than Whites to consume alcohol (Figure 9.3).

Vega et al., in their study of perinatal substance use among 30,000 women, assessed alcohol exposure at the time of delivery, employing

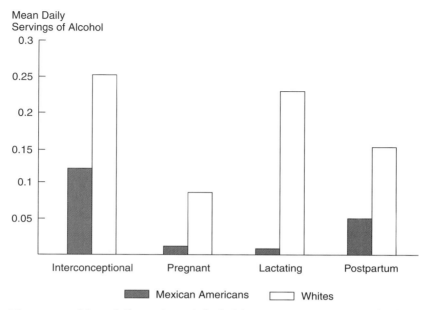

Figure 9.3. Mean daily servings of alcohol for Mexican-American and White women by reproductive stage. Source: Guendelman and Abrams (1994 [46]).

urine toxicology screens.[45] The study found that, in comparison with White women, positive alcohol screens were more likely among Latinas (6.1% vs. 6.9%; Figure 9.4). (A woman was considered positive for alcohol use if she had drunk at least 6 ounces of beer, 2 ounces of wine, or 0.5 ounces of distilled spirits in the period immediately before she was admitted as a maternity patient or had drunk larger quantities of alcohol more than a few hours before admission.) The high prevalence rates of alcohol use for both foreign- (6.7%) and native-born (7.3%) Latinas may suggest cultural prescriptions to use alcohol prior to delivery to better cope with labor. Available evidence based on self-reports supports Guendelman and Abrams's findings that Latina women, especially the Mexican born, are lower consumers of alcohol generally than White women.[49,51-54]

A study of Southeast Asian women participating in the San Diego Comprehensive Perinatal Program revealed low prevalence of alcohol consumption.[49] Furthermore, urine toxicology screens of Asian women at delivery administered in the study by Vega et al. showed fewer positive screens for alcohol compared to Whites (5.1% vs. 6.1%). Anecdotal information suggests that alcohol intake may be restricted to the time of

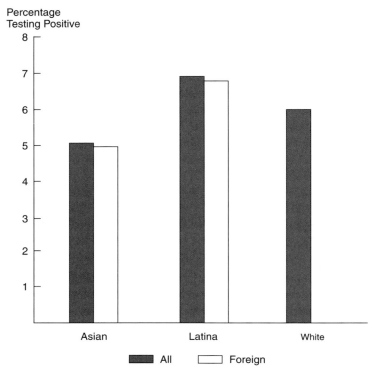

Figure 9.4. Alcohol use of Asian, Latina, and White maternity patients.
Source: Vega et al. (1993 [45]).

delivery. For instance, cultural prescriptions among Cambodian women appear to favor alcohol use both prior to and following childbirth in order to "strengthen the blood." [55]

While important, it does not appear that alcohol has nearly as strong an impact on low birthweight and infant mortality as cigarette smoking.[10] However, the low prevalence rates of alcohol consumption during pregnancy in immigrant groups does suggest a reproductive health advantage.

Illicit Drugs

Prenatal use of controlled substances has been correlated with fetal growth retardation, perinatal death, and pregnancy and delivery complications.[56-60]

In the study by Vega et al.,[45] significantly fewer Latinas tested positive for any drug at the time of delivery than did White women (2.8%

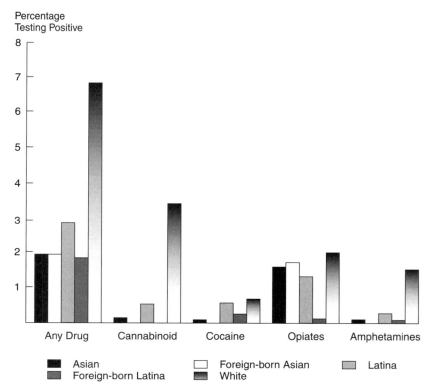

Figure 9.5. Drug use of Asian, Latina, and White maternity patients. Source: Vega et al. (1993 [45]).

vs. 6.8%; Figure 9.5). Asians were also more likely to have lower prevalence rates than Whites for licit and illicit drugs, *except for* opiates (Figure 9.5). As was the case with Latinas, Asian women who were foreign born (which includes the vast majority of Southeast Asians) had much lower prevalence rates of substance use compared to native-born Asians. The only exception was opiate use, which was slightly higher among the foreign born (1.5% vs. 1.3%) and similar for foreign-born Asians and Whites.

Overall, foreign-born Asian and Latina women in this Vega et al. study were far less likely to consume addictive substances than White women during pregnancy, except for alcohol among Latinas. These findings indicating low consumption have been supported by recent studies conducted by Rumbaut and Weeks[49] and Newman et al.[61] in San Diego.

Although few pregnant women engage in drug abuse, it appears that those who do are generally in poorer health and obtain limited prenatal care.[48] The much lower prevalence of illicit drug use among immigrants suggests another health advantage.

DIETARY INTAKE

A nutritious diet helps to meet the changing needs of the pregnant woman and her fetus. Specific nutrients such as calcium, zinc, protein, iron, and vitamins C, A, and E and folic acid have been related to pregnancy outcomes,[38,62] and there is no evidence of substantial differences in nutritional requirements among various ethnic groups. Guendelman and Abrams compared the intake of the previously named eight nutrients between White women and Mexican-American women of reproductive age, using data from two Health and Nutrition Examination Surveys.[63] For the purpose of comparison, these analyses are extended here to examine the different nutrient intakes of Mexican-American pregnant women in the Hispanic HANES (n = 79), White women in the second HANES (n = 72), and a sample of pregnant Southeast Asian women who participated in a Prenatal Nutrition Project at the University of California at San Diego between similar reference periods (1978–90). The latter were studied by Newman et al., who reported results based on 91 Cambodian, 37 Laotian, and 59 Vietnamese women.[61] For all groups, dietary intake was elicited by participant recall of food and beverage consumption during the preceding 24-hour period.

As indicated in Table 9.5, the five study groups did not differ significantly with respect to age or mean number of live births. However, they differed markedly with respect to height, weight, and body mass index (BMI). White women were the tallest, while Mexican Americans had the highest BMI. All three Southeast Asian groups were shorter and lighter and had a lower BMI than either Mexican-American or White women. Despite these differences, the energy intake among the groups was similar (Table 9.6).

A comparison of the mean daily intake of each nutrient relative to the recommended daily allowance (RDA) standards for pregnant women shows that the mean intake of protein was above the RDA for all ethnic groups (Table 9.6). Yet the protein intake was significantly higher for Southeast Asian women (particularly the Vietnamese) in comparison with Mexican-Americans and White women. Mexican-American and White women did not differ significantly in their intake of any of the eight nutrients, and the mean daily intake of vitamins C and A, iron, and zinc relative to the RDA was similar across all ethnic groups. Aside from

TABLE 9.5   MEAN (STANDARD DEVIATION) SOCIAL
AND PHYSICAL CHARACTERISTICS OF PREGNANT
MEXICAN-AMERICAN, SOUTHEAST ASIAN, AND NON-
LATINA WHITE WOMEN

	Mexican-American (n = 74)	Cambodian (n = 91)	Laotian (n = 37)	Vietnamese (n = 59)	Non-Latina White (n = 75)
Age (yr)	25ª (6)	27ª (6)	25ª (5)	26ª (5)	26ª (5)
Height (cm)	159ᶜ (7)	153ᵇ (5)	149ª (5)	152ᵇ (7)	164ᵈ (6)
Weight (kg)	64ᶜ (11)	50ᵇ (8)	48ª,ᵇ (7)	47ª (7)	62ᶜ (12)
Body mass index	25.5ᵈ (4.4)	21.4ᵇ (3.1)	21.7ᵇ (2.9)	20.3ª (2.8)	23.3ᶜ (4.2)
Previous live births	1.6ª (1.6)	2.3ª (1.8)	2.3ª (2.4)	1.6ª (1.6)	1.2ª (1.6)

NOTE: Groups sharing a same-letter superscript are not significantly different from each other at $\alpha = .05$.
SOURCES: Mexican-American data from NCHS, Hispanic Health and Nutrition Examination Survey, 1982–84; Cambodian, Laotian, and Vietnamese data from Newman, Norcross, and McDonald Prenatal Nutrition Project, University of California, San Diego, 1978–90; non-Latina White data from NCHS, Second National Health and Nutrition Examination Survey, 1976–80.

protein, then, the findings do not show a better diet for immigrant compared to nonimmigrant pregnant women. (Because the RDAs are estimated to exceed the nutrient requirements of most individuals, intakes below the RDA for a given group are not necessarily inadequate, but they do suggest an increased likelihood of poor dietary intake.) In fact, compared with non-Southeast Asian women, Cambodian women showed a lower intake of folate, vitamin E, and calcium.

These findings were not adjusted for socioeconomic status. White women in the HANES sample had higher incomes than the immigrant groups in either study, and it is possible that after controlling for income, Southeast Asian women, all of whom were at or under 200% of the poverty level in the Newman et al. study, would have had better nutrient intake than Whites. Clearly, more research, utilizing larger samples and controlling for socioeconomic status, is needed to compare the nutrient intake of Southeast Asian and White women.

Somewhat more information is available for Mexican Americans. As with drug and alcohol use, the nutrient intake of Mexican-born women seems to be far better than the intake of U.S.-born women of Mexican descent. According to Guendelman and Abrams in their study of generational differences in nutrition,[63] Mexican-born immigrants had significantly higher absolute intake and higher average intake relative to RDA standards for protein, vitamins (A, C, E, and folic acid), and calcium than did second-generation Mexican Americans and Whites (Table 9.7).

TABLE 9.6 MEAN (STANDARD DEVIATION) NUTRIENT
INTAKE AS PERCENTAGE OF RECOMMENDED DIETARY
ALLOWANCE FOR PREGNANT MEXICAN-AMERICAN,
SOUTHEAST ASIAN, AND NON-LATINA WHITE WOMEN

Nutrients	Mexican-American (n = 76)	Cambodian (n = 24)	Laotian (n = 24)	Vietnamese (n = 20)	Non-Latina White (n = 72)
Energy (Kcal)	1,901 [a] (796)	1,750 [a] (755)	1,630 [a] (576)	1,932 [a] (753)	1,988 [a] (812)
	Percentage of Recommended Dietary Allowance				
	(n = 79)	(n = 91)	(n = 37)	(n = 59)	(n = 72)
Protein	135 [a] (66)	173 [b] (76)	176 [b] (76)	187 [b] (86)	134 [a] (67)
Vitamin C	166 [a] (151)	178 [a] (140)	205 [a] (201)	168 [a] (143)	172 [a] (164)
Folate	72 [b] (62)	46 [a] (29)	54 [a,b] (31)	55 [a,b] (35)	68 [b] (55)
Vitamin A	177 [a] (376)	129 [a] (88)	199 [a] (239)	190 [a] (225)	184 [a] (175)
Vitamin E	83 [b] (85)	44 [a] (36)	59 [a,b] (47)	77 [b] (84)	92 [b] (125)
Iron	41 [a] (23)	45 [a] (23)	46 [a] (21)	46 [a] (18)	44 [a] (26)
Calcium	79 [c] (42)	42 [a] (28)	51 [a,b] (31)	67 [b,c] (43)	97 [c] (53)
Zinc	77 [a] (43)	78 [a] (41)	81 [a] (50)	82 [a] (46)	93 [a] (120)

NOTE: Groups sharing a same-letter superscript are not significantly different from each other at α = .05.
SOURCES: Mexican-American data from NCHS, Hispanic Health and Nutrition Examination Survey, 1982–84; Cambodian, Laotian, and Vietnamese data from Newman, Norcross, and McDonald Prenatal Nutrition Project, University of California, San Diego, 1978–90; non-Latina White data from NCHS, Second National Health and Nutrition Examination Survey, 1976–80.

TABLE 9.7 MEAN DIETARY INTAKE AND MEAN NUTRIENT ADEQUACY RATIOS (NARS) FOR MEXICAN- AND U.S.-BORN MEXICAN-AMERICAN AND NON-LATINA WHITE WOMEN

	Mexican-Born Mexican-American (n = 475)	U.S.-Born Mexican-American (n = 898)	Non-Latina White (n = 2,326)
Protein			
Mean intake, g (SE)	74.3[c] (1.7)	68.3[b] (1.6)	63.9[a] (0.84)
NAR (SE)	0.92[e] (0.009)	0.88[d] (0.006)	0.89[d] (0.004)
Vitamin A			
Mean intake, IU (SE)	6,347.4[b] (432.2)	4,240.8[a] (228.0)	4,596.5[a] (179.8)
NAR (SE)	0.71[f] (0.017)	0.61[d] (0.015)	0.66[e] (0.008)
Vitamin C			
Mean intake, mg (SE)	104.1[b] (4.7)	84.1[a] (3.9)	87.9[a] (2.5)
NAR (SE)	0.78[e] (0.014)	0.69[d] (0.012)	0.71[d] (0.008)
Vitamin E			
Mean intake, Alpha TE (SE)	7.9 (0.5)	7.3 (0.3)	7.5 (0.2)
NAR (SE)	0.70 (0.020)	0.68 (0.012)	0.70 (0.007)
Folic acid			
Mean intake, mg (SE)	266.5[b] (12.2)	205.5[a] (5.2)	200.2[a] (3.9)
NAR (SE)	0.82[e] (0.020)	0.75[d] (0.010)	0.77[d] (0.006)
Calcium			
Mean intake, mg (SE)	778.8[b] (23.8)	644.5[a] (32.5)	677.7[a] (16.3)
NAR (SE)	0.70[f] (0.024)	0.57[d] (0.014)	0.61[e] (0.009)

NOTE: Data expressed as mean percentage of intake relative to the Recommended Daily Allowance for that nutrient specific to the woman's reproductive state. The NARs were truncated at 1.0.

NOTE: Groups sharing a same-letter superscript are not significantly different from each other at $\alpha = .05$.

SOURCES: Data for Mexican- and U.S.-born Mexican Americans from NCHS, Hispanic Health and Nutrition Examination Survey, 1982–84; data for non-Latina Whites from NCHS, National Health and Nutrition Examination Survey, 1976–80.

Although this study did not follow women through their pregnancies, the results suggest that nutrition may help to explain the much lower rate of low birthweight among first-generation Mexican-American women than among U.S.-born women of Mexican descent.[64,65] Large epidemiological studies are needed to examine the association between dietary intake, weight gain during pregnancy, and pregnancy outcomes among newcomer populations to help us further unravel the epidemiological paradox.

KIN NETWORKS AND FAMILY STABILITY

The role of social factors in explaining the paradox is even more poorly understood than that of health and nutrition habits. Nevertheless, some social factors related to family and social networks seem to provide clues to better reproductive health, even though we do not understand the mechanisms by which they affect pregnancy outcomes.

Close kin networks may confer protection to the pregnant woman and compensate for income deficits by improving access to informational and psychosocial support.[66-69] These resources may translate into more knowledge about healthy pregnancies, the encouragement of positive behaviors, and less stress during pregnancy, all of which more directly affect perinatal morbidity and mortality. They may also alter hormonal and immunological responses associated with pregnancy complications.[70]

Research on Latinos and Southeast Asians has described the centrality of the family in both cultures. Latinos tend to have close kin networks and emphasize the collective needs of the family over individual needs.[71-74] Indeed, the family has been described as the single most important institution for Mexican Americans.[75,76] Kinship in this case comprises not only relatives but also the Latino *compadre* system, which establishes "coparents," in the Catholic tradition, who share broader, less formalized obligations toward the children.[77] Recent evidence further suggests that women of Mexican descent appear to have more social network contacts outside of the family[66] compared with Whites as well as enhanced access to psychosocial and informational social support. As noted, these factors may contribute to favorable pregnancy outcomes by making more resources available to the pregnant woman, thereby compensating for economic deficits.

Family studies conducted in Mexico suggest that children in poor families have a high economic and moral value.[78] They are considered one of the few sources of personal achievement and pride. Children are the main reason for marrying, a compensation for any unsatisfactory or broken marriage and a source of companionship and economic support.[78]

Family is similarly important for each of the Southeast Asian groups.[79] After an extensive review of the literature on Southeast Asians, Frye concluded that kinship solidarity is the "lifeline" in these cultures.[80] Much as Mexicans do, Southeast Asians view the individual as "subservient to the kinship-based group." Yet the specific character of Southeast Asian families and traditions varies. Vietnamese have extended patrilineal family systems, Laotians and Cambodians rely more on nuclear family supports, and Hmong have a clan system.

Despite the heterogeneous family structures of Southeast Asians, pregnant women in these cultures consistently tend to receive positive social support from family and kin, as demonstrated by spousal approval of the pregnancy and familial monitoring of the health, diet, and lifestyle of the pregnant woman.[14] These immigrant subgroups also seem to share with Mexican Americans the cultural belief that having a child demonstrates one's femininity and that fertility signifies womanhood and a main source of marital satisfaction.[81,82] In addition, community assistance from refugee programs in terms of child care, chores, and financial aid represents significant, though dwindling, support.

Family stability also appears to influence reproductive health. For instance, a study by Ramsey et al.[69] showed that women who lived alone were at highest risk of having smaller babies, while living with extended family was correlated with higher birthweights. Living with a husband further increased the likelihood of having a heavier baby.[68] These effects might be mediated by such factors as higher income, better nutrition, and less stress.

Compared with Whites, Mexican Americans have a higher proportion of husband-wife families and lower rates of divorce and separation.[68] Family stability among Mexican Americans appears to be highest among ever-married women who have the lowest educational level and highest use of the Spanish language. Similarly, among Southeast Asian women, the prevalence of unwed mothers is extremely low. Hopkins and Clarke found that within each Southeast Asian subgroup, less than 1% of mothers were unmarried, compared with over 17% in the general U.S. population.[83]

Family stability may play a role in the case of teenage pregnancies as well. Scientific and popular understanding have linked births to teenage mothers (under 18 years) with poverty, welfare dependency, and a host of other social problems, including alienation from family. But teenage pregnancy among Mexican Americans and Southeast Asians appears to follow a different pattern. In both groups, pregnancy at a young age appears to be more common and more culturally acceptable than among Whites, and teenage mothers are often cared for and supported by extended family. While it has been reported that Southeast Asian cultures consider birth out of wedlock to be a disgrace,[84-85] early marriage in these groups is encouraged and creates a context for culturally acceptable teenage births.[86] In fact, although it does not appear that childbearing begins at an earlier age among Southeast Asians than in other populations, Southeast Asian teens are more likely than their White counterparts to have short birth intervals and low contraceptive use. Hence, teen births in these populations may pose risks not because they signal lack of family supports but because of low socioeconomic status and biological considerations.

Few studies have directly tested the relationship between family networks, family stability, and pregnancy outcomes. The prevalence of strong and stable family networks in immigrant populations suggests that these factors might help to explain the paradox of favorable pregnancy outcomes among at-risk populations.

THE EFFECT OF ACCULTURATION ON PREGNANCY RISKS AND OUTCOMES

A corollary to the protective sociocultural hypothesis is the acculturation hypothesis. According to the latter, as immigrants spend more time in the United States or move to the second generation, their healthy behaviors, norms, and attitudes change, resembling those of the White nonimmigrant population or of high-risk groups with which they come into contact. Shifts in health risks coupled with changes in sociodemographic characteristics that occur with acculturation affect pregnancy outcomes.

As discussed in the previous section, alcohol, illicit drugs, and tobacco use are low and family stability is high among recent immigrants. They also adhere to a traditional diet, which seems healthful. With acculturation, healthy behaviors among Mexican Americans are worse: alcohol, tobacco, and drug use during pregnancy increase, and the quality of the diet decreases (Figures 9.1, 9.4, and 9.5; Table 9.7). These shifts could explain the increased prevalence of low birthweight and infant mortality in Mexican Americans who are second generation and beyond (Table 9.4).

Furthermore, teen pregnancies under 18 years increase in the second generation for women of Mexican descent. While 4.6% of Mexican-born mothers are teens, this rate more than doubles to 11.6% among U.S.-born Mexican-American mothers.[65] Reynoso et al. found that acculturated pregnant Mexican-American teenagers engaged in sexual behavior at an earlier age than less acculturated teens and reported that they were more likely to consider single parenthood as an option.[87]

In addition to a loss of protective behaviors, changes in socioeconomic status that occur with acculturation to U.S. society may further affect pregnancy outcomes. Although Mexican immigrants are considered to be of low socioeconomic status in the United States, it has been amply documented that average family earnings are significantly improved over those in Mexico, and a large proportion of newcomers are able to accumulate small savings and send remittances back home.[35] In contrast, U.S.-born women of Mexican descent do not appear to enjoy a similar sense of getting ahead in society. Subjective feelings of poverty and discrimination have been shown to negatively affect birth outcomes,[11] and many of these women become stalled in poverty and feel oppressed by social discrimination.[88] Another insidious influence in ethnic communities is the "corporate targeting" of these groups in alcohol and tobacco advertising. Evidence shows an association between tobacco and alcohol advertisements and an increase in risky behaviors.[89-90] A higher consumption of alcohol and cigarettes among native-born Mexican Americans is consistent with this evidence.

Recent findings suggest that it may not take a whole generation for changes in the reproductive risk profile of Mexican Americans to become apparent. Guendelman and English found that within five years of moving to this country, there was notable deterioration in the perinatal health of Mexican-born women living in California. Long-term residents had fewer planned pregnancies and were more likely to smoke than newcomers who had lived in the country for five years or less. After controlling for smoking, planned pregnancy, and maternal age, long-term immigrants living in the United States for more than five years were more likely to have pregnancy complications and to deliver preterm and low-birthweight infants than newcomers.[91]

Among Southeast Asians, whose immigration to this country is a much more recent phenomenon, more than 95% of women are foreign born.[92] The health effects of acculturation in the second generation and beyond, therefore, remain to be seen, but we can begin to examine the effects of acculturation in the first generation. Preliminary findings suggest that unlike Mexican immigrants, risky behaviors decrease and birth outcomes improve with increased length of stay among Southeast Asians.

Studies by Rumbaut and Weeks[5] and Li et al.[50] indicate that the health status of recent cohorts of Southeast Asian immigrants has not improved, as measured by the prevalence of hepatitis B and tuberculosis. However, Li et al.'s analysis of consecutive births to the same parents from 1984 to 1987 showed that low birthweight declined more than expected during this period among Southeast Asian immigrants. A decline in low birthweight over a five- to six-year period was also observed in trend analyses of Washington, Massachusetts, and San Diego County births to Southeast Asians.[7,26,50] Yip et al. found a similar improvement in low birthweight rates among low-income Southeast Asian refugees at a national level between 1980 and 1989.[93]

Although these researchers suggest that initial observations of low birthweight may have been skewed by health and nutritional deficiencies in refugees coming out of relocation camps, the reduction in low birthweight may also be related to an increased number of years of residency in the United States. Increased acculturation in the Li et al. study allowed for a change in paternal occupational status from student to employed that was associated with a 27% reduction in the low-birthweight prevalence, independent of maternal age, infant sex, and prior gravidity.[50] As with Mexican Americans, this move into employment among refugees presumably leads to an improvement in socioeconomic status that may be associated with good pregnancy outcomes. Another possibility is that a relatively stable yet declining smoking prevalence during the 1984–86 study period in the Washington State Southeast Asian population may account for these improved outcomes. (The number of births to smokers during pregnancy decreased by 0.6%.) Whether these effects are sustained in the second generation will require investigation in the future.

Changing dietary habits may also alter perinatal health. However, studies of adolescents indicate that while Southeast Asians adopt some U.S. nutritional habits such as drinking more milk and soft drinks, they abstain from a lot of nutritionally weak foods.[94] The adherence to a traditional diet may help to preserve favorable birth outcomes in this population.

These preliminary findings indicating differing effects of acculturation on pregnancy risks and outcomes by race/ethnicity suggest that acculturation is mediated by highly contextual factors. The process of acculturation, in which individuals acquire ways of living, values, attitudes, and behaviors from another culture, is complex and segmented and therefore unlikely to be solely a function of time spent in the United States. Future studies assessing the impact of acculturation on birth outcomes should examine the effects of years of residency as well as the age of entry into the United States, the extent of English language use, changes in socioeconomic status, the presence of extended kin networks, family stability and support, community receptivity to immigrant families, and shifts in traditional roles for women.

CONCLUSION

The rapidly growing Mexican-American and Southeast Asian populations in California are quite heterogeneous in terms of social and cultural backgrounds. Despite the diversity, both within and across immigrant groups, these populations share a socioeconomic disadvantage compared to White Californians.

Although research has linked low socioeconomic status with a host of health risk factors and adverse outcomes, this relationship does not necessarily hold when examining the pregnancy outcomes of these immigrant women. As this chapter has shown, Mexican-American and Southeast Asian immigrants have favorable pregnancy outcomes despite their socioeconomic disadvantages. This health paradox is more accentuated among foreign-born women, who are even poorer than their U.S.-born counterparts. There is strong evidence to suggest that immigrants bring to the United States values, attitudes, and health behaviors that may protect them from adverse pregnancy outcomes. Among the protective factors, the very low use of addictive substances stands out as an important contributor to healthy outcomes. Other protective factors such as good nutrition, a strong sense of family and social support, and a positive attitude toward childbearing show strong potential for contributing to favorable pregnancy outcomes.

These protective factors may buffer immigrant women from the stresses of poverty or else directly contribute to positive outcomes by bolstering the immune and hormonal systems. Although several studies have focused on the relationship between these factors and pregnancy outcomes in other populations, remarkably few studies have focused on immigrant Latina and Southeast Asian women. Large epidemiological studies are needed to examine the relationship between pregnancy outcomes and healthy diets, weight gain during pregnancy, healthy habits, family stability, teenage pregnancy within a supportive family system, and networks that provide informational and emotional support and reinforce healthy behaviors among immigrants.

As this chapter demonstrates, the pregnancy outcomes of immigrant women vary according to nativity and increased exposure to American society. Although certain risk factors associated with pregnancy outcomes—such as education, income, and access to prenatal care—improve among U.S.-born, second-generation Mexican Americans, many protective factors become eroded. Compared with first-generation Mexican-American women, the pregnancy outcomes of second-generation women are less favorable.

While it is too early to examine generational changes in birth outcomes among the more recently arrived Southeast Asian population, we can begin to explore the effects of acculturation among foreign-born Southeast Asian women. Research suggests that they may be buffered from many of the negative effects of acculturation, as demonstrated by their improving birth outcomes in recent years. This response contrasts with that of Mexican immigrants who appear to show a marked deterioration in risks and pregnancy outcomes after only five years of residing in the United States. Such differentials may be a result of the different ways in which immigrants adapt to our society. More research is needed to examine the modes of immigrant adaptation and its effect on pregnancy outcomes. We must determine whether the differentials observed between the two immigrant groups are a product of a different community receptivity to these populations or a different sociocultural orientation that immigrants bring to our society.

Recognizing that tremendous gaps in knowledge exist, some preliminary conclusions can be drawn regarding what immigrants can teach us about having healthy babies.

This health paradox demonstrates—contrary to the implications of earlier epidemiological studies—that poverty does not necessarily coincide with unhealthy lifestyles and that a lack of economic resources does not always mean a lack of human and social resources. If we grasp the significance of this paradigm shift, we may be in a better position to design health promotion policies that address immigrants' needs by emphasizing their sociocultural assets rather than assuming—and often blaming them for—their deficits.

With the advent of California's "majority-minority" population in the 21st century and the increasingly negative stereotypes placed on immigrants, as well as the cutbacks in social programs for the poor, it is incumbent on health care providers, public health planners, and policy makers to recognize the positive health and social aspects of immigrant communities. Such awareness is important in order not only to preserve the health and healthy lifestyles of immigrant women and their children but also to learn ways of transferring this knowledge to promote health in other communities with a high incidence of infant mortality and low-birthweight babies. In recognition of these positive and protective factors and the benefits that they provide to all communities, the following steps are recommended:

· Health-media messages reinforcing these protective values and behaviors must be disseminated broadly in ethnic communities to counteract the influences of alcohol, tobacco, and food industry advertising.
· Educational strategies must encourage a sense of pride and confidence in the sociocultural assets that immigrant families and communities possess.
· State funding must be maintained to support primary care facilities for both legal and undocumented immigrants.
· Research and evaluation opportunities must be expanded to assess the best ways to apply the protective knowledge and skills of Southeast Asian and Mexican-American populations to other at-risk populations.

The reproductive health of California's large immigrant populations is a compelling area for future research and the development of new health promotion strategies. Through increased attention to these groups, we can more fully understand how to optimize maternal and child health for all Americans.

NOTE

The author gratefully acknowledges Ann Banchoff for assistance in preparing this manuscript, Beate Herrchen for providing valuable birth cohort file data, and Paul English and Christopher Grover for helpful comments on an earlier draft of this chapter. Thank you also to Lora Santiago for clerical support.

REFERENCES

1. Haan, H., Kaplan, G., and Syme, L. 1989. Socioeconomic status and health: Old observations and new thoughts. In *Pathways to Health: The Role of Social Factors,* edited by J. P. Bunker, D. S. Gumby, and B. H. Kehrer. Pp. 76–133. Palo Alto, Calif.: Henry J. Kaiser Foundation.
2. Syme, L., and Berkman, L. 1976. Social class, susceptibility, and sickness. *American Journal of Epidemiology,* 104, 1–8.
3. Institute of Medicine, Committee to Study the Prevention of Low Birthweight. 1985. *Preventing Low Birthweight.* Washington, D.C.: National Academy Press.
4. California State Department of Finance Demography Research Unit. Data from federal fiscal year 1992–93 (personal communication).
5. Rumbaut, R. G., and Weeks, J. R. 1989. Infant health among Indochinese refugees: Patterns of infant mortality, birthweight and prenatal care in comparative perspective. *Research in the Sociology of Health Care,* 8, 137–196.
6. Levy, S. 1995. *California Population Characteristics.* Palo Alto, Calif.: Center for Continuing Study of the California Economy.
7. California Department of Health Services, Center for Health Statistics. 1993. *California Birth Cohort File.*
8. California Department of Health Services. 1994, February. *Analysis of Health Indicators for California's Minority Populations.* Sacramento: Author.
9. California Department of Health Services, Center for Health Statistics. 1987. *California Birth Cohort File.*
10. Shiono, P. H., Behrman, R. E. 1995. Low birthweight: Analysis and recommendations. *Future of Children,* 5(1), 4–18.
11. Cramer, J. C. 1995. Racial and ethnic differences in birthweight: The role of income and financial assistance. *Demography,* 32(2), 231–247.
12. Shiono, P. H., Klebanoff, M. A., Graubard, B. U., et al. 1986. Birthweight among women of different ethnic groups. *Journal of the American Medical Association,* 255(1), 48–52.
13. Williams, R. L., Binkin, N. J., and Clingman, E. J. 1986. Pregnancy outcomes among Spanish-surname women in California. *American Journal of Public Health,* 76, 387–391.
14. Weeks, J. R., and Rumbaut, J. R. 1991. Infant mortality among ethnic immigrant groups. *Social Science and Medicine,* 33(3), 327–334.
15. Center for Health Policy Research, George Washington University, and the School of Public Health, University of California, Berkeley. 1995. *Mortality Rates among Infants of Mexican Descent in the United States: Evaluating the Validity of Current Estimates.* Washington, D.C.: Author.
16. Selby, M. L. 1984. Validity of the Spanish surname infant mortality rate as a health status indicator of the Mexican American population. *American Journal of Public Health,* 74(9), 998–1002.
17. Teller, C., and Clyburn, S. 1974. Texas population in 1970: Trends in infant mortality. *Texas Business Review,* 40, 240–246.
18. Palloni, A. 1978. Application of an indirect technique to study group dif-

ferentials. In *Demography and Racial and Ethnic Groups,* edited by F. Bean and W. P. Frisbie. New York: Academic Press.

19. Guendelman, S., and Jasis, M. 1992. Giving birth across the border: The San Diego-Tijuana connection. *Social Science and Medicine,* 34(4), 419–425.

20. Yu, E. S. H., and Liu, W. T. 1992. U.S. national health data on Asian Americans and Pacific Islanders: A research agenda for the 1990s. *American Journal of Public Health,* 82(12), 1645–1652.

21. Becerra, J., Hogue, C., Atrash, H., and Perez, N. 1991. Infant mortality among Hispanics: A portrait of heterogeneity. *Journal of the American Medical Association,* 265(2), 217–221.

22. Rogers, R. G. 1989. Ethnic differences in infant mortality: Fact or artifact? *Social Science Quarterly,* 70(3), 642–649.

23. Powell-Griner, E., and Streck, D. 1982. A closer examination of neonatal mortality rates among the Texas Spanish surname population. *American Journal of Public Health,* 72(9), 993–999.

24. Lambert, D. A., and Strauss, L. T. 1987. Analysis of unlinked infant death certificates from the NIMS project. *Public Health Reports,* 102(2), 201–204.

25. Guendelman, S., Chavez, G., and Christianson, R. 1994. Fetal deaths in Mexican American, Black, and White non-Hispanic women seeking government-funded prenatal care. *Journal of Community Health,* 19(5), 319–330.

26. Gann, P., Nghiem, L., and Warner, S. 1989. Pregnancy characteristics and outcomes of Cambodian refugees. *American Journal of Public Health,* 79(9), 1251–1257.

27. Copper, R., Goldenberg, T., DuBard, M., Davis, R., and the collaborative group on preterm birth prevention. 1994. Risk factors for fetal death in white, black and Hispanic women. *Obstetrics and Gynecology,* 84, 490–495.

28. Haub, C., and Yanagishita, M. 1992. *1992 World Population Data Sheet.* Washington, D.C.: Population Reference Bureau.

29. Population Reference Bureau. 1994. UN World Population Prospect 1994 Revision Annex Table A28. Washington, D.C.: Population Reference Bureau.

30. Kasl, S., and Berkman, L. 1983. Health consequences of the experience of migration. *Annual Review of Public Health,* 4, 69–90.

31. Dinerman, I. 1982. *Migrants and Stay-at-Homes: A Comparative Study of Rural Migration from Michoacan, Mexico.* Monograph Series no. 5. La Jolla, Calif.: Center for U.S.-Mexican Studies, University of California, San Diego.

32. Hull, D. 1979. Migration, adaptation, and illness: A review. *Social Science and Medicine,* 13A, 25–36.

33. Frisbie, W. P., and Bean, F. D. 1989. Mexican immigration to the United States: Trends and implications. *International Review of Comparative Public Policy,* 1, 65–95.

34. Portes, A. 1983. International labor migration and national development. In *U.S. Immigration and Refugee Policy: Global and Domestic Issues,* edited by M. M. Kritz. Lexington, Mass.: Lexington Books.

35. Massey, D. 1990. Social structure, household strategies, and the cumulative causation of migration. *Population Index,* 56, 3–26.

36. Guendelman, S. 1987. The incorporation of Mexican women in seasonal migration: A study of gender differences. *Hispanic Journal of Behavioral Sciences,* 9(3), 245–264.

37. Rumbaut, R. G., Chavez, L. R., Moser, R. J., et al. 1988. The politics of migrant health care: A comparative study of Mexican immigrants and Indochinese refugees. *Research in the Sociology of Health Care,* 7, 143–202.

38. Institute of Medicine. 1990. *Nutrition during Pregnancy.* Washington, D.C.: National Academy Press.

39. Abel, E. L. 1980. Smoking during pregnancy: A review of effects on growth and development of offspring. *Human Biology,* 50, 593–625.

40. Wright, J. T., Waterson, E. J., Barrison, I. G., et al. 1983. Alcohol consumption, pregnancy, and low birthweight. *The Lancet,* 1, 663–665.

41. Mills, J. L., Grabaud, B. I., Harley, E. E., et al. 1984. Maternal alcohol consumption and birthweight: How much drinking in pregnancy is safe? *Journal of the American Medical Association,* 252, 1875–1879.

42. Finnegan, L. P. 1988. Drug addiction and pregnancy: The newborn. In *Drugs, Alcohol, Pregnancy and Parenting,* edited by I. J. Chasnoff. Pp. 59–71. Boston: Kluwer Academic Press.

43. Oro, A. S., and Dixon, S. D. 1987. Perinatal cocaine and methamphetamine exposure: Maternal and neonatal correlates. *Journal of Pediatrics,* 111, 571–578.

44. Kramer, M. S. 1987. Determinants of low birthweight: Methodological assessment and meta-analysis. *Bulletin of the World Health Organization,* 65, 663–737.

45. Vega, W. A., Kolody, B., Hwang, J., and Noble, A. 1993. Prevalence and magnitude of perinatal substance exposures in California. *New England Journal of Medicine,* 329, 850–854.

46. Guendelman, S., and Abrams, A. 1994. Dietary, alcohol and tobacco intake among Mexican American women of childbearing age: Results from the HHANES data. *American Journal of Health Promotion,* 8(5), 363–372.

47. Camilli, A., McElroy, L., and Reed, K. 1994. Smoking and pregnancy: A comparison of Mexican American and non-Hispanic white women. *Obstetrics and Gynecology,* 84, 1033–1037.

48. Chomitz, V. R., Cheung, L. W. Y., and Lieberman, E. 1995. The role of lifestyle in preventing low birthweight. *The Future of Children,* 5(1), 121–138.

49. Rumbaut, R. G., and Weeks, J. R. 1994. Unraveling a public health enigma: Why do immigrants experience superior perinatal health outcomes? Paper presented at the 122nd annual meeting of the American Public Health Association, Washington, D.C., November 1.

50. Li, D., Ni, H., Schwartz, S. M., and Daling, J. R. 1990. Secular change in birthweight among Southeast Asian immigrants to the United States. *American Journal of Public Health,* 80(6), 685–688.

51. Caetano, R., and Medina Mora, M. E. 1988. Acculturation and drinking among people of Mexican descent in Mexico and the United States. *Journal of Studies on Alcohol,* 49(5), 462–471.

52. Markides, K. S., Ray, L. A., Stroup-Benham, C. A., and Trevino, F. 1990.

Acculturation and alcohol consumption in the Mexican American population of the southwestern United States: Findings from the HHANES 1982–84. *American Journal of Public Health,* 80(Suppl.), 42–46.

53. Gilbert, M. J., and Cervantes, R. C. 1986. Patterns and practices of alcohol use among Mexican American women: A comprehensive review. *Hispanic Journal of Behavioral Sciences,* 8, 1–60.

54. Holck, S. E., Warren, C. W., Smith, J., and Rochat, R. 1984. Alcohol consumption among Mexican American and Anglo women: Results of a survey along the U.S.-Mexico border. *Journal of Studies on Alcohol,* 45, 149–154.

55. D'Avanzo, C. E., and Frye, B. 1994. Culture, stress and substance use in Cambodian refugee women. *Journal of Studies on Alcohol,* 55, 420–426.

56. Zelson, C., Rubio, E., and Wasserman, E. 1971. Neonatal narcotic addiction: 10-year observation. *Pediatrics,* 48(2), 178–189.

57. Fricker, H., and Segal, S. 1978. Narcotic addiction, pregnancy, and the newborn. *American Journal of Diseases of Children,* 132, 360–366.

58. Lifschitz, M., Wilson, G., Smith, E., et al. 1983. Fetal and postnatal growth of children born to narcotic-dependent women. *Journal of Pediatrics,* 102, 686–691.

59. Robins, L. N., Mills, J. L., Krulewitch, C., and Herman, A. A. 1993. Effects of in utero exposure to street drugs. *American Journal of Public Health,* 83, 12.

60. Oleske, J. 1997. Experiences with 118 infants born to narcotic-using mothers. *Clinical Pediatrics,* 16, 418–423.

61. Newman, V., Norcross, W., and McDonald, R. 1991. Nutrient intake of low-income Southeast Asian pregnant women. *Journal of the American Dietetic Association,* 91, 793–799.

62. Abrams, A., and Berman, C. 1993. Women, nutrition and health. *Current Problems in Obstetrics, Gynecology and Fertility,* 1, 3–61.

63. Guendelman, S., and Abrams, B. 1995. Dietary intake among Mexican American women: Generational differences and a comparison with white non-Hispanic women. *American Journal of Public Health,* 85, 20–25.

64. Guendelman, S., Gould, J., Hudes, M., and Eskenazi, B. 1990. Generational differences in perinatal health among the Mexican American population: Findings from HHANES 1982–84. *American Journal of Public Health,* 80(Suppl.), 61–64.

65. California Department of Health Services, Center for Health Statistics. 1987. *California Birth Cohort File.*

66. Shain, R. 1991. Racial/ethnic differences in adverse pregnancy outcomes. Paper presented at the NICHD Workshop on Infant Mortality and Low Birthweight, Bethesda, Maryland, April 25–26.

67. Cramer, J. C., Bell, K., and Vaast, K. 1991, March. Race, ethnicity, and the determinants of low birthweight in the U.S. Paper presented at the 1991 annual meeting of the Population Association of America, Washington, D.C.

68. Frisbie, W. P., and Bean, F. D. 1995. The Latino family in comparative perspective: Trends and current conditions. In *Racial and Ethnic Families in the United States,* edited by C. Jacobson. Pp. 29–71. New York: Garland.

69. Ramsey, C., Abell, T., and Baker, L. 1986. The relationship between family

functioning, life events, family structure and the outcome of pregnancy. *Journal of Family Practice*, 22, 521–526.

70. McClean, D. E., Hatfield-Timajchy, K., Wingo, P. A., and Floyd, R. L. 1993. Psychosocial measurement: Implications for the study of preterm delivery in black women. *American Journal of Preventive Medicine*, 9(Suppl. 6), 39–81.

71. Keefe, S. E., Padilla, A. M., and Carlos, M. L. 1979. The Mexican American extended family as an emotional support system. *Human Organization*, 38, 144–152.

72. Swicegood, G., Bean, F. D., Stephen, E. H., and Opitz, W. 1988. Language usage and fertility in the Mexican-origin population of the United States. *Demography*, 25(1), 17–33.

73. Bean, F. D., Russell, L. C., and Marcum, J. P. 1977. Familism and marital satisfaction among Mexican Americans: The effects of family size, wife's labor force participation, and conjugal power. *Journal of Marriage and the Family*, 39, 759–776.

74. Triandis, H. C., Kashima, Y., Hui, H., et al. 1982. Acculturation and biculturalism indices among relatively acculturated Hispanic young adults. *Interamerican Journal of Psychology*, 16, 140–149.

75. Alvarez, D., and Bean, F. D. 1976. The Mexican American family. In *Ethnic Families in America*, edited by C. H. Mindel and R. N. Haberstein. Pp. 271–291. New York: Elsevier.

76. Murillo, N. 1976. The Mexican American family. In *Chicanos: Social and Psychological Perspectives*, edited by C. Hernandez. Pp. 15–25. St. Louis: Mosby.

77. Branch, M. P., and Paxton, P. P. 1976. *Providing Safe Nursing Care for Ethnic People of Color*. New York: Appleton-Century-Crofts.

78. De Oliveira, O. 1992. *Trabajo, Fecundidad y Condicion Femenina en Mexico*. El Colegio de Mexico.

79. Rumbaut, R. G., and Weeks, J. R. 1986. Fertility and adaptation: Indochinese refugees in the United States. *International Migration Review*, 20(2), 428–465.

80. Frye, B. A. 1995. Use of cultural themes in promoting health among Southeast Asian refugees. *American Journal of Health Promotion*, 9(4), 269–280.

81. Manderson, L., and Matthews, M. 1981. Vietnamese behavioral and dietary precautions during pregnancy. *Ecology of Food and Nutrition*, 11, 1–8.

82. Kunstadter, P., Kunstadter, S. L., Podhisita, C., and Leepreecha, P. 1993. Demographic variables in fetal and child mortality: Hmong in Thailand. *Social Science and Medicine*, 36(9), 1109–1120.

83. Hopkins, D. D., and Clarke, N. G. 1983. Indochinese refugee fertility rates and pregnancy risk factors, Oregon. *American Journal of Public Health*, 73(11), 1307–1309.

84. D'Avanzo, C. E. 1992. Bridging the cultural gap with Southeast Asians. *Maternal and Child Health Nursing*, 17, 204–208.

85. Faller, H. S. 1992. Hmong women: Characteristics and birth outcomes, 1990. *Birth*, 19(3), 144–150.

86. Swenson, I., Erickson, D., Ehlinger, E., et al. 1986. Birthweight, Apgar scores, labor and delivery complications and prenatal characteristics and older mothers. *Adolescence,* 21(83), 711–722.

87. Reynoso, T. C., Felice, M. E., and Shragg, G. P. 1993. Does American acculturation affect outcome of Mexican-American teenage pregnancy? *Journal of Adolescent Health,* 14, 257–261.

88. Kreiger, N., Rowley, D., Herman, A., et al. 1993. Racism, sexism and social class: Implications for studies of health, disease. *American Journal of Preventive Medicine,* 9(Suppl.), 82–122.

89. Maxwell, B., and Jacobsen, M. 1989. Targeting Hispanics. In *Marketing Disease to Hispanics.* Pp. 27–46. Washington, D.C.: Center for Science in the Public Interest.

90. Mitchell, O., and Greenberg, M. 1991. Outdoor advertising of addictive products. *New Jersey Medicine,* 88, 331–333.

91. Guendelman, S., and English, P. 1995. The effect of United States residence on birth outcomes among Mexican immigrants: An exploratory study. *American Journal of Epidemiology,* 142(Suppl.), S30–S38.

92. U.S. Department of Commerce, Economics and Statistics Administration, Bureau of the Census. 1992. 1990 Census of Population. *General Population Characteristics. California.* Volume 6. Pp. 1–3. Washington, D.C.: Author.

93. Yip, R., Scanlon, K., and Trowbridge, F. 1992. Improving growth status of Asian refugee children in the United States. *Journal of the American Medical Association,* 267(7), 937–940.

94. Story, M., and Harris, L. J. 1988. Food preferences, beliefs, and practices of Southeast Asian refugee adolescents. *Journal of School Health,* 58(7), 273–276.

RACE AND HEALTH

*Implications for Health Care
Delivery and Wellness Promotion*

INTRODUCTION: RACE AND HEALTH

"Race" has been defined as "a subdivision of the human species, characterized by a more or less distinctive combination of physical traits that
are transmitted in descent" and "health" as "the general condition of
the body or mind with reference to soundness and vigor."[1] There is no
obvious reason for these "concepts" to be linked. However, large differences have been noted in the state of "health" between the various racial
groups for many years. Racism and the lack of quality of health care are
not unique to African Americans, but because the author is most familiar with their impact on this group, the discussion to follow will emphasize these issues as they relate to them. The author believes that this discussion addresses concerns that are universal and should be of value to
all Americans who are forced to live with people with skin of a different
color than their own and/or to vote on issues related in any way to race
and ethnicity.

African Americans have always had a lower survival rate than Whites
in this country. Evidence has also always existed suggesting that "nongenetic" explanations have been the dominant causes. For example,
based on a study conducted in 1908, Irish and Italian men living in New
York City actually had a higher mortality rate than Black men living
at that time.[2] Furthermore, for many years it has been known that discrepancies in survival within racial groups varied more by residence
(rural vs. urban) than between races.[3] It is also noteworthy that recent

studies have demonstrated that White men in the Soviet Union currently have a substantially shorter life expectancy than all American men.[4]

Despite the kinds of data noted here, a body of literature has been perpetuated for many years in this country arguing that "race" is a biologic phenomenon associated with some less-than-desirable health consequences. James H. Jones summarized the position of prominent 19th-century physicians in his book *Bad Blood:*[5,6]

> Vociferous advocates of black inferiority such as Dr. Josiah Clark Nott of Mobile and Dr. Samuel A. Cartwright of New Orleans published numerous articles during the 1840s and 1850s on diseases and physical properties thought to be peculiar to blacks. Drs. Nott and Cartwright were merely the best known of a group of southern physicians who helped inflame the controversy over slavery. Among the diseases said to be unique to blacks were Cachexia Africana (dirt-eating) and Struma Africana ("Negro consumption"). Influenced by these physicians, slave holders who wished to treat their bondsmen without benefit of professional help begged southern doctors to write medical manuals on the treatment of blacks. Their requests went unanswered. Instead, physicians simply continued to assert that blacks were medically inferior to whites without offering a plausible medical explanation based on racial differences. Their observations were perfect for polemics but useless for the care of sick blacks.

It was in fact this type of thinking that led to the Tuskegee syphilis experiments. Researchers from the U.S. Public Health Service in the 1930s justified studying untreated syphilis in Blacks because they believed that they knew the natural history of syphilis in Whites (based on an old Scandinavian study) and wanted to prove the hypothesis that syphilis was different in Blacks. Since this atrocity, numerous other papers have been published that imply that being a member of the Black race has a detrimental/adverse effect on the length of survival. Implicit in many of these studies is the suggestion that race is a "real biologic factor," meaning that it must be considered as a separate factor from tumor- or treatment-related factors.

For more than 20 years there has existed clear documentation of an excess cancer mortality in Black Americans compared to White Americans.[5] This excess mortality experienced by Black Americans is associated with a disproportionate financial burden because of the lower incomes, higher unemployment, and the inadequacy of health care resources that are currently available to this community. The impact of the excess mortality rate and the financial burden are magnified by the increased incidence of common cancer sites among Black Americans.

There is no definitive explanation for the discrepancy in survival. Are these differences in health state due to intrinsic genetic tendencies associated with "race," or does belonging to a racial group impact health by "nongenetic" mechanisms?

The assumption that there are major differences in biologic behavior related to race continues to be a theme of medical doctors even today. For example, in the July 1997 issue of the prestigious peer-reviewed *Journal of Urology*, Moul et al. published a paper titled "Black Race Is an Adverse Prognostic Factor. . . ."[7] Later, in an even more widely read journal, *Cancer*, these investigators published an article describing an equation that could be used to predict the risk of failing a radical prostatectomy that incorporated "Black race" as an unfavorable biologic parameter.[8] Both of these papers included relatively small numbers of patients, and neither provided an in-depth discussion of alternative explanations. The successful publication of these papers, despite their failure to discuss other explanations, suggests that the reviewers were in agreement with the authors. Clearly there appears to be a critical mass of researchers who believe that "race" has an intrinsic impact on health. As a result of this established dogma, some researchers have found it difficult to publish papers opposing this notion.

For example, in the 1980s a paper was published in *Cancer* describing the poor outcome of Blacks (n = 92) treated for laryngeal cancer at Harlem Hospital. In response to this paper, I submitted a paper representing a 20-year experience from a Veterans Administration hospital including more than 300 patients demonstrating that the long-term survival in Blacks and Whites was identical.[2] In our paper, I explained that based on the details provided, the care delivered appeared to have been suboptimal in the previously published paper. A major criticism of our paper (resulting in a rejection by *Cancer*) was that we would need "1200 patients to prove that Blacks did not do worse." Since there has never been a paper published in the world's literature on laryngeal cancer that included more than approximately 600 patients, we were placed into an obvious "catch-22" situation. The reviewers believed that the burden of proof should lay on our shoulders and that, until proven otherwise, race should be considered a significant independent determinant of outcome. But is this true?

The answer to this question has a number of implications for the delivery of health care. First, the recognition of genetic differences could allow specific populations to be targeted for the delivery of certain types of health care. After accepting such occurrences as "fact," interventions could be designed to meet the unique needs of these populations. Cost-effective guidelines could be developed for prevention, early detection, and treatment specifically for these populations. Furthermore, social resources might be allocated to support basic research devoted to defining the genetic defects and mechanisms resulting in a worse state of health. Conversely, resources would not be allocated to support basic research devoted to identifying the genetic defects if there was no "genetic defect" to detect. Instead, "nongenetic" causes such as diet, lifestyle, environment, or lack of access to health care might need to be addressed. But do we really want to know?

DO WE REALLY WANT TO KNOW?

Before discussing data assessing the merits of genetic and nongenetic causes, there are several questions that should be answered. First, since race has "been around forever," why do these questions still persist? Is this due to lack of data, or could it be that "we" really do not want to know? Stephen J. Gould recognized this issue and began his book *The Mismeasure of Man* with the following quote from Charles Darwin's *Voyage of the Beagle:*[9]

> If the misery of our poor be caused not by the laws of nature, but by our institutions, great is our sin.

If the basis for the excess mortality among certain racial groups is an intrinsic characteristic of the group, some might consider this a sign of "racial inferiority." Although such a possibility would say nothing about the moral, creative, humanitarian, or other more important features of an individual, members of such a racial group are still likely to be defensive. Conversely, if the excess mortality rate is entirely due to various types of social injustices (such as racism and discrimination, resulting in lack of education, underemployment, and poor access to care, resulting in a fatalistic self-destructive lifestyle), the moral and financial implications would be staggering.

To understand the development of the notion of some sort of inherent tendency for Blacks to be "genetically less healthy," it is best to assess the sources of this belief. Therefore, it is important to look back at the history of events in the history of this country that might have had an impact on the health status of and beliefs about African Americans. The financial implications (liabilities) should also be most obvious if viewed from this context.

RACE AND HEALTH IN A HISTORICAL CONTEXT: MOSTLY A BLACK-AND-WHITE ISSUE?

Just as the issue of "racism in America" is usually perceived as largely a "Black versus White" issue, the issue of "race and health" is often seen in a similar context. For example, annual reports sponsored by the federal government compare outcomes between Blacks and Whites and routinely ignore other groups.[5] It is a simple matter to find 20 to 30 publications comparing outcomes between Black women and White women with breast cancer, but similar studies for other groups are lacking. This reality may result from the several facts. First, Hispanics are generally considered as an ethnic group, not as a race. When Hispanics are placed into one of the major three groups (Blacks, Whites, and Asians), they are for the most part considered "White." Second, for Asians, including Pacific Islanders, and Native American Indians, the details surrounding the impact of racism on their health is both complex and heterogeneous. This is not to suggest that the health issues for these groups are any less important but rather that (1) they are not as well documented, (2) for most health outcome end points (e.g., death due to cancer) the differences are not as large and in some cases favor the Asian populations, (3) differences in social status have not been as clearly enforced by the laws of the land, and (4) over the last 400 years fewer individuals belonging to this "racial group" have been impacted by racism.

The circumstances surrounding the arrival of African people to this country are likely to explain some of the problems in health status seen today. Between 1501 and 1870, it has been estimated that between 9.5 and 14.6 million African people were brought to America in bondage.[10] Furthermore, it is believed that nearly as many African people died, resisting capture, via suicide, or en route, due to hardships. The mortality rates at sea alone have ranged from as high as 33% to as low 12%.[11] It is obvious that the first generation of African Americans had a very short life expectancy. Harley has summarized selected historical events reflecting social events of note in the history of African Americans, and some of these are listed in Table 10.1.[12] Harsh punishments and intolerance were the rule, and it was more than 250 years before the first Black man (who was a slave at the time) was licensed as a physician. This being the

TABLE 10.1 TIME LINE OF SELECTED EVENTS IMPACTING THE HEALTH OF AFRICAN AMERICANS (1492–1997)

Years	Event	Comments
1492	Pedro Alonzo Nino, a navigator of the *Santa Maria,* arrives with Christopher Columbus.	
1502	Portugal lands its first cargo of enslaved Africans in the Western Hemisphere.	
1501 to 1870 (369 years)	Slavery delivered between 9.5 and 14.6 million African people to the Americas, and nearly as many are thought to have died, resisting capture, via suicide, or en route due to hardships.	After 369 years of slavery, and other acts of violence, what reparations would be due these people and their offspring?
1692	Virginia enacts law making it lawful to kill a runaway slave in the course of apprehension.	
1693	Philadelphia: Law permitting Whites to "take up" any Black found without a pass.	
1762	James Derham becomes the first Black man licensed to practice medicine in the United States and 21 years later purchases his freedom.	
1809	New York law sanctions marriage within the Black community.	Married Blacks were not legally recognized as such before this law.
1810	19% of the U.S. population is Black, but only 9% are free.	
1863	The Emancipation Proclamation goes into effect, freeing slaves held in states in rebellion against the Union, *but not in portions of Louisiana, Eastern Virginia, West Virginia, or border states (3).*	Although slaves were freed, they were not able to vote and continued to be systematically oppressed.
1866	The first Civil Rights Act is passed over President Andrew Johnson's veto, declaring Blacks free and nullifying "Black codes."	"Black codes" restrict the rights of freedmen/women.
1868	14th Amendment is passed, granting Blacks "full citizenship and equal rights."	
1890	U.S. Supreme Court allows states to segregate public facilities and control of elections.	
1896	"Separate but equal" facilities ruled constitutional.	

(continues)

Years	Event	Comments
1898–1910	Louisiana, Georgia, North Carolina, Virginia, Alabama, and Oklahoma adopt the "grandfather clause."	Males could vote only if their fathers or grandfathers were eligible to vote.
1932	Tuskegee experiments begun.	
1940	U.S. Congress passes Selective Training and Service Act.	Includes an antidiscrimination clause and a 10% quota system to ensure racial integration.
1957	Civil Rights Act of 1957 passed, authorizing the federal government to bring civil suits on the behalf of citizens.	First Civil Rights Act since 1875.
1964	U.S. Congress passes the Civil Rights Act and establishes the Equal Opportunity Commission (EEOC).	This law was passed to offset hundreds of years of systematic discrimination and racism, but it failed.
1971	National Cancer Act and SEER program established.	SEER created to collect, analyze, and disseminate data.
1994	Black-White Breast Cancer Study: Race not an independent prognostic factor.	Having a high poverty index, lack of insurance, and increased body mass index, and being divorced, separated, or never married associated with a poor outcome.
1994	RTOG 9202 demonstrates that Blacks have more advanced prostate cancer.	More advanced prostate cancer by virtue of higher PSAs not in the clinical stage.
1995	Proposition 209 goes into effect in California, banning Affirmative Action to compensate for past discrimination.	How many years of affirmative action compensate for 369 years of slavery and many years of systematic discrimination and oppression?
1996	RTOG 9412 and the A2 demographic studies.	Both demonstrate that Blacks continue to have lower incomes, less education, and more advanced disease.
1997	CALGB 8541, based on a prospective randomized trial including 1,500 women; race not an independent factor.	Black women continue to have an excess mortality rate from breast cancer.
1997	CA Journal published demonstrating 59% five-year survival for Whites versus 44% for Blacks.	This 1.4-times greater risk of cancer death is the largest recorded since 1960.
1997	Courts rule against "set-aside programs" in Philadelphia for city works programs.	Similar programs struck down in Columbus, Ohio, and Miami.

case, it should not be surprising to find that individuals who were denied participation in traditional medicine would have poor health as assessed by this traditional medicine.

Of note, although the Emancipation Proclamation was passed in 1863 freeing some slaves, it did not apply in portions of Louisiana, Eastern Virginia, West Virginia, or border states. Moreover, freed men and women continued to be systematically oppressed. Consequently, three years after the Emancipation Proclamation, "Black codes" (which systematically restricted the rights of freed men and women) were passed over the veto of the U.S. president.

Two years later the 14th Amendment granted African Americans full citizenship and equal rights. However, 30 years later "separate but equal" was ruled constitutional and "grandfather clauses" (allowing males to vote only if one's father or grandfather voted) were upheld in a number of states (1898–1910). Finally, after 369 years of slavery and 87 years of systematic discrimination, the Civil Rights Act of 1957 was passed. Later the U.S. Congress passed the Civil Rights Act of 1964.

In 1971 the National Cancer Act establishing the SEER (Surveillance Epidemiology End Result) program was created to collect, analyze, and disseminate data useful in the diagnosis and treatment of cancer.[1] These SEER data are published annually and are considered to be the "gold standard" by physicians throughout this country. From 1973 to 1990 information on approximately 1.6 million cases has been collected. Approximately 9.6 percent of the population of the United States is included in the geographic areas making up the database for the SEER program.[1] Since the natural histories of treated and untreated cancers of various types have been well studied, this disease will be considered in some detail to assess the prognostic significance of race.

RACE, CANCER SURVIVAL, AND SEER DATA

A close look at the primary cancer sites for which differences between White and Black Americans are most apparent is required to identify the causes for the survival discrepancies. Five-year survivals based on SEER data for all cancer sites among Blacks and Whites is shown in Figure 10.1. Although the five-year relative survival rate is 54.5% for White patients, it is only 39.4% for Blacks.[1] These data suggest that if you are Black and diagnosed as having cancer, your risk of dying from cancer within five years is 50% higher than for Whites. Equally alarming is the fact that the percentage change in the mortality from 1973 to 1990 increased 16% for Blacks compared to 6% for Whites. These data under-score the magnitude of the cancer health care crisis for African Americans in this country. A similar comparison for cancer outcome differences for two of the most common cancer sites in men and women is discussed in the following.

Figure 10.2 compares the outcome for Black and White men with carcinoma of the prostate. Only 64.4% of Black men diagnosed with prostate cancer were alive at five years compared to 79.4% of White men. This marked difference in survival appears to be a continuing trend with a greater increase in the mortality in Blacks compared to Whites from 1973 to 1990. Of further interest, a much greater increase in the per-centage change in incidence was noted among Whites. This trend prob-ably reflects the more frequent use of the serum marker PSA (prostate-specific antigen) to detect otherwise occult disease in this population. In other words, although the risk of prostate cancer is lower among White men than among Black men, more of the former are systematically be-ing screened.

Figure 10.3 compares the outcome for breast cancer by race. Again a lower survival is noted for Black women compared to White women, with 64.2% and 80.5%, respectively, alive at five years. A 21.4% increase in the percentage change in mortality was noted for Blacks compared to 2% for Whites during this same time period (1973–1990).

The tendency for Black Americans to present with more advanced disease is one of the common explanations offered for these difference in survival.[13] However, even after correcting for the stage of disease, many studies still report an excess mortality rate among Blacks.[1,13–15] For selected sites, differences in socioeconomic status (SES) have also been proposed as an explanation for differences in survival.[14,16,17] However, some studies failed to demonstrate an effect due to SES when the quality of care was comparable.[18,19] Furthermore, a biologic mechanism explain-ing how SES affects outcome is lacking. The possibility that differences in cancer-related mortality might be due to factors such as the quality of the medical care received has not been adequately evaluated. Several studies document differences in initial treatment, patterns of care, the intensity of services provided, as well as a tendency for racial bias in the inpatient setting.[20–24] These last two observations support the notion that lifestyle and nongenetic factors may be the overwhelming determinant of the health status for most people. The fact that recent studies continue to demonstrate changes in mortality in both races as a reflection of lifestyle changes provides additional support for the truism that "you are what

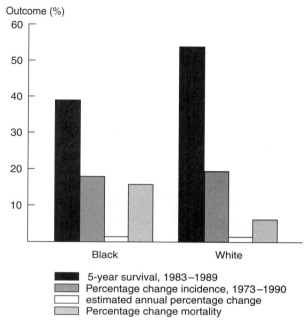

Figure 10.1.   SEER race data, all sites.

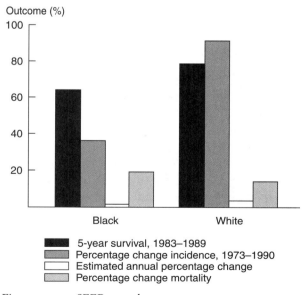

Figure 10.2.   SEER race data, prostate cancer.

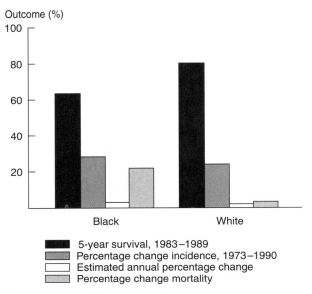

Figure 10.3. SEER race data, breast cancer.

you do" (eat, drink, smoke, exercise), while our genetic makeup is trying to help us survive.

RACE AND HEALTH CARE POLICIES
AND THE CURRENT BELIEF CONSTRUCT

It is clear that Blacks have a lower survival than Whites for a number of common cancers. In response to these kinds of data, in late 1993 the National Cancer Institute (NCI) mandated that cooperative groups conducting large prospective randomized trials involving cancer treatment must include in their study design mechanisms to address the issue of race and cancer outcome (if the published literature suggests that race or gender might affect outcome).[25] This mandate represents a major health care policy decision that could potentially impact the design and implementation of most randomized trials conducted in the United States because for most of the common cancer sites there is a discrepancy in survival between Blacks and Whites.

In addition to explicitly affecting cancer research protocol design policies, the published literature supporting the intrinsic importance of

TABLE 10.2   CURRENT BELIEF
CONSTRUCT THAT DIRECTS
HEALTH CARE POLICY RESEARCH

Conclusions	Results
Cancer survival differences exist for Blacks and Whites.	Race is assumed to be an independent prognostic factor. More data are generated to prove that differences exist.
The burden of proof to the contrary rests on others attempting to disprove.	Biologic basis is assumed for the observed differences in survival by race.
This "biologic" phenomenon should be studied further.	Cancer researchers are funded to study the "racial biology."
There is nothing you can do about a person's race but . . .	. . . perhaps understanding the molecular basis of cancer will be directly helpful (to researchers).

race has tainted the beliefs of many epidemiologists and health care providers. The current belief construct implied by much of the published literature on race and survival from cancer is shown in Table 10.2. Race is attributed independent prognostic significance for survival from cancer. This belief construct is supported by numerous publications demonstrating differences in cancer survival by race, without data to explain the differences. Otherwise, why have data not been repeatedly published comparing the survival of janitors and physicians or of policemen and preachers? The mind-set of expecting to see racial differences frames the comparisons that are made.

This mind-set is contrary to what should be acknowledged as our social norm. Consistent with our social norms opposing racial stereotypes, race should be implicated only as a diagnoses by exclusion. In other words, only after other plausible explanations have been ruled out should race be implicated. If the survival differences noted were attributed to differences in the stage at presentation or to the quality of cancer care received, race should not be the focus of investigation.

AN ALTERNATIVE BELIEF
CONSTRUCT AND EXTENT OF DISEASE BIAS

An alternative belief construct to explain the observed differences in survival by race is summarized in Table 10.3. The implications for this al-

TABLE 10.3   AN ALTERNATIVE
BELIEF CONSTRUCT FOR DIRECTING
CANCER RESEARCH POLICIES

Beliefs	Implications
Cancer survival differences between Blacks and Whites can be explained by differences in the extent of disease at diagnosis and quality of care.	Race is *not* an independent prognostic factor.
The burden of proof to the contrary rests on others attempting to prove that race is a prognostic factor.	"Racism" is *not* perpetuated by "science."
Differences in outcomes should be studied further to identify causes.	Research should focus on differences in the knowledge, behavior, and environment as well as on access and the quality of care.
There is something that you can do about lack of jobs, education, environmental factors, and quality of health care. Lack of health is a symptom of social diseases.	Intervention is *directly helpful* to the people being studied and experiencing the excess mortality. Social changes improve health.

ternative belief construct for future research funding and patient care are also included in this table. This belief construct hinges on the notion that the observed differences in survival can be explained by factors other than race.

An epidemiologic phenomenon that I have chosen to call "extent of disease bias" (EDB) may explain much of the reported survival differences. Staging systems represent somewhat arbitrary ways to separate patients in prognostic groups for the purposes of comparison.[26,27] Historically, these systems usually were primarily based on the size of the tumor as determined by palpation and usually referred to as the "T" stage, with categories 1 through 4.[27] These systems typically also depend on the extent of lymph node involvement, defined by size, location, and number.[27–30] The break points for these staging systems typically reflected whether it was believed that a tumor could be completely resected.

Extent of disease bias results from two major types of shortcomings of the current staging systems. First, the currently used staging systems are overly crude in the degree of absolute separation or "the degree of fineness of separation" of distinct prognostic groups. Second, the current staging systems are designed primarily to answer a question of the relative probability of cure rather than the duration of survival among those patients who are not curable. This shortcoming reflects "the disproportionate predictive priorities" of the current staging systems.

THE EXTENT OF DISEASE BIAS (EDB) MODEL

Figures 10.4 to 10.6 compare two hypothetical populations with differences in the distribution of the extent of disease at presentation. Population A is composed of a cohort of relatively well educated individuals, of higher socioeconomic status, who tend to present with earlier-stage disease. Cohort B is composed of individuals of lower socioeconomic status, with less education and a high percentage being uninsured, who tend to present with more advanced disease. In this model it is assumed that for each population of cancer patients there is a "bell-shaped" distribution of disease-specific survivals that correlates with the extent of disease. This disease-specific survival distribution is a direct reflection of, and consequently is proportional to, the extent of disease. The term "extent of disease" as used in this model takes into account the volume of the tumor and the degree to which the tumor has spread. Extent of disease also includes the fact that with time, biologic changes tend to occur in the aggressiveness of tumors, which may not be manifested as differences in the tumor volume or extent of spread.

Figure 10.4 compares the distribution of cancer in populations A and B using a relatively "crude" staging system, with early, intermediate, and advanced disease corresponding to stages 1, 2, and 3, respectively. Of note, a larger percentage of individuals in population B have stage 3 disease and fewer have stage 1, while a similar percentage of members from both populations have stage 2 disease. It would seem appropriate to most observers that a survival comparison of patients with stage 2 disease from populations A and B would be valid. This may not be the case, however.

Figure 10.5 compares the same groups using a "superstaging" system composed of 12 stage categories instead of three. Figure 10.6 is a "magnified view" of the intermediate extent of disease group. This intermediate extent of disease group corresponds to superstages 5 to 8 and the "crude" stage 2 group. Using the superstaging system it is now apparent that more group B members belonging to the intermediate extent of disease group have superstage 8 and that more group A members have superstage 5. Because of these differences, group B members would be expected to do worse than group A members. An analysis using crude staging would suggest that group membership had independent prognostic significance. In contrast, an analysis using the superstaging system is likely to demonstrate that group membership has *no* prognostic significance independent of the true extent of disease (see Figures 10.5 and 10.6).

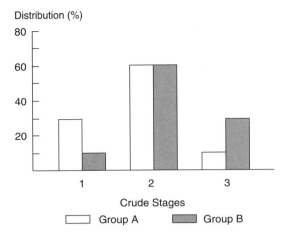

Figure 10.4. Extent of Disease Bias Model: Example of distribution differences in two populations of patients with cancer.

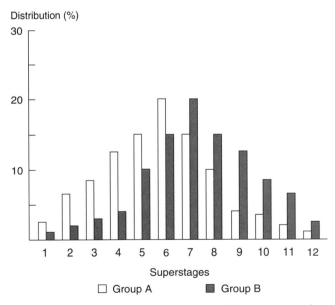

Figure 10.5. Extent of Disease Bias Model: Comparing distribution differences in two populations with cancer using superstaging.

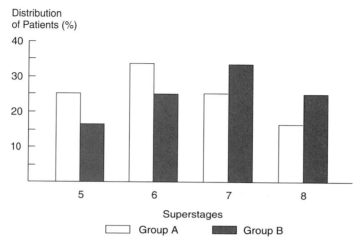

Figure 10.6. Extent of Disease Bias Model Example: Superstages 5 to 8 versus crude stage 2.

SEER DATA AND THE EDB MODEL

Examples taken from published literature demonstrating the potential for EDB for Blacks and Whites with prostate and breast cancer are shown in Figures 10.7 and 10.8. Note that in both the examples shown the distribution of disease is similar to that of populations A and B in the EDB crude staging model. The extent of disease in cancer patients is not naturally divided into three or four distinct groups. Rather, there is a continuum. The less precisely populations are defined, the more likely patients with extensive disease will be "lumped" with patients with less extensive disease. Therefore, differences in the distribution characteristics in two populations can confound an analysis of outcome.

Examples of the Potential for EDB from (Non-SEER-Based) Cancer Treatment Literature

In addition to SEER data, numerous other examples of distribution differences between Blacks and Whites exist in the medical literature.[13,14,26] The same pattern is seen in all these studies: The distribution of cancer in Blacks is "right shifted." The term "right shifted" refers to the relative displacement of the overall shape of the extent of disease distribution toward more advanced stages for Blacks compared to less advanced disease for Whites. The "cruder" the staging system used, the more biased the interpretation is likely to be.

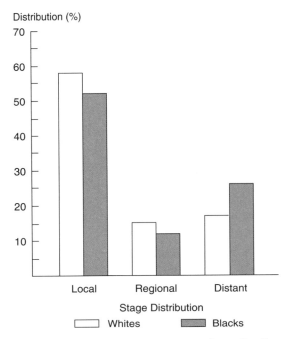

Distribution (%)

Stage Distribution

☐ Whites   ■ Blacks

Figure 10.7.   SEER prostate cancer: Stage distribution data, 1983 to 1987.

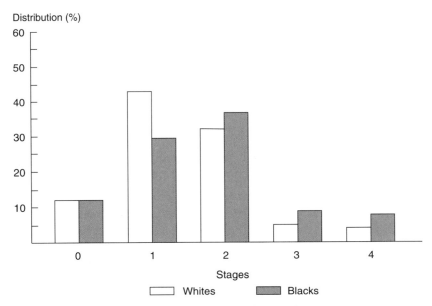

Distribution (%)

Stages

☐ Whites   ■ Blacks

Figure 10.8.   SEER breast cancer: Stage distribution data, 1990.

Examples of how the degree of fineness of separation within a given stage can affect prognosis are available throughout the cancer literature. Rosen et al., for example, reported that within the category of patients with T1 No Mo breast carcinoma (stage I), significant differences in prognosis exist based on the size of the primary tumor.[28] For example, patients with a primary breast tumor less than 1.0 centimeter had an 83% relapse free survival (RFS) at 10 years compared to a 73% RFS for patients with primaries 1.1 to 2.0 centimeters. This represents an excess relapse risk of 59% at 10 years. Differences of this magnitude are common in the series, which report breast cancer survival differences between Blacks and Whites. If the distribution of the extent of breast cancer was such that a larger percentage of Black women had lesions in the 1.1- to 2.0-centimeter range and a larger percentage of Whites had lesions in the range less than or equal to 1.0 centimeter, it is possible that despite "correcting for stage," an analysis might suggest that there were survival differences due to race.

DISPROPORTIONATE PREDICTIVE PRIORITIES

The current staging systems are designed primarily to predict surgical curability.[27-30] Patients who are not curable tend to be lumped into a category that is composed of a heterogeneous group of individuals with a poor long-term prognosis. Although such patients uniformly have a poor long-term prognosis, there can be significant differences in short-term survival. These differences can significantly affect the overall survival curve because a large number of patients fall into this category. Examples can be found in the literature where the differences in survival for patients belonging to the same stage may vary from less than 6 weeks to 6 months to a few years.[29,30] Thus, the current staging systems have disproportionate predictive priorities in the sense that with an increase in the extent of disease, the staging system becomes progressively less discriminating in terms of identifying various prognostic subgroups.

An example of these phenomena is the ability of the current staging systems used to predict the outcome for the average patients with lung cancer. Although most patients who present with lung cancer do not have curable disease (overall five-year survival is about 10%), the staging system is biased in favor of subcategories of patients who are considered potentially surgically resectable.[30] The most widely used staging system is characterized by having four out of six of the major substaging categories dedicated to the small percentage of patients who are considered to be candidates for surgical resection with curative intent. Since only approximately 10% are alive at five years, it is obvious that this staging system is not designed to be of prognostic value for the subgroups to which the typical patient belongs. For example, Albain et al. demonstrated that among patients with metastatic lung cancer (all the same stage), the survival is noted to have been highly variable.[29] In this retrospective analysis a subgroup of patients could be identified with a one-year survival of 27%, while another subgroup could be identified with an expected one-year survival of only 7%. Even larger differences in the range of survivals have been noted among subgroups of patients presenting with certain other types of cancer, such as metastatic prostate and breast cancer. Since these are the two most common primaries occurring in men and women, we will use data for these sites to demonstrate the existence of EDB. Awareness of EDB may allow biases that might result from it to be minimized in future epidemiologic studies.

BREAST CANCER AND EDB: RETROSPECTIVE STUDIES

Although SEER data and numerous studies report a lower survival for Black women with breast cancer, several recent studies strongly suggest that race is not an independent prognostic factor.[13,14,16,18,26,31–42] A detailed analysis of this issue was reported by Roach and Alexander.[26] These authors reviewed the available published literature comparing the survival of Blacks to Whites with breast cancer treated from 1968 to 1988. The five-year survival for Blacks was less than or equal to that of Whites in all studies (difference range about 0 to 19%). However, in 11 of the 18 studies (61%), the reported differences in five-year survival between Blacks and Whites was less than or equal to 3%. We generated a "reliability scoring scale" based primarily on the level of staging sophistication used (crude staging resulted in lower scores) and the likelihood that the quality of care was comparable. Next the relationship between the reliability score and survival was analyzed. Those studies reporting large differences in five-year survival generally had low reliability scores, while those with high scores tended to have small differences in survival.

BREAST CANCER DATA FROM PROSPECTIVE RANDOMIZED TRIALS

Using patients treated on phase III prospective randomized trials avoids potential bias due to differences in the initial staging workup and treatment; thus, assessments of outcome by race are likely to be more accurate.[40-43] Such trials involve recruiting patients with a specific type and stage of cancer to be randomly assigned to receive either the best conventional treatment or a "newer" type of treatment that is believed to possibly be better. Such trials ensure well-defined guidelines for staging, eligibility, and uniformity in treatment and follow-up. These trials are also designed to stratify or balance patients for other factors that could confound the outcome of the study. Three cooperative groups conducting large phase III randomized trials have recently completed analysis of breast cancer treatment outcome by race. The Southwest Oncology Group (SWOG), the Cancer and Leukemia Group B (CALGB), and the National Surgical Adjuvant Breast Program (NSABP) all found that race was not a significant independent prognostic factor for survival from breast cancer.[41-43] Thus, based on the data from the major cooperative groups doing prospective randomized trials, race has been shown not to be a significant independent prognostic factor. These data must be viewed as the most accurate data available on which to judge the significance of race and survival from breast cancer.

The findings of these studies are consistent with the EDB model. However, there are some differences in the presentation of breast cancer in Black and White women that remain unexplained. For example, it is well known that breast cancer is less common in Black women, and some studies suggest that there is an earlier age of onset.[44-46] These differences may be due to the average age of first pregnancy, diet, intrinsic genetic differences, or other factors yet to be defined. Table 10.4 summarizes the findings reached following a prospective study of Black and White women with breast cancer that demonstrated that poverty, martial status, health insurance status, and body mass but not race correlated with death due to breast cancer.[46] Failure to account for differences in these areas may explain at least a portion of the impression reached by some researchers that race was likely to be an independent prognostic factor.

PROSTATE CANCER AND EDB:
RETROSPECTIVE STUDIES

A number of retrospective studies have been published addressing the prognostic significance of race and survival from prostate cancer.[12,13,15,17,18,23,47-53] Austin et al. conducted a retrospective study including 914 patients (867 Whites, 47 Blacks) treated with radiation

TABLE 10.4   SOCIODEMOGRAPHY AND
THE RELATIVE RISK OF DYING OF BREAST
CANCER AMONG BLACK AND WHITE WOMEN

Factor	Relative Risk[a]
Poverty index > 400 (high income)	$0.6 \times (0.4-0.7)$
Divorced, separated	$1.6 \times (1.2-2.2)$
Never married	$1.6 \times (1.0-2.5)$
No health insurance	$2.3 \times (1.5-3.5)$
High body mass index ("overweight")	$2.2 \times (1.5-3.2)$

[a]Unadjusted hazard ratios (95% confidence intervals), modified from Eley et al. (1994 [46]).

therapy.[15] The data were obtained from the Connecticut SEER Tumor Registry and included patients with locally advanced disease (stage T_2–T_4) who were treated from 1973 to 1987. According to these authors, after multivariate analysis controlling for stage and grade, Blacks had a lower survival. Natarajan et al. also noted a lower overall survival for Blacks with prostate cancer.[49] They reported no differences for patients with early stage (T_1) prostate cancer and less than a 10% difference in the five-year survival for patients with stages T_2 and T_4 prostate cancer but larger differences for patients with T_3 lesions. Neither the cause specific survival, the comparability of the quality of care, nor an adjustment for the distribution of other known prognostic factors is possible in these two studies. Perez et al. reported similar findings for patients with more advanced disease.[50] The small number of Blacks included in two of these studies and the mixed nature of the results in the larger study make it difficult to draw definitive conclusions from these studies.

A number of other investigators have reported race to be of no independent significance after adjustment for other prognostic factors.[51-53] In contrast to the series reporting a difference in survival as a function of race, either all these series were likely to have provided a similar quality of care (single institution study or as part of a randomized trial) or an adjustment was made for socioeconomic status (perhaps a predictor for quality care). This is important because of studies showing that Blacks tend to be treated less aggressively.[18]

DATA FROM PROSPECTIVE
RANDOMIZED TRIALS: PROSTATE CANCER

The largest prospective database available for assessing the outcome following definitive radiotherapy for clinically localized prostate cancer is possessed by the Radiation Therapy Oncology Group (RTOG). Using this database Roach et al. evaluated the prognostic significance of race among 1,294 patients who participated in three prospective randomized trials conducted between 1976 and 1985.[54] One hundred and twenty (9%) of the patients were coded as Black, while 1,077 (83%) of the patients were coded as White. Two of the three studies (RTOG 7706 and 8307) revealed that race was not of prognostic significance for disease-free or overall survival. Protocol 7506 revealed that the median survival for Blacks was somewhat shorter (5.4 years vs. 7.1 years, $p = 0.02$). But a higher percentage of Blacks treated on 7506 had an abnormally elevated serum acid phosphatase compared to Whites ($p = 0.006$), and the time to distant failure (primarily spread to bone) tended to be shorter ($p = 0.07$). These findings suggest that Blacks treated on 7506 may have had more extensive disease at presentation. Based on these prospective randomized trials, it is most likely that the lower survival noted for Black Americans with prostate cancer reflects the tendency for Blacks to present with more advanced disease.

Based on the available literature, the preponderance of evidence suggests that after adjustment for the extent of disease, when treatment is comparable, there are no differences in survival from early stage prostate cancer that can be attributed to race.[51-54] For more advanced disease, it is likely that the survival differences reflect differences in the distribution of disease at the time of diagnoses that are not accounted for in the staging system used.[54,55] Since many of the patients treated for prostate cancer are staged clinically and not pathologically, accurately determining the true extent of disease in prostate cancer patients is more difficult than for breast cancer. These inaccuracies in staging, and the differences in the disease distribution in these two populations, result in EDB. Additionally, there are a multitude of socioeconomic differences that might explain differences in outcome.[56] For example, in a large demographic study we noted clear differences in income status and the educational level of Blacks and Whites treated on phase III randomized trials. Clearly, having less support and a poorer understanding of your disease is not likely to be beneficial.

OTHER PRIMARY CANCER SITES IN ADULTS AND OUTCOME FOR CHILDHOOD CANCERS

In addition to breast and prostate cancer studies, data from prospective randomized trials and retrospective reviews of a number of other cancer sites fail to support the independent prognostic significance of race.[57-61]

For example, race was not an independent prognostic factor for survival among patients who participated in lung, brain, or esophageal cancer trials conducted by the RTOG.[57–59] The Southwest Oncology Group evaluated the prognostic significance of race and survival from multiple myeloma, a hematologic malignancy that is known to occur more frequently in Blacks (two to one, compared to Whites) and to be associated with a higher mortality rate in Blacks.[60] This study included 614 patients who were treated on a prospective randomized trial comparing two different chemotherapy regimens. There was no difference in survival by race, and the authors concluded that "the observed differences in mortality between blacks and whites cannot be attributed to differences in survival . . . given comparable care."

A large study of childhood cancers reported by investigators from the St. Jude Children's Research Hospital demonstrated rather conclusively that with "equal access to effective contemporary" care, Black children have the same outcomes as White children. This study included more than 5,000 Black and White children treated for cancer between January 1962 and June 1992. These investigators noted that in the early years, Blacks had a lower survival rate largely due to more advanced disease at the time of diagnosis, but in more recent years there was no difference in outcome by race.[61] Thus, as with adults, the preponderance of evidence suggests that race is not an independent prognostic factor for survival from childhood cancer.

IMPLICATIONS OF EDB

Following an extensive review of the available published data, race does not appear to be a major independent prognostic factor for survival from cancer. Instead, an epidemiologic phenomenon, EDB, may explain all or much of the apparent discrepancy in survival. This phenomenon is due to two related factors. First, the available staging systems are crude measures of the true extent or severity of disease. These staging systems are designed primarily to predict whether patients are curable and not specifically to predict the duration of survival. This limitation is most obvious when applied to patients with advanced cancer. Second, differences in the extent of disease distribution in different populations create bias when the groups are compared. This bias persists despite crudely correcting for stage. The EDB tends to create the general impression that race is an independent prognostic factor for survival from cancer. Careful analysis of the available epidemiologic studies fails to support this assertion when EDB is considered. In other words, race does not appear to be a "real biologic factor" for predicting survival from cancer. There are a number of implications resulting from this conclusion.

The assumption that race is an independent factor (without an adequate scientific basis) technically can be considered as "racist," just as assuming that Black children score lower on standardized tests because of race is racist. The assumption that race is an independent prognostic factor deprives the "victims" of the opportunity to rectify the real health care problems. If the major problem is actually quality of care, efforts should be directed there. Differences in socioeconomic status and the variations in practice patterns and health outcomes by region of the country create enough doubt about the importance of race to require that any study that proposes to demonstrate differences in outcome by race be reviewed very critically for several reasons.[7,20,22-24] First, the bulk of the literature suggests that such a study is likely to be flawed even if the source of the flaw is unclear. Second, thus far, the designation of race as a major health care variable has not resulted in the improvement of care for anyone. Those who have benefited the most from such practices have been health care researchers funded to do research on racial differences. Finally, nothing can be done about an individual's race.

If socioeconomic factors (lack of education, unemployment, and poor-quality health care) are the most important factors, money currently spent studying cancer outcome as a function of race might be better spent addressing these issues.[62-64] Studies may also be considered to address the possibility of higher levels of environmental carcinogens in Black communities. Such studies would force us to study the impact of racism on health care delivery as a social disease. The political implications arising from these issues may not be as popular as acknowledging that "Blacks do worse," as has been done for more than 20 years. Awareness of EDB may allow a more accurate assessment to be made of the impact of lack of education, environmental exposures, socioeconomic status, and other factors, such as diet, that may be associated with differences in survival from cancer.[64]

RACE AND CARDIOVASCULAR
DISEASE AND OTHER CAUSES OF DEATH

It is clear from the previous discussion that the preponderance of evidence suggests that race is not likely to be an independent prognostic

TABLE 10.5   RECENT SELECTED
STUDIES ON CARDIOVASCULAR
DISEASES AND CARE DELIVERED BY RACE

Author (Reference Number)	Journal	Topic	Conclusions
Fang et al., 1996 (65)	*New England Journal of Medicine*	Study of the relationship between the place of birth and the cardiovascular mortality among non-Hispanic Black and White residents of New York City	Although Blacks born in the South had substantially higher age-adjusted rates of death from cardiovascular causes, both Caribbean- and northeastern-born Blacks $\geq$65 years had lower rates.
Krieger and Sidney, 1996 (66)	*American Journal of Public Health*	Association between blood pressure and self-reported experiences of racial discrimination and responses to unfair treatment	Black-White differences in blood pressure were reduced by accounting for reported experiences of racial discrimination and responses to unfair treatment.
Ayanian et al., 1993 (67)	*Journal of the American Medical Association*	Likelihood of coronary revascularization procedures among Medicare Part A enrollees	Whites more likely to receive such procedures.
Peterson et al., 1994 (68)	*Journal of the American Medical Association*	Assessment of cardiac catheterization or revascularization procedures among Blacks and Whites admitted with an acute myocardial infarction to Veterans Administration hospitals	Blacks 33%, 42%, and 54% less likely to undergo cardiac catheterization, undergo coronary angioplasty, and receive coronary bypass surgery, respectively, than Whites.
Kahn et al., 1994 (69)	*Journal of the American Medical Association*	Comparison of hospital care among elderly Black or poor Medicare recipients using a representative sample from 9,932 patients	Patients who are Black or poor have worse processes of care and greater instability at discharge.

TABLE 10.5 *(continued)*

Author (Reference Number)	Journal	Topic	Conclusions
Geronimus et al., 1996 (70)	*New England Journal of Medicine*	Study of the excess mortality among Blacks and Whites under the age of 65.	The probability of reaching age 65 was only 62% for Blacks compared to 77% for Whites, but there were large variations nationally such that Blacks from the Queens-Bronx had a higher likelihood of reaching age 65 than Whites from the lower east side, Detroit, the Appalachians, and northeastern Alabama.

factor for survival from cancer and that the differences in the extent of disease at diagnosis explain much or all of the apparent survival differences. What about other major causes of death? As stated earlier, even in the early 1900s it was clear that nongenetic factors dominated as causes of excess mortality in this country. What about more recent observations? Table 10.5 summarizes a selected series of recent articles published in the most prestigious journals in this country.[65–70] These articles seem to convey the same message: Race is not a major independent determinant of excess mortality.

What about cardiovascular diseases, the number one cause of death? Fang et al. reported that the risk of death from cardiovascular disease appears to depend more on place of birth than on race.[65] But how does one explain the differences seen in the incidence and severity of disease? The study by Krieger et al. may shed light on this matter.[66] They reported that experiencing racial discrimination was associated with having a higher blood pressure. Several studies suggest that Whites tend to be treated more aggressively than Blacks with the same severity of disease.[67] Recent studies have also shown that race was shown to influence the quality of hospital care received for cardiovascular illness regardless of whether patients were treated covered by Medicare or were treated within the Veterans Administration system.[68,69] Still other studies demonstrate that, when assessed by all-cause mortality, regional variations throughout the United States have been noted to exceed the variations between races.[70] These data suggest that it is likely that "nongenetic causes" explain most or all of the observed differences in the health status of the various races and that Blacks and the poor in general receive inferior care in this country.[65-72]

CONCLUSIONS ABOUT RACE AND SCIENCE

Herein data have been presented that support the notion that an epidemiologic phenomenon, EDB, is likely to explain the lower survival rates noted for some "races" with cancer of several common sites. Race also does not appear to be an independent prognostic factor for survival from cardiovascular disease or overall mortality when adjustments are made for other confounding variables. It should not be assumed that biologic differences exist between people of different races unless there are very strong data to support this assumption. This conclusion provides a basis for designing strategies for addressing the problem of excess mortality seen in Blacks.

In addition to the fact that the overview of available medical data really does not support the notion that race is an independent prognostic factor, there is another major reason to doubt the notion that race has major independent significance. "Race" is not a true scientific biologic construct but rather a political construct for the purposes of conveniently dividing people. Recent review articles published in mainstream journals leave little to no doubt of this fact.[73-77] For example, Paul Hoffman, in an editorial written for *Discover* magazine, summarized his findings of a series of review articles on race by several authorities:[73-76]

> On average there is a 0.2 percentage difference in the genetic material between any two randomly chosen people on Earth. Of diversity, 85 percent will be found within any local group of people—say, between you and your neighbor. More than half (9 percent) of the remaining 15 percent will be represented by differences between ethnic and linguistic groups within a given race (for example, between Italians and French). Only 6 percent represents differences between races (for example, between Europeans and Asians). And remember—that's 6 percent of 0.2 percent. In other words, race accounts for a minuscule 0.012 percent difference in our genetic material.

With such a small portion of our genetic makeup, why should anyone expect race to determine one's risk of dying of breast cancer, prostate cancer, hypertension, gunshot wounds, having a lower I.Q., and being unemployed? Clearly there are genetic differences, such as the incidence of sickle cell anemia in different populations. However, this mutation was acquired to provide resistance to malaria and, as is typical of similar mutations, was selected for a survival advantage early enough in life so as to increase one's chances of procreation. None of the major common illness discussed previously are likely to be affected by natural selection because they occur too late in life to provide any advantages during natural selection. The bottom line appears to have been well put by Sharon Begley in *Newsweek* magazine when she wrote, referring to the conclusions of the Human Genome Diversity Project, that

> genetic variation from one individual to another of the same "race" swamps the average differences between racial groupings. The more we learn about humankind's genetic differences, says geneticist Luca Cavalli-Sforza of Stanford University, who chairs the committee that directs the biodiversity project, the more we see that they have almost nothing to do with what we call race.[77]

Even today, research directed at continuing to prove the superiority of the "White race" continues to be funded.[78] Although in this "free country" it may be reasonable to continue to allow privately funded racist research, it is inappropriate to continue to use taxpayer dollars to do so. Such research only serves to divide us as a nation. The mentality behind this type of race-based research was used to justify slavery some 400 years ago and the Tuskegee experiments more than 50 years ago.

BLAME, DO NOT COMPENSATE AND BAN: RACE HEALTH AND PROPOSITION 209

The response of our society to its past moral and ethical failures to address the health needs of some of its people has been to first deny any responsibility for it. Blame the victims of race, and then do not compensate them—not only that, outlaw compensation and accuse them of "reverse discrimination." Carl T. Rowan brought attention to this issue in his book *The Coming Race War in America: A Wake-Up Call,* when he wrote,

> White male paranoia has become epidemic. This despite the fact that the median net worth of black households in this country is $4,604, or just one tenth the median net worth of white families—$44,408. The comparable figure for Hispanics is $5,345.[79]

The passage of Proposition 209 in California is but one example of how well-meaning people can be mislead into supporting an unjust cause that will hinder compensation for past wrongs—this, despite, as Rowan also points out,

> On talk shows and elsewhere I am frequently asked why "blacks get all the college scholarships." The General Accounting Office reports that 96 percent of all the scholarship money in America goes to whites has done little to wipe out white cries of persecution.[79]

The passage of Proposition 209 in California is likely to do more to continue to widen the gap between "the haves and the have-nots" and consequently to do more to widen the gap between the state of health for Blacks and Whites in California. The matter of Proposition 209 brings to mind the letter written to the clergymen on April 16, 1963, from a Birmingham jail by Martin Luther King Jr.:

> There are some instances when a law is just on its face and unjust in its application. For instance, I was arrested Friday on a charge of parading without a permit. Now there is nothing wrong with an ordinance which requires a permit for a parade, but when the ordinance is used to preserve segregation . . . it becomes unjust.[80]

Much of what is currently believed about race in this country grows out of the same mentality that supported segregation then and race-based research now. This mentality is largely responsible for the state of health of African Americans today. In what is considered his last, and most radical, Southern Christian Leadership Conference (SCLC) presidential address, Martin Luther King Jr. raised the question in the title of his presentation: "Where Do We Go from Here?"[81]

FUTURE DIRECTIONS: "WHERE DO WE GO FROM HERE?"

I have argued that "race" is not inexplicably related to health but that racism and poverty are. The history of racial oppression of African Americans in this country is old, deep, and solidly entrenched in our literature, our science, and our culture.[82] Racism and poverty have locked the vast majority of this population not in chains but in a complex superstructure whose roots reach back into the 1500s but whose branches still blossom and provide fruit of despair. This fruit of despair brings to mind the saying from the *Tao Te Ching of Lao Tzu*:

> The best lock has no bolt, and no one can open it.
> The best knot uses no rope, and no one can untie it.[83]

What can be more effective than "scientific proof" of racial differences as an explanation for being less healthy, less intelligent, and less hard working, even if this "scientific proof" is not valid?

When attempting to answer the question of where we go from here, Martin Luther King Jr. had this to say:

> One night, a juror came to Jesus and he wanted to know what he could do to be saved. Jesus didn't get bogged down in the kind of isolated approach of what he shouldn't do. Jesus didn't say, "Now Nicodemus, you must stop lying." He didn't say, "Nicodemus, you must stop cheating if you are doing that." He didn't say, "Nicodemus, you must not commit adultery." He didn't say, "Nicodemus, now you must stop drinking liquor if you are doing that excessively." He said something altogether different, because Jesus realized something basic—that if a man will lie, he will steal. And if a man will steal, he will kill. So instead of just getting bogged down in one thing, Jesus looked at him and said, "Nicodemus, you must be born again."

Here I would contend that similarly America needs to be "born again" with regard to its attitude toward race. We must end racist conjecture. Dr. King went on reflecting on the words of Jesus, saying,

> He said, in other words, "Your whole structure must be changed." A nation that will keep people in slavery for 244 years will "thingify" them—make them things. Therefore they will exploit them, and poor people generally, economically. And a nation that will exploit economically will have to have foreign investments and everything else, and will have to use its military might to protect them. All of these problems are tied together. What I am saying today is that we must go from this convention and say, "America, you must be born again!"

> . . . let us go out with a "divine dissatisfaction." Let us be dissatisfied until America will no longer have a high blood pressure of creeds and an anemia of city of wealth and comfort. . . . Let us be dissatisfied until those that live on the outskirts of hope are brought into the metropolis of daily security . . . and every family is living in a decent sanitary home.[81]

So, too, let us be dissatisfied as long as the risk of dying of cancer is 50% greater for Blacks compared to Whites. It is not due to race. We must end racism by first acknowledging this fact. Only then can we break the link between "race" and "health."

NOTE

The author would like to acknowledge Marion Malack and Pamalar Lewis for editorial support and Dr. Deborah Roach for her patience. A special thanks to

Martin Luther King Jr., whose words of wisdom inspired me to confront the issue of race.

REFERENCES

1. *The Random House College Dictionary.* Revised ed. 1975. New York: Random House.
2. Roach, M., Alexander, M., and Coleman, J. 1992. The prognostic significance of race on survival from laryngeal carcinoma. *Journal of the National Medical Association* 84, 668–674.
3. Jones, James H. 1981. *Bad Blood: The Tuskegee Syphilis Experiment.* New York: The Free Press, 34.
4. Nortzon, F. C., Komarov, Y. M., Ermakov, S. P., et al. 1998. Causes of declining life expectancy in Russia. *Journal of the American Medical Association* 279, 793–800.
5. National Cancer Institute. 1993. SEER cancer statistics review: 1973–1990. In NIH Publication 93-2789. Bethesda, Md.: National Cancer Institute.
6. Jones, James H. 1981. *Bad Blood: The Tuskegee Syphilis Experiment.* New York: The Free Press, 38.
7. Moul, J. W., Douglas, T. H., McCarthy, W. F., and McLeod, D. G. 1996. Black race is an adverse prognostic factor for prostate cancer recurrence following radical prostatectomy in an equal access health care setting. *Journal of Urology* 155, 1667–1673.
8. Bauer, J. J., Connelly, R. R., Sesterhenn, I. A., et al. 1997. Biostatistical modeling using traditional variables and genetic biomarkers for predicting the risk of prostate carcinoma recurrence after radical prostatectomy. *Cancer* 79, 952–962.
9. Gould, Stephen J. 1996. *The Mismeasure of Man.* 2nd ed. New York: W. W. Norton.
10. Franklin, J. H., and Moss, A. A. 1994. *From Slavery to Freedom: A History of African Americans.* 7th ed. New York: McGraw-Hill, 41.
11. Curtin, P. D. 1969. *The Atlantic Slave Trade: A Census.* Pp. 275–276. Madison: University of Wisconsin Press.
12. Harley, S. 1995. The timetables of African-American history. In S. Harley, ed., *A Chronology of the Most Important People and Events in African-American History.* Pp. 226–275. New York: Simon and Schuster.
13. Satariano, W. A., Belle, S. H., and Swanson, G. M. 1986. The severity of breast cancer at diagnosis: A comparison of age and extent of disease in black and white women. *American Journal of Public Health* 76, 779–782.
14. Bassett, M. T., and Krieger, N. K. 1986. Social class and black-white differences in breast cancer survival. *American Journal of Public Health* 76, 1400–1403.
15. Austin, J.-P., Covery, K., and Rotman, M. 1990. Age-race interaction in prostate adenocarcinoma treated with external irradiation. *International Journal of Radiation Oncology Biology Physics* 19(Suppl. 1), 200.

16. Dayal, H., Power, R., and Chui, C. 1982. Race and socio-economic status in survival from breast cancer. *Journal of Chronic Diseases* 27, 675–683.

17. Ernster, V. L., Selvin, S., Sacks, S. T., et al. 1978. Prostatic cancer: Mortality and incidence rates by race and social class. *American Journal of Epidemiology* 107, 311–320.

18. Keirn, W., and Meter, G. 1985. Survival of cancer patients by economic status in a free care setting. *Cancer* 55, 1552–1555.

19. Page, W. F., and Kuntz, A. J. 1980. Racial and socioeconomic factors in cancer survival. *Cancer* 45, 1029–1040.

20. Ruffer, J. E., Barry, E. E., Terry, P., et al. 1991. Lower radiation dose may account for decreased survival of blacks with prostate cancer: Results of the 1978 patterns of care study. *International Journal of Radiation Oncology Biology Physics* 21(1), 212.

21. Diehr, P., Yergan, J., Chu, J., et al. 1989. Treatment modality and quality differences for black and white breast cancer patients treated in community hospitals. *Medical Care* 27, 942–958.

22. Egbert, L. D., and Rothman, I. L. 1977. Relationship between race and economic status of patients and who performs their surgery. *New England Journal of Medicine* 297, 90–91.

23. Flaherty, J. A., and Meagher, R. 1980. Measuring racial bias in inpatient treatment. *American Journal of Psychiatry* 137, 679–682.

24. McWhorter, W. P., and Mayer, W. J. 1987. Black-white differences in type of initial breast cancer treatment and implications for survival. *American Journal of Public Health* 77, 1515–1517.

25. National Institutes of Health. 1994. *National Institutes of Health Guide for Grants and Contracts* 23 (11, March 18), 2.

26. Roach, M., and Alexander, M. 1995. The prognostic significance of race and survival from breast cancer. *Journal of the National Medical Association* 87, 214–219.

27. 1997. *AJCC Cancer Staging Manual.* 5th ed. New York: Lippincott-Raven.

28. Rosen, P. P., Groshen, S., Saigo, P. E., et al. 1989. A long term follow-up study of survival in stage I (T1NoMo) and stage II (T1N1Mo) breast carcinoma. *International Journal of Radiation Oncology Biology Physics* 7, 355–366.

29. Albain, K. S., Crowley, J. J., LeBlanc, M., et al. 1991. Survival determinants in extensive-stage non-small-cell lung cancer: The Southwest Oncology Group experience. *Journal of Clinical Oncology* 9, 1618–1626.

30. Mountain, C. F. 1986. A new international staging system for lung cancer. *Chest* 89, 225S-233S.

31. Mittra, N. K., Rush, B. F., and Verner, E. 1980. A comparative study of breast cancer in the black and white populations of two inner-city hospitals. *Journal of Surgical Oncology* 15, 11–17.

32. Gregorio, D. I., Cummings, K. M., and Michalek, A. 1983. Delay, stage of disease, and survival among white and black women with breast cancer. *American Journal of Public Health* 73, 590–593.

33. Valanis, B., Wirman, J., and Hertzberg, V. S. 1987. Social and biological factors in relation to survival among black vs. white women with breast cancer. *Breast Cancer Research and Treatment* 9, 134–144.

34. Polednak, A. P. 1988. A comparison of survival of black and white female breast cancer cases in upstate New York. *Cancer Detection and Prevention* 11, 245–249.

35. Dansy, R. D., Hessel, P. A., Browde, S., et al. 1988. Lack of a significant independent effect of race on survival in breast cancer. *Cancer* 61, 1908–1912.

36. Sutherland, C. M., and Mather, F. J. 1988. Charity hospital experience with long-term survival and prognostic factors in patients with breast cancer with localized or regional disease. *Annals of Surgery* 207, 569–580.

37. Fields, J. N., Kuske, R. R., Perez, C. A., et al. 1989. Prognostic factors in inflammatory breast cancer. *Cancer* 63, 1232–1255.

38. Cella, D. F., Orav, E. J., Kornblith, A. B., et al. 1991. Socioeconomic status and cancer survival. *Journal of Clinical Oncology* 9, 1500–1509.

39. Axtell, L. M., and Myers, M. H. 1978. Contrasts in survival of black and white cancer patients, 1960–1973. *Journal of the National Cancer Institute* 60, 1209–1215.

40. Farrow, D. C., and Hunt, S. J. M. 1992. Geographic variation in the treatment of localized breast cancer. *New England Journal of Medicine* 326, 1097–1101.

41. Albain, K. S., Green, S., LeBlanc, M., et al. 1992. Proportional hazards and recursive partitioning and amalgamation analyses of Southwest Oncology node-positive adjuvant CMFVP breast cancer data base: A pilot study. *Breast Cancer Research and Treatment* 22, 273–284.

42. Roach, M., III, Cirrincione, C., Budman, D., et al. 1997. Race and Survival from Breast Cancer: Based on Cancer and Leukemia Group B Trial 8541. *The Cancer Journal of Scientific American* 3, 107–112.

43. Dignam, J. J., Redmond, C., Fisher, B., et al. 1997. Prognosis among African-American women and white women with lymph node negative breast carcinoma: Findings from two randomized and clinical trials of the National Surgical Adjuvant Breast and Bowel Project (NSABP). *Cancer* 80(1), 80–90.

44. Krieger, N. 1989. Exposure, susceptibility, and breast cancer risk. *Breast Cancer and Treatment* 13, 205–223.

45. Morabia, A., and Wynder, E. L. 1990. Epidemiology and natural history of breast cancer. *Surgical Clinics of North America* 70, 739–752.

46. Eley, J. W., Hill, H. A., Chen, V. W., et al. 1994. Racial differences in survival from breast cancer: Results of the National Cancer Institute Black/White Cancer Survival Study. *Journal of the American Medical Association* 272, 947–954.

47. Nattinger, A. B., Gottlieb, M. S., Verum, B. S., et al. 1992. Geographic variation in the use of breast-conserving treatment for breast cancer. *New England Journal of Medicine* 326, 1102–1107.

48. Ragaz, J., Jackson, S. M., Plenderleith, I. H., et al. 1993. Can adjuvant radiotherapy (XRT) improve the overall survival (OS) of breast cancer (BR CA) patients in the presence of adjuvant chemotherapy (CT)? 10-year analysis of the British Columbia randomized trial. *Proceedings of ASCO* 12, 70.

49. Natarajan, N., Murphy, G. P., and Mettlin, C. 1989. Prostate cancer in blacks: An update from the American College of Surgeons' patterns of care studies. *Journal of Surgical Oncology* 40, 232–236.

50. Perez, C. A., Garcia, D., Simpson, J. R., et al. 1989. Factors influencing outcome of definitive radiotherapy for localized carcinoma of the prostate. *Radiotherapy and Oncology* 16, 1–21.

51. Roach, M., III, Krall, J., Keller, J. W., et al. 1992. The prognostic significance of race and survival from prostate cancer based on patients irradiated on Radiation Therapy Oncology Group protocols (1976–1985). *International Journal of Radiation Oncology Biology Physics* 24, 441–449.

52. Epstein, J. I., Paull, G., Eggleston, J. C., et al. 1986. Prognosis of untreated stage A1 prostatic carcinoma: A study of 94 cases with extended followup. *Journal of Urology* 136, 837–839.

53. Levine, R. L., and Wilchinsky, M. 1979. Adenocarcinoma of the prostate: A comparison of the disease in blacks versus whites. *Journal of Urology* 121, 761–762.

54. Roach, M., III. Is race an independent prognostic factor for survival from prostate cancer? *Journal of the National Medical Association* 90(11, suppl.).

55. Vijayakumar, S., Winter, K., Sause, W., et al. 1998. Prostate specific antigen levels are higher in African-American patients than whites in a national registration study: Results of RTOG 94–12. *International Journal of Radiation Oncology Biology Physics* 40, 17–25.

56. Chamberlain, R., Winter, K., Vijayakumar, S., et al. 1998. Radiation Therapy Oncology Group demographic analysis of subjects in multicenter clinical trials. *International Journal of Radiation Oncology Biology Physics* 40, 9–15.

57. Graham, M. V., Geitz, L. M., Byhardt, R., et al. 1992. Comparison of prognostic factors and survival among black and white patients treated with radiation therapy for non-small cell lung cancer. *Journal of the National Cancer Institute* 84, 731–735.

58. Simpson, J. R., Scott, C. B., Curran, W. J., et al. 1993. Race, gender and socioeconomic status of brain tumor patients entering multicenter clinical trials—A report from the Radiation Oncology Group. *International Journal of Radiation Oncology Biology Physics* 26, 239–244.

59. Streeter, O. E., Martz, K. L., Gaspar, L. E., et al. 1999. Does race influence survival for esophageal cancer? An analysis of patients treated with chemoradiation on RTOG 85–01. *International Journal of Radiation Oncology Biology Physics* 44(5), 1047–1052.

60. Modiano, M. R., Villar-Werstler, P., Crowley, J., et al. 1996. Evaluation of race as a prognostic factor in multiple myeloma: An ancillary of Southwest Oncology Group Study 8229. *Journal of Clinical Oncology* 14, 974–977.

61. Pui, C.-H., Boyett, J. M., Hancock, M. L., et al. 1995. Outcome of treatment for childhood cancer in black as compared with white children: The St. Jude Children's Research Hospital experience, 1962 through 1992. *Journal of the American Medical Association* 273, 633–637.

62. Gabel, L. L., and Weddington, W. H. 1993. Obligation and opportunity: Family practice research regarding race and quality of care. *Family Practice Research Journal* 13(2), 101–104.

63. Weddington, W. H., Gabel, L. L., Peet, G. M., et al. 1992. Quality of care and black American patients. *Journal of the National Medical Association* 84(7), 569–575.

64. Gorey, K. M., and Vena, J. E. 1994. Cancer differentials among U.S. blacks and whites: Quantitative estimates of socioeconomic-related risks. *Journal of the National Medical Association* 86(3), 209–215.

65. Fang, J., Madhavan, S., and Alderman, M. 1996. The association between birthplace and mortality from cardiovascular causes among black and white residents of New York. *New England Journal of Medicine* 335(21), 1545–1551.

66. Krieger, N., and Sidney, S. 1996. Racial discrimination and blood pressure: The CARDIA Study of young black and white adults. *American Journal of Public Health* 86, 1370–1378.

67. Ayanian, J. Z., Udvarhelyi, S., Gatsonis, C. A., et al. 1993. Racial differences in the use of revascularization procedures after coronary angiography. *Journal of the American Medical Association* 269(20), 2642–2646.

68. Peterson, E., Wright, S. M., Daley, J., and Thibault, G. E. 1994. Racial variation in cardiac procedure use and survival following acute myocardial infarction in the Department of Veterans Affairs. *Journal of the American Medical Association* 271, 1175–1180.

69. Kahn, K. L., Pearson, M. L., Harrison, E. R., et al. 1994. Health care for black and poor hospitalized medicare patients. *Journal of the American Medical Association* 271, 1169–1174.

70. Geronimus, A. T., Bound, J., Waidmann, T. A., et al. 1996. Excess mortality among blacks and whites in the United States. *New England Journal of Medicine* 335, 1552–1558.

71. Hafner-Eaton, C. 1993. Physician utilization disparities between the uninsured and insured: Comparisons of the chronically ill, acutely ill and well non-elderly populations. *Journal of the American Medical Association* 269, 787–792.

72. Worthington, C. 1992. An examination of factors influencing the diagnosis and treatment of black patients in the mental health system. *Archives of Psychiatric Nursing* 6(3), 195–204.

73. Hoffman, P. 1994. The science of race. *Discover: The World of Science* 15(4, Special Issue), 4.

74. Gould, S. J. 1994. The geometer of race. *Discover: The World of Science* 15(4, Special Issue), 64–69.

75. Gutin, J. A. 1994. End of the rainbow. *Discover: The World of Science* 15(4, Special Issue), 70–75.

76. Diamond, J. 1994. Race without color. *Discover: The World of Science* 15(4, Special Issue), 82–89.

77. Begley, S. 1995. Three is not enough. *Newsweek,* February 13, 67–69.

78. Miller, A. 1994/1995. The Pioneer Fund: Bankrolling the professors of hate. *Journal of Blacks in Higher Education,* no. 6(winter), 58–61.

79. Rowan, C. T. 1996. *The Coming Race War in America.* Boston: Little, Brown, 17.

80. King, Martin Luther, Jr. 1991. Historic essays: *Letter from Birmingham City Jail* (written April 16, 1963). In *A Testament of Hope: The Essential Writings and Speeches of Martin Luther King, Jr.,* edited by James M. Washington. San Francisco: HarperCollins, 294.

81. King, Martin Luther, Jr. 1991. Famous sermons and public addresses: *Where Do We Go From Here?* (written April 1967). In *A Testament of Hope: The Essential Writings and Speeches of Martin Luther King, Jr.,* edited by James M. Washington. San Francisco: HarperCollins, 251.

82. Morrison, T. 1993. *Playing in the Dark: Whiteness and the Literary Imagination.* New York: Vintage Books.

83. Brown, B., trans. 1995. *The Tao Te Ching of Lao Tzu.* New York: St. Martin's Press, Saying 27.

■

11

Kathy Sanders-Phillips

HEALTH PROMOTION
IN ETHNIC MINORITY FAMILIES

The Impact of Exposure to Violence

INTRODUCTION

Health, as defined by the World Health Organization, is "physical, mental and social well-being, not merely the absence of disease or infirmity" (Breslow, 1972). This goal calls for the enhancement of both the extent and the quality of life for people in all countries. Unfortunately, the goal is far from being met in many low-income ethnic minority groups in the United States, where poor health outcomes and significantly shorter life spans are associated with ethnic minority status.

There is increasing evidence that the health behaviors of low-income ethnic minorities are significantly influenced by their economic and social environments, which often include a legacy of poverty and disadvantaged social status; daily life experiences in stressful, unpredictable, and unsafe environments; lack of adequate health insurance and access to medical care; and little knowledge of prevention (Syme and Berkman, 1976; McGinnis, 1986; Vega et al., 1988; U.S. Department of Health and Human Services, 1991; Minkler, 1992; Wallerstein, 1992; Franke, 1997). In particular, violence has become a chronic stressor in many ethnic minority communities, where homicide is a leading cause of death (U.S. Department of Health and Human Services, 1986). Exposure to high levels of community violence can result in feelings of alienation and powerlessness, which limit the ability of low-income ethnic minorities to obtain health services and engage in health promotion behaviors (Bullough, 1972).

Health behavior does not develop in a vacuum. It is largely determined by the social context in which it occurs (Berkanovic, 1976; Ehrhardt et al., 1995). There is growing awareness in the field of public health of the critical interplay between the social environment, health behaviors, and health and of the need for a social ecological approach to health promotion (Freudenberg, 1978; Stokols, 1992; Bloom, 1993; Lillie-Blanton et al., 1993; Williams et al., 1994). This approach acknowledges the individual's role in influencing health outcome while recognizing the important role of the environment in determining healthful behavior and health outcome. Environments may impact health behaviors and outcomes by operating as stressors or as sources of safety or danger. The benefits of a well-designed health promotion program may go unrealized if these environmental stressors are not addressed (Stokols, 1992). Developing health promotion programs for low-income ethnic minorities may require recognition of the underlying role that exposure to violence can play in influencing psychological functioning and health behaviors. This chapter reviews literature on the impact of exposure to violence on psychological functioning, health promotion behaviors, and risk behaviors in urban ethnic minority communities. Psychological and behavioral responses to community violence are reviewed, and the impact of exposure to violence on health behaviors is examined, with particular emphasis on the impact of psychosocial stressors, such as exposure to violence on health decisions and behaviors of women. Recommendations are made for future research on the impact of exposure to violence on health behaviors and for the development of health promotion programs that acknowledge and address the potential role of exposure to violence in precipitating unhealthy behaviors in ethnic minority communities.

VIOLENCE IN LOW-INCOME
ETHNIC MINORITY COMMUNITIES

The violence that occurs in many ethnic minority communities takes several forms. Family violence, which refers to violence occurring in the home, and community violence, which is defined as violence occurring in the community or neighborhood outside of the home (U.S. Department of Health and Human Services, 1986; Osofsky, 1995) are the most common forms. Both types of violence may involve homicide and sexual assault, but community violence also includes aggravated assault, burglary, and robbery (Resnick et al., 1986, 1993).

Ethnic minority communities are disproportionately impacted by violence, and African American and Latino males are at particularly high risk for death or injury due to violence. Homicide is a leading cause of death for African American males between the ages of 15 to 44 and for African American females between the ages of 15 to 24 (Centers for Disease Control, 1990; Hammond and Yung, 1993). Until age 70, homicide is second only to heart disease in its contribution to excess deaths among African Americans (U.S. Department of Health and Human Services, 1986). Age-adjusted rates of homicide among Latinos are approximately three to four times higher than those for White males (Smith et al., 1986; Tardiff and Gross, 1986; Centers for Disease Control, 1990), and foreign-born Latinos are at higher risk for homicide than native-born Latinos (Sorenson and Shen, 1996). Although less data are available for Native Americans and Asians, statistics indicate that accidents, which may be related to violence, are the third-leading cause of death for Native Americans, followed by homicides as the seventh-leading cause of death (Dinges and Joos, 1988). Homicide is the eighth-leading cause of death for Asian American males and fourteenth for females (Gall and Gall, 1993).

Nonfatal injuries due to violence have been estimated to be at least 100 times more frequent than homicides (O'Carroll, 1988). Statistics from the National Crime Survey (Christofel, 1990) indicate that approximately 1.2 million crimes of violence are not reported to law enforcement. Like homicide, nonfatal violence is higher among low-income ethnic minority groups. African American males have higher rates of injury due to violence than any other male group, and they outnumber African American females by three to one (Guyer et al., 1989). Latinos have the second-highest rates of injury due to violence (Sumner et al., 1986; Guyer et al., 1989; U.S. Department of Justice, 1991).

Family violence, which includes violence against spouses, domestic homicide (i.e., the killing of one spouse by another), and other forms of violence, is also higher in ethnic minority populations (U.S. Department of Health and Human Services, 1986; Bell and Chance-Hill, 1991). African American women are more likely than African American men to be murdered by a family member or an intimate partner (Humphrey and Palmer, 1986; Wilbanks, 1986; Harlow, 1989). Both African American and Latino children may be overrepresented among sexual abuse victims (Kersher and McShane, 1984; Cupoli and Sewell, 1988). School violence, as measured by the number of robberies and assaults in high schools, is also higher in urban ethnic minority communities (U.S. Department of Health and Human Services, 1986; Sheley et al., 1992). Higher rates of aggravated assaults and illegal drug use, which are associated with high rates of violence, have also been reported for ethnic minority communities (Dawkins and Dawkins 1983; Lester, 1986; Mercy et al., 1986; Bell, 1987; Weiszet al., 1991; Elliot, 1993).

Members of ethnic minority groups are also more likely to witness violence in their daily lives. Much of the violence is witnessed by children, and, in one study, shootings are cited as the most serious danger in the lives of mothers and children living in a low-income ethnic minority community (Dubrow, 1989). In other studies, more than a quarter of urban schoolchildren had witnessed a person being shot, and almost a third had seen a person stabbed (Garbarino et al., 1991a and 1991b; Freeman et al., 1992; Lorion and Saltzman, 1993). Among low-income elderly living in urban communities, fear of victimization and personal safety accounts for the largest percentage of variance in quality of life for African Americans versus White Americans (Harel, 1986).

EXPOSURE TO VIOLENCE AND
HEALTH PROMOTION BEHAVIOR

There is increasing evidence that exposure to violence negatively impacts health promotion behaviors and may increase risk behaviors, particularly in low-income African American and Latino groups. In a sample of low-income African American women and Latinas living in an urban community, having a family member killed or murdered was a significant predictor of health promotion behaviors (Sanders-Phillips, 1996a). That is, women who had a family member killed or murdered were less likely to be engaging in health promotion behaviors, including eating a daily breakfast, sleeping seven to eight hours per night, abstaining from alcohol and tobacco, and exercising at least once per week. Women with a family member beaten by another family member were less willing to change their eating habits to include more healthful foods (Sanders-Phillips, 1994a). Exposure to violence is also related to practicing unsafe dieting and eating foods high in fats among adolescents (Orpinas et al., 1995) and is a predictor of lack of a regular health care provider and delays in seeking medical care among ethnic minority patients (Rask et al., 1994). Exposure to violence is also related to poor health perceptions, functional limitations, chronic disease, and somatic symptoms in ethnic minority groups (Golding, 1994).

Risk behaviors such as the use of illegal drugs and alcohol are also associated with exposure to violence. Illicit drug use is strongly related to assault by a mate, and tobacco and alcohol use are associated with assault by a member of the family of origin (Berenson et al., 1992). Among Latinos, physical abuse is related to higher levels of tobacco use, while both physical and sexual assault are strongly related to alcohol use among African Americans (Berenson et al., 1992). Exposure to violence is also related to higher levels of current, lifetime, and intended drug and alcohol use among children (Lorion and Saltzman, 1993).

There may be specific relationships between exposure to violence and pregnancy-related risk behaviors in women. Stevens-Simon and Reichert (1994) found that adolescent pregnancy was predicted by a history of childhood sexual abuse. Illegal substance use during pregnancy is also significantly related to exposure to violence (Martin et al., 1996). Exposure to psychosocial stressors, which includes exposure to community violence, is related to behavioral risk factors during pregnancy, including chronic medical disease, poor weight gain, alcohol use, and illegal drug use (Orr et al., 1996). Among African American women, exposure to psychosocial stressors is associated with the birth of low-birthweight infants. Zapata et al. (1992) have also shown that among pregnant women in Chile, exposure to community violence, in the form of political violence, was also related to lower-birthweight infants.

Exposure to violence has also been found to impact AIDS prevention and risk behaviors in men and women. Lemp et al. (1994) reported higher levels of AIDS risk behaviors for men exposed to sexual violence. Exposure to community and family violence has been correlated with a greater number of sexual partners among African American males (Durant et al., 1994b). Rotheram-Borus et al. (1996) found a relationship between exposure to sexual violence and increased sexual risk behaviors in adolescents who were also more likely to use alcohol and illegal drugs. Several investigators have reported that exposure to sexual violence is related to HIV and STD sexual risk behaviors and increased alcohol consumption in women (Glaser et al., 1991; Wyatt, 1992; Irwin et al., 1995; Zeiler et al., 1996) and adolescent girls (Orpinas et al., 1995). Kavanaugh et al. (1992), although not specifically examining exposure to violence, found that African American women in an AIDS prevention program experienced high levels of alienation and powerlessness associated with urban life that impacted AIDS-related health behaviors.

These findings strongly suggest that exposure to violence is related to greater involvement in risk behaviors and decreased involvement in health promotion behaviors. In an effort to identify the mechanisms by which exposure to violence may impact health behaviors, a literature review of studies examining relationships between experiences of violence, psychological functioning, and perceptions of health and well-being was conducted. The databases searched were PsychLIT, Medline, Social Citation Index, Sociofile, and Social Work Abstracts using "health," "trauma," "violence," "alienation," and "powerlessness" as key words.

PSYCHOLOGICAL RESPONSES TO VIOLENCE

Although rates of violence have escalated in all segments of our society (Rosenberg and Fenley, 1991), it is the chronic, pervasive, and random nature of the violence that distinguishes life in urban ethnic minority communities from life in other communities. The violence is life threatening and unpredictable and occurs in public places populated by innocent bystanders (Bell and Jenkins, 1991). It has become a chronic stressor that affects quality of life (Cohen et al., 1982; et al., 1991; Garbarino et al., 1991; Sluzki, 1993). Chronic danger, which is defined as regular and persistent attacks of violence that disrupt day-to-day life, requires significant adjustments, including alterations of personality and major changes in patterns of behavior, that allow for interpretation of the danger and accommodation to the realities of community life (Sonnenberg, 1988; Garbarino et al., 1991; Lorion and Saltzman, 1993; Sluzki, 1993). Exposure to chronic danger affects interpersonal, cognitive, psychological, and behavioral functioning on a day-to-day and long-term basis (Lorion and Saltzman, 1993).

Individuals who have been victims of violence may show symptoms of posttraumatic stress disorder, which is characterized by recurrent memories and dreams of the event, illusions, hallucinations, dissociative flashbacks, and intense psychic pain (Sonnenberg, 1988; Davidson and Smith, 1990; Singer et al., 1996). In the long term, victims of violence may continue to experience fear, terror, and a sense of helplessness (Sonnenberg, 1988; Davidson and Smith, 1990). There is often a diminished interest in significant life activities, a feeling of being detached or estranged from others, a restriction of the ability to feel intensely, and a pessimistic sense regarding the future (Sonnenberg, 1988). Symptoms of depression and anxiety are also common among victims of violence (Freeman et al., 1992; Singer et al., 1996).

Those who witness violence may experience all or some of these symptoms. Children who have witnessed violence show higher levels of anxiety and often manifest a sense of futurelessness characterized by a belief that they will not reach adulthood (Hughes, 1988; Bell and Jenkins, 1991; Martinez and Richter, 1993). Adult witnesses to violence also report feeling that the end of life will come soon (Sonnenberg, 1988) and experience pervasive feelings of fear, vulnerability, and hopelessness (Lorion and Saltzman, 1993). Acting-out behaviors, particularly in adolescents, and self-destructive behaviors are common (Bell and Jenkins, 1991). Women and girls are likely to experience depression, anxiety, and sleep problems in response to community violence, while men and boys experience distress and behavioral problems (Lorion and Saltzman, 1993; Martinez and Richter, 1993).

The cumulative experience of exposure to violence and victimization may have significant effects on psychological functioning. Hinton-Nelson et al. (1996) found that African American adolescents who had witnessed violence but who had not experienced violence had higher levels of hope for the future than those who were victims, although feelings of hopelessness were apparent in both groups. Hope was defined as the ability to move toward a goal in life and develop plans to meet that goal. The experience of victimization was related to lower levels of hope and predictions that one's own death would be violent, while exposure to violence was correlated with predictions that one's death would be nonviolent. Durant et al. (1994a, 1995) also found that adolescents who were exposed to high levels of family and community violence did not expect to live to the age of 25. These findings suggest that individuals in communities of high violence tend to predict a cause of death that is consistent with their environment (Hinton-Nelson et al., 1996). Exposure to chronic violence significantly impacts impulse control and risk-taking behavior (Gardner, 1971; Lorion and Saltzman, 1993). Individuals exposed to chronic violence may show a level of passivity and emotional withdrawal, coupled with difficulties in controlling aggressive impulses, that interfere with learning (Gardner, 1971). Since exposure to chronic violence reinforces the conclusion that achieving lasting or socially approved outcomes is unlikely, socially unacceptable, risky, but rewarding behavior may become highly attractive (Garbarino et al., 1991; Lorion and Saltzman, 1993). In addition, community residents may become desensitized to the threat and consequences of violence and pursue opportunities for risk taking and confrontation with danger (Garbarino et al., 1991; Lorion and Saltz-man, 1993). Without hope for a future, some may attempt to gain control over their lives through repeated encounters with life-threatening situations.

POWERLESSNESS, ANOMIE, ALIENATION, AND HEALTH PROMOTION BEHAVIORS

While few studies have specifically examined the relationship between exposure to violence and health promotion behaviors, a number of studies have examined relationships between experiences of violence, subsequent feelings of alienation, anomie, and powerlessness and perceptions of health and well-being. Other investigators have examined relationships between feelings of alienation, anomie, and powerlessness and health promotion behaviors. Collectively, the findings suggest that exposure to violence influences perceptions of control over life and over one's health outcome. Exposure to violence, and the resulting feelings of alienation, anomie, and powerlessness, may specifically impact health promotion and risk behaviors, particularly in low-income urban populations.

Based on the existing literature, a conceptual model of relationships between exposure to violence and health behaviors in low income, urban, ethnic minority communities is presented in Figure 11.1. In this model, exposure to violence serves as an intervening variable that may partially explain relationships between low-income, urban, ethnic minority status; decreased health promotion behaviors; and increased risk behaviors. As illustrated, low-income, urban, ethnic minority status in the United States is associated with exposure to high levels of community and family violence. In turn, exposure to violence may result in feelings of powerlessness, anomie, and alienation that are related to the subsequent development of psychological distress, which may be expressed as hopelessness, decreased self-efficacy, and decreased motivation to seek information. These psychological perspectives may lead to changes in life priorities, including the priority assigned to health, decreased problem-solving skills, and difficulties in social learning that may be necessary for health promotion and disease prevention and decreased utilization of available health services, which may result in decreased health promotion behaviors and increased risk taking regarding health.

Alienation, hopelessness, powerlessness, and anomie are related psy-

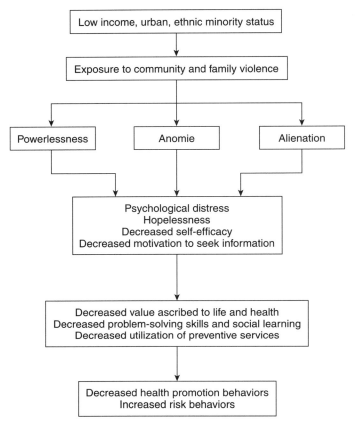

Figure 11.1. Conceptual model of the impact of exposure to violence on health promotion behaviors.

chological constructs that refer to an individual's perceived relationship with the larger society and perceptions of control within that society. Alienation is defined by feelings of powerlessness and social isolation (Morris et al., 1966). It includes feelings that result from rejection of cultural norms for evaluating success and rejection of societal means for achieving success (Wilkerson et al., 1982). Powerlessness is a subjective or perceived expectancy or belief that an individual cannot determine the occurrence of outcomes (Seeman, 1959) and is characterized by feelings that one has no effective control over one's destiny (Morris et al., 1966). Hopelessness is the inability to see or make plans for the future (Hinton-Nelson et al., 1996). In contrast, hope lies in the ability to make linkages between previous desires and to use strategies that meet those needs (Hinton-Nelson et al., 1996). Anomie is a broader concept that includes feelings of alienation, pessimism, distrust, and hopelessness (Cohen et al., 1982). Alienation, hopelessness, powerlessness, and anomie are related to experiences of violence and have been shown to significantly impact health decisions and behaviors.

Cohen et al. (1982) reported that negative feelings about health among both African Americans and Latinos were related to community measures of stress, including poverty, feelings of fear, social problems, and violent crimes. These community stressors resulted in feelings of anomie. In communities of high violence, feelings of powerlessness and anomie may be coupled with a disinclination to worry about events that cannot be controlled (Dubrow and Garbarino, 1989). These feelings are compounded by poor relationships with police (Dubrow and Garbarino, 1989). Community residents are likely to report that they cannot depend on the police or that they fear retaliation if they talk to the police. According to one woman in a low-income housing project plagued by violence, "If identified . . . as a caller (to the police), one's entire family would be in jeopardy" (Dubrow and Garbarino, 1989, p. 9).

Feelings of powerlessness, alienation, and anomie are also associated with poor health behaviors and less preventive care. Feelings of powerlessness and alienation have been associated with increased doctor visits and decreased levels of prenatal care among Mexican Americans (Hoppe and Heller, 1975), lower levels of knowledge among patients regarding their disease (Seeman and Evans, 1962), lower levels of self-initiated preventive care (diet, exercise, alcohol, smoking) and lower levels of belief in the efficacy of early treatment (Seeman and Seeman, 1983), higher rates of pregnancy and lower levels of family planning behavior among low-income women (Groat and Neal, 1967), and low levels of well child care (i.e., immunizations) in low-income mothers, particularly African American mothers (Morris et al., 1966). Alienation, powerlessness, hopelessness, and social isolation significantly decreased the use of preventive services among low-income mothers in Los Angeles, and the effect was most pronounced for African American mothers (Bullough, 1992). Although poverty was a potent predictor of the use of preventive services in this sample, alienation and powerlessness were critical intervening variables in determining health promotion behaviors. More recently, high levels of alienation and powerlessness have been associated with higher rates of AIDS risk behaviors (Kavanaugh et al., 1992).

POWERLESSNESS, ANOMIE,
AND ALIENATION: MECHANISMS OF IMPACT

There are several ways in which exposure to violence, and the resulting feelings of powerlessness, anomie, and alienation, may impact health promotion behaviors. Exposure to violence and perceptions of uncontrollability of aversive and unpredictable events (i.e., powerlessness, helplessness, hopelessness) may result in depression (Green, 1982; Garbarino et al., 1991; Freeman et al., 1992). Depression, in turn, is related to higher levels of smoking and drinking alcohol (Cohen et al., 1991). Other types of psychological distress, including high levels of perceived stress, are related to poor eating habits in the general population and in Mexican Americans (Rakowski, 1988; Vega et al., 1988). These findings suggest that exposure to violence, and subsequent feelings of powerlessness, alienation, and anomie, may result in depression and/or psychological distress that diminish an individual's ability to engage in health promotion behaviors.

Feelings of powerlessness, hopelessness, and alienation may also influence life priorities and affect motivation to seek health promotion and disease prevention information. Motivation to seek information depends on an individual's feelings of powerlessness and the value placed on an outcome (Dodge et al., 1997). High levels of alienation and powerlessness are related to low levels of motivation to seek information, particularly health information, and less value placed on health outcome (Seeman and Evans, 1962; Groat and Neal, 1967). Seeman and Evans and (1962) concluded that "a sense of personal control makes knowledge concerning one's affairs motivationally relevant" and, conversely, that "knowledge acquisition may be irrelevant for those who believe that external forces control the fall of events" (p. 773). "Seeking information is to behave as though it is within one's capacity to control events through knowledge" (Seeman and Evans, 1962, p. 781).

Exposure to violence may also affect social learning and problem-solving skills, resulting in failure to engage in learning that involves planning and control (Seeman and Evans, 1962; Gardner, 1971; Rosenberg, 1987; Ross and Mirowsky, 1989; Spivak and Hausman, 1989; Dodge et al., 1997). Decreased levels of perceived control and problem-solving skills are also related to depression (Ross and Mirowsky, 1989). Thus, the likelihood that a person will seek health information is affected by feelings of control and the value placed on health, and these feelings are significantly impacted by exposure to violence. Perceptions of uncontrollability and a low value for health may also contribute to increased involvement of minorities in high-risk health behaviors. Feelings of powerlessness and alienation also limit the likelihood that an individual will utilize preventive services that may be available and/or that he/she will persist in engaging in health promotion activities (Seeman and Evans, 1962; Mindlin and Densen, 1971; Bullough, 1972; Dubrow and Garbarino, 1989). For example, low-income African American women who lived in violent neighborhoods and reported feelings of powerlessness were less apt to use the services and programs that were available to them (Dubrow and Garbarino, 1989). Similar groups of low-income ethnic minority women were found to initiate health prevention practices but were less likely to persist in these activities over time (Mindlin and Densen, 1971). Both powerlessness and anomie appear to act as psychological deterrents to making the kind of sustained effort that is necessary to be successful in overcoming obstacles or barriers to a desired end (Bullough, 1967). As a result, powerlessness, hopelessness, and alienation may indirectly affect health promotion behaviors by influencing the extent to which barriers such as lack of money or lack of services may be overcome.

Powerlessness may also directly affect health status. Wallerstein (1992) has shown that powerlessness, or lack of control over one's destiny, is an independent risk factor for disease. Powerlessness has been linked to higher rates of physical, mental, and behavioral health problems (Wallerstein, 1992).

Perhaps one of the primary means by which feelings of alienation, powerlessness, and anomie impact health behaviors, particularly in children and adolescents, is via relationships with hopelessness. Ideally, hope is established during infancy in the context of nurturing caretaker-infant interactions (Snyder, 1994). Hope is then cultivated via a child's interactions with the environment and through reinforcement of the perception that they can act to reach their goals and handle impediments to realizing those goals (Hinton-Nelson et al., 1996). According to Hinton-Nelson et al. (1996), life in chronically violent environments may adversely impact parent-child relationships and destroy children's perceptions of links between goals, actions, and achievements. As a result, many of these children perceive that early death is probable, and both children and parents may feel that life cannot be protected (Rinear, 1988). Under these circumstances, hope is understandably diminished, and there is little rationale to pursue goals of health or life. Hopelessness, coupled with the differential access to coping resources that is a characteristic of poverty (Durant et al., 1995), may limit perceived life and health options and decrease motivation to engage in life-enhancing or health promotion behaviors.

PREREQUISITES OF HEALTH
PROMOTION: THE IMPACT OF VIOLENCE

Health promotion behaviors are voluntary, and the factors influencing voluntary behaviors, particularly those undertaken without recommendation by a physician, differ considerably from those influencing other health behaviors (Berkanovic, 1981–82). Although many theories have been proposed to explain the adoption of health promotion behaviors, there is general consensus that anticipation of a negative outcome and the desire to avoid the outcome, or to reduce its impact, creates motivation for self-protection (Weinstein, 1993). The individual must also weigh the expected benefits in risk reduction against the expected costs of acting (Weinstein, 1993). The value ascribed to health also becomes increasingly important as discretion in the use of a service and/or in engaging in a behavior increases (Berkanovic, 1973, 1981–82). Lastly, an individual's belief in his/her ability or likelihood of changing current patterns of behavior (i.e., self-efficacy/perceived behavioral control) will also impact motivation and the degree to which he or she engages in health promotion behavior (Weinstein, 1973; Berkanovic, 1981–82). It is clear that exposure to violence may impact each of these prerequisites of health promotion behavior. It affects one's anticipation of and ability to control negative outcomes, value ascribed to life and health, motivation to weigh costs and benefits of actions, and perceived efficacy and control in determining one's fate. Particularly for ethnic minorities, a sense of efficacy and control are dependent on the nature of their social experiences and the larger social structure and community in which they function (Groat and Neal, 1967; Hughes and Demo, 1989). The larger community both serves as a channel of communication and information and provides for the maintenance of a sense of personal control (Groat and Neal, 1967). However, powerlessness serves as an intervening variable between an individual's social circumstances and his/her social learning (Groat and Neal, 1967). To the extent that one's social environment reinforces the conclusion that individual destiny cannot be controlled, it becomes doubtful that one will engage in self-protective behavior. According to Lorion and Saltzman, "It may make little sense to be careful for oneself or others if physical harm or death are deemed inevitable" (Lorion and Saltzman, 1993, p. 57).

Rainwater (1960) has argued that a sense of stability and trust in the future are essential preconditions for health promotion behaviors. At the very least, health promotion behavior requires planning and a sense of control over one's future or a sense that a future exists. It is clear that exposure to chronic violence can destroy these perceptions.

EXPOSURE TO VIOLENCE
AND EXPERIENCES OF POVERTY

The impact of violence on health behaviors in low-income ethnic minorities may be exacerbated by feelings of powerlessness and anomie that are associated with poverty and ethnic minority status in this country (Berkanovic, 1973; Green, 1982; McLoyd, 1990), regardless of the degree of exposure to violence. A life of poverty is characterized by higher levels of stress, negative life events, and chronic conditions outside of personal control (Liem and Liem, 1978; Kessler, 1979). Chronic poverty severely restricts individual choice in all domains of life, renders a person subject to greater control by others, and weakens an individual's ability to cope with new problems and difficulties (McLoyd, 1990). Thus, those in poverty are more likely to experience feelings of hopelessness, powerlessness, and depression (Green, 1982) that are more severe when catastrophic events are outside of the control of the individual (Liem and Liem, 1978; Kessler and Cleary, 1980).

Even in the absence of violence, the stress of poverty, in conjunction with stressors of ethnic minority status (Ogbu, 1983), may result in feelings of victimization and dissatisfaction (McLoyd, 1990) that influence health behaviors. There is also evidence that poverty is related to decreased access to resources for coping with adversity and increased vulnerability to the long-term effects of violence (Kessler and Magee, 1994). Berkanovic and Reeder (1973) have concluded that both ethnicity and socioeconomic status create different life experiences that are related to value preferences and, subsequently, to variations in health behaviors and use of discretionary health services. The cumulative impact of exposure to violence and poverty may severely limit the motivation, ability, and belief of many low-income ethnic minorities that they can successfully impact their lives and health outcomes.

EXPOSURE TO VIOLENCE, ETHNIC MINORITY
WOMEN, AND HEALTH PROMOTION BEHAVIORS

In the past decade, significant increases have occurred in our knowledge of factors that influence women's health decisions and behaviors as well as barriers to healthy behaviors among women (Brown-Bryant, 1985; Calnan and Johnson, 1985; Makuc et al., 1989; Ruzek et al., 1997b). There is also greater awareness of factors that influence health behaviors in ethnic minority women (Cope and Hall, 1985; Leigh, 1994; Sanders-Phillips, 1994a, 1994b, 1996a, 1996b) and strategies that can be effective in promoting healthier behaviors in ethnic minority women (Eng et al., 1985; Schaefer et al., 1990; Levine et al., 1992; Eng, 1993).

Previous findings indicate that health behaviors are gender specific (Cohen et al., 1982, 1991; Gottlieb and Green, 1984; Rakowski, 1988; Baum et al., 1991; Ruzek et al., 1997a) and impacted by a range of psychosocial factors, including psychological status, exposure to violence, and perceptions of stress. These factors influence health-related self-efficacy and priorities regarding prevention behaviors (Cohen et al., 1982; Broman and Johnson, 1988; Smith, 1992; Sanders-Phillips, 1996a, 1996b) and involvement in health promotion and disease prevention behaviors (Sanders-Phillips, 1994a, 1994b). Although many of the following studies did not examine direct relationships between exposure to violence and health behaviors in women, they demonstrate that women's health behaviors are significantly related to psychological functioning and perceptions of stress. Since exposure to violence is associated with higher levels of stress and depression, it is probable that women's health behaviors are adversely impacted by exposure to violence.

Ferrence (1988) found that women's risk behaviors are significantly related to social status and interactions outside the home, and previous findings indicate that mental health factors may be better predictors of health behaviors for women than men (Lex, 1991). In addition, stressful life events are better predictors of involvement in healthy behaviors for women than for men (Gottlieb and Green, 1984; Rakowski, 1988; Cohen et al., 1991). That is, fewer stressful life events are related to healthier behavior in women, especially in low-income groups. Psychological status, which is related to levels of stressful life events such as exposure to violence, also influences risk behaviors in women (Cohen et al., 1991; Shumaker and Hill, 1991). Poorer health behaviors are more common in women with symptoms of depression (Cohen et al., 1991; Leftwich and Collins, 1994), which is also a correlate of exposure to violence.

Baum and Grunberg (1991) have argued that cigarette smoking, al-cohol, and illegal drug use should be viewed as coping behaviors for women, and Gottlieb and Green (1984) concluded that relationships be-tween stress, alcohol, and smoking in women may be strong enough to justify sex-specific norms for smoking and drinking as coping mecha-nisms for stress. Others have found that both trauma and depression are etiologic factors in women's drug abuse (Fullilove et al., 1992; Singer et al., 1993) and that illegal and prescription drug use among women may serve as forms of self-medication to cope with stresses (Booth et al., 1991). Gender-based differences in the use of substances may be related to differences in perceptions of stress and/or in motivations to regu-late mood through substance use. Thus, women may be at greater risk for coping with stress by altering behaviors that impact health (Baum and Grunberg, 1991).

These results underscore the importance of psychological and social variables to women's risk behaviors and support previous findings that psychological and social factors, such as exposure to violence, are signifi-cant predictors of risk behaviors among all women, particularly ethnic minority women (Rodin, 1986). Increased awareness of relationships between these stressors and unhealthy behaviors may be critical to our understanding of the development of risk behaviors and to the conse-quences of high stress for women. These findings also support the conclu-sion that women's risk behaviors may have common etiologies. Current data also suggest that psychosocial factors may be more important than demographic or biomedical factors in determining health outcomes, especially in low-income ethnic minority groups (Rodin and Ickovics, 1990; Pincus and Callahan, 1995).

In the future, gender-specific models of health behavior are needed that acknowledge the role that factors such as exposure to violence may play in the health and risk behaviors of women. As patterns and profiles of risk factors and illness by gender change, research on psychosocial fac-tors related to women's health will be urgently needed (Rodin and Icko-vics, 1990). Increasing rates of mortality and morbidity for women ap-pear to be related to several factors, including the ability of women to adapt and cope with stress and their perceptions of control (Krieger, 1990; Rodin and Ickovics, 1990; Auerbach and Figert, 1995). Under-standing relationships between psychosocial factors, health and risk behaviors, and health outcomes in women may greatly improve our ability to develop more effective health promotion programs for women. Greater attention to psychosocial factors, such as experiences of violence that may specifically influence health behaviors and outcomes for minority women, may also enhance our theoretical understanding of health and risk behaviors in women.

IMPLICATIONS FOR FUTURE
RESEARCH AND PROGRAM DEVELOPMENT

The findings presented in this chapter identify exposure to violence as a potentially critical intervening variable in explaining the relationship between minority status, poverty, and poor health behaviors. Present data suggest that poor health outcomes are but one of the many problems facing low-income ethnic minority families, perhaps not even the most pressing or immediate problem. In communities with high rates of violence, it is unlikely that health will be a priority in the lives of residents, and they may be less likely to seek health information. Poor ethnic minority families must contend with the cumulative effects of violence, poverty, and stressful life events in urban communities. As Berkanovic (1981–82) notes,

> We need to recognize that health is only one of many values competing for the time and energy of the individual. It may be perfectly rational for one who believes that a course of action is deleterious to his health to take that course of action if some more important values can be realized. In addition to exploring structural factors that go beyond standard demographic characteristics, therefore, perhaps students of health protective behavior might cast a wider net with respect to the social psychological factors that influence such behavior. (p. 235)

Recent studies have attempted to identify racial, demographic, and socioeconomic correlates of health behavior (Martinez and Lillie-Blanton, 1996). To date, however, we know little of the sociodemographic variables related to health promotion that can be modified (Becker, 1979; Berkanovic, 1981–82). Yet, exposure to violence is a sociodemographic variable that can be an important determinant of health promotion behavior, affects attitudes and beliefs about health, and may be modifiable, if health promotion programs are appropriately developed.

Traditional health promotion programs often rely on the diffusion of ideas: They focus on communicating information to a population (Braithwaite and Lythcott, 1989). Unfortunately, this approach often fails to consider the factors that may prevent people from receiving and/ or acting on the information. Health professionals must recognize that providing education regarding health promotion activities may not be effective in changing attitudes or behaviors of ethnic minorities. "It is easy to assume that people will act in accordance with their attitudes and beliefs provided there are no other factors acting to influence their behavior" (Berkanovic, 1981–82, p. 235). Health interventions for low-income ethnic minority groups must address social contexts and quality of life and acknowledge the daily experiences that shape individual perceptions and perceived options. Successful intervention with low-income ethnic minority groups may need to offer ways of reducing and/or coping with life stressors, particularly high levels of chronic violence. The stresses of violence and poverty may be so overwhelming that health promotion programs have limited chance of success unless health is presented as a means of coping with stress and regaining control over one's life. Healthy lifestyles, therefore, must provide a means of coping with life rather than be an added burden, and health promotion programs must empower urban communities to address the stressors that impact their lives and health outcomes.

The concept of increasing a sense of personal or community control and power in order to effect health behavior change is an integral component of the community empowerment model, which emphasizes the importance of reclaiming control over one's life and environment (Gottlieb, 1985; Braithwaite and Lythcott, 1989; Minkler, 1992; Wallerstein, 1992). Empowerment is a social-action process that promotes participation of people, organizations, and communities toward the goals of increased individual and community control, political efficacy, improved quality of community life, and social justice (Wallerstein, 1992, p. 198). Community empowerment models have long recognized the relationship between feelings of alienation, powerlessness, and health behaviors. However, future programs may need to assist communities in reducing levels of community violence before issues of health behavior can be effectively addressed. Or, communities must be assisted in addressing both the level of violence and poor health outcomes. Practical solutions to the realities of violence must be provided, and safe and convenient locations for refuge from the violence and/or for conducting health promotion activities are essential. There is evidence that comprehensive approaches to health promotion, which emphasize community empowerment and address the role of violence in the lives of community residents, can be successful in low-income ethnic minority communities (Minkler, 1992).

For example, as we develop health promotion programs for ethnic minority communities, it will become increasingly important to recognize that violence prevention is indeed a health promotion intervention in ethnic minority communities where there are high levels of interpersonal and community violence. Based on the findings presented in this chapter, high levels of community violence not only impact the well-being of victims of violence but also influence the health behaviors of those who are chronically exposed to it. Thus, health promotion programs targeting urban ethnic minority communities must not only acknowledge that the prevalence of violence influences health behaviors but also must strive to reduce the incidence of violent episodes in the community as a means of improving health behaviors and health outcomes. Perhaps the work of Minkler (1992) best exemplifies this approach. In designing health promotion programs for the elderly poor in San Francisco, "safehouses" where residents could seek refuge from community violence were established to increase a sense of safety among community residents before other health promotion programs were initiated. In this urban community, and in many others, a sense of safety is a prerequisite to healthier individual behaviors.

However, as community-wide violence prevention programs are established, it may also be necessary to address the previous impact of exposure to violence on individual health behaviors. In this regard, lay health advisers have been used successfully to promote health behavior change, especially in ethnic minority groups, and address the social and cultural barriers, such as exposure to violence, to healthy behaviors (Hargreaves et al., 1989; Amezuca et al., 1990). The effectiveness of lay health advisers in helping individuals overcome the cultural and social barriers to healthy behaviors, recruiting individuals to health promotion interventions, and increasing health promotion behaviors has been well documented (Warnecke et al., 1975, 1976; Salber, 1979; Brownstein et al., 1992; Levine et al., 1992). The importance of using lay health advisers who are similar to the target population and who conduct interventions in programs where there is a shared sense of identity has also been stressed (Warnecke et al., 1975; Israel, 1982, 1985). The success of health intervention programs that focus on experiences related to ethnicity (DiClemente and Wingood, 1995) also supports the use of indigenous community workers and underscores the importance of addressing issues such as exposure to violence that may be common in ethnic minority groups.

Finally, in order to develop more effective health promotion programs for urban ethnic minority communities, extensive research on the relationship between exposure to violence and health behavior is also needed. We need to understand how exposure to different types of violence (e.g., murder, domestic violence, physical or sexual abuse) affects health promotion behaviors. Does the time of exposure (i.e., childhood versus adulthood) and/or the level of exposure to violence influence the degree to which health promotion behavior is impacted? Does gender influence the relationship between exposure to violence and health promotion behaviors? And can an individual's response to violence, and the resulting impact on health promotion behaviors, be modified without significant changes in levels of community violence? Answers to these questions are important to our understanding of the relationship between exposure to violence, health promotion behavior, and successful intervention and to the relative need for individual versus community-wide intervention approaches.

Given the growing disparities in health outcomes for many minorities in this country, understanding and examining factors related to ethnic differences in risk factors and health behaviors is crucial. We must move beyond simply identifying ethnic differences in risk and health behaviors to a more comprehensive understanding of what these differences may mean and represent (Martinez and Lillie-Blanton, 1996). Jessor and Donovan (1985), in studying the structure of health and problem behaviors in adolescents, have concluded that risk behaviors are interrelated and can be accounted for by common factors. Their research provides important support for the conclusion that risk behaviors may have common etiologies. It also encourages research on the "risk factors" for the "risk factors" in ethnic minority populations. Orpinas et al. (1995) have also reported evidence of covariation in risk behaviors and suggest that risk behaviors may be linked to psychological and/or environmental factors. These studies provide important support for the conclusion that risk behaviors may have common etiologies. They also encourage research on the "risk factors" for the "risk factors" that impact ethnic minority populations. Link and Phelan (1995) have also emphasized the importance of examining the social conditions that place individuals at risk of risk behaviors.

Martinez and Lillie-Blanton (1996) have also concluded that ethnic differences in health behaviors and outcomes may reflect differences in life experiences and the environments in which these individuals grow and develop. This view is consistent with the findings presented in this chapter on the impact of exposure to violence on health behaviors in ethnic minority populations. Indeed, exposure to community and/or interpersonal violence may be one of the risk factors for other risk factors, such as smoking, lack of exercise, use of alcohol, and use of illegal drugs, that severely compromise the health outcomes of ethnic minorities in this country. Examination of the mediating influence of exposure to violence on health behaviors in urban ethnic minority groups may also increase our understanding of relationships between socioeconomic status and health in ethnic minority groups and help to explain findings linking socioeconomic status to risk factors for chronic disease (Lowry et al., 1996), prevalence of disease in ethnic minority populations (Breen and Figueroa, 1996), and screening behavior in ethnic minority women (Pearlman et al., 1996). Such studies are needed to understand how race and ethnicity interact with other factors in impacting health behaviors and outcomes.

Research in this area may also have significant implications for the planning and development of health promotion and disease prevention programs for urban ethnic minority communities. A recent survey of health officers in economically stressed urban centers in the United States revealed that the five most important public health prevention goals were reducing the incidence of HIV infection and AIDS, improving maternal and infant health, controlling sexually transmitted diseases, reducing violent and abusive behavior, and immunizing against infectious diseases (Greenberg et al., 1995). Current findings suggest that exposure to violence may contribute to the incidence of the other health problems and that controlling violence in urban centers may be an important vehicle for addressing other health problems. Existing data also suggest that failing to address multiple risk behaviors and their common etiologies in comprehensive programs of health intervention and prevention developed for urban communities may result in marginal effects on health outcomes (Orpinas et al., 1995). Health promotion professionals cannot be defeated in their efforts to impact health behaviors and health outcomes among low-income ethnic minority communities. Programs must be developed that acknowledge and incorporate an understanding of levels of violence and respect for realities of life in these communities. We must refocus on the revised definition of health promotion as "a process of enabling people to increase control over and to improve their health" (World Health Organization, 1986) while working to enhance the capability of individuals and communities to effectively respond to challenges posed by the environment (Minkler, 1992). In sum, considerable effort must be made to reestablish health as a priority in the lives of low-income ethnic minority groups exposed to violence and to facilitate a sense of empowerment regarding their life and health outcomes.

REFERENCES

Amezuca, C., McAlister, A., Ramirez, A., and Espinoza, R. 1990. A su salud: Health promotion in a Mexican-American border community. In *Health Promotion at the Community Level,* edited by N. Bracht. Newbury Park, Calif.: Sage Publications.

Auerbach, J. D., and Figert, A. E. 1995. Women's health research: Public policy and sociology. *Journal of Health and Social Behavior* 36, 115–131.

Baum, A., and Grunberg, N. 1991. Gender, stress, and health. *Health Psychology* 10, 80–85.

Becker, M. H. 1979. Psychosocial aspects of health-related behavior. In *Handbook of Medical Sociology,* 3rd. ed., edited by H. Freeman, S. Levine, and L. Reeder. Englewood Cliffs, N.J.: Prentice Hall.

Bell, C. 1987. Preventive strategies for dealing with violence among Blacks. *Community Mental Health Journal* 23, 217–228.

Bell, C. C., and Chance-Hill, G. 1991. Treatment of violent families. *Journal of the National Medical Association* 83, 203–208.

Bell, C. C., and Jenkins, E. J. 1991. Traumatic stress and children. *Journal of Health Care for the Poor and Underserved* 2, 175–188.

Berenson, A. B., San Miguel, V. V., and Wilkinson, G. S. 1992. Violence and its relationship to substance use in adolescent pregnancy. *Journal of Adolescent Health* 13, 470–474.

Berkanovic, E. 1976. Behavioral science and prevention. *Preventive Medicine* 5, 92–105.

———. 1981–82. Who engages in health protective behaviors? *International Quarterly of Community Health Education* 2, 225–237.

Berkanovic, E., and Reeder, L. 1973. Ethnic, economic, and social psychological factors in the source of medical care. *Social Problems* 21, 246–259.

Bloom, M. 1993. Toward a code of ethics for primary prevention. *Journal of Primary Prevention* 13, 173–182.

Booth, M. W., Castro, F. G., and Anglin, M. 1991. What do we know about Hispanic substance abuse? A review of the literature. In *Drugs in Hispanic Communities,* edited by R. Click and J. Moore. New Brunswick, N.J.: Rutgers University Press.

Braithwaite, R., and Lythcott, N. 1989. Community empowerment as a strategy for health promotion for Black and other minority populations. *Journal of the American Medical Association* 261, 282–283.

Breen, N., and Figueroa, J. B. 1996. Stage of breast and cervical cancer diagnosis in disadvantaged neighborhoods: A prevention policy perspective. *American Journal of Preventive Medicine* 12, 319–326.

Breslow, L. 1972. A quantitative approach to the World Health Organization definition of health: Physical, mental and social well-being. *International Journal of Epidemiology* 1, 347–355.

Broman, C. L., and Johnson, E. H. 1988. Anger expression and life stress among Blacks: Their role in physical health. *Journal of the National Medical Association* 80, 1329–1334.

Brown-Bryant, R. 1985. The issue of women's health: A matter of record. *Family and Community Health* 7, 53–65.

Brownstein, J. N., Cheal, N., Ackermann, S. P., et al. 1992. Breast and cervical cancer screening in minority populations: A model for using lay health educators. *Journal of Cancer Education* 7, 321–326.

Bullough, B. 1967. Alienation in the ghetto. *Journal of Sociology* 72, 469–478.

———. 1972. Poverty, ethnic identity, and preventive health care. *Journal of Health and Social Behavior* 13, 347–359.

Calnan, M., and Johnson, B. 1985. Health, health risks and inequalities: An exploratory study of women's perceptions. *Sociology of Health and Illness* 7, 55–75.

Centers for Disease Control. 1990. Homicide among Black males—United States, 1978–1987. *Morbidity and Mortality Weekly Report* 39, 869–873.

Chatman, L. M., Billups, M. D., Bell, C. C., and Priest, M. L. 1991. Injury: A new perspective on an old problem. *Journal of the National Medical Association* 83, 43–48.

Christofel, K. K. 1990. Violent death and injury in U.S. children and adolescents. *American Journal of Diseases in Children* 144, 697–706.

Cohen, P., Struening, E., Muhlin, G., et al. 1982. Community stressors, mediating conditions and wellbeing in urban neighborhoods. *Journal of Community Psychology* 10, 377–391.

Cohen, S., Schwartz, J. E., Bromet, E. J., and Parkinson, D. K. 1991. Mental health, stress, and poor health behaviors in two community samples. *Preventive Medicine* 20, 306–315.

Cope, N., and Hall, H. 1985. The health status of black women in the U.S.: Implications for health psychology and behavioral medicine. *Sage* 2, 20–24.

Cupoli, J., and Sewell, P. 1988. One thousand fifty-nine children with a complaint of sexual abuse. *Child Abuse and Neglect* 12, 151–162.

Davidson, J., and Smith, R. 1990. Traumatic experiences in psychiatric outpatients. *Journal of Traumatic Stress* 3, 459–475.

Dawkins, R., and Dawkins, M. 1983. Alcohol use and delinquency among Black, White and Hispanic offenders. *Adolescence* 18, 798–809.

DiClemente, R., and Wingood, G. 1995. A randomized controlled trial of an HIV sexual risk-reduction intervention for young African-American women. *Journal of the American Medical Association* 274, 1271–1276.

Dinges, N. G., and Joos, S. K. 1998. Stress, coping, and health: Models of interaction for Indian and native populations. In *Behavioral Health Issues among American Indians and Alaska Natives: Explorations on the Frontiers of the Biobehavioral Sciences*.

Dodge, K. A., Lochman, J. E., Harnish, J. D., et al. 1997. Reactive and proactive aggression in school children and psychiatrically impaired chronically assaultive youth. *Journal of Abnormal Psychology* 15, 37–51.

Dubrow, N., and Garbarino, J. 1989. Living in the war zone: Mothers and young children in a public housing development. *Child Welfare* 68, 3–20.

Durant, R. H., Cadenhead, C., Pendergrast, R. A., et al. 1994a. Factors associated with the use of violence among urban Black adolescents. *American Journal of Public Health* 84, 612–617.

Durant, R. H., Getts, A., Cadenhead, C., et al. 1995. Exposure to violence and victimization and depression, hopelessness, and purpose in life among adolescents living in and around public housing. *Developmental and Behavioral Pediatrics* 16, 233–237.

Durant, R. H., Pendergrast, R. A., and Cadenhead, C. 1994b. Exposure to violence and victimization and fighting behavior by urban Black adolescents. *Journal of Adolescent Health* 15, 311–318.

Ehrhardt, A. A., Exner, T. M., and Seal, D. W. 1995. The effectiveness of AIDS prevention efforts. *HIV prevention: State-of-the-science*. Commissioned by the Office of Technology Assessment. Compiled and produced by the American Psychological Association Office on AIDS.

Elliot, B. A. 1993. Community responses to violence. *Primary Care* 20, 495–502.

Eng, E. 1993. The Save Our Sisters Project: A social network strategy for reaching rural Black women. *Cancer* 72, 1071–1077.

Eng, E., Hatch, J., and Callan, A. 1985. Institutionalizing social support through the church and into the community. *Health Education Quarterly* 12, 81–92.

Ferrence, R. G. 1988. Sex differences in cigarette smoking in Canada, 1900–1978: A reconstructed cohort study. *Canadian Journal of Public Health* 79, 160–165.

Franke, N. V. 1997. African American women's health: The effects of disease and chronic life stressors. In *Women's Health: Complexities and Differences*, edited by S. B. Ruzek, V. L. Olesen, and A. E. Clarke. Columbus: Ohio State University Press.

Freeman, L. N., Mokros, H., and Poznanski, E. 1992. Violent events reported by normal urban school-aged children: Characteristics and depression correlates. *Journal of the American Academy of Adolescent Psychiatry* 32, 419–423.

Freudenberg, N. 1978. Shaping the future of health education: From behavior change to social change. *Health Education Monographs* 6, 373–377.

Fullilove, M. T., Lown, A., and Fullilove, R. E. 1992. Crack 'hos and skeezers: Traumatic experiences of women crack users. *Journal of Sex Research* 29, 275–287.

Gall, S. B., and Gall, T. L., eds. 1993. *Statistical Record of Asian Americans*. Detroit: Gale Research.

Garbarino, J., Kostelny, K., and Dubrow, N. 1991a. *Children and Youth in Dangerous Environments: Coping with the Consequences of Community Violence*. San Francisco: Jossey-Bass.

———. 1991b. What children can tell us about living in danger. *American Psychologist* 46, 376–383.

Gardner, G. E. 1971. Aggression and violence—the enemies of precision learning in children. *American Journal of Psychiatry* 128, 77–82.

Glaser, J. B., Schachter, J., Benes, S., et al. 1991. Sexually transmitted diseases in post pubertal female rape victims. *Journal of Infectious Diseases* 164, 726–730.

Golding, J. M. 1994. Sexual assault history and physical health in randomly selected Los Angeles women. *Health Psychology* 13, 130–138.

Gottlieb, B. 1985. Social networks and social support: An overview of research, practice, and policy implications. *Health Education Quarterly* 12, 5–22.

Gottlieb, N., and Green, L. 1984. Life events, social network, life-style, and health: An analysis of the 1979 national survey of personal health practices and consequences. *Health Education Quarterly* 11, 91–105.

Green, L. 1982. A learned helplessness analysis of problems confronting the Black community. In *Behavior Modification in Black Populations: Psychosocial Issues and Empirical Findings,* edited by S. M. Turner and R. T. Jones. New York: Plenum.

Greenberg, M., Schneider, D., and Martell, J. 1995. Health promotion priorities of economically stressed cities. *Journal of Health Care for the Poor and Underserved* 6, 10–21.

Groat, H. T., and Neal, A. G. 1967. Social psychological correlates of urban fertility. *American Sociological Review* 32, 945–949.

Guyer, B., Lescohier, I., Gallagher, S. S., et al. 1989. Intentional injuries among children and adolescents in Massachusetts. *New England Journal of Medicine* 321, 1564–1589.

Hammond, W. R., and Yung, B. 1993. Psychology's role in the public health response to assaultive violence among young African-American men. *American Psychologist* 48, 142–154.

Harel, Z. 1986. Older Americans act related homebound aged: What difference does racial background make? *Journal of Gerontological Social Work* 9, 133–143.

Hargreaves, M. K., Baquet, C., and Gamshadzahi, A. 1989. Diet, nutritional status, and cancer risk in American Blacks. *Nutrition and Cancer* 12, 1–28.

Harlow, C. 1989. Female victims of violent crime. Bureau of Justice Statistics Special Report NCJ-126826. Washington, D.C.: U.S. Department of Justice.

Hinton-Nelson, M. D., Roberts, M. C., and Snyder, C. R. 1996. Early adolescents exposed to violence: Hope and vulnerability to victimization. *American Journal of Orthopsychiatry* 66, 346–353.

Hoppe, S., and Heller, P. 1975. Alienation, familism and the utilization of health services by Mexican-Americans. *Journal of Health and Social Behavior* 16, 304–314.

Hughes, H. 1988. Psychological and behavioral correlates of family violence in child witnesses and victims. *American Journal of Orthopsychiatry* 58, 77–90.

Hughes, M., and Demo, D. H. 1989. Self-perceptions of Black Americans: Self-esteem and personal efficacy. *American Journal of Sociology* 95, 132–159.

Humphrey, J., and Palmer, S. 1986. Race, sex and criminal homicide: Offender-victim relationships. In *Homicide among Black Americans,* edited by D. Hawkins. Lanham, Md.: University Press of America.

Irwin, K. L., Edlin, B. R., Wong, L., et al. 1995. Urban rape survivors: Characteristics and prevalence of human immunodeficiency virus and other sexually transmitted infections. *Obstetrics and Gynecology* 85, 330–336.

Israel, B. A. 1982. Social networks and health status: Linking theory, roles and practice. *Patient Counseling and Health Education* 4, 65–77.

———. 1985. Social networks and social support: Implications for natural helper and community level interventions. *Health Education Quarterly* 12, 65–80.

Jessor, J. E., and Donovan, R. 1985. Structure of problem behavior in adolescence and young adulthood. *Journal of Consulting and Clinical Psychology* 53, 890–904.

Kavanaugh, K. H., Harris, R. M., Hetherington, S. E., and Scott, D. E. 1992. Collaboration as a strategy for acquired immunodeficiency syndrome prevention. *Archives of Psychiatric Nursing* 6, 331–339.

Kersher, G., and McShane, M. 1984. The prevalence of child sexual abuse victimization in an adult sample of Texas residents. *Child Abuse and Neglect* 8, 495–501.

Kessler, R. 1979. Stress, social status, and psychological distress. *Journal of Health and Social Behavior* 20, 259–272.

Kessler, R., and Cleary, P. 1980. Social class and psychological distress. *American Sociological Review* 45, 463–478.

Kessler, R. C., and Magee, W. J. 1994. Childhood family violence and adult recurrent depression. *Journal of Health and Social Behavior* 35, 13–27.

Krieger, N. 1990. Racial and gender discrimination: Risk factors for high blood pressure. *Social Science and Medicine* 30, 1273–1281.

Leftwich, M. J. T., and Collins, F. L. 1994. Parental smoking, depression, and child development: Persistent and unanswered questions. *Journal of Pediatric Psychology* 19, 557–570.

Leigh, W. 1994. The health status of women of color. Joint Center for Political and Economic Studies.

Lemp, G., Hirozawa, A., Givertz, D., et al. 1994. Seroprevalence of HIV and risk behaviors among young homosexual and bisexual men. *Journal of the American Medical Association* 272, 449–454.

Lester, D. 1986. *The Murderer and His Murder: A Review of Research*. New York: AMS Press.

Levine, D. M., Becker, D. M., and Bone, L. R. 1992. Narrowing the gap in health status of minority populations: A community-academic medical center partnership. *American Journal of Preventive Medicine* 8, 319–323.

Lex, B. W. 1991. Some gender differences in alcohol and polysubstance users. *Health Psychology* 10, 121–132.

Liem, R., and Liem, J. 1978. Social class and mental illness reconsidered: The role of economic stress and social support. *Journal of Health and Social Behavior* 19, 139–156.

Lillie-Blanton, M., Anthony, J., and Schuster, C. 1993. Probing the meaning of racial/ethnic group comparisons in crack cocaine smoking. *Journal of the American Medical Association* 269, 993–997.

Link, B. G., and Phelan, J. 1995. Social conditions as fundamental causes of disease. *Journal of Health and Social Behavior* 36(Suppl.), 80–94.

Lorion, R. P., and Saltzman, W. 1993. Children's exposure to community violence: Following a path from concern to research to action. *Psychiatry* 56, 55–65.

Lowry, R., Kann, L., Collins, J. L., and Kolbe, L. J. 1996. The effect of socioeconomic status on chronic disease risk behaviors among US adolescents. *Journal of the American Medical Association* 276, 792–797.

Makuc, D. M., Fried, V. M., and Kleinman, J. 1989. National trends in the use of preventive health care by women. *American Journal of Public Health* 79, 21–26.

Manson, S. M., and Dinges, N. G., eds. 1988. American Indian and Alaska native mental health research. *Journal of the National Center Monograph Series* 1, 9–64.

Martin, S. L., English, K. T., Clark, K. A., et al. 1996. Violence and substance abuse among North Carolina pregnant women. *American Journal of Public Health* 86, 991–998.

Martinez, P., and Richter, J. E. 1993. The NIMH community violence project: II. Children's distress symptoms associated with violence exposure. *Psychiatry* 56, 22–35.

Martinez, R. M., and Lillie-Blanton, M. 1996. Why race and gender remain important in health services research. *American Journal of Preventive Medicine* 12, 316–318.

McGinnis, J. 1986. The 1985 Mary E. Switzer Lecture: Reaching the underserved. *Journal of Allied Health* 15, 293–305.

McLoyd, V. C. 1990. The impact of economic hardship on Black families and children: Psychological distress, parenting, and socioemotional development. *Child Development* 61, 311–346.

Mercy, J., Goodman, R., Rosenberg, M., et al. 1986. Patterns of homicide victimization in the City of Los Angeles. *Bulletin of the New York Academy of Medicine* 62, 427–445.

Mindlin, R., and Densen, P. 1971. Medical care of urban infants: Health supervision. *American Journal of Public Health* 61, 687–697.

Minkler, M. 1992. Community organizing among the elderly poor in the United States: A case study. *International Journal of Health Services* 22, 303–316.

Morris, N. M., Hatch, M. H., and Chipman, S. S. 1966. Alienation as a deterrent to well-child supervision. *American Journal of Public Health* 56, 1874–1882.

O'Carroll, P. W. 1988. Homicides among black males 15–24 years of age, 1970–1984. *Morbidity and Mortality Weekly Report* 37(SS-1), 53–60.

Ogbu, J. 1983. Minority status and schooling in plural societies. *Comparative Education Review* 27, 168–190.

Orpinas, P. K., Basen-Engquist, K., Grunbaum, J. A., and Parcel, G. S. 1995. The co-morbidity of violence-related behaviors with health-risk behaviors in a population of high school students. *Journal of Adolescent Health* 16, 216–225.

Orr, S. T., James, S. A., Miller, C. A., et al. 1996. Psychosocial stressors and low birthweight in an urban population. *American Journal of Preventive Medicine* 12, 459–466.

Osofsky, J. 1995. The effects of exposure to violence on young children. *American Psychologist* 50, 782–788.

Pearlman, D. N., Rakowski, W., Ehrich, B., and Clark, M. A. 1996. Breast cancer screening practices among Black, Hispanic, and White women: Reassessing differences. *American Journal of Health Promotion* 12, 327–337.

Pincus, T., and Callahan, L. F. 1995. What explains the association between socioeconomic status and health: Primary access to medical care or mind-body variables? *Advances: The Journal of Mind-Body Health* 11, 4–36.

Rainwater, L. 1960. *And the Poor Get Children.* Chicago: Quadrangle Books.

Rakowski, W. 1988. Predictors of health practices within age-sex groups: National survey of personal health practices and consequences, 1979. *Public Health Reports* 103, 376–386.

Rask, K. J., Williams, M. V., Parker, R. M., and McNagny, S. E. 1994. Obstacles predicting lack of a regular provider and delays in seeking care for patients at an urban public hospital. *Journal of the American Medical Association* 271, 1931–1933.

Resnick, H., Falsetti, S., Kilpatrick, D., and Freedy, J. 1986. Assessment of rape and other civilian trauma-related post-traumatic stress disorder: Emphasis on assessment of potentially traumatic events. In *Stressful Life Events,* edited by T. W. Miller. Madison, Conn.: International Universities Press.

Resnick, H., Kilpatrick, D., Dansky, B., et al. 1993. Prevalence of civilian trauma and posttraumatic stress disorder in a representative national sample of women. *Journal of Consulting and Clinical Psychology* 61, 984–991.

Rinear, E. 1988. Psychological aspects of parental response patterns to the death of a child by homicide. *Journal of Traumatic Stress* 1, 305–322.

Rodin, J. 1986. Aging and health: Effects of the sense of control. *Science* 233, 1271–1276.

Rodin, J., and Ickovics, J. 1990. Women's health: Review and research agenda as we approach the 21st century. *American Psychologist* 45, 1018–1034.

Rosenberg, M. 1987. Children of battered women: The effects of witnessing violence on their social problem-solving abilities. *The Behavior Therapist* 10, 85–89.

Rosenberg, M. L., and Fenley, M. A., eds. 1991. *Violence in America: A Public Health Approach.* New York: Oxford University Press.

Ross, C. E., and Mirowsky, J. 1989. Explaining the patterns of depression: Control and problem solving—or support and talking. *Journal of Health and Social Behavior* 30, 206–219.

Rotheram-Borus, M. J., Mahler, K. A., Koopman, C., and Langabeer, K. 1996. Sexual abuse history and associated multiple risk behavior in adolescent runaways. *American Journal of Orthopsychiatry* 66, 390–400.

Ruzek, S. B., Clarke, A. E., and Olesen, V. L. 1997a. What are the dynamics of differences? In *Women's Health: Complexities and Differences,* edited by S. B. Ruzek, V. L. Olesen, and A. E. Clarke. Columbus: Ohio State University Press.

Ruzek, S. B., Olesen, V. L., and Clarke, A. E., eds. 1997b. *Women's Health: Complexities and Differences.* Columbus: Ohio State University Press.

Salber, E. J. 1979. The lay health advisor as a community health resource. *Journal of Health Politics, Policy and Law* 3, 469–479.

———. 1994a. Correlates of healthy eating habits in low-income Black women and Latinas. *Preventive Medicine* 23, 781–787.

———. 1994b. Health promotion behavior in low-income Black and Latino women. *Women and Health* 21, 71–83.

———. 1996a. Correlates of health promotion behaviors in low-income, Black and Latino women. *Journal of Preventive Medicine* 12, 450–458.

———. 1996b. The ecology of urban violence: Its relationship to health promotion behaviors in Black and Latino communities. *American Journal of Health Promotion* 10, 88–97.

Schaefer, N., Falciglia, G., and Collins, R. 1990. Adult African-American females learn cooperatively. *Journal of Nutrition Education* 22, 240D.

Seeman, M. 1959. On the meaning of alienation. *Sociological Review* 24, 783–791.

Seeman, M., and Evans, J. 1962. Alienation and learning in a hospital setting. *American Sociological Review* 27, 772–782.

Seeman, M., and Seeman, T. 1983. Health behavior and personal autonomy: A longitudinal study of the sense of control in illness. *Journal of Health and Social Behavior* 24, 144–160.

Sheley, J., McGee, Z., and Wright, J. 1992. Gun-related violence in and around inner city schools. *American Journal of Diseases of Childhood* 146, 677–682.

Shumaker, S. A., and Hill, D. R. 1991. Gender differences in social support and physical health. *Health Psychology* 10, 102–111.

Singer, L., Arendt, R., and Minnes, S. 1993. Neurodevelopmental effects of cocaine. *Clinics in Perinatology* 20, 245–262.

Singer, M. I., Anglin, T. M., Song, L., and Lunghofer, L. 1996. Adolescents' exposure to violence and associated symptoms of psychological trauma. *Journal of the American Medical Association* 273, 477–482.

Sluzki, C. 1993. Toward a model of family and political victimization: Implications for treatment and recovery. *Psychiatry* 56, 178–187.

Smith, J., Mercy, J., and Rosenberg, M. 1986. Suicide and homicide among Hispanics in the Southwest. *Public Health Reports* 101, 265–270.

Smith, T. 1992. Hostility and health: Current status of a psychosomatic hypothesis. *Health Psychology* 11, 139–150.

Snyder, C. R. 1994. *The Psychology of Hope: You Can Get There from Here.* New York: The Free Press.

Sonnenberg, S. M. 1988. Victims of violence and post-traumatic stress disorder. *Psychiatric Clinics of North America* 11, 581–590.

Sorenson, S., and Shen, H. 1996. Homicide risk among immigrants in California, 1970 through 1992. *American Journal of Public Health* 86, 97–100.

Spivak, H., Hausman, A., and Prothrow-Stith, D. 1989. Practitioner's forum: Public health and the primary prevention of adolescent violence—The violence prevention project. *Violence and Victims* 4, 203–212.

Stevens-Simon, C., and Reichert, S. 1994. Sexual abuse, adolescent pregnancy, and child abuse: A developmental approach to an intergenerational cycle. *Archives of Pediatrics and Adolescent Medicine* 148, 23–27.

Stokols, D. 1992. Establishing and maintaining healthy environments: Toward a social ecology of health promotion. *American Psychologist* 47, 6–22.

Sumner, B., Mintz, E., and Brown, P. 1986. Interviewing persons hospitalized with interpersonal violence-related injuries: A pilot study. In *Report of the Secretary's Task Force on Black and Minority Health, Volume 5.* Washington, D.C.: U.S. Department of Health and Human Services.

Syme, S., and Berkman, J. 1976. Social class, susceptibility and sickness. *American Journal of Epidemiology* 18, 635–643.

Tardiff, K., and Gross, E. 1986. Homicide in New York City. *Bulletin of the New York Academy of Medicine* 62, 413–426.

U.S. Department of Health and Human Services. 1986, January. Homicide, suicide, and unintentional injuries, volume 5. In *Report of the Secretary's Task Force on Black and Minority Health.* Washington, D.C.: U.S. Department of Health and Human Services.

U.S. Department of Health and Human Services, Public Health Service, Health Resources and Services Administration. 1991. *Health Status of Minorities in Low Income Groups.* DHHS Publication HRS-D-DV 85-1, 3rd ed.

U.S. Department of Justice. 1991. Criminal victimization, 1990. Special Report NCJ-122743. Washington, D.C.: Bureau of Justice Statistics.

Vega, W., Sallis, J., Patterson, T. R., et al. 1988. Predictors of dietary change in Mexican-American families participating in a health behavior change program. *American Journal of Preventive Medicine* 4, 194–199.

Wallerstein, N. 1992. Powerlessness, empowerment, and health: Implications for health promotion programs. *American Journal of Health Promotion* 6, 197–205.

Warnecke, R. B., Graham, S., Mosher, W., et al. 1975. Contact with health guides and use of health services among Blacks in Buffalo. *Public Health Reports* 90, 213–222.

Warnecke, R. B., Graham, S., Mosher, W., and Montgomery, E. 1976. Health guides as influentials in central Buffalo. *Journal of Health and Social Behavior* 17, 22–34.

Weinstein, N. D. 1993. Testing four competing theories of health-protective behavior. *Health Psychology* 12, 324–333.

Weisz, J., Martin, S., Walter, B., and Fernandez, G. 1991. Differential prediction of young adult arrests for property and personal crimes: Findings of a cohort follow-up study of violent boys from North Carolina's Willie M. program. *Journal of Child Psychology and Psychiatry* 32, 783–792.

Wilbanks, W. 1986. Criminal homicide offenders in the U.S.: Black vs. White. In *Homicide among Black Americans,* edited by D. Hawkins. Lanham, Md.: University Press of America.

Wilkerson, J., Protinsky, H. O., Maxwell, J. W., and Lentner, M. 1982. Alienation and ego identity in adolescents. *Adolescence* 17, 133–139.

Williams, D., Lavizzo-Mourey, R., and Warren, R. 1994. The concept of race and health status. *Public Health Reports* 109, 26–41.

World Health Organization. 1986. Report of the working group on concept and principles of health promotion, 1984. *Health Promotion* 1, 73–76.

Wyatt, G. E. 1992. The sociocultural context of African American and White American women's rape. *Journal of Social Issues* 48, 77–91.

Zapata, B. C., Rebolledo, A., Atalah, E., et al. 1992. The influence of social and political violence on the risk of pregnancy complications. *American Journal of Public Health* 82, 685–690.

Zeiler, S., Wotbeck, B., and Mayer, K. 1996. Sexual violence against women living with or at risk for HIV infection. *American Journal of Preventive Medicine* 12, 304–310.

12

Theodore G. Ganiats
and William J. Sieber

VALUING FUTURE HEALTH IN SOCIAL
POLICY AND HUMAN HEALTH BEHAVIOR

As shown throughout this volume, promoting human wellness involves a wide variety of themes. These themes are usually operationalized through either large groups (e.g., health policy) or on a more micro level (e.g., an individual's behavior). Sometimes this involves formal programs (The Great American Smokeout, Medicare approval of screening mammography). At other times wellness is promoted by supporting an individual's decision to change behavior. Those of us interested in promoting human wellness decide where best to place our efforts.

To make sound decisions, whether they be related to health policy or with an individual patient or client, we must consider all relevant factors. Therefore, an examination of both the methodologies used in quantitative health policy analysis and an individual's choices and the behavior resulting from these choices is essential. Quantitative health policy analysis, an explicit method of evaluating benefits and harms, serves as a policy tool for government and health policy agencies. One element of this tool is particularly influential; in fact, analysis can actually present health policy agencies with conflicting conclusions depending on how an analyst values future health outcomes. Similarly, we argue that the valuation of future health outcomes affects an individual's behavior, but the major models of human health behavior do not account for this time preference.

In this chapter, we explore how the valuing of future health affects both policy analysis and individual health behavior. We begin with a review of the basic principles of quantitative health policy analysis, paying special attention to the concept of discounting (a method of determining the present value of a future outcome). We follow with a review of research on the psychology of discounting. Finally, we provide an overview of two major psychological theories that deal with health behaviors and demonstrate that these theories fail to account for individual differences in the valuation of future health outcomes. In the final part of the chapter, we discuss possible effects of adding time preference to both levels of analysis and propose areas for future research and theory development.

QUANTITATIVE HEALTH POLICY ANALYSIS

A legislature dictates which health care benefits to offer Medicaid recipients. An insurance company decides which benefits to offer its various health plan subscribers. A hospital develops rules that dictate how and when to use various hospital resources. These are the realities of health care policy, manifestations that touch each of us at one time or another.

Policy formulation reflects a host of decision-making techniques. Sometimes political action groups work to ensure that certain health benefits are legislated. Sometimes experts convene and arrive at a consensus. Another method is to list the goals of a health system and then rank programs, giving the greatest weight to those most likely to meet system goals.

This last method, the quantitative approach to health policy formulation, has several advantages over alternatives. It is less susceptible to special interests, and it is more likely to optimize the health of the target population. In addition, when health care resources are limited, the quantitative approach is most likely to optimize their use.[1]

Modeling Health and Resource Use

Examining one such quantitative approach demonstrates the principles of quantitative analysis in health policy development. In the General Health Policy Model, a pioneering effort in health policy formulation,[1-3] any health program has two outcomes: health status and resource use. Using this model, an analyst assumes that the goal of the health care system is to improve health, measured as both life expectancy and quality of life (alternatively stated as "adding years to life and life to years").[1,4]

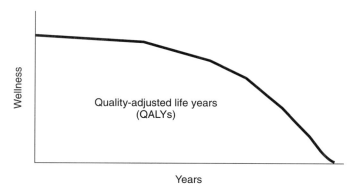

Figure 12.1. The time-wellness graph in which quality of life and time are combined to produce a new health outcome: the quality-adjusted life-year (QALY).

The system achieves this goal by implementing programs that use health care resources, usually described in dollars. If there are budget constraints, the goal is pursued through the efficient use of limited resources.

An analyst estimating resource use evaluates how much the program costs (e.g., in terms of medications, hospitalization, and complications) and how much the program saves (perhaps measuring decreased future health care, decreased risk of future infection, and increased productivity by returning to work). Similarly, when evaluating health, an analyst estimates how the program improves quality of life (decreased symptoms or increased functioning), decreases quality of life (side effects from medications or complications from surgery), and affects mortality.

The resources consumed and saved are merely opposite sides of the same economic coin. Together, they reflect the net resource utilization. In contrast, the two components of health care outcomes are fundamentally different: Quality of life and life expectancy are not directly additive. These two components of health can, however, be combined to create a single health outcome measure for quantitative analysis.

Figure 12.1 shows the integration of quality of life and life expectancy on a single graph, with "time" on the horizontal axis and "wellness," or quality of life, on the vertical axis. The healthier the person, the higher the line; the longer the person lives, the longer the line. To see how well a program succeeds in meeting the goal of prolonging life while increasing quality of life, one merely measures the area displayed under this "time-wellness" plot. Larger areas depict longer, more healthy lives. The area is in the units of the "quality-adjusted life year" (QALY).[5]

Rationing: New Name, Familiar Choices

Each of us hopes for high QALYs. While a quantitative approach to health policy can lead to rationing, such rationing is not a new threat to health care. Our present system relies on rationing to allocate health resources. When a patient needs admission to a full intensive care unit (ICU), a physician decides who will be denied an ICU bed. Because of the short supply of organs for transplantation, organs are routinely rationed among transplant candidates. During the Persian Gulf War, a shortage of gamma globulin required physicians to decide not who needed the gamma globulin but who needed it most. Rationing is a fact of life in health care. A quantitative approach to policy simply illuminates choices related to rationing—choices that are frankly uncomfortable and politically sensitive. This is why we must scrutinize the tenets and perspective of any system used to set health policy.

Perspective: A Societal Vantage Point

Any health policy analysis assumes some perspective. Think of it as varying according to where you sit. Behind a corporate desk, the perspective may be purely financial, aimed at maximizing profit regardless of the health outcome. From a kitchen table, a patient with excellent health insurance may be most concerned with health benefits since his wallet is not involved. As a society, we usually choose a balance between these two perspectives. We want to optimize health for all, but we set limits when resources are strained. The first part of this chapter represents this group perspective; we will assume that the group wishes to use societal resources to improve the average health of the population.

DISCOUNTING: TODAY'S
REWARDS VERSUS TOMORROW'S REWARDS

So far, the description of the quantitative approach to health care has been straightforward: We add benefits (positive health outcomes and dollars saved), subtract costs (adverse health outcomes and dollars spent), and evaluate the balance. In practice, however, this is an oversimplification.

Psychologists have long recognized that people have a time preference for outcomes. Simply stated, time preference recognizes that most

TABLE 12.1   DISCOUNT
MULTIPLIERS FOR VARIOUS YEARS
AT 5% AND 10% DISCOUNT RATES

Years	5% Discount Rate	10% Discount Rate
1	0.952	0.909
2	0.907	0.826
3	0.864	0.751
4	0.823	0.683
5	0.784	0.621
10	0.614	0.386
15	0.481	0.239
20	0.377	0.149
25	0.295	0.092
30	0.231	0.057
40	0.142	0.022

of us prefer a present reward over a future reward of equal value. Similarly, we usually prefer a future penalty over a present penalty of equal weight. Adjusting for this time preference is a standard element of current quantitative health policy analysis. This adjustment is called "discounting." [5]

A simple example illustrates discounting. As a lottery winner, would you choose a $10,000 cash prize today or in one year? Most of us would choose cash today. Even if the future award were adjusted for inflation (e.g., if inflation were 5%, the $10,000 would grow to $10,500), most of us would still prefer our winnings now. This choice implies that we value a future dollar less than a present one. In other words, we discount the value of future dollars.

The process of calculating the present value of future dollars by discounting is, mathematically, the opposite of calculating the future value of present dollars with interest. For example, $10,000 invested at 5% interest will be worth $10,500 ($10,000 + 0.05 × $10,000) after one year. In contrast, if the discount rate is 5%, then $10,000 a year from now is currently valued at $9,500 ($10,000 − [0.05 × $10,000]). Just as compound interest offers dramatic returns after a few years, the compounded effects of discounting can have a marked effect on an economic analysis; the further into the future the outcome occurs, the greater the impact of discounting.

Table 12.1 demonstrates this effect. The discount multiplier for 25 years at a 5% discount rate is 0.295. Someone with a 5% discount rate for future dollars would consider $10,000 received in 25 years to have a current value of 0.295 × $10,000, or $2,950. In other words, this person would be indifferent to receiving $2,950 today or $10,000 in 25 years.

Discounting's Economic Rationale

Why do most of us demonstrate this positive time preference for money, preferring $10,000 in our pockets to comparable funds in a year (even after adjusting for inflation)? The answer is multifactorial.[5-14] First, we could invest the money and earn more than inflation. Second, we could spend money in hand and enjoy the benefits of the dollars now rather than in the future. Third, many of us do not trust the future. Maybe we are not sure that we will be alive in one year and want to enjoy the money now. Maybe we suspect that the source of the $10,000 may default on the dollars owed.

The second and third factors indicate that our preference for today's dollar is not simply a matter of its investment potential. They demonstrate other human factors at work. Thus, discounting is based on multifactorial preferences for present over future dollars.

Economists, while comfortable with the concept of discounting, do not agree on what this discount rate should be. In cost-effectiveness research, proposed discount rates vary from 0% to 20%.[5,11,15,16] Typically, analysts use a discount rate that approximates the prevailing interest earned on investments, and the recent consensus report suggests a discount rate of 3%. Consideration of the previously noted human factors suggests that this is a low estimate.

Discounting Future Health

In a quantitative health policy analysis, one usually assumes that the economic and health discount rates are equal.[5,6,15] This assumption causes an apparent prevention program paradox: While most prevention programs are intuitively cost-effective, many do not fare well in a traditional cost-effectiveness analysis. The explanation for the paradox is clear—prevention programs generate expenditures today, but related health outcomes occur in the future. The ratio of full-valued present dollar costs to discounted future health benefits creates the unfavorable cost-effectiveness ratios so often calculated for prevention programs.

Table 12.2 shows the effect of discounting on cost-effectiveness in two prevention programs. It demonstrates that discounting has the expected, and at times marked, effect on the calculated cost-effectiveness of pre-

TABLE 12.2   EFFECT OF
DISCOUNTING HEALTH OUTCOMES
ON THE COST-EFFECTIVENESS
OF SELECTED PREVENTION PROGRAMS

Program	Cost-Effectiveness (Discounted)	Cost-Effectiveness (Undiscounted)
Universal neonatal hepatitis B immunization	$38,632 per life-year[a]	$3,066 per life-year[a]
Universal adult hepatitis B immunization	$257,418 per life-year[a]	$54,524 per life-year[a]
Neonatal circumcision (Assumption A[b])	$67,402 per QALY	$33,156 per QALY
Neonatal circumcision (Assumption B[b])	N/A (it costs dollars and decreases QALYs)	$8,161 per QALY

[a] Future years of life were not quality adjusted in this study.
[b] The exact assumptions are not important to illustrate the point here. The reader is referred to the original article for the details.

vention programs. This calculation can also affect health policy. For example, if we are willing to spend up to $70,000 to extend life by one year (a reasonable assumption given current health policy), the adult hepatitis B immunization program is cost-effective (at $54,000 per life-year) if we do not discount future health. In other words, if we are willing to spend up to $70,000 in order to get one life-year, then we would find a program costing only $55,000 per life-year to be acceptable. On the other hand, the undiscounted program (at $257,000 per life-year) costs more than $70,000 per life-year and should not be considered cost-effective. In the Assumption B circumcision example, the procedure moves from "charlatan" territory (spending money for diminished health) to a highly cost-effective procedure, depending on whether the analyst discounts future health outcomes. These illustrations offer a graphic demonstration that discounting is not an esoteric topic but is central to cost-effectiveness analysis.

The most often quoted rationale for keeping the economic and health discount rates the same is the work of Keeler and Cretin.[6] They state that if the health discount rate is lower than the monetary discount rate, then no particular program should ever be implemented because the program will become more cost-effective by postponing it for one year. This is the result of the dollar numerator decreasing faster, under the influence of the larger discount rate, than the health outcome denominator: The calculated ratio must be smaller (i.e., more cost-effective) with each successive year. Others note that by keeping the monetary and health discount rates equal, we ensure that the future relationship between the valuation of health and dollars remains constant and the same as today.[5]

These arguments may not be valid since there are significant differences between dollars and health. For example, dollars can be invested and grow in value over time. Health not only cannot be invested but in most people remains constant or slowly decreases over time. In addition, wealth can be spent to obtain some other commodity, but you cannot "spend" health. In fact, health and wealth are so fundamentally different that no evidence suggests that people uniformly discount them at a similar rate.

Further investigation reveals other flaws in the arguments for keeping economic and health discount rates identical. In the argument by Keeler and Cretin, health care programs are postponed because next year they will be more efficient. The math may be correct, but the argument is not relevant. Society does not limit its health resources to only the most efficient program. Instead, we put resources into programs that have an acceptable level of cost-effectiveness. Today's cost-effective program may be more cost-effective next year, but it is still acceptable compared with current (as opposed to future) alternatives. We implement sufficiently efficient programs this year, even if they would be more efficient next year.[17]

The second argument, that the two rates must be equal to preserve a constant relation between dollars and health, is also flawed.[18] There is no a priori reason to insist on this constancy. A nation's health and its wealth may be dynamic. A change in either may modify the relationship between the valuation of future health and future dollars. For example, there may be a general perception that the health of the nation is improving but the economy is stable. Here the ratio of the present value of future health to the present value of future dollars may be greater than the ratio of today's valuation of present health to today's valuation of present dollars. If this is the case, the discount rate for future health should be less than the discount rate for future dollars. The converse, of course, holds if the general sense is that the prospects for future health are declining. In addition, there is evidence that as a country's wealth increases, its residents spend more of the gross national product on health care.[19] This implies that the monetary valuation of health is not an inherent constant but can vary as a function of gross national product. Without constant health valuation, there is no reason to believe that health and economic discount rates remain equal.

Most research on the psychology of discounting (see the next section), though applicable to individual human behavior, has limited usefulness

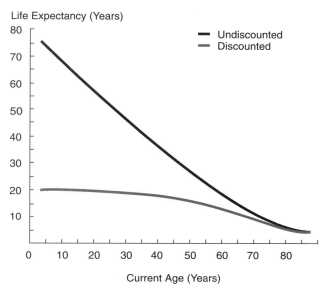

Figure 12.2. Example of a paradox: The effect of discounting life expectancy.

for health policy. For example, most studies assess the discount rate of individuals as opposed to that of a population. This approach may have less relevance in health policy, where population-based data may be more important than data that can be applied to only one individual. Another limitation of current research is that most attempts to assess an individual's discount rate are time consuming and not easily applied to large populations. There are elements of the present research that is limited from both the individual health behavior and the health policy perspectives. For example, there is a tendency in current research to dismiss individuals who claim a negative discount rate for health (i.e., those who prefer future health to present health). Finally, this research tends to focus on graduate students and not patients. The implications of this focus are not clear, but it is reasonable to assume that the preferences of a graduate student will differ from those of a patient with a serious acute or chronic condition. For example, it is unlikely that graduate students would display the dynamic inconsistency that Christensen-Szalanski found in pregnant women.[30]

Finally, Figure 12.2 shows the effect of discounting health outcomes over time and highlights another apparent paradox induced by current models. The current discounting model tells us that the more distant in the future an outcome occurs, the less it is valued. Applying this premise to current life expectancy in the United States, we can see that the 73-year life expectancy of a newborn has a present value of 20 years, while the 5.3-year life expectancy of an 85-year-old is valued as 4.7 years. In other words, according to the current discounting model, the life expectancy of a newborn is valued only 15 years longer (20 years − 4.7 years)—only about four times as long—than the life expectancy of an 85-year-old.

PSYCHOLOGY OF DISCOUNTING

Thus far, this chapter has focused on the impact of discounting on the methods used in quantitative health policy analysis. While discounting can have a major effect on a cost-effectiveness analysis, it may also have a direct effect on individual behavior. Research in economics and psychology has identified several important characteristics of discounting in economics.[21]

High Rates Subjects often report very high discount rates. While this is certainly possible, it does fly in the face of current economic practice. Perhaps more significantly, applying these high discount rates to the health outcomes of a prevention program all but ensures that the program will not be cost-effective (our earlier discussion demonstrated the accrual of discounted future benefits while consuming resources in the undiscounted present).

Dynamic Inconsistency Our discount rates can change as the time to the reward varies.[21–23] For example, one may prefer $200 in eight years over $100 in six years (discount rate < 41%). Six years from now, the same person might prefer $100 right away instead of doubling the money in two years (discount rate > 41%).[21]

Magnitude Effect Some investigators have found that discount rates are lower for large magnitude outcomes.[22–24] For example, someone may prefer $10 now over $15 in a year but may prefer $15,000 in a year over $10,000 now, even though both involve the same relative change.

Sign Effect The framing of a question may be important since discount rates may be lower for losses than for gains.[23–26]

Sequence Effect Investigators have found that discount rates are not additive. Subjects confronted with a series of decisions (each with its own discount rate) often do not make the same choice as when the decision is presented as a single problem.[25,27,28]

In contrast to this body of research in economic discounting, little work has been done to address the psychology of discounting health outcomes.[14,20,29,30] There is some evidence that dynamic inconsistency exists,[20] although this is not a universal finding.[29] In one example, Christensen-Szalanski studied labor anesthesia preferences among pregnant women.[20] A month before and a month after delivery, the women wanted to avoid anesthesia; during labor, however, many of these same women were much more favorably disposed toward anesthesia. Like economic outcomes, the psychology of discounting health outcomes is likely multifactorial.

DISCOUNTING AND MODELS OF HEALTH BEHAVIOR

A person's time preference affects his choices, and these choices in part determine health behavior. It is therefore surprising to find that dominant psychological models of health behavior fail to consider time preference. In this section we illustrate this failing by highlighting two major psychological models of individual health behavior. We then offer directions for incorporating the concept of discounting into future work in the field.

Over the past two decades, two models have dominated the psychological literature on explaining individual health behavior. The Health Belief Model[31,32] postulates that before an individual engages in a health-promoting behavior, several factors influence the initiation of action. The model has served as the theoretical basis for hundreds of health education research studies and helped in the formulation of innumerable interventions. The Transtheoretical Model[33,34] uses stages of change to help identify where an individual is in the change process and match the processes most effective in each of these stages with the individual to maximize further change. It has been used primarily in designing proactive interventions, particularly assisting in the cessation of behaviors such as cigarette smoking. Better understanding of each of these models and how discounting may affect each model's ability to predict health behavior is needed.

The Health Belief Model has been used across the health continuum, from prevention to detection to illness behavior. It is appealing to a wide range of professionals in designing and evaluating interventions to alter health behavior. The Health Belief Model was developed in an effort to explain the widespread failure of people to participate in programs to prevent or detect disease [35] but was later extended to address compliance with medical regimens. [31] In this model health behavior is seen as resulting from a combination of several necessary factors: an individual's perceived susceptibility to illness, perceived severity of the illness, perceived benefits of action to reduce vulnerability (i.e., health-promoting behavior), and an evaluation of potential barriers to the proposed action. Lastly, a relevant stimuli is required to trigger health action (i.e., perceived body dysfunction, advice from a physician), though this is the least understood component of the model. More recently, Bandura's concept of self-efficacy has been incorporated into the model to help better explain individual differences observed in taking action to improve one's health. However, what is missing is the importance (or value) of the health benefit of taking such action. [36]

There are components of the Health Belief Model that address this issue indirectly. Namely, perceived illness severity is used as a measure of the aversiveness of the outcome should no change occur in health behavior. This aversiveness may measure motivation to act. However, a more direct measure of the value that an individual places on the health gain at some time in the future may be a more accurate predictor of behavior than rating of disease severity without reference to time. A second component of the model, perceived benefits of action to reduce vulnerability, assesses the perceived effectiveness of the behavior change in reducing the noxious outcome (i.e., disease). Again, the expected efficacy of the behavior on an outcome is not directly related to the value of the outcome. While two individuals may rate the efficacy of a behavior in producing an outcome to be equal, they may differ greatly in how valuable that outcome is. For example, even though a person may see the "severity" of cancer to be significant and the perceived benefit of action (i.e., quit smoking) as being effective in reducing the vulnerability to cancer, the value of life without cancer may be very different for a 70-year-old male with other multiple health problems as compared to the value of a cancer free life as rated by a 30-year-old adult with no other health problems. Also, while a behavior change may be seen as effective in producing some outcome, significant differences in the delay in which benefits are realized may affect the value of that outcome. For example, greater motivation to quit smoking would exist if benefits were derived within a matter of days or hours as compared to describing only those benefits derived from years of abstinence. Adding the value of the outcome (accounting for discounting) to the Health Belief Model may better assess the motivation of an individual to engage in a health-promoting behavior. Discounting of health may vary between individuals—as well as across time for the same individual—in predictable ways and thus add to our understanding of why some individuals engage in health-promoting behavior under some circumstances while others do not.

The Transtheoretical Model emerged from a comparative analysis of leading theories of psychotherapy and behavioral change. Most of the early research on this model compared cigarette smokers who successfully stopped cigarette smoking as a result of a structured smoking cessation program to those who were unsuccessful.[37] This research, and several studies that followed, revealed that behavioral change unfolds through a series of stages. Innumerable studies have used this model to explain the success (and failure) of specific programs designed to promote healthy behavior. The stages described in this model have been labeled precontemplation, contemplation, preparation, action, and maintenance. Precontemplation is used to describe that period in which a person has no intention to change behavior in the next six months, contemplation involves an intent to change behavior within six months, and preparation involves the intent to change behavior within 30 days and may include some initial change in health behavior. The action stage is defined as having implemented some behavior change within the previous six months, while maintenance is defined as overt behavior change having lasted for more than six months. Prochaska et al. confirmed that the Transtheoretical Model also generalized across 12 problem behaviors, including cessation of negative behavior (e.g., smoking) as well as the acquisition of positive behavior (e.g., exercise, mammography screening).[38] This model proposes that people are at different stages in the change process and that matching different processes with the stage in which an individual is at should maximize transition to a more advanced stage of behavior change. Recent studies have demonstrated that this matching does maximize treatment effectiveness (e.g., reference 39).

While matching of the stages to intervention types has shown to be effective, less is known about facilitating transition between stages, particularly from precontemplation to contemplation to preparation.[40] While these authors argue that research is needed to determine the consistency of the crossover (one stage to the next) occurring prior to the action stage, gathering evidence suggests that many people transition to the next stage when the pros of changing the behavior outweigh the cons. In a number of studies, the ratio of pros to cons (or benefits to harms) of performing a certain behavior predicts subsequent behavior. Initial suggestions are that interventions designed to help a person progress from precontemplation to contemplation should target increasing the pros of changing and that only later should the focus be on reducing the negatives of changing. The value of a health outcome may play a significant role in a person's view of the pros of behavior change. That is, while improved health is often assumed to be a valuable benefit of behavior change, differences in the value assigned to health may differ significantly between individuals and over time.

Variables that affect the value of health need to be better understood. For example, most exercise programs are designed for people who have decided to exercise (e.g., preparation or action stage), yet most people do not exercise, and few have little interest in starting.[41,42] This may reflect the fact that the cons of beginning an exercise program (e.g., aches, effort) outweigh the pros of exercising (e.g., improved cardiovascular health) because the health outcome is placed in the future where its value is discounted. Namely, if the benefits of exercise focused on are primarily experienced within six months of initiating the exercise program, the value of this benefit is likely to be more motivating than if the benefits focused on would not be realized for five years. One reason we believe that people differ in their engaging in health behavior is that the value of the health benefit differs between individuals and is affected by how far in the future it is to be realized. Transition from one stage in the Transtheoretical Model to the next may be more the result of changing values placed on future health than of reducing barriers to change. Clearly, more must be known about how individuals differ in their perception of benefits (i.e., future health) before we can examine when the balance between the pros and cons favors behavior change.

While these two models have dominated the field of health psychology and have been successfully used to understand the process by which individuals change behavior, both models do not clearly address the motivational component of change. Namely, people change behavior because the pros of change outweigh the cons, and in fact there has been an unchallenged assumption that for individuals to change, they must value health in the future (when change will supposedly result in better health). However, how people value health in some distant future is anything but clear.

SOME FUTURE CONSIDERATIONS

It is apparent that the scientific inquiry into time preference has been somewhat neglected. Most health policy research has focused on the limited view of the normative model that future health and future financial outcomes must be discounted at the same rate. Much of the research in the field assumes the normative stance. Further, a large amount of the research focuses on populations that are not representative of the population at large. Major psychological models of human health behavior similarly neglect or minimize the issue of time preference—all of this despite the importance of time preference in individual and group decision making.

Work is needed on the appropriate discount rate for policy analysis, especially of prevention programs. The current recommendations of the U.S. Department of Health and Human Service's Panel of Cost Effectiveness in Health and Medicine[43] are that future health and financial outcomes be discounted at the same rate. While this is the current state of the art, it may not be the final word. Prevention programs are disadvantaged by this approach since the bulk of the expenses (both dollar investments and adverse health effects) occur in the undiscounted present, while benefits (cost savings and improved health) accrue in the discounted future. If in fact people do discount preventive care, this approach is appropriate. However, prevention specialists argue, and the growing number of people living a healthier lifestyle support, that prevention programs may be valued higher than treatment programs.

This point can be illustrated with a discussion of routine Papanicolaou (Pap) smears. The chance that a woman will benefit from any one Pap smear is quite small, as are the risks associated with that Pap smear. Still, women routinely disrupt their daily routines to have this test performed; for these women the chance of future health benefits outweighs the certainty of the current inconvenience. The benefits also include other factors, such as the peace of mind afforded by a negative examination. In many ways these benefits increase with time, so discounting these benefits may be counter to the patient's true preferences. If the analyst does not discount future outcomes, the future benefits of the Pap smear would be magnified. This perspective would vastly improve the apparent cost-effectiveness of most prevention programs. More work is needed in this area before we pursue any single direction.

Several directions may be pursued in incorporating the concept of discounting into attempts to account for individual behavior change. First, exploration of the best assessment methodology to assess a person's value of future health will need to be developed. Discounting rates can be derived for an individual at present through a rather elaborate and laborious task. Pursuit of establishing discount rates for groups of people may be a worthwhile avenue to pursue. Second, once assessment technologies are developed, the value that an individual places on a health outcome could be assessed in addition to the other components of the Health Belief Model. Given that health benefits may be experienced at various intervals of delay from the change in behavior, assessing the value of the health outcome when it is to be realized would be especially important. Discounting the value of a future heath outcome may be found to be a stable individual trait or more prone to influence by situational variables; this may prove a fertile area for future research. Third, understanding how a health outcome is valued may illuminate why some behavior change strategies are more effective than others. Research has focused on motivation to change behavior but rarely incorporated differences in perceived value of a health outcome as a component of that motivation. Fourth, once valuing (discounting) of health outcomes is better understood, interventions could be tailored for individuals who have high discount rates by focusing more on immediate/short-term benefits, whereas interventions for individuals who discount future health less drastically may make use of motivational strategies that focus on long-term health benefits of behavior change. Identification of these individual differences or the circumstances that influence the phenomenon of discounting may provide valuable information for the designers of health education/intervention programs.

CONCLUSION

Time preference affects health policy and the study of individual health behavior. In the current economic climate, health care will undergo a radical revision. The values in decision making regarding expenditures for prevention, clinical practice, and what constitutes "basic health care" are being addressed. By better understanding all key elements affecting health policy and behavior, such as time preference, we can best promote human wellness.

NOTE

Prepared in part for the 1994 University of California/Health Net Wellness Lecture Series under a grant from Health Net. Parts previously published in the *American Journal of Preventive Medicine*. Used with permission.

REFERENCES

1 Chen, M., and Bush, J. W. 1976. Maximizing health system output with political and administrative constraints using mathematical programming. *Inquiry* 13, 215–227.

2. Fanshel, S., and Bush, J. W. 1970. A health status index and its application to health services outcomes. *Operations Research* 18, 1021–1066.

3. Kaplan, R. M., Anderson, J. P., and Ganiats, T. G. 1993. The Quality of Well-being scale: Rationale for a single quality of life index. In *Quality of Life Assessment: Key Issues in the 1990s*, 2nd ed., edited by S. R. Walker and R. M. Rosser. Pp. 65–94. London: MTM Press.

4. World Health Organization. 1984. Health promotion: A discussion document on the concepts and principles. (!CP/HSR 602(mo1) ed.) Copenhagen: WHO Regional Office Europe.

5. Weinstein, M. C., Fineberg, H. V., Elstein, A. S., et al. 1980. *Clinical Decision Analysis*. Philadelphia: W. B. Saunders.

6. Keeler, E. B., and Cretin, S. 1983. Discounting of life-saving and other nonmonetary effects. *Management Science* 29, 300–306.

7. Udry, J. R., and Morris, N. M. 1971. A spoonful of sugar helps the medicine go down. *American Journal of Public Health* 61, 776–785.

8. Sox, H. C., Blatt, M. A., and Higgins, M. C. 1988. *Medical Decision Making*. Boston: Butterworths.

9. Warner, K. E., and Luce, B. R. 1982. *Cost-Benefit and Cost-Effectiveness Analysis in Health Care: Principles, Practice, and Potential*. Ann Arbor, Mich.: Health Administration Press.

10. Sackett, D. L., Haynes, R. B., and Tugwell, P. 1985. *Clinical Epidemiology—A Basic Science for Clinical Medicine*. Boston: Little, Brown.

11. Grabowski, H. G., and Hansen, R. W. 1990. Economic scales and tests. In *Quality of Life Assessments in Clinical Trials*, edited by B. Spilker. Pp. 61–70. New York: Raven Press.

12. Wheeler, J. R. C., and Smith, D. G. 1988. The discount rate for capital expenditure analysis in health care. *Health Care Management Review* 13, 43–51.

13. Messing, S. D. 1973. Discounting health: The issue of subsistence and care in an undeveloped country. *Social Science and Medicine* 7, 911–916.

14. Lipscomb, J. 1989. Time preference for health in cost-effectiveness analysis. *Medical Care* 27(Suppl.), S233–S253.

15. Russell, L. B. 1987. *Evaluating Preventive Care: Report on a Workshop.* Washington, D.C.: The Brookings Institution.
16. Barnum, H. 1987. Evaluating healthy days of life gained from health projects. *Social Science and Medicine* 24(10), 833–841.
17. Ganiats, T. 1992. On sale: future health care—The paradox of discounting. *Western Journal of Medicine* 156(5), 550–553.
18. Ganiats, T. G. 1994. Discounting in cost-effectiveness research. *Medical Decision Making* 14(3), 298–300.
19. Schieber, G. J., and Poullier, J. P. 1989. International health care expenditure trends. *Health Affairs* 8, 169–177.
20. Chapman, G. B., and Elstein, A. S. 1995. Valuing the future: Temporal discounting of health and money. *Medical Decision Making* 15(4), 373–386.
21. Thaler, R. 1981. Some empirical evidence on dynamic inconsistency. *Economic Letters* 8, 201–207.
22. Benzion, U., Rapoport, A., and Yagil, J. 1989. Discount rates inferred from decisions: An experimental study. *Management Science* 35(3), 270–284.
23. Loewenstein, G., and Prelec, D. 1992. Anomalies in intertemporal choice: Evidence and interpretation. *Quarterly Journal of Economics* 107(2), 573–597.
24. Loewenstein, G. 1987. Anticipation and the valuation of delayed consumption. *Economic Journal* 97, 666.
25. Loewenstein, G. F. 1988. Frames of mind in intertemporal choice. *Management Science* 34(2), 200–214.
26. Elster, J. 1985. Weakness of the will and the free-rider problem. *Economics and Philosophy* 1, 231.
27. Loewenstein, G. F., and Sicherman, N. 1991. Do workers prefer increasing wage profiles? *Journal of Labor Economics* 9, 67–84.
28. Rose, D. N., and Weeks, M. G. 1988. Individual's discounting of future monetary gains and health states. *Medical Decision Making* 8, 334.
29. Redelmeier, D. A., and Heller, D. N. 1993. Time preference in medical decision making and cost-effectiveness analysis. *Medical Decision Making* 13(3), 212–217.
30. Christensen-Szalanski, J. J. J. 1984. Discount functions and the measurement of patients' values: Women's decisions during childbirth. *Medical Decision Making* 4, 47–58.
31. Becker, M. H., ed. 1974. The health belief model and personal health behavior. *Health Education Monographs* 2.
32. Janz, N. K., and Becker, M. H. 1984. The health belief model: A decade later. *Health Education Quarterly* 11, 1–47.
33. Prochaska, J. O. 1979. *Systems of Psychotherapy: A Transtheoretical Analysis.* Pacific Grove, Calif.: Brooks-Cole.
34. Prochaska, J. O., and DiClemente, C. C. 1984. *The Transtheoretical Approach: Crossing the Traditional Boundaries of Therapy.* Homewood, Ill.: Dow-Jones/Irwin.
35. Rosenstock, I. M. 1996. Why people use health services. *Milbank Memorial Fund Quarterly* 44(3), 94–124.

36. Bandura, A. 1986. *Social Foundations of Thought and Action: A Social Cognitive Theory*. Englewood Cliffs, N.J.: Prentice Hall.
37. DiClemente, C. C., and Prochaska, J. O. 1982. Self change and therapy change of smoking behavior: A comparison of processes of change in cessation and maintenance. *Addictive Behavior* 7, 133–142.
38. Prochaska, J. O., Velicer, W. F., Rossi, J. S., et al. 1994. Stages of change and decisional balance for 12 problem behaviors. *Health Psychology* 13, 39–46.
39. Perz, C. A., DiClemente, C. C., and Carbonari, J. P. 1996. Doing the right thing at the right time? The interaction of stages and processes of change in successful smoking cessation. *Health Psychology* 15, 462–468.
40. Velicer, W. F., Rossi, J. S., and Prochaska, J. O. 1996. A criterion measurement model for health behavior change. *Addictive Behaviors* 21, 555–584.
41. Marcus, B. H., Banspach, S. W., Lefebvre, R. L., et al. 1992. Using the stages of change model to increase the adoption of physical activity among community participants. *American Journal of Health Promotion* 6, 424–429.
42. Marcus, B. H., and Owen, N. 1992. Motivational readiness, self-efficacy and decision-making for exercise. *Journal of Applied Social Psychology* 22, 3–16.
43. Gold, M. R., Siegel, J. E., Russell, L. B., and Weinstein, M. C., eds. 1996. *Cost-Effectiveness in Health and Medicine*. New York: Oxford University Press.

PART THREE

WELLNESS PROMOTION PRACTICE: TOWARD MORE COMPREHENSIVE APPROACHES

P art 3 extends the discussion of innovative wellness promotion strategies into the realm of making recommendations for practice. Minkler (chapter 13) discusses some of the issues that have been inadequately addressed in past wellness programs, including the role of social inequities in determining health status, the empowerment of communities to participate in health planning, and the unanticipated consequences of health promotion efforts. She provides a specific example of a program wherein the health behaviors of elderly residents in a high-crime neighborhood are enhanced by increasing their sense of personal security through community-level changes. The needs of the elderly also are addressed by Duxbury (chapter 15) and Beck (chapter 16), with the former discussing the pros and cons of cancer screening and the latter focusing on the prevention of disability through comprehensive assessment techniques. The arguments put forth by Duxbury against population-wide prostate cancer screening provide an illustration of Minkler's point concerning the unanticipated consequences of health promotion, while Beck's description of the need to include social and environmental assessments in concert with medical assessments to effectively prevent disability in the elderly exemplifies one possible effect of a "person-centered" approach on clinical practice.

Within the context of educational institutions, Slavin and Wilkes (chapter 17) present an approach toward restructuring the medical school curriculum to promote a person-centered approach among phy-

sicians, and Nader (chapter 18) highlights the value of establishing partnerships between universities and communities to promote wellness.
The model curriculum described by Slavin and Wilkes centers around
problem-based learning and encourages medical students to look beyond
vital statistics to familial, social, and environmental influences on health.
The partnerships depicted by Nader illustrate how these different levels
of influence can be incorporated into wellness interventions targeted
toward school-age children. Together, these chapters speak to the piv-
otal role that educational institutions can play in community wellness
promotion.

Finally, Zhu and Anderson (chapter 14) provide an example of an intervention that melds the clinical and public health approaches into an
integrated program to promote smoking cessation. The Smokers' Helpline combines the intensity of the clinical approach with the accessibility and low cost associated with the public health approach to achieve
meaningful and cost-effective change at the population level. Moreover,
the way that the program was conceived and the feature that allows callers to choose from a menu of preferred services reflect Minkler's point
concerning the value of involving communities in the planning of
programs that are designed to promote their health. Altogether, part 3
serves to illustrate some of the ways that nontraditional perspectives
may lead to highly effective health promotion practice.

13

Meredith Minkler

HEALTH PROMOTION
AT THE DAWN OF THE 21ST CENTURY

Challenges and Dilemmas

Recent discussions of the challenges facing health promotion in the United States have focused heavily on the advantages and disadvantages of managed care and where health promotion and disease prevention may fit in our rapidly evolving health care system. Although such deliberations are important, little attention has been devoted in these discussions to how we as a society can make the necessary changes to significantly improve the health of the American people.[1] This larger question goes well beyond the nature of our medical care system, and it raises difficult challenges, beginning with how we as a nation should be defining health promotion in the first place.

This chapter begins by briefly examining the dominant vision of health promotion in the United States, its policy level implementation, and its more recent evolution and expansion. I then highlight just a few of the health promotion challenges and paradoxes we face, as health professionals and as a society, at the dawn of a new century. These challenges include, first, the need to continue to broaden the focus of our health promotion efforts in order to better address the profound role of social inequities in influencing health status; second, the importance of giving more than lip service to the rhetoric of empowerment and community participation for health by fully embracing them as a framework for health planning; third, the need to recognize and address some of the unanticipated consequences of our health promotion efforts, for example, in unwittingly reinforcing prejudice against the elderly and disabled and in inadvertently encouraging the tobacco industry to become even more aggressive in its targeting of youth, people of color, and Third World nations; and fourth, the need to reframe the continuing public health debate between individual autonomy and the common good. I will argue in particular that we need to broaden and considerably deepen our definition of the common good to stress societal interdependence and not merely the collective rights of individual citizens within a society.

Although this chapter can do little more than scratch the surface in these areas, it is put forward in the hope of contributing to a dialogue that will help us think about the challenges we face in health promotion in some new and different ways. Toward this end, the chapter closes with a brief discussion of the recent Canadian framework for health promotion as a means of illuminating potentially useful avenues for further expanding the vision and the reality of health promotion in the United States.

THE DOMINANT VISION OF HEALTH PROMOTION IN THE UNITED STATES

Before looking at where we might head as a society in terms of health promotion, it is important to look at where we are and where we have come from. The dominant view of health promotion in the United States today emerged in the 1970s in response to a growing disillusionment with the limits of medicine, pressures to contain health care costs, and a social and political climate emphasizing self-help and individual control over health.[2,3] It is a vision that sees individual behavior as in large part responsible for the health problems we face as a society. In the words of J. K. Iglehart, editor of the journal *Health Affairs,* this vision suggests that "most illnesses and premature death are caused by human habits of living *that people choose for themselves*" (emphasis added).[4]

Ironically, this traditional approach to heath promotion has tended to be disease oriented rather than health oriented. As Wallack and Montgomery[5] have pointed out, it defines health primarily as the absence of disease and sees disease as being associated largely with known and controllable risk factors such as cigarette smoking, poor diet, and heavy drinking. The individual is seen as the appropriate focus for intervention to control risk factors, with those interventions typically consisting of providing knowledge and skills for changing unhealthy behaviors.[5] This vision of health promotion was given institutional expression in Canada, with the publication of the Lalonde Report[6] in 1974, and in the United

States, in the Surgeon General's report *Healthy People.*[7] Both of these documents, it should be noted, discussed the role of broader environmental factors in influencing health and did not limit themselves to a discussion of individual lifestyle or personal behavior issues. The Surgeon General's report, for example, argued persuasively that "we are killing ourselves" not only by "our own careless habits" but also by polluting the environment and permitting harmful social conditions to exist.[7] Despite their efforts to address some of these broader issues, however, the major contributions of both the Lalonde and the Surgeon General's reports lay in calling attention to the often substantial role individuals can play in modifying their personal behaviors and in other ways improving their health status.[8–10]

In the United States, the Surgeon General's report was followed by the development of clearly articulated and measurable "Objectives for the Nation."[11] Developed by the U.S. Public Health Service with the Office of Health Information and Promotion (OHIP) playing a facilitating role, the "Objectives" were designed to help address more specifically the broad goals set forth in *Healthy People.* They made a major contribution in focusing attention on prevention and health promotion and in providing clear performance indicators and serving as a stimulus to action. The listing of activities for achieving each objective was extremely thorough and included strategies on the levels of institutional change, legislation, and policy and not merely in the realm of personal behavior change. This broad approach further was in keeping with the view of health promotion put forward at this time by OHIP Director Lawrence Green and his colleagues,[12] who defined health promotion as "any combination of health education and related organizational, political and economic interventions designed to facilitate behavioral and environmental changes conducive to health."

In reality, however, implementing this broad vision, particularly in an era of fiscal conservatism, proved difficult indeed. Moreover, as Green[13] has noted, the sharp distinction drawn in U.S. policy between health promotion (focused mainly on behavior and lifestyle issues) and health protection (concerned more with the physical environment) led to a narrower interpretation of health promotion in the United States than in many European nations, which argued that both physical and social environmental factors lay within the purview of health promotion.

In the United States, fully a third of "Objectives" and a special section within *Healthy People* were devoted to health protection with a focus on environmental concerns within such domains as toxic agent control and occupational health and safety. As noted earlier, many of the interventions proposed under these categories were far-reaching in scope, yet the very process of creating a dichotomy between health promotion and protection may have had the effect of limiting our vision with respect to a broader view of health promotion. In Green's[13] words, "We Americans allowed our health promotion terrain to be restricted to lifestyle determinants of health, but we also allowed lifestyle to be interpreted too narrowly as pertaining primarily if not exclusively to the behavior of those whose health is in question."

As a consequence, most of the programs that grew out of the early push for health promotion in the United States tended to focus primarily on the level of personal behavior change. The programmatic emphasis on individual *responsibility* for health, in short, frequently was not accompanied by attention to individual and community *response-ability*,[14] or the capacity of individuals and communities to build on their strengths and respond to their personal needs and the challenges posed by the environment.

Expanding the Vision

Health promotion in the United States has evolved in important new directions since the early 1980s. Although most work-site health promotions continue to operate primarily on the level of the individual,[15] many have significantly broadened their focus. Education on parenting skills, prenatal care, and interpersonal communications is frequently included in U.S. work-site health promotion programs in addition to the more traditional smoking cessation classes and related interventions aimed at modifying objective risk factors. The "Education for Action" training program, through which workers in hospitals and other settings around the nation have been helped to identify and address unsafe working conditions, provides an illustration of the broader approach to work-site health promotion that has gained popularity.[16]

In the community, innovative health promotion efforts, like the school-based Adolescent Social Action Program (ASAP) in Albuquerque, New Mexico, are including empowerment education and community development in both their methodology and their raison d'être.[17] A university-community partnership, ASAP involves dozens of public schools in an effort to address alcohol and substance abuse problems on multiple levels while creating the conditions in which youth can become empowered to make healthier choices in their own lives. In the area of HIV prevention, projects like Stop AIDS in San Francisco, California, similarly are stressing both community development and individual behavior change. Participants in Stop AIDS education and support groups, for example, are asked as part of their involvement to commit themselves both to practicing safer sex and to doing community organizing around the epidemic.[18]

On another level, statewide legislative initiatives, such as California's Proposition 99, which put a 25-cent tax on cigarettes and allocated 20% of the revenue generated to tobacco education and anticigarette advertising, increasingly are seen as being within the purview of health promotion activities. Finally, as will be noted later, unprecedented new efforts to drastically curtail the power and privileges of the tobacco industry nationwide currently are being attempted and have achieved considerable public support. Such developments are encouraging and have helped widen the scope of health promotion in the United States in important new ways. For the most part, however, even these broader efforts have failed to address the profound influence of broad social inequities on health.

Addressing Social Inequities

The need for developing health promotion programs that address the role of social inequalities in influencing health status is well documented. A voluminous body of evidence, for example, has demonstrated that social class is one of the major risk factors, and perhaps even *the* major risk factor for disease.[19-22] Studies have shown that there is a clear gradient in social class and mortality rates: Not only do people in the highest socioeconomic groups have the lowest mortality rates, but these rates increase at each correspondingly lower rung of the socioeconomic ladder.[21] As Syme[22] has noted, the evidence linking social class and illness is indeed so powerful that researchers routinely control for socioeconomic status in their studies of variables influencing health since this single factor would otherwise overshadow most of their other findings.

The need for addressing social inequities in the design and implementation of our health promotion programs is illustrated in a case study from San Francisco's Tenderloin district. Twenty years ago, my students and I began a project in the Tenderloin to help reduce social isolation and powerlessness and thereby improve the physical and mental health of some of the neighborhood's 8,000 low-income elderly residents. The health problems in this area were daunting. Approximately 40% of the elderly residents were malnourished or undernourished, for example, and although cooking in their rooms was not allowed, they often resorted to illegal hot plates since they could not afford to eat out.[23] Many of the Tenderloin residents with whom we worked wanted to improve their diets. But they lived on small, fixed incomes in a neighborhood that afforded little access to fresh fruits and vegetables. Many residents wanted to get more exercise, but they lived in tiny, cramped rooms in an area with the highest crime rate in the city. Taking a brisk walk may be anything but health promoting in such an environment!

For residents of neighborhoods like the Tenderloin, the primary challenge often is not that of having individuals "take more responsibility" for their health" but rather of improving their "response-ability," by ensuring an adequate income, access to nutritious foods, and, for those with significant functional impairments, access to such coping resources as homemaker services, meals on wheels, and senior escorts. Services like these routinely are made available to the disabled in Canada and western Europe. However, they are effectively rationed in this country by our grossly inadequate funding for such programs and by the fact that they are easy targets for the budget axe in times of fiscal retrenchment.[23]

Health promotion efforts that fail to address the social context within which people live not only minimize the possibility of success but also risk violating the ethical admonition to "do no harm." Already alienated individuals may experience an even greater sense of powerlessness when they try to change health-related behaviors and fail, for example, and this in turn may have negative health consequences[24] (see chapter 11). While continuing to acknowledge the critical need for individuals to take more responsibility for their health, a major challenge at the turn of the century, then, is to develop health promotion efforts that include an equally compelling emphasis on changing those broader social and environmental conditions that so often constrain individual choice in matters related to health. Part of incorporating broader contextual considerations into the policies and programs we design involves placing a far greater emphasis on the principles of community participation and empowerment, and it is to these related areas that I now turn.

Community Participation and Empowerment

Empowerment is a much used and abused term, and it has often been coopted by conservative policy makers who have used the rhetoric of empowering communities as a rationale for cutting back on needed health and social services. But if power is "the ability to predict, control and participate in one's environment,"[25] then empowerment is the process by which people and communities are enabled to take such power and act effectively in transforming their lives and their environments.[26] Borrowing from earlier feminist conceptualizations of power, it suggests that we reframe old notions of "power over" with newer visions of "power to" or "power with."[27]

The concepts of community empowerment and participation reflect a commitment to such precepts as the common good and shared responsibility for health. Acting on these concepts means enabling communities to participate, in equal partnership with health professionals, in setting the health agenda defining their health problems and helping to develop the solutions to address those problems.

This focus is critical. Sociologist John MacKinlay is reported to have remarked that professionals frequently suffer from an unfortunate malady known as "terminal hardening of the categories."[28] We get the kinds of answers we are comfortable dealing with because we ask the kinds of questions that will give us those answers. We conduct behavioral risk surveys, for example, that will carefully document heart disease as a major community health problem but will, in all likelihood, miss the fact that very different sorts of issues, like drugs or violence, may be the major health concerns of residents.[28]

In contrast, an empowering approach to health promotion would "start where the people are" by having them set the health agenda and then work to address the issues they collectively have identified. Such an approach validates the community's ability to assess its needs and strengths and builds on the latter in helping to increase the problem solving ability of both individuals and the larger community. The results can be dramatic. The Tenderloin project referred to earlier is illustrative.

When my students first formed the Tenderloin Senior Organizing Project (TSOP), they organized support groups among the elderly residents of several deteriorating Tenderloin hotels and asked participants what their major health concerns were. In hotel after hotel, the residents responded, "Crime," and the students politely said, "You misunderstood, we were asking about health problems." The residents held their ground, pointing out that they could not safely go outdoors without being mugged and therefore could not get to the doctor's office, go for a walk, or get an evening meal. Crime, they argued, was their biggest health problem.[23]

The students and project staff listened. Then they helped the residents organize a community-wide meeting on the subject of crime and enlist the support of the mass media. They helped garner resources so that the residents could start an interhotel coalition, the Tenderloin Tenants for Safer Streets. Members of this grassroots coalition subsequently met with the mayor and demanded and got increased beat patrol officers in the neighborhood. The students and staff also helped, but always in the background, as residents began the Safehouse Project, recruiting 40 local merchants and agencies to be places of refuge where residents could go for immediate aid if they were being followed or just needed to sit down because of shortness of breath.

Residents' organizing on crime prevention was given much of the credit for an 18% drop in the crime rate that occurred in this neighborhood in the first 12 months of their mobilization.[23] Their organizing efforts also translated into some effective individual-level behavior change. For example, residents' new found feelings of power, self-efficacy, and improved self-esteem led some to successfully quit smoking and cut down on problem drinking.[23]

Had the students and staff of the Tenderloin Senior Outreach Project failed to pay attention to and support the community's definition of need, they might still be running support groups in hotel lobbies one morning a week—if indeed they were still welcome at all. Instead, by trusting the people to determine and act on their own health agenda, they were able to contribute to something that has had a real and lasting impact on the health of that community.

The Tenderloin project is but one of a number of examples that could be cited of health promotion efforts that have actively involved local communities in identifying and addressing their health problems and in the process building on and reinforcing community strengths. The earlier mentioned ASAP program in New Mexico, through which youth, many of them Native American and Hispanic, are helped to identify and then creatively address substance abuse problems in their community, is an example of another such effort and one that has demonstrated measurable successes in terms of increasing participants' perceptions of high-risk behaviors and their sense of social responsibility.[17] The Black Women's Health Project (BWHP), founded in 1981 and based in Oakland, California, is another example of an empowering approach to health promotion. A national network of approximately 100 self-help groups in approximately two dozen states, the BWHP helps African American women gain information, skills, and access to resources while enabling them to work together to identify and analyze health-related concerns and to collectively address these issues.[29] On a smaller scale, an innovative health promotion action research project in an automotive parts plant in Michigan involved workers, in partnership with researchers, in a Stress and Wellness Committee that identified sources of stress in the workplace and then designed and sought implementation of strategies on a variety of levels to address these concerns.[30]

Projects like these share a commitment to helping communities identify their needs and then working with them in developing health promotion programs and approaches that truly meet those needs. Implementing such a commitment, however, is often far from easy. As Gail Siler-Wells[31] points out, "Behind the euphemisms of empowerment and community participation lay the realities of power, control and ownership." The very real structural distinctions that exist between professionals and communities, and our very location as professionals in health agencies and bureaucracies, confer a certain power that includes the power to set the health agenda.[31]

As we enter a new decade and a new century, new and innovative ways must be developed to better enable individuals and communities to take the power they need to bring about health improvements. Professionals committed to facilitating this process may be aided by applying a tool developed by community organizers Herbert and Irene Rubin[32] and called the DARE criteria for empowerment. The DARE criteria would have us answer the following set of questions with respect to any health promotion project in which we are engaged:

Who Determines the goals of the project?

Who Acts to achieve them?

Who Receives the benefits of the actions?

Who Evaluates the actions?

The more we can answer these questions by responding, "The community," the more likely our health promotion projects are to be contributing to true community empowerment and self-determination.[33]

Public health departments, hospitals, and other health institutions also can contribute to community participation and empowerment by forming what Ron Labonte[34] describes as "authentic partnerships" with communities and ensuring that our "community based" projects are not merely "community placed."[34] Such authentic partnerships will take on particular relevance, moreover, as new and complex areas such as violence prevention become an increasing part of public health practice.

A problem such as violence presents a whole new set of challenges, in part because it is widely viewed in this society as a problem to be addressed through law enforcement and criminal justice rather than through efforts directed at economic development, human welfare, and public health. The statistics, of course, tell a different story. As Michael McGinnis and William Foege[35] have demonstrated, firearms rank sixth (after tobacco, diet and exercise, and so on) as an actual cause of death in the United States. And although the overall homicide rate in this country began to decline in the early 1990s,[36] we continue to rank first—by a wide margin—among the advanced industrialized nations.[37] When we turn our attention to youth violence, an even more disconcerting picture emerges. For despite recent declines, and whether as victims, perpetrators, or witnesses, young people aged 15 to 24 continue to experience disproportionately high rates of violence. A recent comparison of the overall firearms-related deaths among children under 15 in 26 advanced industrialized countries revealed the U.S. rate to be 12 times higher than that of all the other countries combined (1.66 vs. 0.14).[38] The firearms-related homicide rate in U.S. children was almost 16 times that of the other nations combined (0.94 vs. 0.06)[38] (see Figure 13.1).

Facts and statistics like these provide compelling evidence that the public health system should be a major force in violence prevention efforts.

The suggestion that health professionals and their institutions take on violence as a major public health problem is in no way meant to underplay the critical need for broad societal-level economic and social change if we are truly to make a lasting impact on the violence that plagues our nation. With many of the new jobs created at or below minimum wage and with the gap between rich and poor greater today than at any time since World War II and continuing to expand rapidly,[39] it is not hard to understand the increase in violent crime, particularly among unemployed and underemployed youth for whom drug trafficking and related violence may be very lucrative. Similarly, with handguns and semiautomatics within easy reach of our nation's most vulnerable children, and with violence endemic on our movie and television screens, it is unlikely that significant and lasting change can be made at the community level without dramatic changes on our societal landscape.

However, communities can and do have a vital role to play, and by working in partnership with communities, local health departments can lend their resources, skills, and credibility to a frontline attack on violence.

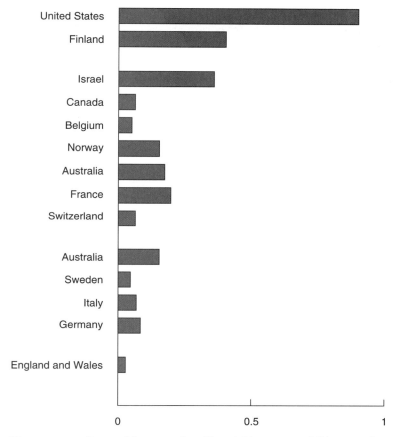

Figure 13.1.   Rates of firearm-related homicides among children aged
<15 years in 26 industrialized countries. Rates are per 100,000 children
aged <15 years and for one year during 1990–1995. In this analysis,
Hong Kong, Northern Ireland, and Taiwan are considered countries.
Source: Adapted from *Morbidity and Mortality Weekly Report*, February 7, 1997, Figure 1, p. 104.

A powerful illustration of an empowering and collaborative approach
to violence prevention that links health institutions to local communities was developed by Deborah Prothow-Stith and her colleagues[40] at
Harvard's School of Medicine and Massachusetts General Hospital. Offered to youth in high-risk neighborhoods through local housing projects, schools, churches, and YMCAs, the project teaches young people
new ways of coping with their anger and aggressive feelings. But it also
has them explore the root causes of violence in racism, poverty, and a
culture where, in Prothow-Stith's words, the most popular heroes have

"Rambo hearts and Terminator heads."[41] Although this program has been hailed as a success in terms of primary prevention and increasing individual and community responsibility in relation to violence prevention, part of its strength lies in its continued efforts to mobilize other sectors, including government, business, and the mass media, in order to develop broad-based and multilevel attacks on the problem of violence.[38,41] These efforts appear to have paid off. Breaking down the traditional turf lines between police, the courts, schools, churches, and nonprofit health and youth agencies, the city of Boston has developed an ambitious combination of after-school activities, job training, police reorientation toward knowing and valuing their neighborhoods, and other violence prevention efforts. The "Boston model" of crime prevention indeed has been credited with the fact that the city recently experienced an unprecedented 29-month period without a single murder among its children and adolescents.[42]

On a still larger scale, the Violence Prevention Initiative (VPI) of The California Wellness Foundation has been credited with helping to create a new social and political climate for promoting handgun control and other measures that can help reduce violence on a statewide basis.[43] Initiated in 1993 with a five-year, $35 million endowment, the VPI was designed to reduce the state's high youth violence rates through a multipronged grant-making program that included community action programs, public education, research, and policy development. A central piece of this ambitious effort—the successful mobilization of a statewide effort to pressure for the banning of handguns—is described in detail by Lawrence Wallack in chapter 19. In his words, the VPI has left "a large footprint . . . in the legislative landscape" and has paved the way for continued dramatic policy changes in a state where murder remains one of the top two killers of children and youth.[44]

Empowering community and multisectoral approaches to violence prevention like those described here well illustrate how expanding our definition of health promotion and disease and injury prevention and working in broad partnerships on a wide variety of levels can help address one of the most critical public health problems of our times.

Avoiding Prejudice against the Elderly and Disabled in Our Health Promotion Efforts

I have discussed so far the need to devote greater attention in our health promotion efforts to the social determinants of health and to do this in part by taking more seriously the notion of community empowerment for health. While we move in these broader directions, however, we face another challenge as we enter a new century—that is, to reexamine the health promotion efforts already under way in our country to better understand the ways in which these programs and approaches may unwittingly reproduce and transmit such problematic aspects of our dominant culture as gerontophobia and handicappism or stigmatization of and prejudice against the elderly and the disabled.[45]

With some notable exceptions, the elderly largely have been ignored in most private- and public-sector health promotion efforts. The high costs of such failure are painfully evident. Helen Schauffler and her colleagues at the University of California, Berkeley, School of Public Health,[46] for example, conducted the first study ever to demonstrate a relationship between risk factors for heart disease and Medicare payments. They discovered that three triggers for heart disease—high blood pressure, high cholesterol, and cigarette smoking—are costing Medicare at least $16.6 billion per year in extra medical services, yet the program does almost nothing to prevent these conditions (see Figure 13.2).

Although Medicare's failure to cover much health promotion and disease prevention for the elderly reflects in large part a more generalized reluctance in both public- and private-sector health insurance plans to cover such services,[47] it may also reflect the widespread belief that such programs have little to offer the elderly, who are deemed "resistant to change" anyway and whose "productive years" are largely behind them.[48] Recent changes in the Medicare program take an important step forward in providing coverage for colorectal screening and annual mammograms, increased payments for preventive injections, and coverage of glucose monitoring and other costs associated with the management of diabetes.[49] But while our health promotion efforts must include even greater efforts toward the prevention of unnecessary disability and functional impairment, a challenge for the decades ahead is to find ways of doing so that do not in the process stigmatize and devalue those elders who are or may become disabled.

The renewed emphasis on individual responsibility for health in this country has been accompanied by the reemergence of a Victorian-era notion that healthy old age is a just reward for a life of self-control and "right living."[50] Such a notion opens the door to victim blaming of those elders who dare to become chronically ill or disabled. In David Lewin's words, "Good health has become a new ritual of patriotism, a market place for the public display of secular faith in the power of will."[51]

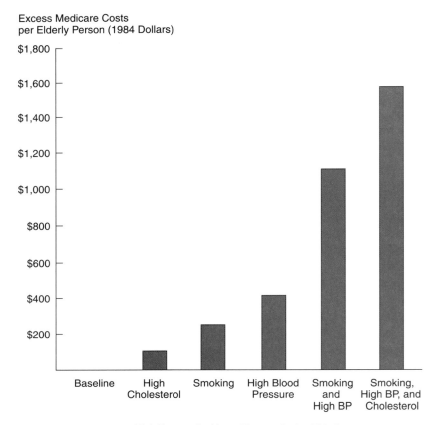

Excess Medicare Costs
per Elderly Person (1984 Dollars)

Risk Factors for Heart Disease in the Elderly

Figure 13.2.   Increased Medicare costs per elderly person per year associated with risk factors for heart disease. Source: Schauffler et al. (1993 [46]).

Within such a vision, where is there a place for the 85-year-old man with a disabling respiratory ailment or for the obese and severely arthritic elderly woman in a wheelchair?

The unwitting tendency of some health promotion efforts to foster this kind of stigmatization can also be seen in many recent injury prevention campaigns. Once again, we are faced with a paradox. On the one hand, it is critical that health promotion include an emphasis on injury prevention, and it is heartening, too, that this has expanded to include such controversial areas as handgun control. On the other hand, we must be concerned when the messages of our prevention campaigns build on and contribute to fear of disability and in the process further stigmatize those who are already disabled.

As Caroline Wang[52] has pointed out, health promotion approaches to injury prevention that carry the implicit or explicit message, "Don't let this happen to you!" often inadvertently stigmatize people with disabilities, suggesting that they are "inherently flawed" and undesirable. In her words,

> If the public health perspective rightly contends that *becoming* disabled is an unacceptable risk in our society, it paradoxically often fails to acknowledge the stigmatizing notion that *being* disabled is an unacceptable status in our society.[52]

Heeding the physicians' admonition to "first, do no harm," those of us concerned about health promotion and injury and disease prevention must ensure that the campaigns we design and the messages we transmit through them do not further contribute to the handicappism and gerontophobia that already plague our society.

The Continuing Challenge of the Tobacco Industry

In some of the most critical arenas within health promotion, such as alcohol and tobacco, the very success of some of our health promotion efforts is raising new problems and challenges we have only begun to tackle. Recent developments in the area of tobacco marketing and advertising provide an excellent case in point.

Accounting for over 416,000 deaths per year, cigarette smoking has been called by the Centers for Disease Control and Prevention "the most devastating preventable cause of disease and premature death this country has ever experienced."[53] Yet despite this reality, some impressive strides have been made. Smoking rates overall have dropped from 40% of the population in 1965[54] to about 23% in 1998.[55] Public health measures such as increased excise taxes, mandatory warning labels on cigarette packages, restrictions on tobacco advertising, mass-media campaigns, and public and private antismoking rules and ordinances have been given much of the credit for these declines.[56]

The very success of health promotion efforts in the area of tobacco control, however, has contributed inadvertently to aggressive new efforts by cigarette manufacturers to find new markets at home and abroad and to take steps to increase their ebbing legitimacy. In the United States, increased targeting of people of color, women, and young people has been one consequence, with direct advertising appeals supplemented by tobacco companies' sponsorship of baseball games, tennis matches, and cultural events like Cinco de Mayo parades.[57] Although recently cut back as a result of the tobacco settlement, such efforts have paid off. Among 8th-, 10th-, and 12th-graders, for example, the proportion of youth who smoke daily increased by almost 50% between 1991 and 1996, with 20% of 12th-graders now smoking on a daily basis.[58,59]

To improve their public image, leading tobacco companies also have become major donors to both large and small nonprofit organizations including, ironically, the Partnership for a Drug Free America.[60] Such money often comes with strings attached. Shortly after accepting $150,000 from Phillip Morris, for example, New York City's Coalition for the Homeless was asked to help kill a bill mandating antismoking ads by pressuring the city council to focus on more important issues like homelessness.[60] In a time of dwindling public and private funding for a plethora of good organizations and worthy health and social causes, the tobacco companies' substantial role in financing raises troubling ethical dilemmas.[33]

A combination of developments in the late 1990s seriously damaged the already waning credibility of the tobacco industry and greatly increased political and popular support for stiff new tobacco taxes and other antismoking measures. The release and wide publicizing of credibility harming tobacco industry memos and other secret documents, public revulsion at new evidence of the industry's sophisticated efforts to hook teens and to increase the addictive content of cigarettes, state-level efforts to sue tobacco companies as a means of recovering Medicaid costs for smoking-related illnesses, and one cigarette manufacturer's break with the rest of the industry in acknowledging the addictive nature of nicotine were among the events signaling a potential watershed in antitobacco mobilization in the United States.[61] Health promotion efforts such as the well-financed Campaign for Tobacco Free Kids and the earlier mentioned California Tobacco Control Program (which was credited with having helped a million smokers quit the habit in its first three years of operation)[62] also began playing an important role in discouraging smoking, especially among youth.

Major legislative events have further helped change the tobacco landscape. After months of heated debate between tobacco industry representatives, state attorneys general, and other parties, a proposed $368.5 billion "tobacco settlement" was announced in June 1997 that called for sweeping changes in the regulation, sale, and advertising of tobacco.[61,63] The settlement was quickly opposed by a plethora of anti-tobacco forces, including the American Lung Association and the American Public Health Association, which argued that it "let the tobacco industry off the hook" far too easily. The proposed settlement, for example, would have hindered the Food and Drug Administration's (FDA's) ability to regulate nicotine for the next 12 years despite the fact that this regulatory power had already been granted by a federal court.[63] In the ensuing months, President Clinton charged Congress with passing tough national tobacco legislation that would include a combination of industry payments and penalties that would increase the cost of a pack of cigarettes by up to $1.50 over the next 10 years. A comprehensive plan to dramatically reduce youth smoking, expanded efforts to restrict access and limit the appeal of cigarettes, and the granting of full authority to the FDA to regulate tobacco products were among the key elements proposed.[64] The national tobacco settlement finally reached in 1998 involved payments to 46 states totaling about $206 billion over the next 25 years. Under the settlement, more than 14,000 cigarette billboards were removed, outdoor advertising was banned on public transit and in many public arenas, and such popular cartoon figures as Joe Camel were permanently retired. Of even greater importance, the settlement prohibited the industry from lobbying against tobacco control laws and ordinances.[65]

The tobacco settlement led to a 45-cent-per-pack increase in the price of cigarettes between 1998 and 1999, with a corresponding decline in total cigarette consumption of 7.5% over the same period.[65] As some analysts have noted, however, "the welcome fall in consumption resulting from the price increase may turn out to be temporary unless it is followed up with serious efforts to dissuade kids from smoking."[65] With just 8% of the tobacco settlement monies to states so far going to anti-smoking efforts and the great bulk of the funds being used for road construction, tax cuts and the like,[66] early hopes for dramatic declines in youth smoking appear unlikely to be realized.

We continue to face other ethical challenges when the activities of American cigarette manufacturers are viewed within a global context. The use of tobacco worldwide has increased dramatically since the mid-1960s, with much of this increase occurring in Third World countries. While cigarette smoking now is declining by 1.4% annually in industrialized nations, moreover, the habit continues to grow by 1.7% per year in the developing nations, where tobacco accounted for more than

1.2 million deaths annually by 1995.[65] In many Third World nations, smoking has only recently become widespread, and daily consumption is lower than in the developed world largely for economic reasons. Yet as large cohorts of young smokers age and as personal disposable income increases in these nations, substantial increases in daily consumption are anticipated, unless effective tobacco control measures are put into place.[66–68]

In a provocative and troubling article "Advertising for All by the Year 2000," Wallack and Montgomery[5] demonstrate how dwindling markets and increasing advertising bans at home have made Third World nations one of the most "promising frontiers" for our nation's tobacco industry. The United States is the world's largest tobacco exporter, with our cigarette exports growing 260% from 1986 to 1996 and two-thirds of cigarettes manufactured in the United States now sold internationally.[63,69] American tobacco companies also rank among the leading advertisers in many Third World nations,[5] and in Asia and Latin America, researchers have documented an association between increased cigarette advertising and both general increases in smoking and specific increases among women and children.[70] Tobacco consumption already accounts for a substantial proportion of overall mortality in many Third World countries, and estimates suggest that by 2025, seven out of every 10 tobacco-related deaths will occur in the Third World.[69,71]

The policy implications raised by these realities are profound and suggest the need for action on multiple levels. Working through groups like the World Health Organization (WHO), for example, we might promote a massive international antitobacco advertising campaign while at home we continue to press for national tobacco legislation along the lines described previously. We further must require that U.S.-manufactured cigarettes that are marketed in other nations be held to the same standards in terms of warning labels, nicotine content, and the like as those sold domestically. Such efforts are essential if we are to achieve real success in dramatically reducing smoking rates at home while preventing the realization of the WHO's dire projection that tobacco will be the world's leading cause of death by 2020.[71]

Rethinking "The Public Good"

A final challenge for broadening the focus of health promotion as we begin a new century is perhaps the most difficult, for it involves rethinking conceptualizations of health issues that are deeply embedded in both

Western and uniquely American value systems. Health-related behaviors such as cigarette smoking frequently are discussed in terms of the tension between individual autonomy and the public or community good. This debate has been badly constrained, however, because our dominant notions of justice are impoverished.[70,72] In Larry Churchill's[72] words, they are based on "a moral heritage in which answers to the question 'what is good?' and 'what is right?' are lodged definitively in a powerful image of the individual as the only meaningful level of moral analysis."

When the ethical notion of public or community good is invoked in arguments for mandatory motorcycle helmet use, for example, "common good" frequently is operationalized in terms of the economic rights of law-abiding citizens. Public or community good, in short, is defined as my right not to pay for your foolish or risky behavior.[2] Economic arguments of this sort may have a place. But when we limit our conceptions of the public or common good in this way—when we suggest that "the public good is nothing more . . . than the protection of every individual's private rights,"[73]—we miss the broader meaning of community. In Dan Beauchamp's[74] words,

> By ignoring the communitarian language of public health, we risk shrinking its claims. We also risk undermining the sense in which health and safety are a signal commitment of the common life—a central *practice* by which the body-politic defines itself and reaffirms its values.

Motorcycle helmet laws, for example, are not simply "championing some individuals over others" but rather are upholding "the public or community interest" over the interests of individuals or groups.[75] Such laws ideally are saying that when one of us engages in risky behavior, our collective well-being is affected because we are all part of the same community.

Broadening our concept of the public good to embrace a sense of our intimate interdependence, a notion that we are indeed "all in this together," will not be easy. For in the words of Dan Callahan,[76] the dominant culture in America "does not speak easily the language of community." If we are to move toward broader, more community-oriented policies in the name of health promotion, however, our vision of public good must become considerably more than the rights and obligations of the collection of individuals who happen to occupy the same geographic space.

Contrary to witnessing an enhanced notion of the common good, unfortunately, the late 1990s heralded several new measures that further restricted America's sense of community. The 1996 welfare reform bill, for example, abolished the nation's 60-year-old commitment to an entitlement of aid for low-income families with dependent children and by some estimates may move an estimated 1.1 million additional children into poverty.[77] The Personal Responsibility and Work Opportunity Reconciliation Act, as this measure was named, also called for the elimination of food stamps, SSI (Supplemental Security Income), and a range of other benefits for some 800,000 of the nation's legal immigrants.[78] Although many of the proposed cuts were subsequently restored through the Balanced Budget Act, new measures on the state and federal levels continue to capitalize on growing anti-immigrant sentiment and threaten to constrain still further notions of the common good.

The Canadian Framework for Health Promotion

As this chapter has attempted to demonstrate, addressing social inequities, taking seriously the rhetoric of community participation and empowerment, confronting the unanticipated consequences of our health promotion efforts, and rethinking and broadening our notion of the common good constitute major challenges for those concerned with broadening the vision and the reality of health promotion in the United States. Moreover, although health promotion has moved in important new directions since the rebirth of interest in this approach in the 1970s, recent setbacks, including importantly the failure to enact health care reform legislation and the passage of a punitive and potentially health-compromising welfare reform bill, suggest that much remains to be done.

As we grapple with these and other challenges to health promotion during this unique historical period, a new conceptual framework must be developed that incorporates such underlying principles as a commitment to social justice, empowerment, and a broader notion of the common good. Toward this end, it is useful to review WHO's vision of health promotion and specifically how that vision has been crafted into a conceptual framework for health promotion policy and its implementation in Canada.

WHO radically revised its notion of health promotion in the mid-1980s, defining it as "a process of enabling people to increase control over, and to improve their health."[79] It went on to state that health promotion represents "a mediating strategy between people and their environments, synthesizing personal choice and social responsibility in health."[79] The principles set forth by WHO as underlying this alternative vision of health promotion included acting on the determinants or causes of health, eliciting high-level public participation, and using a variety of approaches that go well beyond lifestyle education and that include legislation, organizational change, and community development.[79,80]

The Canadian approach to health promotion that was developed in the mid-1980s and refined over the subsequent decade provides an illustration of how such a broadened vision may constitute a useful framework for action. After a period of considerable preoccupation with healthy lifestyles and individual responsibility for health, the Canadian government undertook a massive restructuring of its approach to health promotion. Two important points stand out in the Canadian approach. First, the number one challenge set forth for health promotion is reducing inequities between low- and high-income groups, and this is not framed in terms of individual responsibility but of broader societal responsibility.[81] Second, three levels of concern are set forth—health challenges, health promotion mechanisms, and implementation strategies—and on each of these levels there is attention to the role of broad institutional or environmental change (see Figure 13.3). Self-care, for example, is advocated within a framework that devotes considerable attention to the creation of healthy environments within which positive personal health behaviors can flourish. Canadian legislation on smoking is among the toughest in the world, with many provinces having developed "healthy public policies" on tobacco that have included changing their policies on marketing, crop substitution, and smoking in the workplace at the same time that they urge individuals to quit the habit.

In several Canadian provinces, premier's councils on health have been established through which government leaders in the different sectors provide advice on health promotion and work together in jointly setting goals for helping to address the social determinants of health.[80] In the Northwest Territories, land claims and the development of First Nation's People's rights have been discussed as part of a broadly defined health agenda.[82] Finally, across the nation, hundreds of cities have designated themselves "healthy communities," stressing intersectoral planning, high-level community participation, and reciprocity between the individual and the broader society.[83]

Hard outcome data that would indicate whether the new Canadian approach to health promotion has resulted in actual declines in morbidity and mortality are not yet available. Further, as Irving Rootman[84] and Lawrence Green[85] predicted, increased government perceptions of a need for cutbacks in social spending have led to some redesign of so-

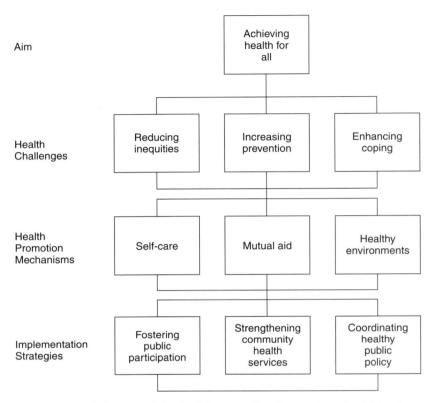

Figure 13.3.   A framework for health promotion. Source: Epp (1986 [79]).

cial programs in ways that are constricting the implementation of health promotion, in much the same way that occurred in the United States under the Reagan and Bush administrations. Although the Canadian Public Health Association's [86] recent "Action Statement for Health Promotion in Canada" reaffirmed the importance of continuing to use the Ottawa Charter as "the framework that defines health promotion in Canada," it went on to note that the current climate of increasing poverty, environmentally harmful global economic practices, and cuts in the very health and social programs that have defined Canadians "as a caring people" present a stark contrast to "the optimistic days when the Ottawa Charter was first written." [86] The Action Statement went on to reaffirm those visions and values deemed essential to health promotion, among them an "explicit value base" that includes a commitment to respecting individual liberties but giving priority to the common good, giving priority to people whose living conditions place them at greater risk, and pursuing social justice "to prevent systemic discrimination and to reduce health inequities."[86]

As noted earlier, even health promotion efforts that are firmly grounded in a values base like this one may stumble as a result of continuing budget cuts, growing power differentials between rich and poor, and the structural distinctions that continue to exist between communities and health and social service professionals. At the same time, however, the Canadian framework for health promotion and the values and principles underlying it stand as an important example of a vision that offers a balanced concern for personal behavior change within the context of broader social change. In its attention to broader environmental issues, moreover, the Canadian approach explicitly addresses the connection between health promotion and the roots of public health in concerns for social justice and improved social and economic conditions as a vital part of public health.

The classic illustration of this connection lies in the well-known story of Rudolph Virchow,[87] the founder of cellular pathology, who in 1848 was asked by his superiors to provide recommendations on what to do about a typhus epidemic that was raging in an impoverished area in eastern Prussia. After visiting the area and studying the situation, Virchow prepared a report in which he spoke of the need for land reform, redistribution of wealth and income, and only later of some medical reforms. The report was met with displeasure, and Virchow was accused of proposing a political rather than a medical solution to the epidemic. His often-cited reply was that "medicine is a social science and politics nothing more than medicine on a large scale."[87]

Taking a cue from Virchow, health promotion and the ways in which we define and operationalize it must be seen in inherently political and multidisciplinary terms if we are to be successful in meeting the profound challenges to the public's health that we face in this last decade of the 20th century. As health professionals, we must ask ourselves what our own responsibilities are in relation to health promotion programs and activities. Do we contribute to social equity, or do we reinforce existing inequities? Do we advance the concept of individual and community empowerment, or do we merely use the language of community partnerships and empowerment to blur hierarchical distinctions without changing the status quo?[33] Do our health promotion activities inadvertently contribute to problems such as gerontophobia and handicappism? Do they, in Marshall Becker's[88] words, equate "being ill" with "being guilty?" And finally, is our notion of community good broad enough to reflect an appreciation of our intimate interdependence? With Larry Churchill,[72] are we able to see individual freedoms and social bonds as complementary rather than opposing forms of human well-being?

The story is told of a traveler, hopelessly lost on a dusty dirt road, who stops a local farmer and asks, "Is this the road to Baduka?" The farmer replies, "Mister, if I was going to Baduka, I wouldn't start from here." The dominant American self-image stressing individualism, self-reliance and progress, and the "ethical individualism" to which it predisposes us[72] makes our starting point on the road to a broader approach to health promotion a difficult one indeed. But as we enter a new century and a new millennium, the time is ripe for considerably broadening the ways in which we think about and approach health promotion.

REFERENCES

1. U.S. Department of Health and Human Services, Public Health Service, Centers for Disease Control. 1993. Public health in the new American health system. Discussion paper, Bethesda, Maryland.

2. Leichter, H. M. 1991. *Free to Be Foolish: Politics and Health Promotion in The United States and Great Britain.* Princeton, N.J.: Princeton University Press.

3. Walker, S. N. 1994. Health promotion and prevention of disease and disability among older adults: Who is responsible? *Generations* (spring), 45–50.

4. Iglehart, J. K. 1990. From the editor: Special issue on promoting health. *Health Affairs* 9(2), 4–5.

5. Wallack, L., and Montgomery, K. 1992. Advertising for all by the year 2000: Public health implications for less developed countries. *American Journal of Public Health Policy* 13(2), 76–100.

6. Lalonde, M. 1974. *A New Perspective on the Health of Canadians.* Ottawa: Government of Canada.

7. U.S. Surgeon General. 1979. *Healthy People: The Surgeon General's Report on Health Promotion and Disease Prevention.* Washington, D.C.: Department of Health and Human Services.

8. Hancock, T. 1986. Lalonde and beyond: Looking back at "A new perspective on the health of Canadians." *Health Promotion* 1, 93–100.

9. Terris, M. 1984. Newer perspectives on the health of Canadians: Beyond the Lalonde report. *Journal of Public Health Policy* 5, 327–337.

10. Newbauer, D., and Pratt, R. 1981. The second public health revolution: A critical appraisal. *Journal of Health Politics, Policy and Law* 6(2), 327–337.

11. U.S. Surgeon General. 1980. *Health promotion Disease prevention: Objectives for the nation.* Washington, D.C.: Department of Health and Human Services.

12. Green, L. W., Kreuter, M., Deeds, S. G., and Partridge, K. B. 1980. *Health*

Education Planning: A Diagnostic Approach. Palo Alto, Calif.: Mayfield Publishing.

13. Personal communication from L. W. Green, May 17, 1988.

14. Personal communication from E. Zimmerman, October 16, 1980.

15. Stokols, D., Pelletier, K., and Fielding, J. 1996. The ecology of work and health: Research and policy directions for the promotion of employee health. *Health Education Quarterly* 23(2), 137–158.

16. Weinger, M., and Wallerstein, N. 1990. Education for action: An innovative approach to training hospital employees. In *Essentials of Modern Hospital Safety,* edited by W. Charney and J. Schirmer. New York: Lewis Publishers.

17. Wallerstein, N., Sanchez-Merki, V., and Dow, L. 1997. Freirian praxis in health education and community organizing: A case study of an adolescent prevention program. In *Community Organizing and Community Building for Health,* edited by M. Minkler. Pp. 195–211. New Brunswick, N.J.: Rutgers University Press.

18. Wohlfeiler, D. 1997. Community organizing and community building around gay and bisexual men: The Stop AIDS project. In *Community Organizing and Community Building,* edited by M. Minkler. Pp. 230–244. New Brunswick, N.J.: Rutgers University Press.

19. Berkman, L., and Syme, S. L. 1976. Social class—Susceptibility and sickness. *American Journal of Epidemiology* 104, 1–8.

20. Kaplan, G. A., Haan, M., Syme, S. L., et al. 1987. Socioeconomic status and health. *American Journal of Epidemiology* 125, 989–998.

21. Marmot, M. G., Rose, G., and Hamilton, P. J. S. 1978. Employment grade and coronary heart disease in British civil servants. *Journal of Epidemiology and Community Health* 32, 244–249.

22. Syme, S. L. 1990. Control and health: An epidemiological perspective. In *Self Directedness: Cause and Effects throughout the Life Course,* edited by J. Rodin, C. Schooler, and K. W. Schaie. Pp. 213–229. Hillsdale, N.J.: Lawrence Erlbaum Associates. New York: Wiley (in association with the Commission of European Communities).

23. Minkler, M. 1997. Community organizing among the elderly poor in San Francisco's Tenderloin District: A case study. In *Community Organizing and Community Building for Health,* edited by M. Minkler. Pp. 244–258. New Brunswick, N.J.: Rutgers University Press.

24. Minkler, M. 1994. Challenges for health promotion in the 1990s: Social inequities, empowerment, negative consequences, and the common good. *American Journal of Health Promotion* 8(6), 403.

25. Kent, J. 1970. *A descriptive approach to community.* Unpublished report, Denver, Colorado.

26. Miller, M. 1985. *Turning Problems into Actionable Issues.* San Francisco: Organize Training Center.

27. French, M. 1986. *Beyond Power: On Women, Men and Morals.* London: Abacus.

28. Labonte, R. 1994. Health promotion and empowerment: Reflections on professional practice. *Health Education Quarterly* 21(2, summer), 253–268.

29. Avery, B. Y. 1990. Breathing life into ourselves: The evolution of the Black

Women's Health Project. In *Black Women's Health Book,* edited by E. C. White. Pp. 4–10. Seattle: Seal Press.

30. Schurman, S. J., and Israel, B. 1995. Redesigning work systems to reduce stress: A participatory action research approach to creating change. In *Job Stress Intervention: Current Practices and New Directions,* edited by G. Keiter, S. Sauter, J. Hurrell, and L. Murphy. Pp. 235–263. Washington, D.C.: American Psychological Association.

31. Siler-Wells, G. L. 1989. Challenges of the Gordian knot: Community health in Canada. In *International Symposium on Community Participation and Empowerment Strategies in Health Promotion,* edited by J. Warren Salmon and Eberhard Goepel. Pp. 42–55. Bielefeld, Germany: Center for Interdisciplinary Studies, University of Bielefeld.

32. Rubin, H., and Rubin, I. 1992. *Community Organizing and Development.* 2nd ed. New York: Macmillan.

33. Minkler, M., and Pies, C. 1997. Ethical issues in community organizing and community participation. In *Community Organizing and Community Building for Health,* edited by M. Minkler. Pp. 120–136. New Brunswick, N.J.: Rutgers University Press.

34. Labonte, R. 1997. Community, community development and the forming of authentic partnerships: Some critical reflections. In *Community Organizing and Community Building for Health,* edited by M. Minkler. Pp. 88–102. New Brunswick, N.J.: Rutgers University Press.

35. McGinnis, J. M., and Goege, W. H. 1993. Actual causes of death in the United States. *Journal of the American Medical Association* 270(18), 2207–2212.

36. Trends in rates of homicide—United States, 1985–1994. 1996. *Morbidity and Mortality Weekly Report* 45(22, June 7), 460–464.

37. Rachuba, L., Stanton, B., and Howard, D. 1995. Violent crime in the United States: An epidemiologic profile. *Pediatric and Adolescent Medicine* 149, 953.

38. Rates of homicide, suicide and firearm-related death among children—26 industrialized countries. 1997. *Morbidity and Mortality Weekly Report* 46(5, February 7), 101–105.

39. Thurow, L. 1996. *The Future of Capitalism.* New York: William Morrow.

40. Prothow-Stith, D. 1995. The epidemic of youth violence in America: Using public health prevention strategies to prevent violence. *Journal of Health Care for the Poor and Underserved* 6(2), 95.

41. Prothow-Stith, D. 1995. Violence prevention with youth. Keynote presentation for the Annual Conference of the American Journal of Health Promotion, Orlando, Florida, March 20.

42. Tucker, C. 1997. Boston shows how to deal with teens. *San Francisco Chronicle,* December 20, A20.

43. RAND and Stanford Center for Research in Disease Prevention. 1997, June. *The California Wellness Foundation Violence Prevention Initiative Mid-Initiative Assessment, Volume 1.* Santa Monica, Calif.

44. California Department of Health Services. 1997. Injury deaths for homicides by age and cause, California 1995. Sacramento, May 22.

45. Robertson, A., and Minkler, M. 1994. The new health promotion movement: A critical examination. *Health Education Quarterly* 21(3), 295–312.
46. Schauffler, H. H., D'Ogostino, R. B., and Kannel, W. B. 1993. Risk for cardiovascular disease in the elderly and associated Medicare costs: The Framingham Study. *American Journal of Preventive Medicine* 9(3), 146–154.
47. Davis, K., Bialek, R., Parkinson, M., et al. 1990. Paying for preventive care: Moving the debate forward. *American Journal of Preventive Medicine* 6(4), 7–30.
48. Minkler, M., and Pasick, R. 1986. Health promotion and the elderly: A critical perspective on the past and future. In *Wellness and Health Promotion of the Elderly,* edited by K. Dychtwald. Pp. 39–54. Rockville, Md.: Aspen Systems Corporation.
49. Lynch, M., and Minkler, M. 1998. The restructuring of Medicare and Medicaid and its impacts on the elderly: A conceptual framework and analysis. *Critical Gerontology: Perspective from Political and Moral Economy,* edited by M. Minkler and C. L. Estes. Pp. 185–201. Amityville, N.Y.: Baywood Publishing.
50. Cole, T. 1988. The specter of old age: History, politics and culture in an aging America. *Tikkun* 3(5), 14–18,93–95.
51. Levin, D. 1987. *Pathologies of the Modern Self.* New York: University Press.
52. Wang, C. 1982. Culture, meaning and disability: Injury prevention campaigns in the production of stigma. *Social Science and Medicine* 3(5), 1093–1102.
53. U.S. Department of Health and Human Services, Office on Smoking and Health. 1989. *Smoking, Tobacco and Health: A Factbook.* Washington, D.C.: General Accounting Office.
54. U.S. Department of Health and Human Services, Office on Smoking and Health. 1991. *Trends in Cigarette Smoking Prevalence in the United States, 1965–1991.* Washington, D.C.: U.S. Government Printing Office. (data from the National Health Interview Surveys, 1965–1991, compiled by the Office on Smoking and Health)
55. State-specific prevalence of current cigarette and cigar smoking—U.S. 1998. 1998. *Morbidity and Mortality Weekly Report* 45(48, November), 1034–1039.
56. U.S. Department of Health and Human Services, Office on Smoking and Health. 1989. *Reducing the Health Consequences of Smoking: 25 Years of Progress: A Report of the Surgeon General.* Washington, D.C.: U.S. Government Printing Office.
57. Warner, K. E. 1986. *Selling Smoke: Cigarette Advertising and Public Health.* Washington, D.C.: American Public Health Association.
58. U.S. Department of Health and Human Services. 1996. *National Survey Results on Drug Use from the Monitoring the Future Study, 1975–1995. Volume 1: Secondary School Children,* Table 3, 60. Washington, D.C.: U.S. Department of Health and Human Services.
59. Johnston, D. C. 1997. Anti-tobacco groups push for higher cigarette taxes. *New York Times,* April 3, A1, A18.

60. Quindlen, A. 1992. Good causes, bad money. *New York Times,* November 15, A1.
61. Humphrey, H. H., III. 1997. Let's take the time to get it right. *Public Health Reports* 112, 378–385.
62. Skolnick, A. 1994. Anti-tobacco advocates fight "illegal" diversion of tobacco control money. *Journal of the American Medical Association* 271(18), 1387–1389.
63. Tobacco deal: Public health advocates say proposal falls short. 1997. *The Nation's Health,* July, 1, 24.
64. Clinton responds. 1997. *The Nation's Health,* October, 7.
65. National Association of Attorneys General. 1999. Tobacco settlement proceeds to be released to states, tobacco sales down during first year since settlement. PRNewsire, November 12.
66. National Association of Attorneys General. 1999. Tobacco wars, still. *Washington Post,* December 29, A26.
67. World Health Organization, Tobacco or Health Program. 1996. The tobacco epidemic: A global public health emergency. *Tobacco Alert: Special Issue. World No-Tobacco Day, 1996.* Geneva, Switzerland: World Health Organization.
68. Lee, G. A. 1995. Mixed review for environment study: Growing population, cigarette production marked '94. *Washington Post,* May 21, A5.
69. Brown, L. 1997. *State of the World, 1997.* New York: WorldWatch Institute.
70. Chapman, S., and Wong, W. 1990. *Tobacco Control in the Third World: A Resource Atlas.* Penang, Malaysia: International Organization of Consumers Unions.
71. Kadlec, D. 1997. How tobacco firms will manage. *Time,* June 30, 29.
72. Churchill, L. 1987. *Rationing Health Care in America: Perceptions and Principles of Justice.* Notre Dame, Ind.: University of Notre Dame Press.
73. Levy, L. 1957. *The Law of the Commonwealth and Chief Justice Shaw.* Cambridge, Mass.: Harvard University Press.
74. Beauchamp, D. E. 1985. *Community: The Neglected Tradition of Public Health.* Hastings-on-the-Hudson, N.Y.: The Hastings Center.
75. Wickler, D. 1987. Who should be blamed for being sick? *Health Education Quarterly* 14(1), 11–25.
76. Callahan, D. 1987. *Setting Limits: Medical Ethics in an Aging Society.* New York: Simon and Schuster.
77. Edelman, P. 1997. The worst thing Bill Clinton has done. *Atlantic Monthly,* March, 43–58.
78. Families USA. 1996. *Hurting Real People: The Human Side of Medical Cuts.* Washington, D.C.: Families USA.
79. World Health Organization. 1984. *Report of the Working Group on the Concept and Principles of Health Promotion.* Copenhagen: World Health Organization.
80. World Health Organization. 1986. *Ottawa Charter for Health Promotion.* Copenhagen: World Health Organization.
81. Epp, J. 1986. *Achieving Health for All: A Framework for Health Promotion.* Ottawa: National Health and Welfare, Government of Canada.

82. Yazdanmehr, S. 1994. Northwest Territories. In *Health Promotion in Canada,* edited by A. Pederson, I. Rootman, and M. O'Neill. Pp. 226–243. Toronto: W. B. Saunders.

83. Pederson, A., Rootman, I., and O'Neill, M., eds. 1994. *Health Promotion in Canada.* Toronto: W. B. Saunders.

84. Personal communication from I. Rootman, January 12, 1994.

85. Green, L. W. 1994. Canadian health promotion: An outsider's view from the inside. In *Health Promotion in Canada,* edited by A. Pederson, I. Rootman, and M. O'Neill. Pp. 314–326. Toronto: W. B. Saunders.

86. Canadian Public Health Association. 1996, July. *Action Statement for Health Promotion in Canada.* Ottawa: Canadian Public Health Association.

87. Taylor, R., and Rieger, A. 1985. Medicine as a social science: Rudolf Virchow on the typhus epidemic in Upper Silesia. *International Journal of Health Services* 15(4), 547–559.

88. Becker, M. 1986. The tyranny of health promotion. *Public Health Review* 14, 15–23.

14

Shu-Hong Zhu and
Christopher M. Anderson

BRIDGING THE CLINICAL AND PUBLIC HEALTH APPROACHES TO SMOKING CESSATION

California Smokers' Helpline

INTRODUCTION

Smoking is a major risk factor for heart disease, lung cancer, and strokes and is the most important preventable cause of premature death in the United States.[1] In California alone, over 42,000 deaths each year are attributable to smoking.[2] However, studies have consistently shown that smokers who achieve long-term cessation significantly reduce their risk of disability and early death.[3] For that reason, efforts to persuade smokers to quit and to help them with the process have been encouraged on both the federal and state levels.[4,5] In recent years, in particular, many states have launched aggressive antismoking campaigns. With revenues from a voter-approved tobacco tax initiative (Proposition 99), California has developed one of the most comprehensive tobacco control programs in the country, with a budget that includes funding for a variety of smoking cessation interventions.[6-9]

Such interventions have been said to fall into two categories: the clinical approach, with its emphasis on depth of intervention, and the public health approach, which emphasizes broad-based interventions.[10,11] The clinical approach is characterized by intensive, multisession interventions; small populations; and high quit rates. The public health approach, on the other hand, is characterized by brief, low-cost interventions; large populations; and relatively low quit rates. There are many studies and service programs that fall within one framework or the other, but programs that successfully combine the intensity of the clinical approach with the breadth of the public health approach are few.

One that does attempt to bridge the two approaches is the California Smokers' Helpline, a telephone-based program that was established as a statewide service in August 1992. Because it is telephone based, the Helpline is accessible to nearly all smokers in the state and is thus in a position to play a strong public health role as both a referral agency and a clearinghouse for cessation materials. In addition, the Helpline also provides intensive, multicomponent, multisession behavioral modification counseling for any who need it. Though intensive, this telephone counseling intervention is focused and brief in its approach, emphasizing cost-efficiency in its design. In this way, the California Smokers' Helpline strives to put the benefits of a strong clinical program within reach of a much broader population than more traditional programs have been able to do.

OBSTACLES IN THE HELP-SEEKING PROCESS

One problem with the traditional clinical approach to smoking cessation is that although psychologically intensive programs are effective in helping smokers quit smoking,[12] few smokers use them.[13,14] One national survey has shown that only 10% of smokers who tried to quit smoking used a program to help them do so.[14] The reason for this is unclear; one reasonable guess would be that the remaining 90% do not want any help. But surveys have also shown that most smokers are worried about the prospect of quitting smoking. According to the 1990 California Tobacco Survey, 77.6% of smokers believe they are addicted to cigarettes, and 85.9% consider it important that there be programs to help smokers quit.[15] Moreover, there is a striking difference in help-seeking patterns among ethnic groups, with smokers of ethnic minority backgrounds less than half as likely as White smokers to seek help to quit.[16]

Even smokers who want to quit and who believe they need help may not know where to find that help. For example, a 1990 survey conducted in San Diego County asked 1,049 smokers to name "up to three programs that are helpful for people who want to quit smoking." Surprisingly, only 39.4% of smokers were able to name any program at all relating to smoking cessation. Furthermore, non-White smokers were even less aware of available programs (31.3%) than White smokers were (41.2%), suggesting one reason why minority smokers are less likely to seek help.[17]

Even if smokers do know where help can be found, they must still weigh the costs and benefits of obtaining that help. A decision-making model would suggest that only when the perceived benefits outweigh the perceived costs will smokers take action to attend a program.[18] Attendance fees are not the only cost involved. Smokers may weigh less tangible costs as well, such as time away from home, scheduling difficulties, child care and transportation problems, and loss of anonymity. All of these costs must be weighed against the uncertain benefits of success in quitting. For those smokers who would like help quitting, these costs may lessen the perceived accessibility of that help.

INCREASING THE ACCESSIBILITY
OF SMOKING CESSATION SERVICES

As part of an effort to redress this problem, the Tobacco Control Section of the California Department of Health Services began funding the California Smokers' Helpline in August 1992. Smokers from across the state are referred to the Helpline through a variety of means, including media advertisements and physician referral. When they call, they are offered a range of services according to their preference and their readiness to quit. Smokers who are not yet ready to quit are sent materials designed to spur them along, while those who do feel ready but who prefer to quit on their own receive self-help quit kits. Smokers who would like more intensive help can enroll in the Helpline's free telephone counseling program.

The first way in which the Helpline increases the accessibility of smoking cessation services is by educating smokers on where they can get help to quit. The Helpline is aggressively promoted by the media component of the state's Tobacco Control Section, which includes the Helpline's toll-free numbers in ads urging smokers to quit. These ads, in the six languages in which Helpline services are provided, appear on television, radio, and billboards and in newspapers across the state. The Helpline also provides detailed information about its services to health care providers and volunteer organizations so that they have a dependable referral source. Moreover, the Helpline publicizes other cessation programs by sending each caller a descriptive list of all the available programs in his or her area. In these ways, public awareness of help for smoking cessation is enhanced.

The Helpline also reduces many of the costs associated with getting help to quit smoking. The first of these is the actual financial cost. Supported by revenues from the state tax on cigarettes and other tobacco products, the Helpline offers help at no charge to the caller.

As mentioned previously, there are other less tangible costs that smokers may incur from traditional programs, including having to wait for cessation classes to form, taking time away from home to attend them, and the effort and expense of arranging for transportation and child care. Even the potential benefit of social support from attending group sessions may be outweighed, for some, by the prospect of facing a roomful of strangers. Some smokers face geographic or language barriers as well. The Helpline reduces all of these costs by enabling smokers to get help without leaving home and by providing services in six of the state's most common languages—English, Spanish, Mandarin, Cantonese, Vietnamese, and Korean. (The Helpline also has a TDD line for the hearing impaired and has recently added a line for smokeless tobacco users.)

The Helpline is also able to increase its accessibility by stretching its resources. The program operates out of a single site, minimizing overhead costs. Also, it employs a stepped-care approach;[19] that is, instead of attempting to provide every caller with its most intensive form of assistance—telephone counseling—it presents a variety of options, including simply receiving materials in the mail or attending one of the cessation groups noted on the referral list. The Helpline lets each caller select the services that he or she feels would be most useful. By allowing callers to "serve themselves" from a menu of different approaches, the Helpline is able to spread its resources among a greater number of people. In just over four years of operation, the Helpline has served more than 41,000 smokers in this way, an average of more than 10,000 people a year. An additional 2,300 nonsmokers have also called the Helpline to get help for their friends and families.

In many cases, it is smokers' own ambivalence that limits their access to programs. A study conducted in southern California when the Helpline was funded to provide counseling only in San Diego County may illustrate this point. In response to calls from more than 700 Los Angeles smokers who said they were planning to quit within a month, the Helpline sent self-help materials and a directory of all the smoking cessation programs in the Los Angeles area. Five weeks later, the Helpline staff called them back and asked if they had attended any of the programs in the directory. Only 6.2% had done so. Given that the first time they called they had appeared motivated to get help to quit, the low rate at which they actually did so suggests that, as a group, they experienced considerable ambivalence about using the available programs. It seems reasonable to suppose that many in the group found the idea of committing to a program—and thus of being obliged to take action to quit smoking—to be an uncomfortable prospect.[17]

To counteract this ambivalence and reduce the resulting attrition, the Helpline tested a proactive approach with its counseling clients. As part of a larger study, more than 3,000 smokers who said they were ready to quit within a week and who opted for telephone counseling were told by intake personnel that they would receive a packet of quitting materials in a few days, at which time they should call back to begin the counseling. Subjects were then randomized into two groups. Members of one group were left to call back as instructed; about 34.2% eventually did so and received counseling. In contrast, members of the other group were contacted directly by a counselor. In this group, 74.7% received counseling, demonstrating that a proactive approach to providing service can have a strong counteractive effect on clients' ambivalence.[20]

WHO SEEKS HELP FROM
THE CALIFORNIA SMOKERS' HELPLINE?

With respect to the population that uses the Helpline, two demographic dimensions deserve special attention. One is its ethnic diversity, and the other is the active participation of rural smokers.

Table 14.1 indicates the ethnic diversity of the population using the Helpline. As the table shows, the 1993 California Tobacco Survey (CTS) found that smokers of ethnic minority backgrounds were underrepresented among those who sought help in general to quit smoking. Hispanic/Latino smokers, for example, accounted for 18.5% of the smokers in California but only 9.4% of those who sought help to quit. African-American smokers made up 7% of the state's smokers but only 4.3% of those who sought help. Asian-American smokers were likewise underrepresented (5% vs. 2.6%).

On the other hand, ethnic minority smokers were about as well represented among Helpline users as among smokers in general. Hispanic/Latino smokers accounted for 18.2% of Helpline users, a proportion approaching their representation among the state's smokers. African-American smokers were actually overrepresented among Helpline users (11.4% vs. 7%). Asian-American smokers were still underrepresented (2.6% vs. 5%). Taken as a group, however, smokers of ethnic minority

TABLE 14.1   SMOKERS IN CALIFORNIA,
SMOKERS WHO SOUGHT ASSISTANCE,
AND SMOKERS WHO CALLED
THE HELPLINE, BY ETHNICITY

	Smokers in California, 1992–1993 (%)	Sought Help ≤ 12 Months Prior to 1993 CTS (% [±95% CI])	Called the Helpline, 8/92–8/96 (% [±95% CI])
N	4,078,306	3,425	39,903
White	67.4	78.9 (4.9)	62.3 (0.5)
Hispanic	18.5	9.4 (3.4)	18.2 (0.4)
Black	7.0	4.3 (3.0)	11.4 (0.3)
Asian	5.0	2.6 (1.9)	2.6 (0.2)
Others	2.0	4.8 (3.5)	5.4 (0.2)

NOTE: Because only adult smokers participated in the 1993 CTS, Helpline callers under 18 are excluded from this analysis.
SOURCES: 1993 California Tobacco Survey and the California Smokers' Helpline. Adapted from Pierce et al. (1994 [8]) and Zhu et al. (1995 [16]).

backgrounds were better represented among Helpline users (37.6%) than among smokers seeking help in general (21.1%).

The fact that the Helpline's services are available in several languages, each with its own 1-800 number, contributes to its success in recruiting minority smokers. The high proportion of Hispanic callers, for example, is due largely to the Helpline's Spanish line. In fact, 71% of all Hispanic callers use that line. Conversely, the low percentage of Asian callers may be due in part to the relatively late addition of the Asian lines, 19 months after the English and Spanish lines.

Through targeted advertising and ethnic networks, the promotion of the Helpline also encourages minority participation. Because the Helpline is not tied to any particular local base, it can be selectively promoted in underserved communities wherever they occur in the state. This feature makes the Helpline particularly useful as part of a larger public health effort to reduce the smoking prevalence wherever it is especially high.

Much of this effort is spent in rural and mixed areas, where the population is low but the smoking prevalence is higher than the state average. As Table 14.2 illustrates, the likelihood of using the Helpline varies according to the urbanization of the state's 58 counties: smokers from rural counties have been disproportionately active participants in the program. (For this analysis, the classification of counties developed by the California Senate Committee on Local Government was used.)[21] This may reflect the relative scarcity in rural areas of programs to help people

TABLE 14.2   SMOKERS IN CALIFORNIA
AND SMOKERS WHO CALLED
THE HELPLINE, BY TYPE OF COUNTY

	Smokers in California (%)	Called the Helpline 8/92–8/96 (% [±95% CI])
N	4,078,306	41,232
Rural	7.2	11.5 (0.3)
Mixed	17.5	16.0 (0.4)
Urban	75.1	72.5 (0.4)

NOTE: Percentages for the state of California are estimated from the smoking prevalence rates at the time of the 1993 survey.
SOURCE: 1993 California Tobacco Survey and California Smokers' Helpline.

quit smoking and suggests that there is a real need in such areas for this kind of assistance.

Interestingly, the most significant means of reaching and encouraging rural smokers to call is not—as it is with urban smokers—the mass media. Across the state, the mass media were responsible for the majority of the Helpline's callers (60.9%), while health care providers referred an additional 15.7%. But as illustrated in Table 14.3, there were substantial differences by type of county in terms of how smokers learned of the Helpline. In rural counties, health care providers were responsible for 43.3% of referrals, while the media accounted for only 18.1%. The situation was reversed in urban counties, where the media accounted for 72.6% of referrals and health care providers only 7.7%. Mixed counties fell somewhere in the middle. This pattern suggests that where intensive media advertising of an important public health service becomes impractical, there are physicians, nurses, and other community health advocates who are willing to take up the slack. In fact, the active participation of these individuals in the promotion of the Helpline is further evidence that the program addresses a scarcity of needed services in their communities. Appropriately, in counties where the smoking prevalence is high and where programs are few, rural health care professionals have been playing an important role in directing smokers to accessible help.

THE EFFECTIVENESS OF TELEPHONE COUNSELING

The greater accessibility of the Helpline format, especially among ethnic minority groups and in geographic areas that are relatively underserved

TABLE 14.3   HOW HELPLINE CALLERS HEARD
ABOUT THE PROGRAM, BY TYPE OF COUNTY

	Rural (%)	Mixed (%)	Urban (%)	Total (%)
N	4,715	6,588	29,834	41,232
Mass media	18.1	38.4	72.6	60.9
Health care provider	43.3	32.3	7.7	15.7
Family/friend	14.6	12.2	8.9	10.1
Nonprofit organization	8.7	5.5	2.2	3.5
Other	14.7	10.8	7.8	9.1
Don't remember	0.7	0.8	0.9	0.8

SOURCE: California Smokers' Helpline.

by smoking cessation programs, is a key issue from a public health stand-point. But to justify large-scale application, the Helpline's interventions also had to be shown to help people actually quit smoking. The telephone counseling services offered by the Helpline are, in fact, directly based on interventions that in an earlier randomized trial were shown to work.

This trial was conducted in San Diego County before the California Smokers' Helpline was established. More than 3,000 smokers who said they were ready to quit within a week were randomized into three groups. The first group received only a self-help quit kit. The second group received the quit kit plus one 50-minute session of telephone counseling preparatory to quitting. The third group received the quit kit, the prequit session, and up to five additional 20-minute sessions in the first month after quitting.

The self-help condition served as a control for the two counseling conditions, although the self-help treatment was in itself a minimal intervention. Therefore, any effect attributable to the addition of counseling on top of the self-help treatment is a conservative estimate of the intervention's total effect.

The rationale for testing the single counseling intervention was to discover whether a minimal counseling intervention could produce an effect. Given the frequent real-world scenario in which smokers show up for a first session and then disappear, it was important to see whether just one contact with a counselor could help smokers quit. If so, the effect of the single counseling treatment would in itself argue for a real-world application of telephone counseling.

To maximize the likelihood of its success, it was crucial that the prequit session be thoughtfully planned and executed. The design of the counseling was based on a combination of the principles of motivational interviewing for inducing behavior change and those of the cognitive-behavioral approach to treating substance abuse.[22–24] The motivational interviewing approach is intended to create a collaborative counselor-client relationship through which the client's motivation to change is enhanced. The cognitive-behavioral approach focuses on restructuring the client's beliefs about smoking and quitting and emphasizes the development and implementation of coping strategies.[24] The role of the counselor in this conception, then, is to promote the motivation to change and to help the client develop competence in self-management. The Helpline developed a structured counseling protocol that embodies these principles.

The structured counseling protocol was intended to help the counselor conduct a comprehensive session in a brief and focused manner.[25] The session was to cover a wide range of clinical issues, including smoking and quitting history, nicotine dependence, motivation to quit, self-efficacy, social and environmental influences, anticipating difficult situations, planning effective coping strategies, and committing to a quit date. All these areas were to be covered in about 50 minutes.

Similarly, if the multiple counseling condition was to achieve a greater effect than that of single counseling, the follow-up sessions would have to be conducted in a therapeutic manner. Like the single counseling intervention, multiple counseling was also conceived as a brief intervention: The total time spent per smoker was intended to be short enough that, if proven effective, the treatment could later be applied in a public health setting, where efficiency and brevity are central concerns.[26] For this reason it was decided that follow-up counseling should entail no more than five 20-minute postquit sessions to be scheduled in the most efficient manner possible. Thus, the total time spent per client would be under three hours.

The question of how best to schedule the follow-up sessions turned out to be critical. In most traditional multisession interventions for smoking cessation, the sessions are held weekly. Though convenient for the clinician, the weekly schedule is not necessarily optimal from a therapeutic standpoint. Why this is so can be seen by considering the shape of a typical relapse curve for smoking cessation, as shown in Figure 14.1. If relapse were a linear function of time, an equal-interval schedule of sessions, such as the traditional weekly schedule, would be most suitable. However, as the shape of the curve in Figure 14.1 makes clear, relapse is in reality a negatively accelerated function of time. In other words, relapse is most likely in the period immediately after quitting and becomes

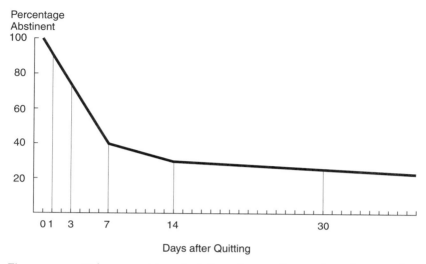

Figure 14.1. Relapse-sensitive scheduling of counseling sessions. Source: Zhu and Pierce (1995 [34]). © 1995, American Psychological Association, Inc.

less so as time goes on. The fact that by the end of the first week over 60% of the smokers have relapsed suggests that if follow-up sessions are to achieve a relapse-prevention effect, they must begin within that first week. For this reason, the Helpline used a new scheduling method that differed from that of traditional group sessions as well as from those used in previous trials of multisession telephone counseling.[27–33] In this method, sessions are arranged according to the probability of relapse: three during the first week of quitting, one at two weeks, and one at one month, as indicated by the vertical lines in Figure 14.1. It was hoped that this arrangement would prove not only to be therapeutic but also to be most efficient in that help would be provided when it is most needed and not when the anticipated return is small. This probabilistic approach to multisession counseling has been dubbed relapse-sensitive scheduling.[34]

An analysis of 12-month abstinence rates for the three experimental groups showed that both counseling conditions were significantly more effective than self-help.[35] Moreover, there was a clear dose-response relation between the intensity of counseling and treatment effect, as multisession counseling was significantly more effective than single-session counseling. The 12-month abstinence rates were 14.7%, 19.8%, and 26.7% for self-help, single counseling, and multiple counseling, respectively. These results are represented in Figure 14.2 as the end points of

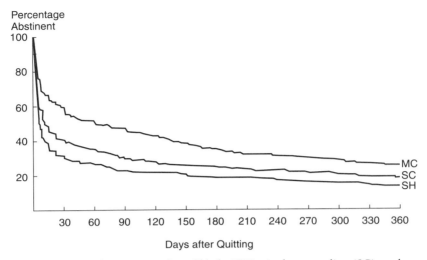

Figure 14.2.   Relapse curves for self-help (SH), single counseling (SC), and multiple counseling (MC). Source: Zhu et al. (1996 [35]). © 1996, American Psychological Association, Inc.

three separate relapse curves. The dose-response relation confirms the consistency of the counseling approach and indicates that the counseling tapped into variables that affect the probability of success.[35,36]

The multisession protocol became the basis for the telephone counseling currently provided by the California Smokers' Helpline. It has been further shaped and refined by the Helpline's collective experience of counseling additional smokers since expanding statewide. Similar statewide telephone counseling services have been established for Massachusetts and Michigan using the same protocol.

BRIDGING THE CLINICAL
AND PUBLIC HEALTH APPROACHES

After decades in which clinical approaches to smoking cessation have dominated, researchers have begun calling for more of a public health perspective in interventions to help people quit smoking.[10,37,38] Although they are needed both as a resource for heavily addicted smokers and as a source of scientific innovation,[39] clinical programs are not sufficient to reach the large number of smokers who are at risk for smoking-related diseases. In contrasting the features of the two approaches to smoking cessation, Lichtenstein and Glasgow have observed that clinical programs may achieve a higher quit rate than public health interventions do; however, because most smokers will not use such programs, the public health approach can actually produce a greater net result in terms of reducing smoking and therefore the incidence of tobacco-related morbidity and mortality.[10] They suggest both the greater incorporation of public health perspectives into clinical interventions and an increased effort to bring interventions to a wider population, in other words, a bridge between the two approaches.

The California Smokers' Helpline is one attempt at such a bridge. On the one hand, the Helpline has developed an intensive and clinically comprehensive program that produces a long-term success rate comparable to that of traditional clinical programs. On the other hand, the Helpline is highly accessible, reaches a broad population, and uses a stepped-care procedure to maximize its reach.

The Helpline's initial research on the efficacy of telephone counseling was designed, from the beginning, to establish its suitability for large-scale, real-world application. In fact, the research was conducted using paraprofessional counselors operating from a single site and drawing smokers from the community at large, just as the larger application would be expected to do. For these reasons, it was easy to translate the results from the study into a program serving smokers statewide. The duplication of the program in Massachusetts and Michigan has likewise been straightforward. For the Massachusetts Smokers' Quitline, the original researchers provided early training and program support. The Smokers' Helpline of Michigan, meanwhile, contracts with the California Smokers' Helpline to provide counseling for Michigan smokers on a per-client basis; all other Helpline services are provided from their headquarters in Lansing. This arrangement suggests the potential for a single counseling center to provide telephone counseling for a multistate region or even for the entire nation.

Just as the Helpline's early research supported a wide application of its findings, that application in turn supports increased research. The size of the Helpline's population allows opportunities for research on smoking and the quitting process that would be difficult to conduct with smaller populations of smokers. For example, a close comparison of hazard functions for relapse for different intervention groups is often infeasible in typical smoking cessation research because of insufficient sample size. But a large sample gives researchers confidence to make such comparisons, providing new information about the differential effects of interventions at different points in time.[35] The size and diversity of the Helpline population also provide opportunities to study sub-groups of smokers in relatively large samples.

THE FUTURE: TELEPHONE COUNSELING AS AN ADJUVANT TO PHYSICIAN ADVICE

The California Smokers' Helpline has made an attempt to blend features of both the clinical and the public health approaches to smoking cessation with the aim of bringing a clinically effective intervention to a large and diverse population. Undoubtedly, more could be done along these lines. One possibility that the Helpline is currently pursuing is to apply telephone counseling to primary care settings.

The role of physicians in helping patients to quit smoking is one of the most active areas of research in smoking cessation. Most smokers visit their doctors at least once a year,[40,41] an occasion that has been called a "teachable moment" because it is then that they are likely to be receptive to advice on behavior changes that could improve their health.[42] The effect per smoker may be quite low, but if all physicians were to start doing this, they would quickly reach the majority of smokers. The overall effect, therefore, could be dramatic. For this reason, there is now a big push to urge physicians to take a more active role in helping to reduce the smoking prevalence.[43] Many creative approaches to physician involvement have been proposed, such as the vital sign approach, in which smoking status is included among the vital signs that physicians assess as part of routine physical checkups.[44] Such approaches are intended to create an impetus for physicians to advise their smoking patients to quit.

There are obstacles to physician involvement, however. Doctors are not reimbursed for providing behavioral modification counseling and, moreover, may feel inhibited by a lack of counselor training.[45] Further, those who are inclined to advise patients on preventive health measures may have little time to do so. In managed care settings, physicians typically have about 15 minutes with each patient, during which time they must diagnose, discuss, and treat the presenting complaint; arrange needed referrals or routine screenings; and respond to other possible concerns of the patient. And given the high attrition rate in smoking cessation clinics, the physicians who refer their patients to them may quickly become discouraged with that strategy.[46]

Telephone counseling may work well as an adjuvant intervention in such a setting.[47,48] The minimum intervention that physicians undertake under this scenario is to ask whether their patients smoke, and if so, to advise them to call the Helpline's toll-free number for help in quitting. Not all patients will call, of course, but those who do will enhance their chances of successfully quitting. Some may feel more confident about quitting simply by knowing that there is free help available should they need it. If they do call and enroll in counseling, the Helpline's proactive counseling procedure helps to keep attrition low. Many health care providers, especially in rural areas, are already working in partnership with the Helpline to get help for smoking cessation to those who might not otherwise seek it. In the future, we hope to expand this base of referring physicians to include more practitioners in urban areas. We are currently developing strategies to increase their participation, including encouraging providers to consider the Helpline a member of their health care team and reinforcing their efforts with feedback about how their efforts are paying off. It is in this sort of collaborative intervention that we expect to see even more synergy between the clinical and the public health approaches.

NOTE

This work was supported by grants 90-10961 and 92-15416 from the California Department of Health Services, Tobacco Control Section. Preparation of this chapter was supported by a grant from The California Wellness Foundation. This chapter follows closely the content of a Wellness Lecture presented in October 1996, when the number of calls to the Helpline had reached 41,000. At the time this volume went to print, the number of first-time calls had surpassed 120,000. For updated information on the demographic distribution of callers to this program, interested readers may wish to consult S.-H. Zhu et al., "A Centralized Telephone Service for Tobacco Cessation: The California Experience" (*Tobacco Control* [Suppl., August 2000]).

REFERENCES

1. U.S. Department of Health and Human Services. 1989. *Reducing the Health Consequences of Smoking: 25 Years of Progress. A Report of the Surgeon General.* DHHS Publication (CDC) 89-8411. Washington, D.C.: U.S. Department of Health and Human Services, Public Health Service, Centers for Disease Control and Prevention, National Center for Chronic Disease Prevention and Health Promotion, Office on Smoking and Health.

2. Centers for Disease Control and Prevention. 1996. *State Tobacco Control*

Highlights—1996. CDC Publication 099-4895. Atlanta: Centers for Disease Control and Prevention, National Center for Chronic Disease Prevention and Health Promotion, Office on Smoking and Health.

3. U.S. Department of Health and Human Services. 1990. *The Health Benefits of Smoking Cessation: A Report of the Surgeon General.* DHHS Publication (CDC) 90-8416. Washington, D.C.: U.S. Department of Health and Human Services, Public Health Service, Centers for Disease Control and Prevention, National Center for Chronic Disease Prevention and Health Promotion, Office on Smoking and Health.

4. U.S. Department of Health and Human Services. 1991. *Healthy People 2000: National Health Promotion and Disease Prevention Objectives.* Washington, D.C.: Public Health Service.

5. Kizer, K. W., Honig, B., Allenby, C., and Deukmejian, G. 1990. *Toward a Tobacco Free California: A Status Report to the California Legislature on the First Fifteen Months of the California Tobacco Control Program.* Sacramento: Department of Health Services.

6. Bal, D. G., Kizer, K. W., Felten, P. G., et al. 1990. Reducing tobacco consumption in California. *Journal of the American Medical Association* 264(12), 1570–1574.

7. Breslow, L., and Johnson, M. D. 1993. California's Proposition 99 on tobacco, and its impact. *Annual Review of Public Health* 14, 585–604.

8. Pierce, J. P., Evans, N., Farkas, A. J., et al. 1994. *Tobacco Use in California: An Evaluation of the Tobacco Control Program, 1989–1993.* La Jolla: University of California, San Diego.

9. Bal, D. G., Russell, C., Motylewski, C., et al. 1995. The California Tobacco Control Program: Lessons learned. In *Tobacco and Health,* edited by K. Slama. New York: Plenum Press.

10. Lichtenstein, E., and Glasgow, R. E. 1992. Smoking cessation: What have we learned over the past decade? *Journal of Consulting and Clinical Psychology* 60(4), 518–527.

11. Lichtenstein, E., and Glasgow, R. E. 1997. A pragmatic framework for smoking cessation: Implications for clinical and public health programs. *Psychology of Addictive Behaviors* 11(2), 142–151.

12. Schwartz, J. L. 1987. *Review and Evaluation of Smoking Cessation Methods: The United States and Canada.* NIH Publication 87-2940. Washington, D.C.: U.S. Department of Health and Human Services.

13. Chapman, S. 1985. Stop-smoking clinics: A case for their abandonment. *The Lancet* 1(8434), 918–920.

14. Fiore, M. C., Novotny, T. E., Pierce, J. P., et al. 1990. Methods used to quit smoking in the United States: Do cessation programs help? *Journal of the American Medical Association* 263(3), 2760–2765.

15. Burns, D., and Pierce, J. P. 1992. *Tobacco Use in California, 1991–1992.* Sacramento: California Department of Health Services.

16. Zhu, S.-H., Rosbrook, B., Anderson, et al. 1995. The demographics of help-seeking for smoking cessation in California and the role of the California Smokers' Helpline. *Tobacco Control* 4(Suppl. 1), S5–S15.

17. Zhu, S.-H., Anderson, C. M., and Pierce, J. P. 1995. Smoking cessation in

California: The importance of assistance to smokers in quitting. Paper presented at the 123rd annual conference of the American Public Health Association, San Diego, November.

18. Von Winterfeldt, D., and Edwards, W. 1986. *Decision Analysis and Behavioral Research*. Cambridge: Cambridge Press.

19. Abrams, D. B. 1993. Treatment issues: Towards a stepped-care model. *Tobacco Control* 2(Suppl.), S17–S29.

20. Zhu, S.-H., Freeman, D., Martinez, E., and Anderson, C. M. 1995. Help-seeking and active helping in smoking cessation. Paper presented at the 16th annual scientific session of the Society of Behavioral Medicine, San Diego, March.

21. California Legislature, Senate Committee on Local Government. 1985. *Rural Counties' Fiscal Problems*. Sacramento: State Capitol.

22. Miller, W. R., and Rollnick, S. 1991. *Motivational Interviewing: Preparing People to Change Addictive Behavior*. New York: Guilford Press.

23. Beck, A. T., Wright, F. D., Newman, C. F., and Liese, B. S. 1993. *Cognitive Therapy of Substance Abuse*. New York: Guilford Press.

24. Marlatt, G. A., and Gordon, J. R. 1985. *Relapse Prevention: Maintenance Strategies in the Treatment of Addictive Behavior*. New York: Guilford Press.

25. Zhu, S.-H., Tedeschi, G., Anderson, C. M., and Pierce, J. P. 1996. Telephone counseling for smoking cessation: What's in a call? *Journal of Counseling and Development* 75(2), 93–102.

26. Glynn, T. J., Boyd, G. M., and Gruman, J. C. 1990. Essential elements of self-help/minimal intervention strategies for smoking cessation. *Health Education Quarterly* 17(3), 329–345.

27. Lando, H. A., Hellerstedt, W. L., Pirie, P. L., and McGovern, P. G. 1992. Brief supportive telephone outreach as a recruitment and intervention strategy for smoking cessation. *American Journal of Public Health* 82(1), 41–46.

28. Ockene, J. K., Kristeller, J., Pbert, L., et al. 1994. The physician-delivered smoking intervention project: Can short-term interventions produce long-term effects for a general outpatient population? *Health Psychology* 13(3), 278–281.

29. Prochaska, J. O., DiClemente, C. C., Velicer, W. F., and Rossi, J. S. 1991. Standardized, individualized, interactive and personalized self-help programs for smoking cessation. *Health Psychology* 12(5), 399–405.

30. Ossip-Klein, D. J., Giovino, G. A., Megahed, N., et al. 1991. Effects of a smokers' hotline: Results of a 10-county self-help trial. *Journal of Consulting and Clinical Psychology* 59(2), 325–332.

31. Orleans, C. T., Schoenbach, V. J., Wagner, E. H., et al. 1991. Self-help quit smoking intervention: Effects of self-help materials, social support intervention, and telephone counseling. *Journal of Consulting and Clinical Psychology* 59(3), 439–448.

32. Curry, S. J., McBride, C., Grothaus, L. C., Louie, D., and Wagner, E. H. 1995. A randomized trial of self-help materials, personalized feedback and telephone counseling with nonvolunteer smokers. *Journal of Consulting and Clinical Psychology* 63(6), 1005–1014.

33. Lando, H. A., Rolnick, S., Klevan, D., et al. 1997. Telephone support as an

adjunct to transdermal nicotine in smoking cessation. *American Journal of Public Health* 87(10), 1670–1674.

34. Zhu, S.-H., and Pierce, J. P. 1995. A new scheduling method for time-limited counseling. *Professional Psychology: Research and Practice* 26(6), 624–625.

35. Zhu, S.-H., Stretch, V., Balabanis, M., et al. 1996. Telephone counseling for smoking cessation: Effects of single-session and multiple-session interventions. *Journal of Consulting and Clinical Psychology* 64(1), 202–211.

36. Howard, K. I., Kopta, S. M., Krause, M. S., and Orlinsky, D. E. 1986. The dose-effect relationship in psychotherapy. *American Psychologist* 41(2), 159–164.

37. Abrams, D. G., Emmons, K., Niaura, R. D., et al. Tobacco dependence: An integration of individual and public health perspectives. In *The Annual Review of Addictions Treatment and Research,* edited by P. E. Nathan, J. W. Langenbucher, B. S. McCrady, and W. Frankenstein. New York: Pergamon Press.

38. Winett, R. A., King, A. C., and Altman, D. G. 1989. *Health Psychology and Public Health: An Integrative Approach.* New York: Pergamon Press.

39. Shiffman, S. 1993. Smoking cessation treatment: Any progress? *Journal of Consulting and Clinical Psychology* 61(5), 202–211.

40. Gritz, E. R. 1988. Cigarette smoking: The need for action by health professionals. *CA—A Cancer Journal for Clinicians* 38(4), 194–212.

41. Gilpin, E., Pierce, J. P., Goodman, J., et al. 1992. Trends in physicians' advice to stop smoking. *Tobacco Control* 1(1), 1–36.

42. Vogt, T. M., Lichtenstein, E., Ary, D., et al. 1989. Integrating tobacco intervention into a health maintenance organization: The TRACC program. *Health Education Research* 4(1), 125–135.

43. U.S. Department of Health and Human Services. 1994. *Tobacco and the Clinician: Interventions for Medical and Dental Practice.* NIH Publication 94-3693. Washington, D.C.: U.S. Department of Health and Human Services, Public Health Service, National Institutes of Health.

44. Fiore, M. C., Jorenby, D. E., Schensky, A. E., et al. 1995. Smoking status as the new vital sign: Effects on assessment and intervention in patients who smoke. *Mayo Clinic Proceedings* 70(3), 209–213.

45. Sexton, M., Stine, J., and Cahill, S. 1994. Smoking intervention by providers of health care for women. In *Tobacco and the Clinician: Interventions for Medical and Dental Practice.* NIH Publication 94-3693. Washington, D.C.: U.S. Department of Health and Human Services, Public Health Service, National Institutes of Health.

46. Lichtenstein, E., and Hollis, J. 1992. Patient referral to a smoking cessation program: Who follows through? *Journal of Family Practice* 34(6), 739–744.

47. Fiori, M. C., Bailey, W. C., Cohen, S. J., et al. 1996, April. *Smoking Cessation.* AHCPR Publication 96-0692. Clinical Practice Guideline 18. Rockville, Md.: U.S. Department of Health and Human Services, Public Health Service, Agency for Health Care Policy and Research.

48. Tsoh, J. Y., McClure, J. B., Skaar, K. L., et al. 1997. Smoking cessation: 2. Components of effective intervention. *Behavioral Medicine* 23(1), 15–27.

15

Andrew Duxbury

DISEASE PREVENTION
VERSUS HEALTH PROMOTION

Pitfalls of Preventive Care
in the Geriatric Population

INTRODUCTION

Rapid gains in medical knowledge, technology, and public health measures through the 20th century have led to a demographic shift unprecedented in human history. A much larger portion of the population is surviving to old age, placing great strains on long-established social structures and concepts. The geriatric age-group, usually defined as those 65 years of age or older, has become one of the fastest-growing segments of our society in terms of both percentage and absolute numbers.[1,2] At the turn of the 20th century, there were approximately five million adults over the age of 65 in the United States, or about 4% of the total population. In 1990, that number had increased to 30 million, or 12.5%. If present trends continue, by the middle of the 21st century, nearly 70 million, or more than 20%, will qualify as members of the geriatric age-group.[3]

This demographic change is forcing our society to grapple with multiple complicated issues related to aging. These include questions of social and medical policy that impact the lives of older adults and their caregivers. One of these questions is, How should our health system approach the subject of preventive health care for the geriatric population? Should the model we use focus on disease prevention, or is this model inadequate to deal with the normal physiologic changes of an aging population? What should be the role of screening for specific disease in a population with high prevalence of disease from the physiologic and functional challenges of the aging process? This chapter looks at some of the issues surrounding these questions and discusses the failings of the traditional disease prevention model of preventive care in coping with geriatric medicine. It also discusses alternative approaches to these problems.

There has been a tendency in American social and medical policy to consider all persons over the age of 65 as a homogeneous entity of "geriatric" individuals. However, such inclusiveness does not allow for the differences that may exist within the older population in terms of life expectancy, functional status, or disease burden. In order to better understand this demographic group, some sort of divisions are helpful. Some authors advocate splitting older adults into three groups based strictly on chronologic age: The "young old," aged 65 to 75, who are physically and physiologically quite similar to younger adults; the "middle old," aged 75 to 85, who are more likely to be impaired physically or functionally from disease; and the "old old," those over the age of 85 who are at the highest risk for severe morbidity.[4-7] Others recommend considering older adults solely on the basis of their functional status, arguing that there is little difference between a robust and healthy 65- and 85-year-old.[8-10] Functional dependence, or an inability to complete basic activities of daily living such as bathing or dressing, affects less than 5% of adults 65 to 75 but approaches 40% in those over 85.[11] Either way, the majority of the "geriatric" age-group is not what most would consider geriatric in either health status or functioning. The poorly functional, often the "old old," bear the brunt of age-related disease and their associated costs, economic and human.

The decline in mortality that has led to a longer life span has not been matched by a decline in morbidity.[12] Older people are in danger of severe physical and functional compromise from both acute and chronic disease states. The medical and social problems of such dependent individuals pose both a direct and an indirect economic burden to society and the health care system. Over the last few decades, Alzheimer's disease, one of the more common diseases of aging, has emerged from relative obscurity to the 16th most costly disease in our health system in direct dollar costs.[13] If indirect costs such as lost productivity of patients and caregivers are factored in, it rises to third, following only heart disease and cancer.[14] The direct costs of dementia care alone are expected to top $100 billion a year by 2040, most of it being spent on functional needs.[15] Good medical practice and old-fashioned common sense say that the afflictions that create this frail, dependent fraction of the elderly population should be minimized, as they drain increasingly scarce health care dollars, often without hope of restoration of premorbid functioning.

Given the intense interest on both local and national levels regarding expenditures for health care, it is time to take a critical look at how our health care system goes about the task of maintaining health. Much of the current focus in gerontology is on so-called successful aging, whereby older individuals maintain lifestyles and health similar to those of younger people. The U.S. medical system is organized around acute interventions; treatment is offered for a specific illness or diagnosis. Thinking is based on the concepts of disease and cure. Preventive measures, when they are offered, fit into this model by obviating the need for a later cure. The evolving specialty of geriatrics, with its emphasis on functional status and health maintenance, requires a new paradigm of "health promotion" in which preventive measures are integrated into the full life cycle including the older age-group. The focus becomes not one of "disease" but rather one of "health."

OLDER ADULTS AND THE HEALTH CARE SYSTEM

The average primary care physician currently spends between 30% and 40% of his or her time with patients in the geriatric age-group. It is estimated that this will increase to at least 50% early in the 21st century, given current population trends.[16,17] The majority of these adults are able-bodied and independent; however, 22% require some assistance from others to remain at home, while another 5% reside in a long-term-care facility.[18] These frail, dependent individuals are more at risk for morbidity and mortality from disease processes.

Medicare, the federal health program for the elderly, has an annual budget of over $170 billion.[19] Its cost has been increasing at roughly 15% a year since its adoption in 1966.[20] At the time of its inception, life expectancy for Americans was roughly 70 years, five years beyond the age for qualification.[20] Life expectancy has increased to age 79 today, and for those who are healthy at age 65, it is now 84 for men and 89 for women.[19] Medicare was designed to allow older Americans access to the acute care model of health service provision prevalent in the United States. It was never intended to be a comprehensive health insurance policy. It pays for services necessary to recover from an acute disease. For the most part, it does not pay for preventive measures, treatments for chronic conditions, or acute conditions after a specified time frame if meaningful recovery is not achieved. Because up to 80% of those over the age of 65 suffer from at least one chronic disease, there is a divergence between the goals of the Medicare program and the health needs of those it serves.

Many frail elderly are in need of chronic care. The need for skilled nursing facilities is expected to increase dramatically in the coming years. In 1964, prior to the creation of Medicare and Medicaid, only about 500,000 older adults lived in skilled nursing facilities. Numbers increased to about 1.5 million by 1990.[21] For persons turning 65 in 1990, it has been estimated that 43% (900,000) will be admitted to a nursing home at least once prior to their death.[22] Medicare pays for less than 5% of nursing home care costs. Most long-term care is, by definition, chronic and therefore outside the scope of Medicare. It is paid for by either state Medicaid programs or private funds.[23] The economic burden to the federal government, states, and private individuals continues to increase and is part of the ongoing debate on health care reform. The combination of Medicare's emphasis on acute health conditions, its lack of payment for chronic health care needs, increasing life expectancy, and medical inflation have led to the ironic result that the elderly spend a larger portion of their income on out-of-pocket health expenses today than they did in 1965, prior to the introduction of Medicare.[24]

Despite the best efforts of the health care system, ultimate mortality for the human race remains at 100%. Death cannot be prevented, only postponed. The system can only try to control the types of disease and other morbid conditions that lead to death. There is some perception by the public that too many of our scarce resources are "wasted" on the elderly. Various studies have shown that the elderly do consume 30% to 35% of health care dollars.[25,26] However, a more detailed analysis shows that the fraction of the elderly in the terminal stages of their life is responsible for the lion's share of these costs. Thirty percent of Medicare dollars are spent on individuals who die within a year; 52% of these are spent in the last 60 days of life.[27] Younger people who die or have catastrophic disease also use large quantities of health care dollars.[28] The bottom line is that a significant portion of the health care costs in this country goes to terminal care of those without hope of meaningful recovery.

HEALTH CARE MAINTENANCE

It is clear that the diseases of the frail elderly pose an increasing burden on society's ability to provide care. The medical specialty of geriatrics sees those patients with chronic health problems and tries to help the patients cope with them without necessarily recommending costly acute care interventions. The ultimate goal is to improve the frail toward a similar status to that of the healthy majority. One of the cornerstones of geriatric health maintenance is the comprehensive geriatric assessment. This is generally a multidisciplinary exam of a patient undertaken to identify not only physical health problems but also functional problems, cognitive problems, and social problems that might affect health status.[10] Treatment plans usually work toward maximizing a patient's functioning in his or her usual environment on the theory that this will keep his or her diseases from being as heavy a burden on the health care system in the future.[29]

Improvement in a patient's ability to meet his or her own self-care activities of daily living is assumed to be a cornerstone of better health. In fact, frailty and an inability to care for one's self are those things most feared by the older population, not death.[30] Research looking for predictors of frail health and disability among older adults has failed to demonstrate any consistent positive predictors. The most consistent risk factor noted has been that of physical inactivity.[12] Inactivity, particularly if related to a disease, often starts a downward spiral from which there is no recovery. Neuromuscular atrophy, decreased aerobic capacity, and a decrease in basal metabolic rate all set in rapidly during bed rest in the geriatric age-group.[31] The misconception that prolonged rest is good for the ill and the elderly adds to their morbidity.[12] Functional assessment is aimed at interrupting this process.

Controlled randomized trials of geriatric functional assessment for frail patients on inpatient geriatric units have shown the benefits of this approach.[32-34] The results are not so clear-cut on ambulatory patients.[35,36] Medicare does not recognize functional assessment as a separate entity distinct from an office visit, so most practicing physicians limit its use.[37] The growth of functional assessment and the spreading of the geriatrics gospel have increased the realization that interventions practiced now on older people may help prevent future burdens on the health care system. Two important concepts have come from this. The first is the idea of a compression of morbidity, eloquently articulated by Fries nearly 20 years ago.[38] As death cannot be prevented, functional healthy life should be extended until the period just prior to death, and then all morbidity should be suffered relatively acutely. Theoretically, this leads to maximal functional life of high quality and an obvious period of sharp, irreversible decline, which should be allowed to run its course without heroic intervention. Second, the ideals of preventive health care,

TABLE 15.1   TYPES OF PREVENTIVE CARE

Primary prevention—Those measures designed to prevent a given disease state from occurring.

Secondary prevention—Those measures designed to interrupt an established disease process prior to the onset of clinical symptoms.

Tertiary prevention—Those measures designed to prevent complications of a symptomatic disease state.

long recognized as beneficial for younger adults, should and can be applied to the older population.

PREVENTIVE HEALTH CARE

Mathematical modeling of Medicare expenditures into the 21st century has shown that a decrease is expected if appropriate preventive health measures convert a majority of the population into healthy low-cost users of the system rather than strictly treating the acute disease states that create high-cost users of the system.[39] These preventive health care measures can be divided into several classes, as shown in Table 15.1.

Many primary and secondary measures of preventive care have been shown to be cost-effective and therefore are the ones most intensely studied.[39] Preventive health care modalities that have been looked at in the geriatric population include primary measures such as vaccination against pneumococcal pneumonia and influenza virus, counseling on proper nutrition, home safety, and cholesterol screening. Secondary measures include blood pressure measurement, smoking cessation strategies, and cancer screening modalities such as mammography or fecal occult blood testing. Many of these are now considered standard in the routine care of the older adult. These preventive measures are usually cast in terms of disease rather than in terms of health.

THE DISEASE PREVENTION MODEL

Most physicians in the United States are indoctrinated by the health care system principles of acute care medicine. The goal is to take a diseased patient and apply an intervention that renders that patient no longer diseased. The physician becomes reactive to the disease of the patient. When issues of preventive care are addressed, they are also usually considered within this acute care framework. The goal of preventive care is "disease prevention." The patient is regarded as a potential repository of a disease state, and the intervention is designed to prevent that disease state from taking place.

The problem with this system is that the emphasis is placed on disease, not the patient and not health. The focus on disease can lead to a "can't see the forest for the trees" blindness on the part of physicians and the health care system. Physicians become so focused on disease that they are unable to deal adequately with information that does not neatly fit into a disease-based model. They tend to neglect pure preventive measures and miss proactive measures, such as discontinuing an unneeded medication.[40] Research by Reed et al. has shown that the disease-based worldview is strongly ingrained in even the youngest practicing physicians. Their survey of family practice residents regarding the follow-up of recommendations from a geriatric functional assessment showed that physicians ordered additional tests for diagnosis 70.3% of the time. They ordered additional medication for treatment 85.4% of the time. They were much less likely to stop a medication (64.3%) or perform preventive measures (54.3%).[41] Clearly, the goals of maximizing function and health in the geriatric population require a more encompassing view than one that deals strictly with "disease."

SCREENING TESTS IN OLDER ADULTS

A major focus of disease prevention in the geriatric age-group is screening tests for serious medical conditions. Some, such as blood pressure screening, are so routine and easily performed that they are considered a normal part of a visit to the doctor. Others, such as screening tests for certain cancers, diabetes, or elevated cholesterol, require special examinations. Medicare, which pays approximately 50% of the health care bill for those over 65, was conceived under the acute care model.[42] Medicare reimburses doctors and hospitals for the care of disease states. It was never designed to be an all-encompassing health program, and screening tests, with certain exceptions, are not covered benefits, as they do not treat acute disease.

Whether a given screening test is worthwhile in a population depends heavily on that test's sensitivity and specificity. Sensitivity is defined as the proportion of patients with a given disease whose test will be positive for that disease. A sensitive test produces few false-negative results. Specificity is defined as the proportion of patients without a specific disease whose test will be negative for that disease. A specific test produces few false-positive results. Insensitive tests are not useful, as they will miss individuals with the disease process, making the costs of implementing a screening program not worthwhile. Nonspecific tests identify too many individuals, and the cost of workup of those without the disease nullifies the cost-benefit of the screening program.[43] Measurements of sensitivity and specificity, along with exhaustive cost-benefit nalysis, are usually acquired and reviewed prior to any new screening procedure being introduced to the medical system.[44] The American medical system, like it or not, is obsessed with cost; no new test or procedure will be covered by private insurance or public funds without demonstrated benefit. The politics of health, however, are often at odds with the economics of health. There is often a push to introduce new screening methodologies to save pain or suffering on the individual level without serious thought to the aggregate effects on the population. Cancer screening is an example.

CANCER SCREENING: AN OVERVIEW

Cancer lends itself to the disease prevention model of preventive care and screening. It is the second-leading cause of death in the elderly, after atherosclerotic cardiovascular disease.[45] Fully 50% of diagnosed cancers occur in the over-65 age-group.[46] Awareness of the disease in older patients is high.[47] The goal of most cancer screening tests is to detect early malignancies prior to regional spread and metastasis, when the chance of curative treatment is high.[48] Therapy for malignancies that have spread remains problematic, particularly in older individuals who may be debilitated from other disease and unable to tolerate radical surgery or chemotherapy.[49] By screening, the clinician hopes to extend additional "well" time to an individual and limit the morbidity and mortality of the disease process, thus fulfilling the goal of compression of morbidity discussed previously.

Difficulties arise in trying to determine just what type of screening is appropriate in the older age-group. Data from controlled trials is limited or nonexistent. Conflicting recommendations are issued by authoritative groups. The American Cancer Society (ACS) is perhaps the best known of these; it issues screening recommendations with periodic updates for most common cancers. Some physicians, however, find the ACS recommendations too burdensome for the average patient.[16,50] Various physicians groups, such as the American College of Physicians[51] and the American Academy of Family Practice,[52] issue their own recommendations, usually less stringent than those of the ACS. Other national groups, such as the United States Preventive Services Task Force, sidestep the issue altogether by leaving screening in the over-65 age-group up to "clinical discretion."[53]

These conflicts can leave the clinician caring for the older patient somewhat confused. Different groups make different recommendations on the basis of the same data. Patients may request specific preventive services, not caring that they may be inappropriate. There may be pressures from colleagues or the makers of equipment used in screening exams for referrals. Authoritative, rational guidelines as to appropriate care of the elderly are not uniformly distributed. The physician often uses the old paradigms of acute care medicine and orders a screening exam, assuaging his or her conscience with a feeling of "it's better to do something than to do nothing." Two of the most common cancer screening exams, mammography and the prostate-specific antigen, can be used to illustrate the pitfalls of preventive care in the elderly, particularly if they are used without thought or rationale.

MAMMOGRAPHY

It is estimated that one out of nine American women will develop breast cancer at some point in her adult life.[54] Currently, an estimated 180,000 women are diagnosed with the disease annually, and 44,000 die.[46] These numbers have steadily increased; some of the increase is due to improved detection; the reason for the rest is less clear. A number of risk factors for breast cancer have been established, including increased age, family history, and not having borne children.[55] Seventy-five percent of cancers, however, occur in the absence of specific definable risk factors placing all women at risk.[56] Despite advances in detection and treatment, mortality rates today are similar to those of 20 years ago.[57] Women in the geriatric age-group are at much higher risk for breast cancer than their younger counterparts. They constitute approximately 14% of the female population but account for 43% of the diagnoses of breast cancer.[58] Breast cancer rates for older women are listed in Table 15.2.

A renewed focus on women's health issues and the commonplace nature of the disease have led to increased public awareness of the problem

TABLE 15.2   BREAST CANCER INCIDENCE
IN OLDER WOMEN

Age	Rate per 100,000 Population
65–69	390.7
70–74	421.8
75–79	461.4
80–84	451.3
85+	411.9

SOURCE: National Institutes of Health (1991 [59]).

and to screening methods for early detection. The most studied of these has been mammography, an X-ray of the breast tissue designed to locate malignant change at an early stage. The lack of change in mortality rates for established disease means that increased detection at an early stage is the major method for improvement of survival. Breast cancer diagnosed prior to hematogenous or lymphatic spread has a five-year survival of more than 80% while decreasing to less than 60% afterward.[60] Numerous studies around the world, including several well-designed controlled clinical trials, have shown positive benefits of routine mammographic screening in terms of improved morbidity and mortality for women between the ages of 50 and 74.[61-66] Absolute data are lacking for women 75 years of age and older, but most authors encourage extrapolation of the results to this population as long as they are healthy with a good life expectancy.[57] The American Cancer Society,[67] National Cancer Institute,[68] American College of Physicians,[51] American College of Obstetricians and Gynecologists,[69] and American Academy of Family Practice[52] all recommend annual mammography after age 50 based on the results of these studies. The American Geriatrics Society[70] and the United States Preventive Services Health Task Force[53] recommend this be changed to biennial mammography in those over 75. These conclusions for extending screening past the age of 75 are based on the facts that the biology of breast cancer in older women appears to be similar to that in younger women and that older women have similar tolerance for curative and palliative procedures as younger women.[58] Mandelblatt et al. have shown cost-benefit for screening up to the age of 85 and beyond, even in the presence of comorbid conditions.[71]

Like all X-ray examinations, mammography is not an inexpensive procedure. Costs range from $40 to $250 for the examination, with an average charge in the United States of $120 to $150. Based on a cost of $115 per exam, Brown predicted a cost of between $40,000 and $60,000 per year of life saved in the geriatric age-group for screening and treatment of breast cancer.[72] One major question that remains to be answered is the lack of resources for the interpretation of mammograms. The number of radiologists skilled in mammography will have to be increased by a factor of nine in order to handle the approximately 47 million annual mammograms that would be produced in this country with full screening of women over 50.[73]

Mammography has a proven track record, but the elderly are among those least likely to receive screening. Risk factors for not receiving screening mammography include age over 65, low income, low educational level, living in a rural area, and ethnic minority status.[74] The goal of the National Cancer Institute is an 80% screening rate of at-risk women by the year 2000.[75] Currently, approximately 35% to 40% of women over age 50 are being screened.[76,77] Massive trial community-based intervention programs have managed to increase this to about 55% in selected areas.[78] The number of women being screened continues to increase, and an individual is nearly nine times more likely to be screened now than in the mid-1980s.[79] Why are women over 65, who bear the brunt of the disease burden, less likely to receive screening, which has been proven to be of benefit? The reasons for this are several. First, physicians are less likely to recommend mammography to older women.[80] Seventy-six percent of women who undergo mammography have the exam at the advice of a physician and not through their own initiative.[77] If an older woman's physician does not recommend the test, it usually is not done. Physicians fail to make the recommendation for many reasons: They assume older women have relatively short life expectancies and screening is not warranted, they are unaware of the data and recommendations that say older women should be screened, and they are less likely to be asked by patients for the procedure.[80,81] Many physicians believe that they recommend the procedure for their older female patients, but review of their records show that their beliefs and their practices are vastly different and that mammography is underutilized.[82] Older patients are less likely to believe that they need screening.[83] Media attention to the disease has focused on the risks to younger women. This youth-oriented approach has lulled many older women into a false sense of security regarding their risks.[84] There is also a tenacious belief, held mainly by older women, that healthy women without risk factors are not in need of mammography. In addition, women over the age of 65 have some inherent distrust of

TABLE 15.3 INCIDENCE OF PROSTATE
CANCER IN OLDER AMERICAN WHITE MEN

Age	Rate per 100,000 Population
65–69	303.0
70–74	487.6
75–79	705.6
80–84	949.5
85+	1,043.9

SOURCE: Morrison et al. (1990 [89]).

a technological screening tool, preferring instead to trust an exam by a physician.[85]

PROSTATE-SPECIFIC ANTIGEN

Cancer of the prostate gland remains a major cause of morbidity and mortality for males in the United States. It is the most commonly diagnosed tumor among men, the second-highest cause of cancer death for men,[46] and the fourth most common cause of death overall.[86] Prostate cancer rates in older men are given in Table 15.3. The death rate from prostate cancer has been slowly increasing since the early part of the 20th century. In 1930, the mortality rate was approximately 14 per 100,000 men, and by 1985 this had increased to 23 per 100,000.[87] More than 50% of men over the age of 70 could be diagnosed with the disease if full screening were performed in this age-group.[88] The American Cancer Society estimates 334,500 new diagnoses and 42,000 deaths for calendar year 1997.[46]

Given the high prevalence of the disease, there is an intense interest in screening and disease prevention. Mortality has changed little over the last 20 years because of the advanced nature of the disease at diagnosis in most men.[90] Approximately two-thirds of newly discovered cases have extended beyond the prostatic capsule or have distant metastases at diagnosis, making them poorly amenable to treatment.[91] The serum enzyme acid phosphatase, discovered in 1936, was linked to prostatic function and recognized as a marker for prostatic cancer in 1948.[92,93] For the next four decades, it became a standard screening test for prostatic cancer. Acid phosphatase, however, had poor diagnostic accuracy for the disease and often reached abnormal levels only after skeletal metastasis had taken place.[94,95] Another indicator was needed.

TABLE 15.4   PROSTATE CANCER STAGING

Stage	Extent of Tumor	Five-Year Survival
A₁	Well-differentiated focal carcinoma—not clinically detectable	>90%
A₂	Diffuse localized carcinoma—not clinically detectable	>90%
B₁	Discrete nodule in single lobe of gland	77%
B₂	Multiple nodules or multiple lobe involvement	77%
C₁	Localized invasion of adjacent tissue; no involvement of seminal vesicles	64%
C₂	Localized invasion with seminal vesicle involvement or >70-g tumor	64%
D₀	Biochemical evidence of metastatic tumor without physical evidence	
D₁	Tumor metastatic to lymph nodes or with hydronephrosis	
D₂	Tumor with distant or bony metastases	Median survival 2.5 years

SOURCE: Garnick (1993 [102]).

Immunologists recognized the high antigenicity of the prostate gland as early as 1960.[96] One of these antigens, originally identified as gamma-seminoprotein and later as protein E and protein p30, has now been characterized as the prostate-specific antigen (PSA).[97] It is a 30,000-dalton glycoprotein of the kallikrein family of serine proteases, produced only in the prostate gland with elevated levels being present in states of hypertrophy or carcinoma.[98] It has been extensively studied, and its structure is well known. The development of radioimmunoassays for the substance has allowed the marketing of commercial tests for measurement of the PSA in serum from patients on a routine basis.[97] The value of the PSA level in a patient's serum has been shown to be proportional to the size of the cancer and its stage.[99–101] Prostatic cancer is usually divided into four stages, as shown in Table 15.4; early-stage cancers can be cured through surgical intervention.[97]

The logarithmic relationship between cancer stage and serum level of PSA, plus the relatively slow doubling time of most prostate cancers, would seem to make them easily amenable to a sensibly designed screening program.[103] Unfortunately, men with benign prostatic hypertrophy (BPH) and no evidence of carcinoma will also have elevated levels of PSA.[104,105] A PSA level of 4 ng/ml, taken as the upper limit of normal, will uncover many false positives from BPH. A PSA level of 10 ng/ml will avoid most of the cases of BPH but will also miss many of the very early stage cancers, which are most likely to be cured by early intervention.[106]

A number of uncontrolled studies of PSA measurement have been done in an attempt to define a benefit for screening of the population. Results have been controversial at best. Studies such as those of Catalona et al.,[106] Brawer et al.,[107] and Labrie et al.[108] have shown that PSA is extremely useful in detecting cancers that would otherwise have been missed by more conventional methods, such as digital rectal examination. There are, however, no controlled studies to show that this earlier detection makes any difference in either morbidity or mortality. Such studies are currently being performed, but because of the indolent nature of the disease, results are not expected until well into the 21st century.[109]

This lack of proven benefit has called the use of PSA as a screening test into question. To complicate the picture further, the very nature of the disease raises serious questions about the utility of screening.[110,111] Population studies suggest that approximately 30% of the male population at age 50 and 50% at age 70 have malignant change in the prostate gland.[88] A vast majority of these cancers remain latent. Only one in about 400 ever progresses to clinical disease.[112] This has led to the old adage that "far more men die with prostate cancer than from prostate cancer." Prostate-specific antigen cannot differentiate which of these cancers will progress to overt disease and which will remain latent. Improved detection will lead to many more men undergoing treatment for a condition that would never have led to any clinical problems. Even the urologic literature has been polarized over the utility of using PSA as a screening test.[113,114] In order to settle the debate, recent work has used sophisticated decision analysis techniques to determine if PSA is a viable screening tool. These studies have shown PSA to be of little to no benefit in the testing of unselected populations.[115,116]

Despite the doubts raised about PSA and the lack of consensus from the medical community on its usefulness, the American Cancer Society adopted recommendations in December of 1992 that all men over the age of 50 undergo annual PSA screening for prostate cancer in addition to the previously recommended digital rectal examination.[117] Their focus of disease prevention argues that elimination of the disease is both necessary and worthwhile. As public awareness of the PSA test has increased, demand by patients has increased; arguments of a statistical or cost-benefit nature are not easily used to mollify an individual who is concerned about his personal risk. The clinician is left torn between the competing imperatives of the patient and of the health care system.

Which should be believed: a public eager to end a potentially lethal disease or a scientific community that is unable to define a benefit from an intervention?

Widespread screening of the male population with PSA is not without substantial risk. The current treatment of choice for early disease, stages A and B, remains either surgical removal through radical prostatectomy or radiation therapy.[109] More advanced disease also usually involves either surgical or chemical castration, as the tumor tends to be androgen dependent.[118] Both prostatectomy, despite improved surgical techniques, and radiation therapy can have significant sequelae.[119] As a screening program, yearly PSA levels would uncover many cases of latent disease, and the estimated iatrogenic morbidity and mortality would increase astronomically.

Questions have also been raised regarding the cost-effectiveness of massive PSA screening. Optenberg and Thompson, in a detailed study from 1988 (see Table 15.5), estimated current costs to the health care system from screening and follow-up to be in the neighborhood of $255 million a year. This would increase to $11.3 billion if the population were screened and all PSA levels over 10 ng/ml were followed up with biopsy and appropriate treatment. If the abnormal level were dropped to 4 ng/ml in order to better detect stages A and B cancers that were more likely curable, the cost to the system would be expected to rise to nearly $28 billion.[120] This study was done using the population between the ages of 50 and 70 as a model. No analysis has been done involving only the geriatric age-group, in which the disease becomes even more common, and morbidity and mortality from surgery or radiation may be increased.

THE HEALTH PROMOTION MODEL

The examples discussed here show that the disease-based model of preventive health care may not provide the whole answer. Mammography has been proven to have a place in the health care of the older patient, but the data on PSA are not convincing, as PSA in particular looks highly problematic with potential rates of iatrogenic disease that are simply unacceptable. Geriatrics, with its emphasis on an integrated approach to the patient, offers an alternative to a disease-based model, namely, one founded on the concept of health. The goal of geriatric care is to maintain an individual at optimum health and functional status. All recommendations for treatment, screening, and other health care measures are

TABLE 15.5   ESTIMATED MORBIDITY
FROM DETECTION AND TREATMENT
OF PROSTATE CANCER

	Current Screening Levels	100% PSA Screening
No. cases impotence	3,354	266,671
No. cases incontinence	908	61,618
No. colostomies	133	10,522
No. treatment deaths	220	20,563
Expense per year	$255 million	$3.8–27.9 billion

SOURCE: Optenberg and Thompson (1990 [120]).

based on their relationship to the ultimate health and function of the patient. This "health promotion" model takes the position that maintaining health is the primary goal of interactions between patient and provider and that treatment of individual disease states will follow from this rather than being exclusive ends in themselves. Patients and their lives are the focus, not their cancers or infections or disabilities.

In order to discuss a model of health promotion, it is important to define health. In the geriatric age-group, health is probably not best defined as "freedom from disease." Most older people have chronic disease burden and continue to lead active normal lives. Health is instead a self-reported feeling of well-being and of being able to function to maximal abilities within a self-selected lifestyle. Work done on health attitudes of older people shows a strong correlation between self-reported perception of health and ultimate morbidity.[121] The older patient needs to be approached with an understanding that disease may not be an overriding concern for him or her. An ability to function and undertake usual activities often is much more important. Patients may choose not to undergo treatment for disease if it would leave them functionally impaired.

These ideas of health and function may best be conceptualized within a framework of basic ecologic principles. Modern biology contains a construct known as niche theory, which is a useful analogy in understanding the approach to the older adult.[122] The basic principles of niche theory are contained in Table 15.6.

In brief, a species and an ecological niche must always fit together hand in glove. If they do not, extinction is the end result. The older adult fits together with a chosen life in a similar fashion. Individuals and lives evolve together over the decades in a symbiotic relationship. When there

TABLE 15.6   PRINCIPLES OF NICHE THEORY

1.   Each species has a unique ecological niche within the ecosystem.

2.   The species has adapted to fill that niche.

3.   A change or mutation in the species requires that the niche also change in accommodation.

4.   A change in the niche from external environmental influences requires a change in species behavior or function in reaction.

is change in the person from disease, and if that change is not reversible, as is often the case in chronic disease, then compensatory change must come in the life to keep the fit together. In geriatrics, maintaining health often becomes a matter of environmental manipulation rather than of curing of the individual. Promoting health in the geriatric population requires an understanding of this dynamic and a willingness to see health as the fit between individual and environment rather than as an absolute disease-free state.

For the health promotion model to work effectively in a primary care practice setting, the following conditions are necessary. First, there must be an expectation on the part of both the physician and the patient that such measures be addressed in an encounter. In addition, communication between physician and patient must be effective. Second, the patient must be motivated to pursue these measures outside the physician's office and to modify lifestyle choices. Patients can be educated and encouraged to become a more active partner in the information loop. Such measures as informational brochures and pocket checklists have proven beneficial to increasing compliance and awareness. Third, the physician must be knowledgeable in the principles of health maintenance and be aware of measures with proven efficacy versus those that are of more dubious value. Fourth, the health care system must regard health maintenance issues as central to health care and place priority on carrying them out and allowing adequate reimbursement.[123]

Health promotion, particularly in the geriatric age-group, would seem to be a rather obvious conclusion and nothing short of common sense. However, it bucks the thinking and teaching of acute care medicine to consider the patient as a complete individual rather than as the sum of diagnostic parts. Most physicians are guilty of thinking of their patients as "the lady with the breast mass" or "the colon cancer in room 302." Simple health promotion interventions for the elderly are still in their infancy. It is well established that 10% of community-dwelling elderly are malnourished and are therefore at greater risk for serious health problems.[124] Nutritional screening, a simple checklist approach to identify those at risk, is just now receiving attention from the medical establishment.[125] Another common health problem of aging, urinary incontinence, costs society approximately $10 billion a year and is present in up to 10% to 20% of the healthy elderly.[126] Many primary care providers remain unfamiliar with diagnostic strategies or basic incontinence management techniques.[127] The chief cause of preventable death in older adults is injury from fall. It is the fifth-leading cause of death and a major source of excess morbidity. Despite its well-known dangers, many physicians are ignorant of fall prevention techniques and many never see their patients walk.[128] Environmental and caregiver evaluation are often overlooked by busy physicians who focus entirely on the patient and medical issues at the expense of a life that is falling apart. Most of these issues fall under the heading of true primary prevention, preventing disease from ever occurring in a well person.

EVALUATION OF PREVENTIVE MEASURES

The precepts of health promotion require that screening examinations, particularly those with the potential of inflicting morbidity, be studied as to their impact on the whole patient, not just the disease process. Rational criteria must be developed for the evaluation of current and future screening procedures to see if they truly fit the needs of the elderly population. Issues such as the effect of a test or service on the caregiver of an older patient are not taken into account under standard methods of evaluation.[44] Cost-benefit analyses by some experts tend to be inherently biased against the elderly, as their life expectancy tends to be shorter than that of younger persons.[129,130] Frame and Carlson published a set of six principles (listed in Table 15.7) for assessing screening exams that have been widely used as a method of determining their benefits.

The Department of Family Practice at the University of Michigan, under the leadership of Klinkman and Zazove, have taken these criteria and modified them to make them more representative of the special needs of the elderly. Their modified criteria are listed in Table 15.8.

The University of Michigan criteria fulfill the goals of health promotion by placing the major focus immediately on the total health of the patient. The shift from the older criteria is subtle. It includes a major stress on the concept of health, a word that does not appear at all in

TABLE 15.7 FRAME AND CARLSON'S CRITERIA FOR EVALUATION OF SCREENING EXAMS

1. The disease must have a significant effect on the quality of life.

2. Acceptable methods of treatment must be available.

3. The disease must have an asymptomatic period during which detection and treatment significantly reduce morbidity or mortality.

4. Treatment in the asymptomatic phase must yield a therapeutic result superior to that obtained by delaying treatment until symptoms appear.

5. Tests that are acceptable to patients must be available at reasonable cost to detect the condition in the asymptomatic period.

6. The incidence of the condition must be sufficient to justify the cost of screening.

SOURCE: Frame and Carlson (1975 [131]).

TABLE 15.8 KLINKMAN ET AL.'S CRITERIA FOR THE EVALUATION OF SCREENING EXAMS

1. The condition must have a significant effect on health.

2. Acceptable methods of preventive intervention or treatment must be available for the condition.

3. For primary preventive services (counseling, chemoprevention, immunizations), the intervention must be effective in preserving health.

4. For other preventive services or interventions:

    a. There must be a period before the individual (or his or her caretaker) is aware of the condition, or of its seriousness or implications, during which it can reliably be detected by providers.

    b. Tests used to identify the condition must be able to reliably discriminate between cases and noncases of the condition.

    c. Preventive services or treatment during this "preawareness" period must have greater effectiveness than care or treatment delayed until the individual or caretaker brings it to the provider's attention.

5. For individuals who are cared for by caregivers, the benefit offered by the preventive service must outweigh any negative effects on the quality of life of caregivers.

6. The relative value of the preventive service or intervention must be determined by a comparison of its costs with its expected health benefits.

SOURCE: Klinkman et al. (1992 [44]).

Frame's criteria. The new criteria are also flexible enough to account for the dependent elderly both at home and in institutions.

The University of Michigan criteria can be applied to the cancer screening modalities discussed previously. Mammography has been shown to be quite effective in women up to 75 years of age, and it meets all six criteria. The evidence is less clear for women 75 and older. The United States Preventive Services Task Force suggests that women who have been regularly screened up to age 75 are unlikely to develop cancer after that age and do not need to be screened further, but hard data are lacking.[52] Women over 75 without previous screening should probably be screened. Prostate-specific antigen does not meet criteria 4a, 4b, or 4c because of its lack of sensitivity and potential for causing new disease related to medical treatment. It may also not meet criterion 6.[112,118,132–135]

HEALTH AND THE OLDER PATIENT

A focus on health requires a different mind-set from a physician. He or she must learn to inquire into a patient's individual health values. He or she must be flexible in approaching disease processes, as the textbook "cures" available for them may not be in the patient's best interest. Those physicians who are unable to see the patient for the disease leave patients with new problems created by failed curative measures, polypharmacy, and suboptimal social situations. It is estimated that 10% of hospital admissions in the over-65 age-group are due to medication reactions of one kind or another.[136] A patient over 65 has a one in three chance of new problem being caused by his or her health care during a hospital stay.[137] The personal and economic costs are staggering. A health-based approach might be able to make substantial inroads into these problems.

As a society, we remain ambivalent about health care for older individuals. The adoption of Medicare was a statement that we believe in the rights of older people to have access to treatment for acute disease processes. Societal thinking on preventive measures is not as clear, as there has been no formal adoption of programs or goals. There is discussion of mass screening for serious disease with the techniques discussed here, but the costs involved are considerable. We must tread very carefully in these times when disease is easily politicized and health conditions compete in the legislative and economic arenas for shrinking pools of public resources. The question we must answer is, Should we place our resources into disease prevention modalities such as PSA where the benefits are ill-defined, or should we put them into health promotion areas? Changing demographics and the advance of technology will continue to push costs up. It is our responsibility to spend society's resources wisely. If we do the studies to validate simple health-based measures such as functional assessment, nutritional screening, and medication review, we might have cheaper weapons with which to fight the disabilities of older age. Why not let the geriatric age-group be healthy and let disease take care of itself? Social programs aimed at keeping older people functional in their own homes or additional training for primary care physicians in geriatric care may not be glamorous but could be closer to what older individuals really need. However, as long as the health care system continues to reimburse procedures and "cures" over caring and compassion, we are likely to be stuck with the system as it now exists. A revolution in the medical thinking process and training are needed to effect true change. The economic reforms currently sweeping the American medical system may begin this process; many HMOs have a wellness focus. However, it may take some time for these policies to penetrate the training system for physicians and lead to a revamping of medical school curricula away from acute-care- and disease-based training.

Care of the geriatric patient requires a sense of the art of medicine as well as of the science of medicine. The goals of health promotion are designed to remove the blinders of disease-based thinking so that the patient is seen as a unique challenge in health maintenance. Preventive medicine is an essential part of the care of the geriatric patient, but physicians can develop an overreliance on their need to "stamp out disease" and use the precepts of preventive care in ways that may not be beneficial to the overall health of their patients. Applying rational criteria to preventive services, such as those from the University of Michigan, helps the physician understand the goals of health promotion. Physicians can and should be taught to look at their older patients in a more holistic light so that they do not pursue disease and "cure" at the expense of the patient. Doing this will help physicians, patients, and society avoid the pitfalls of preventive care.

REFERENCES

1. Siegel, J. S. 1980. Recent and prospective demographic trends for the elderly population and some implications for health care. In *Second Conference on*

the Epidemiology of Aging, edited by S. G. Haynes and M. Feinleib. DHHS (NIH) 80-969. Washington, D.C.: U.S. Government Printing Office.

2. U.S. Bureau of the Census. 1984. Demographic and socioeconomic aspects of aging in the United States. In *Current Population Reports.* Series P-23, No. 138. Washington, D.C.: U.S. Government Printing Office.

3. Spencer, G. 1989. Projections of the population of the United States by age, sex and race: 1988 to 2080. In *Current Population Reports.* Series P-25, No. 1018. U.S. Bureau of the Census. Washington, D.C.: U.S. Government Printing Office.

4. Health and Public Policy Committee, American College of Physicians. 1988. Comprehensive functional assessment for elderly persons. *Annals of Internal Medicine* 109(1), 70–72.

5. Stults, B. M. 1984. Preventive health care for the elderly. *Western Journal of Medicine* 141(6), 832–845.

6. Rubenstein, L. Z., Calkins, D. R., Greenfield, S., et al. 1988. Health status assessment for elderly patients: Report of the Society of General Internal Medicine Task Force on Health Assessment. *Journal of the American Geriatrics Society* 37(6), 562–569.

7. Epstein, A. M., Hall, J. A., Fretwell, M., et al. 1990. Consultative geriatric assessment for ambulatory patients: A randomized trial in a health maintenance organization. *Journal of the American Medical Association* 263(4), 538–544.

8. Rowe, J. W., and Kahn, R. L. 1987. Human aging: Usual and successful. *Science* 237(4811), 143–149.

9. Shock, N. W. 1984. Energy metabolism, caloric intake, and physical activity of the aging. In *Normal Human Aging: The Baltimore Longitudinal Study of Aging.* Pp. 372–390. DHHS (NIH) 84-2450. Bethesda, Md.: U.S. Government Printing Office.

10. Heath, J. M. 1989. Comprehensive functional assessment of the elderly. *Primary Care* 16(2), 305–327.

11. LaCroix, A. Z. 1987. Determinants of health—Exercise and activities of daily living: Health Statistics on Older Persons, United States, 1986. In *Vital and Health Statistics,* Series 3, No. 25, edited by R. J. Havlik, M. G. Liu, M. G. Kovar, et al. DHHS (PHS) 87-1409. Washington, D.C.: U.S. Government Printing Office.

12. Buchner, D. M., and Wagner, E. H. 1992. Preventing frail health. *Clinics in Geriatric Medicine* 8(1), 1–17.

13. Varmus, J. 1995. Disease-specific estimates of direct and indirect costs of illness and NIH support. DHHS (PHS) NIH Office of the Director.

14. Snow, C. 1996. Medicare HMOs develop plan for future of Alzheimer's programming. *Modern Healthcare,* September 23, 67–70.

15. Schneider, E. L., and Guralnik, J. M. 1990. The aging of America: Impact on health care costs. *Journal of the American Medical Association* 263(17), 2335–2340.

16. Murray, J. L. 1989. Health maintenance. *Primary Care* 16(2), 289–303.

17. Cypress, B. K. 1984. Patterns of ambulatory care in internal medicine:

The National Ambulatory Care Survey, United States, January 1980–December 1981. In *Vital and Health Statistics.* Series 13, No. 80. DHHS (PHS) 84-1741. Washington, D.C.: U.S. Government Printing Office.

18. Feller, B. A. 1986. Americans needing home care. In *Vital and Health Statistics.* Series 10, No. 153. DHHS (PHS) 86-1581. Washington, D.C.: U.S. Government Printing Office.

19. U.S. Bureau of the Census. 1996. *Statistical Abstract of the United States: 1996.* Washington, D.C.: U.S. Government Printing Office.

20. National Center for Health Statistics. 1988. *Vital Statistics of the U.S., 1985.* DHHS (PHS) 88-1104. Washington, D.C.: U.S. Government Printing Office.

21. Hing, E., Sekscenski, E., and Strahan, G. 1989. The National Nursing Home Survey: 1985 summary for the United States. In *Vital and Health Statistics.* Series 13, No. 97. DHHS (PHS) 89-1758. Washington, D.C.: U.S. Government Printing Office.

22. Kemper, P., and Murtaugh, C. M. 1991. Lifetime use of nursing home care. *New England Journal of Medicine* 324(9), 595–600.

23. Waldo, D. R., and Lazenby, H. C. 1984. Demographic characteristics and health care use and expenditures by the aged in the United States: 1977–1984. *Health Care Financing Review* 6(1), 1–30.

24. Christensen, S. 1987. Acute health care costs for the aged Medicare population: Overview and policy options. *Milbank Memorial Fund Quarterly* 65, 397–416.

25. Vladeck, B. C., Miller, N. A., and Clauser, S. B. 1993. The changing face of long term care. *Health Care Financing Review* 14(4), 5–23.

26. Estes, C. L. 1988. Cost containment and the elderly: Conflict or challenge? *Journal of the American Geriatrics Society* 36(1), 68–72.

27. Lubitz, J. D., and Riley, G. F. 1993. Trends in Medicare payments in the last years of life. *New England Journal of Medicine* 328(15), 1092–1096.

28. Bayer, R., Callahan, D., Fletcher, J., et al. 1983. The care of the terminally ill: Morality and economics. *New England Journal of Medicine* 309(24), 1490–1494.

29. Kane, R. A., and Kane, R. L. 1981. *Assessing the Elderly: A Practical Guide to Measurement.* Lexington Mass.: Lexington Books.

30. Breslow, L., and Somers, A. 1977. The lifetime health monitoring program: A practical approach to preventive medicine. *New England Journal of Medicine* 296(11), 601–608.

31. Convertino, V. A. 1986. Exercise responses after inactivity. In *Inactivity: Physiological Effects,* edited by H. Sandler and J. Vernikos. Orlando: Academic Press.

32. McVey, L. J., Becker, P. M., Saltz, C. C., et al. 1989. Effect of a geriatric consultation team on functional status of elderly hospitalized patients. *Annals of Internal Medicine* 110(1), 79–84.

33. Rubenstein, L. Z., Josephson, K. R., Wieland, G. D., et al. 1984. Effectiveness of a geriatric evaluation unit: A randomized clinical trial. *New England Journal of Medicine* 311(26), 1664–1670.

34. Campion, E. W., Jette, A., and Berkman, B. 1983. An interdisciplinary geri-

atric consultation service: A controlled trial. *Journal of the American Geriatrics Society* 31(12), 792–796.

35. Rubenstein, L. Z., Stuck, A. E., Siu, A. L., and Wieland, D. 1991. Impacts of geriatric evaluation and management programs on defined outcomes: Overview of the evidence. *Journal of the American Geriatrics Society* 39(Suppl.), 8S-16S.

36. Rubenstein, L. Z., Wieland, D., and Bernabei, R., eds. 1995. Research on comprehensive geriatric assessment. *Aging Clinical and Experimental Research* 7(3, Special Issue), 157–260.

37. Rubenstein, L. Z. 1987. Geriatric assessment: An overview of its impacts. *Clinics in Geriatric Medicine* 3(1), 1–15.

38. Fries, J. F. 1980. Aging, natural death and the compression of morbidity. *New England Journal of Medicine* 303(2), 130–135.

39. Solomon, D. H. 1988. Geriatric assessment: Methods for clinical decision making. *Journal of the American Medical Association* 259(16), 2450–2452.

40. Cohen, H. J., and Feussner, J. R. 1989. Comprehensive geriatric assessment: Mission not yet accomplished. *Journal of Gerontology* 44(6), 175–177.

41. Reed, R. L., Klingman, E. W., and Weiss, B. D. 1990. Comprehensive geriatric assessment recommendations: Adherence of family practice residents. *Journal of Family Practice* 31(4), 389–392.

42. Kane, R. L., Ouslander, J. G., and Abrass, I. B. 1989. *Essentials of Clinical Geriatrics.* 2nd ed. New York: McGraw-Hill.

43. Fletcher, R. H., Fletcher, S. W., and Wagner, E. H. 1982. *Clinical Epidemiology — The Essentials.* Baltimore: Williams and Wilkins.

44. Klinkman, M. S., Zazove, P., Mehr, D. R., and Ruffin, M. T. 1992. A criterion-based review of preventive health care in the elderly: Part 1. Theoretical framework and development of criteria. *Journal of Family Practice* 34(3), 205–224.

45. Baranovsky, A., and Myers, M. H. 1986. Cancer incidence and survival in patients 65 years of age and older. *CA: A Cancer Journal for Clinicians* 36(1), 27–41.

46. Parker, S. L., Tong, T., Bolden, S., and Wingo, P. A. 1997. Cancer Statistics, 1997. *CA: A Cancer Journal for Clinicians* 47(1), 5–27.

47. Cohen, H. J. 1990. Oncology and aging. In *Principles of Geriatric Medicine and Gerontology,* 2nd ed., edited by W. R. Hazzard, R. Andres, E. L. Bierman, and J. P. Blass. Pp. 72–84. New York: McGraw-Hill.

48. Robie, P. W. 1989. Cancer screening in the elderly. *Journal of the American Geriatrics Society* 37(9), 888–893.

49. Oddone, E. Z., Feussner, J. R., and Cohen, H. J. 1992. Can screening older patients for cancer save lives? *Clinics in Geriatric Medicine* 8(1), 51–67.

50. Weisman, C. S., Celentano, D. D., Teitelbaum, M. A., and Klassen, A. C. 1989. Cancer screening services for the elderly. *Public Health Reports* 104(3), 209–214.

51. Eddy, D. M., ed. 1991. *Common Screening Tests.* Philadelphia: American College of Physicians.

52. American Academy of Family Physicians. 1991. *Positions on the Clinical Aspect of Medical Practice.* Kansas City: American Academy of Family Practice.

53. U.S. Preventive Services Health Task Force. 1989. *Guide to Clinical Prevention Services: An Assessment of the Effectiveness of 169 Interventions.* Baltimore: Williams and Wilkins.

54. American Cancer Society. 1991. *Cancer Facts and Figures 1991.* Atlanta: American Cancer Society.

55. Warner, E. A. 1992. Breast cancer screening. *Primary Care* 19(3), 575–588.

56. Strax, P. 1984. Mass screening for control of breast cancer. *CA: A Cancer Journal for Clinicians* 34(1), 65–70.

57. Costanza, M. E. 1992. Breast cancer screening in older women: Synopsis of a forum. *Cancer* 69(7, Suppl.), 1925–1931.

58. Costanza, M. E., Annas, G. J., Brown, M. L., et al. 1992. Breast cancer screening in older women: Supporting statements and rationale. *Journal of Gerontology* (47, Suppl.), 7–16.

59. National Institutes of Health. 1991. *National Cancer Institute Statistics Review 1975–1988.* NIH 91-2789. Bethesda, Md.: U.S. Government Printing Office.

60. Ferguson, D. J., Meier, P., Karrison, T., et al. 1982. Staging of breast cancer and survival rates: An assessment based on 50 years of experience with radical mastectomy. *Journal of the American Medical Association* 248(2), 1337–1341.

61. Shapiro, S., Strax, P., Venet, L., and Rosen, R. 1982. Ten to fourteen year effect of screening on breast cancer mortality. *Journal of the National Cancer Institute* 69(4), 349–355.

62. Tabar, L., Gad, A., Holmquist, U., et al. 1985. Reduction in mortality from breast cancer after mass screening with mammography: Randomized trial from the Breast Cancer Working Group from the Swedish National Board of Health and Welfare. *The Lancet* 2(8433), 829–832.

63. Andersson, I., Aspergren, K., Janzon, L., et al. 1988. Mammographic screening and mortality from breast cancer: The Malmo screening trial. *British Medical Journal* 297(6653), 943–948.

64. Roberts, M. M., Alexander, F. E., Anderson, T. J., et al. 1990. Edinburgh trial of screening for breast cancer: Mortality at seven years. *The Lancet* 335(8684), 242–246.

65. UK Trial of Early Detection Group. 1988. First results on mortality reduction in the UK trial of early detection of breast cancer. *The Lancet* 2(8576), 411–416.

66. Verbeek, A. L. M., Hendriks, J. H. C. L., Holland, R., et al. 1984. Reduction of breast cancer mortality through mass screening with modern mammography: First results of the Nijmegen project, 1975–81. *The Lancet* 1(8388), 1222–1224.

67. American Cancer Society. 1988. *Summary of Current Guidelines for the Cancer-Related Check Up: Recommendations.* Atlanta: American Cancer Society.

68. National Cancer Institute Early Detection Branch. 1987. *Working Guidelines for Early Detection.* Bethesda, Md.: U.S. Government Printing Office.

69. American College of Obstetricians and Gynecologists Committee on Professional Standards. 1989. Report of Task Force on Routine Cancer Screen-

ing. In *Standards for Obstetric/Gynecologic Services.* 7th ed. Washington, D.C.: American College of Obstetricians and Gynecologists.

70. American Geriatrics Society. 1989. Screening for breast cancer in elderly women. *Journal of the American Geriatrics Society* 37(9), 883–884.

71. Mandelblatt, J. S., Wheat, M. E., Monane, M., et al. 1992. Breast cancer screening for elderly women with and without comorbid conditions: A decision analysis model. *Annals of Internal Medicine* 116(9), 722–730.

72. Brown, M. L. 1992. Economic considerations in breast cancer screening of older women. *Journal of Gerontology* 47(Suppl.), 51–58.

73. Monsees, B. S. 1992. Screening mammography: Who will meet the need? *Radiology* 184(1), 30–31.

74. Calle, E. E., Flanders, W. D., Thun, M. J., and Martin, L. M. 1993. Demographic predictors of mammography and pap smear screening in US women. *American Journal of Public Health* 83(1), 53–60.

75. National Cancer Institute. 1986. Cancer control: Objectives for the nation 1985–2000. *National Cancer Institute Monograph* 2, 1–93.

76. Farwell, M. F., Foster, R. S., and Costanza, M. C. 1993. Breast cancer and earlier detection efforts: Realized and unrealized impact on stage. *Archives of Surgery* 128(5), 510–514.

77. Sienko, D. G., Hahn, R. A., Mills, E. M., et al. 1993. Mammography use and outcomes in a community: The greater Lansing area mammography study. *Cancer* 71(5), 1801–1809.

78. Fletcher, S. W., Harris, R. P., Gonzalez, J. J., et al. 1993. Increasing mammography utilization: A controlled study. *Journal of the National Cancer Institute* 85(2), 112–120.

79. Zapka, J. G., Hosmer, D., Costanza, M. E., et al. 1992. Changes in mammography use: Economic, need and service factors. *American Journal of Public Health* 82(10), 1345–1351.

80. Costanza, M. E., Stoddard, A. M., Zapka, J. G., et al. 1992. Physician compliance with mammography guidelines: Barriers and enhancers. *Journal of the American Board of Family Practice* 5(2), 143–152.

81. Mah, Z., and Bryant, H. 1992. Age as a factor in breast cancer knowledge, attitudes and screening behavior. *Canadian Medical Association Journal* 146(12), 2167–2174.

82. Roetzheim, R. G., Fox, S. A., and Leake, B. 1995. Physician-reported determinants of screening mammography in older women: The impact of physician and practice characteristics. *Journal of the American Geriatrics Society* 43(12), 1398–1402.

83. Fuller, S. M., McDermott, R. J., Roetzheim, R. G., and Marty, P. J. 1992. Breast cancer beliefs of women participating in a television promoted mammography screening project. *Public Health Reports* 107(6), 682–690.

84. Baines, C. J. 1992. Women and breast cancer: Is it really possible for the public to be well informed? *Canadian Medical Association Journal* 146(12), 2147–2148.

85. Taplin, S. H., and Montano, D. E. 1993. Attitudes, age, and participation in mammographic screening: A prospective analysis. *Journal of the American Board of Family Practice* 6(1), 13–23.

86. Brawer, M. K., and Lange, P. H. 1989. Prostate-specific antigen and pre-malignant change: Implications for early detection. *CA: A Cancer Journal for Clinicians* 39(6), 361–375.
87. Cooner, W. H., Mosley, B. R., Rutherford, C. L., et al. 1990. Prostate can-cer detection in a clinical urological practice by ultrasonography, digital rec-tal examination and prostate specific antigen. *Journal of Urology* 143(6), 1146–1154.
88. Sheldon, C. A., Williams, R. D., and Fraley, E. E. 1980. Incidental carci-noma of the prostate: A review of the literature and critical reappraisal of classification. *Journal of Urology* 124(5), 626–631.
89. Morrison, A. S., Cole, P., and Maclure, K. M. 1990. Epidemiology of uro-logic cancers. In *Principles and Management of Urologic Cancer,* 2nd ed., edited by N. Javadpour. Pp. 12–31. Baltimore: Williams and Wilkins.
90. Chodak, G. W. 1989. Early detection and screening for prostatic cancer. *Urology* 34(4, Suppl.), 10–56.
91. Murphy, G. P., Natarajan, N., Pontes, J. E., et al. 1982. The national sur-vey of prostate cancer in the United States by the American College of Sur-geons. *Journal of Urology* 127(5), 928–934.
92. Guinan, P., Bhatti, R., and Ray, P. 1987. An evaluation of prostate specific antigen in prostate cancer. *Journal of Urology* 137(4), 686–689.
93. Brawer, M. K. 1990. Laboratory studies for the detection of carcinoma of the prostate. *Urologic Clinics of North America* 17(4), 759–768.
94. Vikho, P., Kontturi, M., Lukkarinen, O., et al. 1985. Screening for carci-noma of the prostate. *Cancer* 56(1), 173–177.
95. Imai, K., Zinbo, S., Shimizu, K., et al. 1988. Clinical characteristics of pro-static cancer detected by mass screening. *Prostate* 12, 199–207.
96. Flocks, R. H., Urich, V. C., Patel, C. A., and Opitz, J. M. 1960. Studies on the antigenic properties of prostatic tissue. *Journal of Urology* 84, 134–143.
97. Oesterling, J. E. 1991. Prostate specific antigen: A critical assessment of the most useful tumor marker for adenocarcinoma of the prostate. *Journal of Urology* 145(5), 907–923.
98. Armbruster, D. A. 1993. Prostate-specific antigen: Biochemistry, analytical methods, and clinical applications. *Clinical Chemistry* 39(2), 181–195.
99. Daver, A., Soret, J. Y., Coblentz, Y., et al. 1988. The usefulness of prostate-specific antigen and prostatic acid phosphatase in clinical practice. *American Journal of Clinical Oncology* 11(Suppl.), S53–S59.
100. Lange, P. H., Ercole, C. J., Lightner, D. J., et al. 1989. The value of serum prostate specific antigen determinations before and after radical prostatec-tomy. *Journal of Urology* 141(4), 873–879.
101. Partin, A. W., Carter, H. B., Chan, D. W., et al. 1990. Prostate-specific antigen in the staging of localized prostate cancer: Influence of tumor differ-entiation, tumor volume and benign hyperplasia. *Journal of Urology* 143(4), 747–752.
102. Garnick, M. G. 1993. Urologic cancer. In *Scientific American Medi-cine,* edited by E. Reubenstein and D. D. Federman. New York: Scientific American.
103. Schmid, H. P., McNeal, J. E., and Stamey, T. A. 1993. Observations on the

doubling time of prostate cancer: The use of serial prostate-specific antigen in patients with untreated disease as a measure of increasing cancer volume. *Cancer* 71(6), 2031–2040.

104. Stamey, T. A., Yang, N., Hay, A. R., et al. 1987. Prostate-specific antigen as a serum marker for adenocarcinoma of the prostate. *New England Journal of Medicine* 317(14), 909–916.

105. Weber, J. P., Oesterling, J. E., Peters, C. A., et al. 1989. The influence of reversible androgen deprivation on serum prostate-specific antigen levels in men with benign prostatic hyperplasia. *Journal of Urology* 141(4), 987–992.

106. Catalona, W. J., Smith, D. S., Ratliff, T. L., et al. 1991. Measurement of prostate-specific antigen in serum as a screening test for prostate cancer. *New England Journal of Medicine* 324(17), 1156–1161.

107. Brawer, M. K., Chetner, M. P., Beatie, J., et al. 1992. Screening for prostatic carcinoma with prostate specific antigen. *Journal of Urology* 147(3, pt. 2), 841–845.

108. Labrie, F., Dupont, A., Suburu, R., et al. 1992. Serum prostate specific antigen as a pre-screening test for prostate cancer. *Journal of Urology* 147(3, pt. 2), 846–852.

109. Garnick, M. B. 1993. Prostate cancer: Screening, diagnosis, and management. *Annals of Internal Medicine* 118(10), 804–818.

110. Hinman, F. 1991. Screening for prostatic carcinoma. *Journal of Urology* 145(1), 126–130.

111. Louria, D. B. 1992. Is digital screening for prostatic cancer effective? *Bulletin of the New York Academy of Medicine* 68(4), 470–475.

112. Roetzheim, R. G., and Herold, A. H. 1992. Prostate cancer screening. *Primary Care* 19(3), 637–649.

113. Hall, R. R. 1996. Screening and early detection of prostate cancer will decrease morbidity and mortality from prostate cancer: The argument against. *European Urology* 29(Suppl. 2), 24–26.

114. Crawford, E. D., and DeAntoni, E. P. 1993. PSA as a screening test for prostate cancer. *Urological Clinics of North America* 20(4), 637–646.

115. Cantor, S. B., Spann, S. J., Volk, R. J., et al. 1995. Prostate cancer screening: A decision analysis. *Journal of Family Practice* 41(1), 33–41.

116. Krahn, M. D., Mahoney, J. E., Eckman, M. H., et al. 1994. Screening for prostate cancer: A decision analytic view. *Journal of the American Medical Association* 272(10), 773–780.

117. Mettlin, C., Jones, G., Averett, H., et al. 1993. Defining and updating the American Cancer Society guidelines for the cancer-related check up: Prostate and endometrial cancers. *CA: A Cancer Journal for Clinicians* 43(1), 42–46.

118. National Conference on Prostate Cancer. 1990. *Cancer* 66(Suppl. 5), 5.

119. Kemp, E. D. 1992. Prostate cancer: Finding and managing it. *Postgraduate Medicine* 92(1), 67–89.

120. Optenberg, S. A., and Thompson, I. M. 1990. Economics of screening for carcinoma of the prostate. *Urological Clinics of North America* 17(4), 719–737.

121. Mossey, J. M., and Shapiro, E. 1982. Self rated health: A prediction of mortality among the elderly. *American Journal of Public Health* 72(8), 800–808.

122. Krebs, C. J. 1994. *Ecology—The Experimental Analysis of Distribution and Abundance*. Pp. 243–254. Menlo Park, Calif.: Addison-Wesley Longman.

123. McCormick, W. C., and Inui, T. S. 1992. Geriatric preventive care: Counseling techniques in practice settings. *Clinics in Geriatric Medicine* 8(1), 215–229.

124. Chandra, R. K., Imbach, A., Moore, C., et al. 1991. Nutrition of the elderly. *Canadian Medical Association Journal* 145(11), 1475–1487.

125. Lipschitz, D. A., Ham, R. J., and White, J. V. 1992. An approach to nutrition screening for older Americans. *American Family Physician* 45(2), 601–608.

126. Sier, M., Ouslander, J. G., and Orzeck, S. 1989. Urinary incontinence among geriatric patients in an acute-care hospital. *Journal of the American Medical Association* 257(13), 1767–1771.

127. Ouslander, J. G. 1990. Causes, assessment, and treatment of incontinence in the elderly. *Urology* 36(Suppl.), 25–35.

128. Wolinsky, F. D., Johnson, R. J., and Fitzgerald, J. F. 1992. Falling, health status, and the use of health services by older adults. *Medical Care* 30, 587–597.

129. Avorn, J. 1984. Benefit and cost analysis in geriatric care: Turning age discrimination into health policy. *New England Journal of Medicine* 310(20), 1294–1301.

130. Welch, H. G. 1991. Comparing apples and oranges: Does cost-effectiveness analysis deal fairly with the old and young? *Gerontologist* 31(3), 332–336.

131. Frame, P. S., and Carlson, S. J. 1975. A critical review of periodic health screening using specific screening criteria: Part 1. Selected diseases of the respiratory, cardiovascular and central nervous systems. *Journal of Family Practice* 2(1), 29–36.

132. Ransohoff, D. F., and Lang, C. A. 1991. Screening for colorectal cancer. *New England Journal of Medicine* 325(1), 37–41.

133. Resnick, M. L. 1988. Background for screening: Epidemiology and cost effectiveness. *Progress in Clinical and Biological Research* 269, 111–120.

134. Thompson, I. M., Ernst, J. J., Gangai, M. P., and Spence, C. R. 1984. Adenocarcinoma of the prostate: Results of routine urologic screening. *Journal of Urology* 132(4), 690–692.

135. Metlin, C., Lee, F., Drago, J., et al. 1991. The American Cancer Society national prostate cancer detection project: Findings on the detection of early prostate cancer in 2425 men. *Cancer* 67(12), 2949–2958.

136. Nolan, L., and O'Malley, K. 1988. Prescribing for the elderly, part 1: Sensitivity of the elderly to adverse drug reactions. *Journal of the American Geriatrics Society* 36(1), 142–149.

137. Steel, K., Gertman, P. M., Crescenzi, C., and Anderson, J. 1981. Iatrogenic illness on a general medical service at a university hospital. *New England Journal of Medicine* 304(10), 638–642.

16

John C. Beck

PREVENTING DISABILITY IN OLDER AMERICANS

The Challenge of the 21st Century

THE GRAYING OF AMERICA

It is often stated that we live in an aging world. This fact represents one of the major success stories of the 20th century but simultaneously presents the 21st century with one of its major challenges. As America and other industrialized societies approach the new century, the aging population is increasing rapidly, causing growing concern in the broader health care community as well as within local, state, and national legislative arenas. In the United States, persons 65 years or older numbered 33.5 million in 1995, representing almost 13% of the of the U.S. population. In that year, the 65- to 74-year age-group (18.8 million) was 8 times larger than in 1900, the 75- to 84-year group (11.1 million) was 14 times larger, and the 85-year group (3.6 million) was 29 times larger.[1,2] The latter, together with centenarians, represent the most rapidly growing age-group. The growth slowed somewhat during the 1990s because of the low birth rate in the 1930s, but the most rapid increase is expected between 2010 and 2030, when the "baby boom" generation reaches age 65. By 2030, about 70 million older persons, more than twice the number in the 1990s, will be in this age-group, representing at least 20% of the population.[1] The group over 75 require more health/social care services than "younger" elderly, and concern is generated because present evidence suggests that there will be an absolute and perhaps also a relative increase in the disability burden that persons of advanced age will place on society.[3] Solutions to this problem will become one of the major issues of the 21st century.

DEFINITION OF HEALTH

Many factors that are substantially different in the elderly than in the young influence health status as well as illness behavior and the utilization of health and social services. Although the World Health Organization's (WHO's) definition of health as "a state of complete physical, mental, and social well-being, and not merely the absence of disease and infirmity" has been criticized as being too broad, the breadth of the first part of the definition is an essential concept to a definition of health in the elderly. Complex relationships exist between physical health, mental health, socioeconomic status, and the environment. Defining and measuring health as well as disability must therefore take into account these complex relationships.

The breadth of the second part of the WHO definition, however, is problematic. The traditional definition of health status as the presence or absence of disease is less usable in the elderly than in other populations because it does not include a critical concept—the impact of chronic disease on function. Impairment of function in terms of basic activities of daily living (ADLs), such as dressing, eating, bathing, and toileting, or instrumental activities of daily living (IADLs), such as shopping, cooking, and housekeeping, or advanced activities of daily living (AADLs), such as recreational exercise, gardening, and participating in social activities, has an important influence on the elderly individual's ability to cope with disease and illness as well as on their need for health and social services. The latter (AADLs) represent physical and social functions that are voluntary, the loss of which may indicate early functional decline. A reasonable, usable definition of health in the elderly therefore necessarily includes the concept of function. Such a definition would, for example, encourage providers to see elderly persons as individuals rather than as members of a homogeneous group. Because of the extreme heterogeneity of functional status at any age over 65, ranging from independence to dependency, it has been obvious for some time that functional impairment is not just a natural consequence of aging, and it deserves evaluation on an individual basis. In addition, evidence is increasing that the processes leading to impairment may be

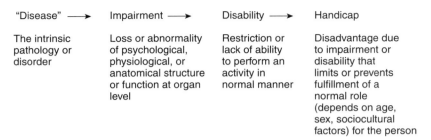

Figure 16.1. International Classification of Impairments, Disabilities, and Handicaps (ICIDH).

modified by intervention(s), with partial reversal or total return to normal function.

MODELS OF THE DEVELOPMENT OF DISABILITY

An understanding of the impact of disease on functioning or the transition from independence to dependency has been aided by the development of new models or conceptual schemes describing this process. The first was developed by the WHO—the WHO International Classification of Impairments, Disabilities and Handicaps (ICIDH) (Figure 16.1).[4] Another somewhat similar scheme was conceived and developed by Nagi,[5-7] and this one embraces a more holistic approach to health and disability. It is becoming the preferred one and was adopted by the Institute of Medicine.[8] I have further modified this model to include the transitional step between independence and dependency. These are illustrated in Figures 16.1 and 16.2, respectively.

More recently, the Disablement Process Model has been developed by Verbrugge and Jette.[9] The model is demonstrated in Figure 16.3. It has been modified to include the independence-dependency concept. It emphasizes the pathway of the development of disability and dependency.[10] In addition, the model identifies factors that are predisposing as well as introduced, that either speed up and slow down the pathway from independence to dependency. It emphasizes that there are always social, psychological, environmental, and other factors that are operating to modify the pathway. The model describes the impacts that chronic and acute conditions have on the functioning of specific body systems as well as the total organism and on people's ability to act in necessary, usual, expected, and personally desired ways in their society. These models permit the development of research addressing the mechanisms involved in

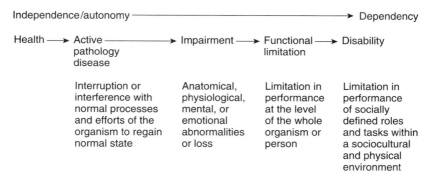

Figure 16.2.   Modified Institute of Medicine model.

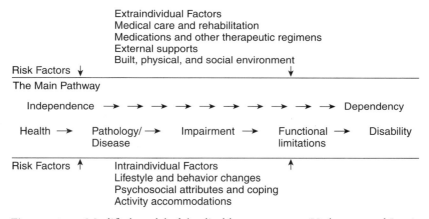

Figure 16.3.   Modified model of the disablement process (Verbrugge and Jette).

these transitions as well as the testing of interventions that might modify these transitions in a potentially beneficial way.

THE NEED FOR DISABILITY PREVENTION

In mid- and late life, chronic conditions dominate, and individuals often accumulate several of them. The most common chronic conditions tend to be nonfatal: For middle-aged and older women, the highest prevalence conditions include arthritis, high blood pressure, chronic sinusitis, tinnitus, hearing impairments, allergic rhinitis, chronic back conditions, varicose veins, hemorrhoids, migraine headaches, cataracts, and visual impairments.[11,12] The only fatal conditions in women's top 15 rankings

TABLE 16.1   COMPARISON OF DATA,
DISABILITY DEFINITIONS, AND PROJECTION
METHODOLOGIES OF RECENT PROJECTIONS
OF THE DISABLED ELDERLY POPULATION

	Jackson et al. (1991 [13])	Manton (1989 [14])	McBride (1989 [17])	Rogers et al. (1990)
Data source	1981–86 LSOA; 1984–86 CLTC	1984 NLTCS; 1985 NNHS	1984 SOA; 1985 NNHS; 1976–80 AHS	1984–86 LSOA
Projections include:				
Community-dwelling	Yes	Yes	Yes	Yes
Nursing home	Yes	Yes	Yes	No
No. of ADLs used in projections	5	6	5	7
Definition of disability	Human assistance	Human assistance (special equipment)[a]	Difficulty	Difficulty
Projections method	Multistate; life table	Static components	Static components	Multistate; life table

[a] Data exclude standby assistance.

of each disease-specific prevalence rate are ischemic heart disease, diabetes, and, at ages greater than 75 years, atherosclerosis. For middle-aged and older men, fatal conditions have higher prevalence rates and ranks than for women, but nonfatal conditions still dominate. It thus seems evident that people mostly live with chronic conditions rather than die from them, and thus symptoms and disabilities are their principal outcomes. It is also important to view disability as a gap between personal capability and environmental demand.

Projections of the size of the disabled elderly population have been made by a number of groups, including our own. Data from the United States demonstrate the disability burden common to developed nations. These projections have varied substantially, depending on how the survey instruments define disability and what criteria are used by investigators to analyze disability[13-17] (Table 16.1). Manton has estimated that from 1985 to 2050, the number of disabled older persons will approximately triple in and out of institutions.[14] The number of community-based older persons with five or more limitations in ADLs will increase

TABLE 16.2   COMPARISON OF PROJECTIONS
OF THE ADL-DEPENDENT ELDERLY (IN 1000S)

	1990	2000	2010	2020	2030	2040
Jackson et al.						
(1991 [13])						
Low-mortality						
assumption	3,617	4,381	5,242	5,819	6,933	9,009
Mid-mortality						
assumption	3,752	4,116	4,631	5,589	7,130	7,907
Manton (1989 [14]) [a]	—	4,086	—	5,675	—	—
McBride (1989 [17])						
Base case	6,200	—	9,000	—	13,800	—
Optimistic mortality	6,200	—	9,900	—	16,300	—
Optimistic mortality						
and health	6,000	—	8,800	—	13,400	—
Rogers et al. (1990) [b]	5,190	6,300	6,662	7,480	9,869	12,014

[a] Assumes that 10% of institutionalized population is ADL dependent.
[b] Age 70 and over.

from 0.8 to 2.6 million; the number of institutionalized older persons will increase from 1.3 to 4.5 million. In our own study, regardless of which mortality assumption is applied, the number of disabled elderly will increase dramatically over the next decade. For example, using the middle mortality assumption, the number that would be ADL-dependent is predicted at 4.1 million in the year 2000. This number would increase to 5.6 million in 2020 and to 7.9 million in 2040 (Table 16.2). The pattern is even more dramatic when a low mortality assumption is involved: 4.4 million in 2000, 5.8 million in 2020, and 9 million in 2040.[13] This increasing number of older persons and concomitant decreasing levels of support lead us to suggest that prevention of functional decline should be explored more vigorously.

There is no conclusive evidence at present as to whether older persons are becoming more or less disabled. Some argue that sociomedical advances have increased life expectancy but not changed the age of morbidity and dependency onset, thus projecting greatly increased numbers of disabled older persons. Others contend that morbidity, compressed into the very last stage of life, will increase the functional life expectancy of older adults and decrease the proportion of older persons requiring long-term care.[18–22]

The concept of functional life expectancy is illustrated in Figure 16.4,

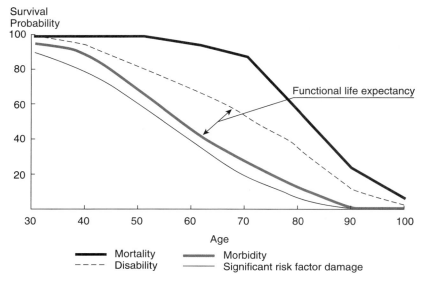

Figure 16.4. Survival curve for persons dying of degenerative disease.

which depicts a set of survival curves representing the risk factors: morbidity (impairments), disability, and mortality patterns typically associated with chronic degenerative conditions such as degenerative joint disease, hypertension, diabetes, or osteoporosis. These conditions produce a much larger impact on disability in the older populations than do many other conditions, and they increase in prevalence with age. Their natural history differs as well, in that impairments of functioning become manifest long after the onset of the disease. The figure demonstrates that the person who is affected with such slowly developing conditions tends to live longer and spend a greater proportion of their life span in a functionally disabled state than those who are not affected. Lifestyle issues such as sedentary lifestyle, poor nutrition, high alcohol consumption, and smoking also fit into this type of model. The concept of functional life expectancy represents the area between the morbidity and disability curves, and an extension of functional life expectancy would imply a movement of the disability curve much closer to that of the mortality curve.

A number of recent reports have contributed further data that add evidence to those who believe that there are progressive declines in chronic disability prevalence rates. The long-accepted theories of Gompertz that mortality rates increase with age at predictable trajectories have been challenged because age trajectories of mortality do not follow predictable curves.[23] In fact, in humans, mortality rates decrease with age. The same group of investigators using the 1982, 1984, 1989, and 1994 National Long Term Care Surveys (NLTCS) has shown substantial declines in prevalence rates of chronic disability. In 1994, the disability prevalence was 3.6% lower than in 1982.[24] Another group has examined the change in the prevalence of disability, from 1982 through 1993, using two longitudinal studies—the Longitudinal Study on Aging (LSOA) and the National Health Interview Survey (NHIS). They also addressed the likelihood of recovering from disability, now a well-established phenomenon. In the NHIS sample, the disability incidence and prevalence rate were lower in more recent years, and the recovery rate was higher. In the LSOA sample, the prevalence rate of disability increased at some dates after 1984. In both these data sets, there was substantial fluctuation in disability prevalence rather than a convincingly clear trend.[25] Two conclusions can be drawn from these and other data. First, the U.S. Bureau of the Census continues to underestimate the U.S. population of older persons, and, second, the controversy as to whether the disability burden will be absolutely or relatively increased remains unresolved.

DEMAND REDUCTION STRATEGIES

The terms *functional impairment* and *disability* imply an increase in the demand for health services (medical/social). These services with respect to the chronic disease burden in older persons are often termed *long-term-care* services and can include community-based, home-based, and institutional services (residential care facilities or nursing homes). (Though many definitions exist of *long-term care,* the implied meaning here is a broad one and includes any aspect of the care of the elderly that is provided over a long period of time. It implies that this care may occur in many settings and that an effective coordination of this care across these various settings is mandatory.) An important policy question is whether these services might actually be reduced. A number of strategies have been considered as nations begin to expand the options and seek improvements in their long-term-care system: (1) increasing provision of formal home-based long-term care (*formal care*), (2) increasing provision of unpaid long-term care in the community (*informal care*), and (3) decreasing the number of older persons developing functional disabilities requiring long-term care.[11,26]

The first strategy, formal home care, can supplement or substitute for informal home care, but home care has almost no effect on institutional placement, and community-based programs have not decreased placement either. Neither method has had a significant effect on functional capacity or other aspects of health. In the few cases in which nursing home use was reduced, program costs have offset any savings.[27-30]

The second strategy, informal home care, has most often involved female spouses or nonworking daughters and may be infeasible in the future because women have entered the paid workforce in increasing numbers. In addition, while two-thirds of the current cohort of older persons with functional limitations live with relatives (United States), the next cohort of older persons will have families half the size of the current older cohort, limiting family support systems even more.[31-34]

The third demand-reduction strategy argues for extending functional life expectancy as a national policy. This strategy has only recently become feasible with increasing evidence that improvement in functional status and delay or prevention in loss of independence can be achieved by the following: (1) primary prevention, or the prevention of a disease or health problem before it occurs; (2) secondary prevention, or the early detection of a disease or problem when it may respond favorably to treatment; and (3) tertiary prevention, or rehabilitation for the residual effect of a disease or problem that has already occurred. Primary prevention aims to avert the onset of pathology, secondary prevention aims at the early detection and management of pathology, and tertiary prevention aims to maintain and restore function. In addition, it includes efforts to avoid the onset of secondary conditions and to sustain or improve the quality of life.

The next sections deal with three possible approaches to delaying or preventing the development of functional impairment and disability. These include (1) comprehensive geriatric assessment (CGA), (2) in-home assessment programs, and (3) the development of a health risk assessment system for the elderly (HRA-E). All address various steps in the Verbrugge-Jette model of the disablement process (Figure 16.3).

COMPREHENSIVE GERIATRIC ASSESSMENT

Comprehensive geriatric assessment (CGA) was developed in the early 1970s and has proliferated since that time. It was defined by a 1987 National Institutes of Health (NIH) Consensus Development Conference as being "a multi-disciplinary evaluation in which the multiple problems of older persons are uncovered, described, and explained, if possible, and in which the resources and strengths of the person are catalogued, need for services assessed, and a coordinated care plan developed to focus interventions on the person's problems."[35] The report of the Technical Committee on Health Services of the 1981 White House Conference on Aging recommended combining assessment with preventive services.[36] Various settings and formats for CGA are reported, including inpatient geriatric consultation, inpatient geriatric evaluation units, ambulatory geriatric assessment clinics, and in-home assessment programs.[37-42] Even in academic practices, the assessment process, settings for CGA, persons targeted, and the personnel involved have not been uniform.[43] Some of the studies evaluating CGA effectiveness have demonstrated significant benefits, including improvements in diagnostic accuracy, placement, functional status, affect, cognition and survival, as well as reduction in medications, use of hospital services, nursing home days, and overall medical costs.[44-46] Each of these benefits, however, has not been demonstrated in every study.[47] In addition, because of cost constraints as well as practicability, the composition of the assessment teams has changed. Often only one health professional type is involved and calls on other health professionals when need arises. The University of California, Los Angeles, Multicampus Program in Geriatric Medicine and Gerontology (MPGMG) has taken a lead role in this area of research from the national perspective.

The CGA, or multidimensional assessment process, has been primarily institution based, and controlled studies have demonstrated important benefits, the most dramatic of which were first documented in in-hospital programs.[44,45] The inconsistent findings reported in some studies of CGA have been postulated as due to the following methodological limitations:

1. Basic flaws in study design

2. Small sample sizes

3. Homogeneous settings of patient populations, such as in the Department of Veterans Affairs (DVA) or in Academic Medical Centers

4. Selection criteria for study populations

5. Patient gender (e.g., 96% males in DVA studies compared to 60% to 80% females in other hospital settings)

6. Different levels and types of care in "control" groups, ranging from usual care by attending physicians to enhanced care similar to CGA

7. Lack of adherence of participants and/or their providers

8. Most recently, training and continuing competence of the professionals responsible for the assessment

In addition, there have been differences in the interventions that make comparisons of studies difficult. These include the timing of the intervention; variable patient length of stay for delivery of the intervention; assessment processes and approaches, such as geriatric assessment units versus consultation teams; strategies aimed at restorative treatment versus prevention of functional decline; and the intervention strategies themselves. Thus, some studies have offered recommendations only, while others have implemented recommendations, and still others have provided specialized follow-up care. The process of care in CGA programs has been termed the "black box" of multidimensional assessment and follow-up.

IN-HOME ASSESSMENT PROGRAMS

A more recent, alternative approach is to provide assessment, referral, and follow-up services in the home. Home outreach strategies take place before the older person seeks medical or other attention for a problem and permit early preventive interventions. Providing CGA in home settings permits insight into a person's living environment (e.g., hazards, accessibility, resources, adequacy, self-care ability, nutritional adequacy, inappropriate medications, and the nature of social relations and support) and provides an excellent social environment for communication, health education, health promotion, and reinforcing self-care activities. A small number of randomized trials of in-home assessment and prevention programs have been undertaken during the past 15 years, most of them outside the United States, with some promising results.[48-52]

Results of the first two randomized trials of in-home assessment were published in 1984, one from the United Kingdom and the other from Denmark. Both demonstrated that individuals visited at regular intervals had lower mortality and made greater use of community services than those who were not visited regularly.[46,47] In addition, the Danish study showed a decrease in hospital days and emergency room visits, whereas the U.K. study showed improved quality of life; neither of these involved CGA as defined by the NIH Consensus Conference.[33] More recent studies tend to confirm these results, although not all findings are consistent. Another U.K. study published in 1990 reported reduction in long-term-care institutionalization,[50] and another study demonstrated improved mood[53] among the subjects who received in-home visits and referrals by community health workers and/or volunteers. A 1992 U.K. study of a home-visit case-finding surveillance program demonstrated reduced mortality and number of hospital days at the three-year follow-up.[48] In 1992, a Canadian study of an in-home, nurse-administered health promotion program demonstrated an increased three-year "living at home" rate.[54] Recently, a group from the Netherlands[55] has reported inconclusive results from a three-year randomized trial of visiting nurse home visits without CGA. They concluded that this type of intervention was effective only for subjects in poor health.

Kaplan, in reexamining data for Alameda County,[56] develops suggestive evidence that early interventions in older persons with chronic disease may alter the risk for loss of independence. He showed convincingly that certain incident chronic diseases, in addition to behavioral, social, and demographic risk factors that are associated with chronic disease (e.g., race, income, hypertension, degenerative disease, smoking, excessive weight, alcohol), are associated with poor physical functioning.[57] His data suggest that interventions reducing or delaying functional impairment associated with chronic diseases and other behavioral and social interventions may modify the impact of these multiple factors on functioning. The data also suggest that these interventions may increase the level of functioning in those who survive with or without disease.

It is also important to recognize that problems in functional impairment are often reversible. In one national study reported in 1988, 35% of those older persons with five or six problems in ADLs who survived two years improved in functioning over that two-year period,[58] confirming earlier studies that we reported in 1984.[59]

A recent meta-analysis of CGA (including in-home assessment programs) has recently been reported by our UCLA faculty. It compared 4,959 subjects allocated to one of five CGA types (determined by location) and 4,912 control subjects. The combined odds ratio (95% confidence interval) of one of the outcomes—living at home—was 1.68 (1.17 to 2.41) for hospital-based units, 1.49 (1.12 to 1.98) for hospital-home assessment services, and 1.20 (1.05 to 1.37) for home-assessment services. The data from this meta-analytic approach demonstrated CGA to be highly effective for improving survival, place of residence, and function in older persons.[49] Figure 16.5 demonstrates the effects on mortality at one year for institutional programs and at the end of the intervention

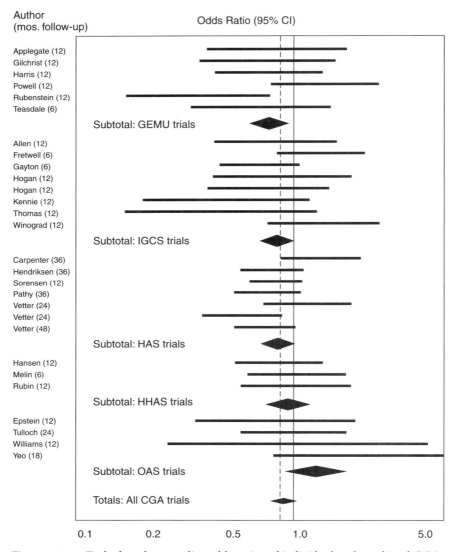

Figure 16.5. End-of-study mortality odds ratios of individual and combined CGA trials. Source: Stuck, A. E., et al., "Comprehensive Geriatric Assessment: A Meta-Analysis of Controlled Trials," *The Lancet* (October 23, 1993). Reproduced with the permission of The Lancet.

period for noninstitutional programs. One critique of this study was the "lumping" of the in-home programs under the rubric of CGA. Some had CGA components, while others were "friendly visitor" visits.

A RANDOMIZED TRIAL OF ANNUAL IN-HOME CGA FOR ELDERLY PEOPLE IN THE COMMUNITY

Of the 13 million Americans aged 75 and over, 91% live at home. Among those elderly with functional impairment, 80% live in the community, and 25% of these live alone. Further, older people are disproportionate users of the health care dollar. Although those age 75 and older account for only 5% of the population, they account for 15% of acute hospital admissions and nearly 25% of hospital days.[60] Clearly, methods to prevent decline and to improve the health status of community-dwelling elderly may be of great importance.

We conducted a three-year randomized controlled trial of annual in-home CGA and follow-up for people in the community who were 75 years of age or older. The 215 people in the intervention group were seen at home by gerontological nurse practitioners (GNPs) who, in collaboration with geriatricians, evaluated problems and risk factors for disability and gave specific recommendations. The 199 persons in the control group received their regular medical and social care.

The program used specially trained GNPs to implement the following program components:

1. Problem and risk identification by in-home comprehensive geriatric assessment

2. Problem solution and recommendations

3. Health education with emphasis on the role of the older person as an active agent in determining his or her own health and well-being (empowerment and self-care)

4. Health promotion and disease prevention

5. Regular quarterly follow-up visits to aid in adherence to the recommendations and to identify new problems

In the yearly in-home CGA and in the shorter follow-up visits every three months, the home setting facilitates shared decision making and allows the GNP to observe the older person's function in his or her own environment. The goal of the first visit was to establish a personal relationship, complete a comprehensive assessment, and develop an initial problem list on which the first recommendations were based. During the visit, the GNPs evaluated the home for safety, including hazards for falls, such as poor lighting, clutter, and uneven surfaces. They inspected home pharmacies for appropriateness, with each prescription checked for type, dosage, instructions, ordering physicians, expiration date, and the potential for drug interactions. They evaluated other potential functional barriers, such as adequacy of transportation, accessibility to the home (e.g., unsafe stairs), the need for assistive devices, and the social support as well as the social networks of the older person.

After having taken action on any urgent problems, the GNP carefully reviewed the baseline findings and the generated problem list with the project geriatricians during regular case conferences and developed an individualized preventive, health educational and health promotional plan to be presented to the older person at the next visit. Each older person's plan was unique and formulated on the basis of the initial home visit. Recommendations were made for those areas in which the team felt the older person could make a positive contribution toward the management or prevention of the problem. Specifically, recommendations were either something the individuals could do for themselves (e.g., a lifestyle change) or something that required referral to a health professional or community service (e.g., seeing a physician for a medication adjustment or contacting a local senior center for a stroke support group).

Measures were taken to maximize client adherence to recommendations. Health education by the GNP provided clients with the knowledge base to understand the recommendations and institute appropriate action. Potential barriers, such as financial or memory deficits, were addressed, and recommendations were prioritized, written down, and limited in number, if necessary, to avoid overwhelming the client. When serious health questions arose, the GNP or project geriatrician contacted the primary care physician by mail or telephone after obtaining permission from the client to do so.

At follow-up visits every three months, the GNP queried the older person about recent physician and community visits, medication changes, episodic illnesses, and falls and then performed a limited assessment to determine how well the client complied with previous recommendations. The GNP noted changes in problem status and consulted the project geriatricians if necessary. The previous recommendations were reinforced, modified if they required it, or supplemented with new ones on the basis of a new finding.

Each subsequent annual home visit, in contrast to the follow-up visit, included a repeat CGA, a review of adherence with the previous year's recommendations, an update of the routine health maintenance record (which was a checklist of preventive care items, such as cancer screening), and a review of the active problems. The GNP encouraged good health behaviors and made additional recommendations for action when indicated. At the final (36-month) visit of the study period, each older person received from the GNP a written summary of that person's personal health priorities and the final recommendations from the team, a copy of his or her individualized health maintenance schedule, and information about community resources if applicable. The last visit included a full CGA and focused on the implications of completing the program and moving to what was hoped would be improved client-initiated use of appropriate health and community services. It is important to emphasize that the GNP did not perform primary care nursing.[61]

The main outcome measure was the prevention of disability, defined as the need for assistance in performing basic ADLs or IADLs, and the prevention of nursing home admissions.

The baseline characteristics of the participants and the results are shown in Tables 16.3 through 16.8. In summary, at three years, 20 people in the intervention group (12% of 170 surviving participants) and 32 in the control group (22% of 147 surviving participants) required assistance in performing the basic activities of daily living (adjusted odds ratio, 0.4; 95% confidence interval, 0.2 to 0.8; P = 0.02). The number of persons who were dependent on assistance in performing the IADLs but not the basic ADLs did not differ significantly between the two groups. Nine people in the intervention group (4%) and 20 in the control group (10%) were permanently admitted to nursing homes (P = 0.02). Acute care hospital admissions and short-term nursing home admissions did not differ significantly between the two groups. In the second and third years of the study, there were significantly more visits to physicians among the participants in the intervention group than among those in the control group (mean number of visits per month, 1.41 in year 2 and 1.27 in year 3 in the intervention group, as compared with 1.11 in year 2 and 0.92 in year 3 in the control group; P = 0.007 and P = 0.001, respectively). It thus appears that a program of this type can delay the development of disability and reduce permanent nursing home stays among the relatively well elderly persons living in the community.

The intervention was not a substitute for usual care (medical and social services) but instead was integrated with such care. It was therefore

TABLE 16.3   BASELINE CHARACTERISTICS
OF THE STUDY PARTICIPANTS, ACCORDING
TO THE ORIGINAL GROUP ASSIGNMENT[a]

Characteristic before Random Assignment	Intervention Group (N = 215)	Control Group (N = 199)
Age—years	81.0 = 3.9	81.4 = 4.2
Women—no. (%)	149 (69)	141 (71)
Living alone—no. (%)	140 (65)	125 (63)
Completed high school—no. (%)	173 (80)	151 (76)
Annual income < $11,000—no. (%)[b]	82 (38)	74 (37)
Mean score for self-perceived health[c]	3.2 = 1.2	3.1 = 1.2
Independence in basic ADL—no. (%)	196 (91)	183 (92)
Depression score[d]	2.8 = 2.7	3.1 = 2.9
Regular exercise— no. (%)	142 (66)	116 (58)
Current nonsmoker— no. (%)	198 (92)	184 (92)
No. of medications	4.9 = 2.8	4.6 = 3.1
No. of visits to physicians in previous month	1.3 = 1.4	1.1 = 1.6
Characteristic at Initial Geriatric Assessment[e]		
Arterial hypertension— no. (%)	67 (33)	—
Poor vision—no. (%)	34 (17)	—
Poor hearing—no. (%)	61 (30)	—
Impaired gait and balance—no. (%)	20 (10)	—
Underweight—no. (%)	14 (7)	—
Overweight—no. (%)	54 (27)	—
In-home hazard— no. (%)	61 (30)	—

[a]Plus-minus values are means (SD). Basic ADL denotes basic activities of daily living (bathing, dressing, feeding, grooming, transferring from bed to chair, and moving around inside the house).

[b]An annual income of $11,000 is considered the poverty line.

[c]The rating scale for self-perceived health ranges from 5 (excellent) to 1 (poor).

[d]The Geriatric Depression Scale, short form, ranges from 0 to 15, with a score above 5 indicating probable depression.

[e]Data are missing for 13 persons who dropped out of the study before the assessment could be performed. Assessments were not performed in the control group. Arterial hypertension was defined as > 160 mm Hg systolic or > 90 mm Hg diastolic. Poor vision was defined as < 20/50 in the better eye. Poor hearing was defined as 1,000 or 2,000 Hz not heard at 40 dB in the better ear. Impairment in gait and balance was defined as a score < 23 on a scale of 0 to 28, with 28 representing the best result (from A. E. Stuck, M. H. Beers, A. Steiner, et al., Inappropriate medication use in community-residing older persons, *Archives of Internal Medicine* 331(1994): 821–827. Underweight was defined as 20% below average body weight and overweight as 20% above average body weight (from A. M. Master, R. P. Lasser, and G. Beckman, Tables of average weight and height of Americans aged 65 to 94 years, *Journal of the American Medical Association* 172(1960): 658–663).

TABLE 16.4   MEAN FUNCTIONAL-STATUS SCORE
AMONG THE SURVIVING PARTICIPANTS AT THREE
YEARS, ACCORDING TO
INTENTION-TO-TREAT ANALYSIS

Functional-Status Score	Intervention Group (N = 170)	Control Group (N = 147)	Difference in Scores (Intervention Group vs. Control Group)	P Value
	Mean (95% CI)			
Basic ADL[a]	96.8	95.4	+1.4	0.1
	(94.8–98.8)	(93.4–97.4)	(−0.3 to +3.1)	
Instrumental ADL[b]	72.3	69.3	+3.0	0.02
	(69.0–75.6)	(66.0–72.6)	(+0.6 to +5.4)	
Basic and instrumental ADL	75.6	72.7	+2.9	0.03
	(73.2–77.9)	(70.2–75.2)	(+0.4 to +5.4)	

NOTE: Data are based on reports by 287 study participants and 30 proxies (in most cases, a spouse or close relative) during the home interview at three years. Data were not available for 45 persons in the intervention group (24 died, 14 refused, and 7 moved away) and 52 in the control group (26 died, 21 refused, and 5 moved away). Results have been adjusted for age, sex, whether the subject lived alone, baseline self-perceived health, and baseline functional status. ADL denotes activities of daily living, and CI denotes confidence interval. All scores are on a scale of 0 to 100, with 100 representing the highest functional status.
   [a] As defined in Table 16.3.
   [b] Instrumental ADLs include cooking, handling finances, handling medication, engaging in "handyman" work, housekeeping, doing laundry, shopping, using the telephone, and using public or private transportation.

not unexpected that, as a result of the detection of new or unrecognized problems and the recommendations by the nurse practitioners, the people in the intervention group consulted their physicians more frequently than the people in the control group. To calculate the overall cost of the intervention, we included the cost of these additional visits to physicians.

   The intervention was not associated with changes in the use of in-home and supportive services. Study participants in the intervention group were more likely than those in the control group to use services promoting socialization, such as college courses for older persons or a friendly-visitor program (Table 16.7).

   In the second and third years, the people in the intervention group had significantly more outpatient visits than those in the control group (Table 16.8). Exploratory subgroup analyses showed that this effect was more pronounced among the study participants with symptoms of depression (P = 0.03). The intervention was also associated with a reduction in the proportion of persons who did not visit a physician in a 12-month period. Nine percent of the study participants in the intervention group, as compared with 16% of those in the control group, did not visit a physician during the third year of follow-up (P = 0.04).

TABLE 16.5 FUNCTIONAL STATUS
(DEPENDENCE OR INDEPENDENCE)
OF THE SURVIVING PARTICIPANTS
AT THREE YEARS, ACCORDING
TO INTENTION-TO-TREAT ANALYSIS

Functional Status	Intervention Group (N = 170)	Control Group (N = 147)	Odds Ratio (95% CI)[a]	P Value
	No. of persons (%)			
Dependent on assistance in basic ADL[b]	20 (12)	32 (22)	0.4 (0.2–0.8)	0.02
Dependent on assistance in instrumental but not basic ADL[c]	39 (23)	28 (19)	1.1 (0.6–2.0)	0.8
Independent[d]	111 (65)	87 (59)	—	—

[a] Odds ratios are based on a polychotomous logistic-regression analysis adjusted for age, sex, whether the subject lived alone, baseline self-perceived health, and baseline functional status, with independent persons as the reference group. The odds ratios are for the intervention group, as compared with the control group. CI denotes confidence interval.
[b] Dependence was defined as requiring assistance in at least one of the basic ADLs (defined in Table 16.3).
[c] Dependence was defined as independence in basic ADL but a need for assistance in at least one of the instrumental ADLs (defined in Table 16.4).
[d] Independence was defined as a need for no assistance in either basic or instrumental ADLs.

The intervention did not have a significant effect on the number of admissions to acute care hospitals or the number of short-term nursing home stays (Table 16.6). Eighteen percent of the study participants in the intervention group and 21% of those in the control group were admitted at least once to an acute care hospital in the first year; 21% and 20%, respectively, were admitted at least once in the second year; and 24% and 25%, respectively, were admitted at least once in the third year. The mean length of stay per acute care admission was 6.3 days in the intervention group and 5.1 days in the control group (P = 0.7, by the polychotomous logistic-regression analysis). With self-reported hospital admissions outside the study area added to the data in Table 16.4, the estimated number of hospital days per 100 subjects per year was 203 for the intervention group and 180 for the control group.

Although there was no overall effect of the intervention on hospital admissions, we performed an exploratory analysis to determine whether the intervention was associated with an increased or decreased number of admissions among certain subgroups of study participants. A poly-

TABLE 16.6   HOSPITAL AND NURSING
HOME ADMISSIONS DURING THE THREE-YEAR
FOLLOW-UP PERIOD, ACCORDING TO
INTENTION-TO-TREAT ANALYSIS

Type of Admission	Intervention Group (N = 215)	Control Group (N = 199)	Adjusted Odds Ratio or Relative Risk (95% CI)[a]	P Value
Permanent nursing home				
No. of persons admitted (%)	9 (4)	20 (10)	OR = 0.4 (0.2–0.9)	0.02
No. of days/ 100 persons/year	128	820		
Acute care hospital				
No. of persons admitted at least once (%)	99 (46)	93 (47)	RR = 1.0 (0.8–1.4)	0.8
No. of days/ 100 persons/year	197	160		
Short-term nursing home				
No. of persons admitted at least once (%)	27 (13)	31 (16)	RR = 0.9 (0.6–1.4)	0.6
No. of days/ 100 persons/year	89	111		

NOTE: Nursing home data are based on information reported by the study participants, with verification from secondary sources. Permanent and short-term admissions are defined in the text. Hospital data are based on systematic reviews of admissions to local hospitals.

[a] Results have been adjusted for age, sex, baseline self-perceived health, and baseline functional status. The odds ratio (OR) is based on a multivariate logistic-regression analysis, and the relative risks (RR) are based on multivariate analyses corrected for overdispersion. The odds ratio and relative risks are for the intervention group, as compared with the control group. CI denotes confidence interval.

chotomous logistic-regression analysis showed that the intervention was associated with a decreased number of short stays (i.e., those lasting one to seven days) among persons with fair or poor self-perceived health (odds ratio, 0.4; 95% confidence interval, 0.2 to 1.0; P = 0.05) and among those with less than a high school education (odds ratio, 0.3; 95% confidence interval, 0.1 to 1.0; P = 0.04). None of the subgroups of the intervention group had significant increases in admissions to acute care hospitals.

We hypothesize that the lack of a significant effect on acute hospital use may reflect a balance between two opposite effects of the intervention. It is likely that among study participants with previously unrecognized or

TABLE 16.7 USE OF COMMUNITY SERVICES DURING THE THREE-YEAR FOLLOW-UP PERIOD, ACCORDING TO INTENTION-TO-TREAT ANALYSIS

Type of Service	Intervention Group (N = 215)	Control Group (N = 199)	P Value
	No. of persons (%)		
In-home and supportive services			
Care management[a]	43 (20)	33 (17)	0.4
Home health care	27 (13)	17 (9)	0.2
Homemaker	24 (11)	28 (14)	0.4
Meals on wheels	23 (11)	18 (9)	0.6
Personal care	20 (9)	24 (12)	0.4
Services promoting socialization			
College courses for senior citizens	45 (21)	23 (12)	0.01
Friendly visitors[b]	23 (11)	7 (4)	0.01
Community transportation	57 (27)	36 (18)	0.04

NOTE: Data are based on reports provided by the study participants at one or more of the interviews conducted every four months during the three-year follow-up period.

[a]Formerly known as case management.

[b]Denotes a home-based program that schedules social visits by volunteers with elderly persons.

TABLE 16.8 MEAN NUMBER OF VISITS TO PHYSICIANS PER MONTH, ACCORDING TO INTENTION-TO-TREAT ANALYSIS

Year	Intervention Group		Control Group		Adjusted Relative Risk (95% CI)[a]	P Value
	No. of Persons	*Mean No. of Visits*	*No. of Persons*	*Mean No. of Visits*		
1	207	1.27	185	1.03	1.1 (1.0–1.3)	0.1
2	199	1.41	180	1.11	1.2 (1.1–1.4)	0.007
3	191	1.27	162	0.92	1.4 (1.1–1.6)	0.001

NOTE: Data are based on Medicare claims data and on records of health maintenance organizations. Persons who had died, moved permanently to nursing homes, or moved out of the area were excluded from the analysis. In addition, 22 persons (8 in the intervention group and 14 in the control group) were excluded because reliable data on the number of visits to physicians were not available.

[a]Relative risks (based on a multivariate analysis corrected for overdispersion) have been adjusted for age, sex, membership in a health maintenance organization, baseline self-perceived health, and baseline functional status. Relative risks are for the intervention group, as compared with the control group. CI denotes confidence interval.

suboptimally managed problems, hospital admissions increased, whereas among other participants, unnecessary admissions were prevented. In addition, our study sample was small and limited these analyses.

The approximate yearly cost of the intervention can be derived from the costs of the program itself, including the costs for personnel (1.0 full-time-equivalent nurse practitioner and 0.1 full-time-equivalent geriatrician per 136 persons), supplies, travel, and overhead (estimated at $48,000 per 100 persons); the marginal costs for the increased number of visits to physicians (estimated at $18,000 per 100 persons); and the marginal savings from the decreased number of permanent-stay nursing home days (estimated at $42,000 per 100 persons), resulting in a net cost of $24,000 per 100 persons. Acute care hospital admissions and short-term nursing home stays are not included in this calculation because they did not differ significantly between the two groups.

The effect of the intervention on health-related outcomes can be summarized in two ways: by estimating the number of disability-free years gained by the intervention (4.1 years per 100 persons per year during the three-year follow-up) or by calculating the number of permanent-stay nursing home days avoided (692 days [820 − 128] per year) (Table 16.6). On the basis of these estimates, the cost for each disability-free year of life gained was approximately $6,000. The cost of preventing one day of a permanent stay in a nursing home was $35.[62]

As compared with the U.S. population of persons 75 years old or older living at home, our study group had a higher educational level, a lower mortality rate, and a lower rate of acute care hospital admissions, with a higher proportion of persons living alone.[63,64] The first three of these factors suggest a higher health status of the study population.

During this study, we had an opportunity to examine the role that the participant's physician played in patient adherence to the recommendations given by the nurse practitioner. Although all physicians in the community had been made aware of the study, we did not wish to involve them directly except in emergency situations. This was because we were focusing our efforts on further improving the participants' ability to deal more effectively with their problems as well as their providers. We examined the factors that led to cooperation of the primary care physician with the community-based prevention program, the relationship between physician cooperation and patient adherence, and patient satisfaction with health care. The providers who were rated as cooperative were more likely to have a positive appraisal of the program (they were younger and had fewer years in practice), and their patients had higher adherence rates to program recommendations. These findings suggest that in implementation of programs of this type, increasing primary care physician cooperation might improve effectiveness.[65] This notion deserves more extensive research and is being addressed in a Swiss study.

Other studies of preventive-type home visits were reported in the literature during the study: a one-time in-home geriatric assessment with follow-up, regular telephone follow-up, or health promotion that may improve outcomes in the elderly. Also, studies show that older persons with congestive heart failure discharged from hospital benefit from regular, intensive home-care surveillance with an improvement in functional status and a reduction in hospital admission rates and duration of hospital stay.[66,67] Improvement in these latter studies probably is related to better adherence with medications and diet, increased exercise, and more effective response to early signs of cardiac decompensation. A study of the long-term effectiveness of comprehensive support and counseling for spouse/caregivers and families of Alzheimer's disease patients has shown a postponement or prevention of nursing home placement.[68] These latter studies, like most of the studies of CGA, have focused on tertiary prevention in persons at high risk for developing disability.

Our own trial also presented an opportunity for examining the process of care linked to the annual home CGA. Detailed data were collected prospectively on the problems detected, the specific recommendations made for these problems, and subject adherence with the recommendations made by the GNP.

These data showed that major independence-threatening problems were identified in all domains of CGA (medical, including mental health, functional, and social/environmental), although the most common problems were medical. New problems appeared at a regular rate—approximately two medical to one social per subject per year.

In the first year, three-quarters of the subjects had at least one major problem identified that was either previously unknown or suboptimally treated. One-third of the subjects had additional major problems identified during the second year. A constant number of recommendations was made each year (11.5 per subject per year). Subject adherence varied by type of recommendation; adherence was better for referrals to a physician than for referrals to a nonphysician professional or community service and lowest for recommendations involving self-care activities, including behavioral change.

The important issue of linking processes of care to outcomes requires larger studies. Such an opportunity presented itself in the EIGER project in Bern, Switzerland, which is a replication of our earlier Santa Monica–based study addressing a whole series of different research questions. The Swiss study enrolled 791 participants (264 randomized to the intervention group) for a three-year intervention, which has just been completed, and preliminary data analyses are under way.[69,70] This study confirms the main findings in the Santa Monica study, namely, that in-home preventive visits can delay or prevent the onset of functional impairment and reduce nursing home use. The Swiss study also demonstrates the ineffectiveness of a "friendly visit" or social contact as the major component of the intervention.

In a further analysis of the Santa Monica database, we have been able to show that more highly functioning persons appear to benefit most. This finding appears to be confirmed in our Swiss project and raises the intriguing question of targeting preventive interventions to a younger and thus more functional and healthier population.

Development of a Health Risk Appraisal System for Older Persons (HRA-E)

To ensure reaching at-risk adults as they age in the community, surveillance needs to be directed toward a high-volume activity with broad outreach. This requirement necessitates that the service be cost-effective (i.e., prevention and treatment must be efficacious), but surveillance needs to be developed at low cost per older person screened. This is in contrast to many programs developed to date and particularly those that are inpatient based and have focused on smaller numbers of frail older persons. It was with this background that a group of senior faculty with expertise in health promotion, disease prevention, epidemiology, and geriatric medicine began developing a health risk appraisal instrument for the elderly (HRA-E) with an aim to reducing the development of functional impairment.[71]

Health risk appraisal in younger persons has been a promising approach for the maintenance of health. It begins with the identification of specific factors in individuals that increase the risk of impairments, disability, and premature mortality and then develops and recommends strategies for minimizing their impact. In the younger workforce, HRA alone has not been a highly effective intervention for bringing about behavior change. Traditionally, HRA is a process that entails (1) data collection about an individual, (2) use of a computerized algorithm to analyze the data, and (3) feedback designed to encourage medical and behavioral action directed toward avoiding premature mortality. In translating this concept into a possible method for the identification of risk factors as persons age, it seemed more relevant to focus on risk factors for functional impairment and disability than on mortality.

The first phase in this project was the development of a prototype HRA-E questionnaire and feedback statements for preliminary testing. We sought to examine risk factors that could impact function, such as vision, hearing, memory, chronic diseases and their consequences, and medications. Risk factors were selected on the basis of the magnitude of the effect and potential impact on functional impairment, the feasibility of assessment, the generalizability of these assessment results, and the potential for risk reduction. Criteria for selection of survey instruments for individual items were the availability of psychometric properties in older adults, the feasibility of data collection in a self-administered questionnaire, the feasibility of self-administration, and the prior or current use in other population-based studies. Included in the initial survey instrument were items addressing functional status, although these would also be used in any more long term study addressing outcomes as important outcome variables. These included basic ADLs, IADLs, and AADLs. This process led to a selection of the domains that were in the first version of the questionnaire or survey instrument.

Algorithms and feedback statements regarding the results of the assessment of each risk factor and important risk factor combinations were developed to provide the participants with a response based on current literature. The algorithms covered all possible combinations of questionnaire responses. Computer software using these algorithms were developed and alpha and beta tested. Thus, each person completing a questionnaire received a computer-generated personalized HRA-E feedback report with a series of statements in each domain, including a generic statement about the problems identified, individually tailored suggestions for actions and the rationale for them, sources for further information and assistance, and a health care summary report, including a section dealing with how more effectively to communicate with physicians or other providers. In addition, a computer-generated summary was developed that could be sent to the health provider when requested by the participant.

The second phase of this project included further development of the questionnaire and refinement of the algorithms and feedback statements for the computer-generated personalized reports to the participants and where applicable, to their physicians. The feasibility of using the questionnaire survey instrument and personal reports were then field tested in three separate populations that reflected the range of settings in which it was envisaged that the HRA-E could be beneficially employed. The objective was to obtain information from individuals affiliated with each of these three groups of older adults that differ in their objectives as a group, their geographic distribution, and the age and gender groups that compose these populations. Although every attempt was made to obtain a representative sample from each group, this was difficult since one of our objectives was to measure the response to a single letter of invitation to a particular participant. Samples of eligible subjects 55 years and older from the American Association of Retired Persons (AARP), a large group practice, and a senior center were extended the invitation to participate. The recruitment strategies varied by site, but the majority of persons 55 years or older received a single letter of invitation. Response rates also varied by site, and the overall response rate was 15%. Those responding affirmatively to the invitation were given a questionnaire and evaluation form, and each person who returned the questionnaire received his or her personal report and a second evaluation form. Four months after receiving the reports, respondents were questioned about interim behavior changes.

Preliminary findings based on early analyses of 1,924 respondents indicate that nearly all participants found the questionnaire easy to complete and were pleased with its overall length. In addition, most participants read their reports, and many planned to take action on the basis of the reports' recommendations. These findings will be presented under the categories of Health Status and Health Risk Factors, Personal Health Habits, Physiological Risk Factors, and Preventive Practices and will be followed by a brief summary of the four-month evaluation. The evaluation is based on data obtained by the participant completing a self-administered questionnaire.

HEALTH STATUS AND HEALTH RISK FACTORS

From 25% to 30% of each of the three groups reported excellent health, 55% to 65% reported good health, and 11% to 16% reported fair to poor health. In the three groups, between 18% and 26% reported fair, poor, or no vision. Fair or poor hearing or deafness was common and ranged from 34% to 36% of each group. Between 20% and 25% of the participants reported at least a single fall in the past 12 months. Positive screens on the memory score, implying possible cognitive impairment, ranged from 8% to 18%, this being in part dictated by the age distribution of the three populations studied.

A positive depression screen (a score less than 66 using the RAND MHI items from the SF-36) was found in 10% to 23% of the samples, and between 15% and 32% of the samples were either isolated or deficient in their social network. A significant percentage of each group, ranging from 10% to 12%, had a positive screen for an adverse drug event to prescription medications, and 10% were taking five or more prescription drugs.

PERSONAL HEALTH HABITS

Two-thirds to three-quarters of each group reported participation in some form of physical activity on most days, 72% to 83% consistently avoided eating high-fat food, and only 5% to 7% were current cigarette smokers. A high proportion, 90% to 98%, always or nearly always wore seat belts. Alcohol consumption patterns revealed that of the combined total of 1,127 older drinkers across the three sites, 23.7% reported alcohol problems using either the Short MAST-6 or the CAGE.

PHYSIOLOGICAL RISK FACTORS

Self-reported systolic blood pressures above 140 occurred in one-third of each group, with almost 10% reporting systolic-diastolic hypertension. Between 20% and 35% of the population reported percentage serum cholesterol levels in excess of 240 milligrams.

PREVENTIVE PRACTICES

More than 95% of the three groups reported having a blood pressure check within the last year, and a similarly high proportion reported receiving cholesterol measurements within the past year. Over 80% of the group reported having a hearing test. Immunization for influenza in the past year was reported by approximately two-thirds of the populations studied, while only 37% to 49% had received pneumonia vaccination at any time. A very high percentage of the women in all groups had mammograms within the past two years (84% to 93%) with slightly lower percentages having had Pap smears (72% to 81%).

EVALUATION

Among the 65% of the participants who submitted an evaluation form immediately after receiving their individualized report, more than 90% had read all of the report, and the remainder had read most of it: 90% found it "very easy" to understand, and the remainder reported it to be "easy." In excess of 90% found the length "right," while 5% found it "too long" and 3% "too short." Ninety-five percent found the format to be "excellent" or "good," and more than two-thirds reported that they intended to take some steps as a result of the report.

Eighty percent of those who completed the questionnaire responded to a third evaluation request four months after receiving their personalized report. Preliminary examination of these data indicate a high response to the recommendations made in the participant report, especially for those recommendations pertaining to preventive health measures. Eighty-five percent of the respondents said that they had either had a blood pressure check or had one scheduled; 61% had or scheduled a cholesterol check. Over half reported having or scheduling a flu shot, and one-fourth reported the same for pneumonia vaccination. Nearly one-quarter reported having or scheduling a colonoscopy/sigmoidoscopy. Seventy-three percent had or scheduled a dental exam, and nearly 60% had or scheduled a vision exam. Only 21% had or scheduled a hearing exam. Twenty-nine percent reported increasing their physical activity levels, while 43% reported decreasing their intake of dietary fat. Rather small numbers reported increasing their seat belt use, decreasing their alcohol intake, or decreasing or quitting smoking since receiving their individualized report, but, as reported previously, many participants were already engaging in healthy behaviors except for alcohol use. On the basis of this experience, a revised health risk assessment for the elderly system has subsequently been developed, and the products of this work to date include the following:

1. A revised questionnaire for comprehensive health risk assessment of older persons

2. Revised software for processing computer-generated, personal reports to participants and their physicians from the returned questionnaire

3. Findings from testing the questionnaire and software in three different populations

4. Favorable experience with the HRA-E on the part of a long-established prestigious physician group

5. A substantial database consisting of information about responses, questionnaire item answers, reports to participants and physicians, participant evaluation of questionnaires and reports, and behavior changes reported four months later

6. A user guide

These products are envisaged for use in further refinement of the instrument and system in order to assess its impact in a randomized controlled trial design on outcomes such as behavior, health status, medical service utilization, and costs and offer a crucial body of information to assess whether this particular strategy of prevention of disability is effective and might be implemented on a large public health scale.

RESEARCH, PRACTICE, AND POLICY ISSUES

Issues of research, practice, and policy are in part addressed in each of this chapter's sections but are more explicitly articulated in this section. However, the magnitude of the problem of loss of independence as the baby boom begins to enter the elder phase of the life span and the importance of testing promising interventions directed at preventing or delaying the onset of functional impairment/disability deserve reiteration.

The disability burden has already been addressed from the national perspective, but the demographic shift is of even greater importance in California. In 1990, there were over three million persons 65 years of age or older, ranking first in the nation and involving 10% of the nation's senior population. It is estimated that California's elderly population will increase by 52% between 1990 and 2010.

Within the elderly population nationally, certain ethnic segments are growing more rapidly than others. The proportion of African Americans 65 years of age and older increased by 26% between 1980 and 1994. Hispanic elders increased by 103% in the same time period. Asian elders represent the greatest increase, from 210,000 to 565,000 (169%) in the 14-year time frame. California reflects this increased diversity and houses the most Hispanic and Asian individuals and the second-most African Americans in the United States.[72] Predictions made on the basis of the relationship of socioeconomic status to health would suggest even higher disability burdens in at least two of these three ethnic groups.

The health care system of the United States, and in particular that of California, is undergoing enormous changes, in part driven by the progressive rise in costs over the last several decades. These changes also reflect an apparent transition in the societal values of health from primarily being a "social good" to being an "economic good."

In addressing the issues relating to the prevention of functional impairment/disability, the implication is one of moving health care policy from "dependency" services to promoting "independence" through preventative strategies. This, too, would necessitate a major culture shift from the traditional treatment paradigm to one focusing on prevention. This change in policy with respect to older persons has actually been legislated in a number of member nations of the European Union in which a variety of "system" or structural problems are interfering with the optimal implementation of these legislative efforts.

In the United States, there is a great deal of rhetoric about prevention, particularly in the emerging managed care organizations. In this country, only a few of the long-established HMOs have moved their rhetorical statements to serious implementation activities. An understanding of the factors involved in the reticence to change is timely. There are serious questions about the effectiveness of prevention efforts and the feasibility of implementing programs for older persons at acceptable costs. These can be addressed only by a concerted research strategy addressing the unresolved issues. The most important of these can be addressed only by long-term studies since the increasing evidence of the effectiveness of disability prevention programs has been obtained in short-term studies of one to three years. In a recent literature review, there are over 1,000 papers addressing risk factors for impairment and disability, and the majority of the identified risk factors are amenable to a preventive intervention.

The remainder of this chapter discusses the future research, practice, and policy issues involved in the three types of intervention strategies discussed in this chapter.

COMPREHENSIVE GERIATRIC ASSESSMENT

Comprehensive geriatric assessment (CGA) in a clinical setting has become an established practice pattern for optimal quality clinical management. Multiple interrelated problems cutting across traditional disease categories are identified, be they physical, cognitive, affective, social, or environmental. Some of these problems fall outside the traditional clinical examination and are often missed by physicians. Moreover, the process of multidimensional assessment underscores the importance of functional status in addressing this issue. The assessment instruments used differ greatly in their usefulness in various clinical settings and are extensively discussed elsewhere.

The unresolved questions from a research and programmatic point of view include the following: (1) How can the populations that respond best to this intervention be identified? (2) What are the adherence issues with recommendations in both the older person and their providers? (3) What is the optimal frequency of the assessment? (4) What is the best way to link process to outcomes? (5) How can this process be most cost-effectively introduced into a prepaid health care system?

IN-HOME PREVENTION PROGRAMS

In addition to the unresolved issues raised in the previous section, the following questions apply specifically to in-home prevention programs: (1) Which professional grouping is most appropriate for carrying out these programs? (2) Where in a seamless health care system for older persons does a program of this type fit best? (3) How much are payors prepared to contribute to a prevention program, and who is responsible for payment? (4) What is the best quality control system to maintain high standards, and where does the responsibility for such a system lie? (5) Who is responsible for developing competency criteria for the providers and supplying them with the appropriate training? (6) How can older persons most effectively be motivated to participate in a program of this type? The issue of how to most effectively develop reliable communication systems between the principals holds for both the CGA and the in-home prevention strategies for delaying or preventing functional impairment (see Figure 16.6). In this figure, GNP refers to gerontologic nurse practitioner; C/A refers to communication/adherence issues as they relate to the nurse practitioners' recommendations for problem solution directed at both the older person and the physician; M.D. (geriatrician) implies that well-trained generalist physicians especially trained in the process of in-home prevention might substitute for a formally trained geriatrician. The lower part of the model suggests that the major out-

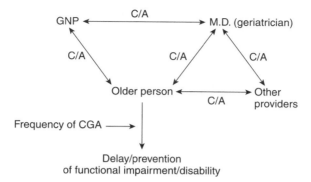

Figure 16.6.   Model of in-home prevention effectiveness.

come measure is a delay and/or prevention of the movement from independence to dependence of the older person.

HEALTH RISK ASSESSMENT SYSTEMS
FOR THE ELDERLY (HRA-E)

The majority of the unresolved questions in the previous two sections hold also for health risk assessment systems for the elderly (HRA-E). In addition, the following represent research questions that primarily confront this particular strategy: (1) What is the effect of HRA-E and immediate feedback on participants and their providers, as compared with more extended interventions targeted at one or both of these groups, on outcomes such as behavioral change, medical care utilization, functional status change, disenrollment from a health plan, satisfaction with care, and cost of the intervention related to estimated outcomes for individuals and for health plans? (2) When is the most opportune time for moving toward a quantitative rather than qualitative risk assessment so that future feedback algorithms might include quantitative statements about risk of functional decline? (3) What is the validity of self-reported information? (4) How can systems of this type be most effectively marketed? (5) How can readiness to change be most effectively determined? (6) What are the most beneficial strategies for bringing about behavioral change and self-care capabilities? (7) How can better strategies be developed to enhance long-term adherence with induced behavioral change? (8) In this era of rapidly changing health care technologies, how can the most appropriate method of administration be addressed, the options being self-administration, interviewer administered, computer assisted, and an in-

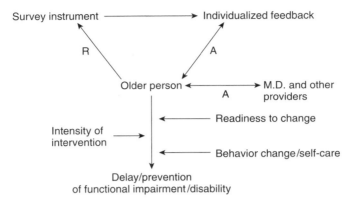

Figure 16.7. Model of HRA-E effectiveness.

teractive mode? These unresolved issues are illustrated in Figure 16.7. In this model, R (accuracy/honesty) refers to the reliability of the information given by the older person in completing the survey instrument; A refers to the adherence of the older person, their physician, and other providers to the individualized feedback resulting from completion of the survey instrument; intensity of the intervention refers to the frequency as well as to the characteristics of the feedback intervention; and readiness to change implies the older person's willingness to take these recommendations and respond to them.

It is important to recognize that effects are often diluted when interventions of these types are applied to large-scale community programs in the real world. Because the interventions comprise many individualized steps, standardizing the intervention to be applied outside the research setting is difficult. Relatively subtle changes in the intervention often result in lower levels of effectiveness.[73] To test an intervention's effect on reducing or preventing disability, we recommend that randomized clinical trials be conducted that are characterized by the identification of the critical risk factors for disability, clarification of the causal mechanisms behind their impact on disability, careful documentation of the components of the intervention process, linking of process to outcome, and delineation of the interplay across time between and among functional limitations and disability.

The recently published book *The Future of Long-Term Care: Social and Policy Issues*[74] contains a summary of a modified Delphi methodology of a large number of experts in the field addressing the issues of what the long-term-care system might look like early in the 21st century.

Implications of this forecasting suggest that emphasis should be placed on the following: prevention of disability; strengthening of the informal care system; improved management and service delivery based on careful evaluative analyses; increasing and enhancing the training of personnel in the field; promoting technology, including the information sciences; rethinking the issue of residential care, particularly long-term institutional care; improving quality by developing better methodologies; and creating an affordable financing system. The following paragraph, taken from this book, is worthy of emphasis: "Long-term care should be shaped by conscious choices about future directions, rather than being fated by seemingly random and uncontrollable events. As society ponders long-term care, it should not squander the future as it has the past."

NOTE

The author wishes to acknowledge many colleagues who have contributed to the studies referred to in this chapter: Cathy A. Alessi, Harriet U. Aronow, Lester Breslow, Christophe J. Bula, Jonathan Fielding, Jerilyn Higa, Christoph E. Minder, Alison A. Moore, Hal Morgenstern, Rosane Nissenbaum, Larry Z. Rubenstein, Andreas E. Stuck, and J. Walhart.

REFERENCES

1. American Association of Retired Persons/Administration on Aging, Program Resources Department. 1995. *A Profile of Older Americans: 1995*. Washington, D.C.: AARP/AOA.
2. Rosenwaike, I. 1985. A demographic portrait of the oldest old. *Milbank Memorial Fund Quarterly* 63(2), 187–205.
3. Lubitz, J., Beebe, J., and Baker, C. 1995. Longevity and Medicare expenditures. *New England Journal of Medicine* 332, 999–1003.
4. World Health Organization. 1980. *International Classification of Impairments, Disabilities, and Handicaps*. Geneva: World Health Organization.
5. Nagi, S. Z. 1991. Disability concepts revisited: Implications for prevention. In *Disability in America: For the National Agenda for Prevention*, edited by A. M. Pope and A. R. Tarlov. Pp. 309–217. Washington, D.C.: National Academy Press (for the Division of Health Promotion and Disease Prevention, Institute of Medicine).
6. Nagi, S. Z. 1965. Some conceptual issues in disability and rehabilitation. In *Sociology and Rehabilitation*, edited by M. B. Sussman. Pp. 100–113. Washington, D.C.: American Sociological Association.
7. Nagi, S. Z. 1979. The concept and measurement of disability. In *Disability*

Policies and Government Programs, edited by E. D. Berkowitz. Pp. 1–15. New York: Praeger.

8. Pope, A. M., and Tarlov, A. R., eds. 1991. *Disability in America: Toward a National Agenda for Prevention.* Washington, D.C.: National Academy Press (for the Division of Health Promotion and Disease Prevention, Institute of Medicine).

9. Verbrugge, L. M., and Jette, A. M. 1994. The disablement process. *Social Science Medicine* 38(1), 1–14.

10. It is important to view disability as a gap between personal capability and environmental demand. The terms "functional limitation" and "disability" are often used interchangeably, and although they are conceptually similar, they refer to different behaviors. Functional limitations refer to an individual capability without reference to situational requirements, while disability refers to the expression of a functional limitation in a social context, that is, the pattern of behavior arising from the loss or reduction of ability to perform expected or specified social role activities because of a chronic disease or impairment.

11. Verbrugge, L. M. 1987. From sneezes to adieux: Stages of health for American men and women. In *Health in Aging: Sociological Issues and Policy Directions,* edited by R. A. Ward and S. S. Tobin. Pp. 17–57. New York: Springer.

12. Verbrugge, L. M. 1990. Pathways of health and death. In *Women, Health, and Medicine in America: A Historical Handbook,* edited by R. D. Apple. Pp. 41–79. New York: Garland.

13. Jackson, M. E., Siu, A. L., Drugovich, M. L., et al. 1991. Alternative projections of the disabled elderly population. Report to the Administration on Aging, Washington, D.C.

14. Manton, K. G. 1989. Epidemiological, demographic, and social correlates of disability among the elderly. *Milbank Quarterly* 67 (Suppl. 2, pt. 1), 13–58.

15. Zedlewski, S., Barnes, R., Burr, M., et al. 1990. *The Needs of the Elderly in the 21st Century* (p. 45). Washington, D.C.: The Urban Institute.

16. Lee, D. J., and Markides, K. S. 1990. Activity and mortality among aged persons over an eight-year period. *Journal of Gerontology* 45(1), S39–S42.

17. McBride, T. 1989. *The Disabled Elderly: Empirical Analysis and Projections into the 21st Century.* Washington, D.C.: The Urban Institute.

18. Gruenberg, E. M. 1977. The failures of success. *Milbank Memorial Fund Quarterly* 55(1), 3–24.

19. Kramer, M. 1980. The rising pandemic of mental disorders associated with chronic diseases and disabilities. *Acta Psychiatrica Scandinavica Supplementum* 62, S285.

20. Fries, J. F. 1980. Aging, natural death, and the compression of morbidity. *New England Journal of Medicine* 303(3), 130–135.

21. Fries, J. F. 1983. The compression of morbidity. *Milbank Memorial Fund Quarterly* 61(3), 397–419.

22. Fries, J. F. 1989. The compression of morbidity: Near or far? *Milbank Quarterly* 67(2), 208–232.

23. Beck, J. C. 1996. Multicampus Program in Geriatric Medicine and Geron-

tology: Preventing disability: Beyond the black box. *Journal of the American Medical Association* 276(21), 1756–1757.

24. Manton, K. G., Corder, L., and Stallard, E. 1997. Chronic disability trends in elderly United States populations: 1982–1994. *Proceedings of the National Academy of Sciences* 94(March), 2593–2598.

25. Crimmins, E. M., Saito, Y., and Reynolds, S. L. 1997. Further evidence on recent trends in the prevalence and incidence of disability among older Americans from two sources: The LSOA and the NHIS. *Journal of Gerontology: Social Sciences* 52B(2), S59–S71.

26. Branch, L. G., and Jette, A. M. 1982. A prospective study of long-term care institutionalization among the aged. *American Journal of Public Health* 72(12), 1373–1379.

27. Kemper, C. 1988. The evaluation of the Long-term Care Demonstration Project: An overview of the findings. *Health Services Research* 23, 161–174.

28. Weissert, W. G., and Hedrick, S. C. 1994. Lessons learned from research on effects of community-based long-term care. *Journal of the American Geriatrics Society* 42, 348–353.

29. Weissert, W. G., Cready, C. M., and Pawelak, J. E. 1988. The past and future of home- and community-based long-term care. *Milbank Quarterly* 66, 309–388.

30. Weissert, W. G., Wan, T. T. H., Livieratos, B., et al. 1980. Cost-effectiveness of homemaker services for the chronically ill. *Inquiry* 17, 230–243.

31. Glick, P. C. 1979. The future marital status and living arrangements of the elderly. *The Gerontologist* 19(3), 301–309.

32. Greenberg, J., and Ginn, A. 1979. A multivariant analysis of the predictors of long-term care placement. *Home Health Care Services Quarterly* 1, 75–79.

33. Gruenberg, E. M. 1977. The failures of success. *Milbank Memorial Fund Quarterly* 55(1), 3–24.

34. Kramer, M. 1980. The rising pandemic of mental disorders associated with chronic diseases and disabilities. *Acta Psychiatrica Scandinavica Supplementum* 62, S285.

35. National Institutes of Health. 1988. Geriatric Assessment Methods for Clinical Decision-making. Consensus Development Conference Statement. *Journal of the American Geriatrics Society* 36, 342–347.

36. White House Conference on Aging. 1981. *Report of the Technical Committee on Health Services*. Washington, D.C.: U.S. Department of Health and Human Services.

37. Barker, W. H., Williams, T. F., Zimmer, J. G., et al. 1985. Geriatric consultation teams in acute hospitals: Impact on back-up of elderly patients. *Journal of the American Geriatrics Society* 33(6), 422–428.

38. Blumenfield, S., Morris, J., and Sherman, F. T. 1982. The geriatric team in the acute care hospital: An educational and consultation modality. *Journal of the American Geriatrics Society* 30(10), 660–664.

39. Lichtenstein, N., and Winograd, C. H. 1984. Geriatric consultation: A functional approach. *Journal of the American Geriatrics Society* 32(5), 356–361.

40. Rubenstein, L. Z., Josephson, K., Wieland, D., et al. 1987. Geriatric assessment on a subacute hospital ward. *Clinical Geriatric Medicine* 3, 131–143.

41. Steel, K., and Hays, A. 1981. A consultation service in geriatric medicine at a university hospital. *Journal of the American Medical Association* 245(14), 1410–1411.

42. Williams, M. E. 1987. Outpatient geriatric evaluation. *Clinics in Geriatric Medicine* 3(1), 175–183.

43. Epstein, A. M., Hall, J. A., Besdine, R., et al. 1987. The emergence of geriatric assessment units: The "new technology of geriatrics." *Annals of Internal Medicine* 106(2), 299–303.

44. Campion, E. W., Jette, A., and Berkman, B. 1983. An interdisciplinary geriatric consultation service: A controlled trial. *Journal of the American Geriatrics Society* 31(12), 792–796.

45. McVey, L. J., Becker, P. M., Saltz, C. C., et al. 1989. Effect of a geriatric consultation team on functional status of elderly hospitalized patients: A randomized, controlled clinical trial. *Annals of Internal Medicine* 110(10), 79–84.

46. Rubenstein, L. Z., Josephson, K. R., Wieland, D., et al. 1984. Effectiveness of a geriatric evaluation unit: A randomized clinical trial. *New England Journal of Medicine* 311(26), 1664–1670.

47. Rubenstein, L. Z., Stuck, A. E., Siu, A. L., and Wieland, D. 1991. Impacts of geriatric evaluation and management programs on defined outcomes: Overview of the evidence. *Journal of the American Geriatrics Society* 39(9, pt. 2), 8S-16S.

48. Vetter, N. J., Jones, D. A., and Victor, C. R. 1984. Effect of health visitors working with elderly patient in general practice: A randomized controlled trial. *British Medical Journal* 288, 369–372.

49. Hendricksen, C., Lund, E., and Stromgard, E. 1984. Consequences of assessment and intervention among elderly people: A three year randomized controlled trial. *British Medical Journal* 289, 1522–1524.

50. Pathy, M. S., Bayer, A., Harding, K., and Dibble, A. 1992. Randomized trial of case finding and surveillance of elderly people at home. *The Lancet* 340, 890–893.

51. Stuck, A. E., Siu, A. L., Wieland, D., et al. 1993. Effects of comprehensive geriatric assessment on survival, residents, and function: A meta-analysis of controlled trials. *The Lancet.*

52. Carpenter, G. I., and Demopoulis, G. R. 1990. Screening the elderly in the community: Controlled trial of dependency surveillance using a questionnaire administered by volunteers. *British Medical Journal* 300, 1253–1256.

53. McEwen, R. T., Davidson, N., Forster, D. P., et al. 1990. Screening elderly people in primary care: A randomized control trial. *British Journal of General Practice* 40, 94–97.

54. Hall, N., DeBeck, P., Johnson, D., and MacKinnan, K. 1992. Randomization trial of health promotion for frail elders. *Canadian Journal of Aging* 11(1), 72–91.

55. VanRossum, E., Frederiks, C. M. A., Philipsen, H., et al. 1993. Effects of preventive home visits to elderly people. *British Medical Journal* 307, 27–32.

56. Berkman, L. F. 1970. *Health and Ways of Living: The Alameda County Study* (pp. 149–178). New York: New York University Press.
57. Kaplan, G. A. 1992. Maintenance of functioning in the elderly. *Annals of Epidemiology* 2(6), 823–834.
58. Manton, K. G. 1988. A longitudinal study of functional changes and mortality in the United States. *Journal of Gerontology* 45, S153–S161.
59. Katz, S., Branch, L. G., Branson, M. H., et al. 1983. Active life expectancy. *New England Journal of Medicine* 309, 1218–1224.
60. Schneider, E. L., and Guralnik, J. M. 1990. The aging of America: Impact on health care costs. *Journal of the American Medical Association* 263(17), 2335–2340.
61. Rubenstein, L. Z., Aronow, H. U., Schloe, M., et al. 1994. A home-based geriatric assessment, follow-up and health promotion program: Design, methods and baseline findings from a 3-year randomized clinical trial. *Aging/ Clinical and Experimental Research* 6, 105–120.
62. Stuck, A. E., Aronow, H. U., Steiner, A., et al. 1995. A trial of annual in-home comprehensive geriatric assessments for elderly people living in the community. *New England Journal of Medicine* 333, 1184–1189.
63. National Center for Health Statistics, Adams, P. F., and Benson, V. 1990. *Current Estimates from the National Health Interview Survey, 1989: Vital and Health Statistics.* Series 10, No. 176. DHHS (PHS) 90-1504. Washington, D.C.: U.S. Government Printing Office.
64. National Center for Health Statistics, Benson, V., and Marano, M. A. 1994. *Current Estimates from the National Health Interview Survey, 1992: Vital and Health Statistics.* Series 10, No. 189. DHHS (PHS) 94-1517. Washington, D.C.: U.S. Government Printing Office.
65. Bula, C. J., Alessi, C. A., Aronow, H. U., et al. 1995. Community physicians' cooperation with a program of in-home comprehensive geriatric assessment. *Journal of the American Geriatrics Society* 43, 1016–1020.
66. Kornowski, R., Zeeli, D., Averbuch, M., et al. 1995. Intensive home-care surveillance prevents hospitalization and improves morbidity rates among elderly patients with severe congestive heart failure. *American Heart Journal* 129, 762–766.
67. Rich, M. W., Beekham, V., Wittenberg, C., et al. 1993. A multidisciplinary intervention to prevent the readmission of elderly patients with congestive heart failure. *New England Journal of Medicine* 333, 1190–1195.
68. Mittleman, M. S., Ferris, S. H., Shulman, E., et al. 1996. A family intervention to delay nursing home placement of patients with Alzheimer disease: A randomized controlled trial. *Journal of the American Medical Association* 276, 1725–1731.
69. Stuck, A. E., Zwahlen, H. G., Neuenschwander, B. E., et al. 1995. Methodologic challenges of randomized controlled studies on in-home comprehensive geriatric assessment: The EIGER project. *Aging/Clinical and Experimental Research* 7(3), 218–223.
70. Stuck, A. E., Stuckelberger, A., Zwahlen, H. G., et al. 1995. Visites préventives à Domicile avex évaluations gériatriques multidimensionnelles chez les 75 ans et plus: Project EIGER. *Medecine et Hygiene* 53, 2385–2397.

71. Breslow, L., Beck, J. C., Morgenstern, H., Fielding, J. E., Moore, A. A., Carmel, M., and Higa, J. 1997. Development of a health risk appraisal for the elderly (HRA-E). *American Journal of Health Promotion* 11(5), 337–343.

72. U.S. Bureau of the Census. 1995, September. *Vital Statistics, Statistical Abstract of the United States 1995.* 115th ed. Washington, D.C.: U.S. Bureau of the Census.

73. Wagner, E. H. 1996. The promise and performance of HMOs in improving outcomes in older adults. *Journal of the American Geriatrics Society* 44, 1251–1257.

74. Binstock, R. H., Cluff, L. E., and von Mering, O., eds. 1996. *The Future of Long-Term Care: Social and Policy Issues.* Baltimore: The Johns Hopkins University Press.

17

Stuart J. Slavin
and Michael S. Wilkes

AN EDUCATIONAL APPROACH TO ENGAGE
HEALTH CARE PROFESSIONALS
IN WELLNESS PROMOTION

Health care in the United States is changing rapidly. The importance of health promotion and disease prevention has been widely recognized. To work effectively in this new paradigm for medical care, physicians and other health care professionals need to acquire a new set of skills, knowledge, and values. David Rogers, M.D., wrote,

• Our nation needs doctors with a broader and more sensitive view of the place and role of medicine in the larger society. Doctors will need more skills with which to assess the efficacy of medical interventions and the relative contribution of medicine to the health of society.
• Our nation needs doctors who are more skillful in doctor-patient relationships. We should introduce a better blend of humanism and science into our health care institutions and the students they graduate.
• Modern physicians should pay more attention to health promotion, disease prevention, and the social, environmental, and emotional factors bearing on health.
• Both the physicians who graduate and the academic medical institutions that produce them should have a strong sense of social responsibility for the health and medical care rendered in their communities.[1]

Unfortunately, the education of health care professionals has not changed rapidly to fulfill this need. In 1991, the Pew Health Professions Commission surveyed health care professionals about perceptions of their educa-

TABLE 17.1   1996 ASSOCIATION
OF AMERICAN MEDICAL
COLLEGES GRADUATION SURVEY

Topic Area	% Rating Inadequate Teaching
Health promotion and disease prevention	25.2
Public health and community medicine	30.3
Role of community health and social service agencies	39.5
Nutrition	53.1
Cross-cultural communication	38.3

tion.[2] Forty-three percent of physicians rated their education in preventing disease as fair or poor, compared to 7% who rated their education in treating disease as fair or poor. Thirty-four percent of nurses surveyed also felt that their education in preventing disease was fair or poor.

Since 1991 there is little evidence of substantial improvement. In the 1996 Medical School Graduation Questionnaire of the Association of American Medical Colleges, medical students were asked if they believed that the time devoted to their instruction in a number of areas was excessive, appropriate, or inadequate.[3] Responses for issues relating to prevention and wellness are shown in Table 17.1.

Strikingly, only 4.1% of medical students felt that the time devoted to education in the basic sciences was inadequate.

New educational initiatives are needed to teach medical students, physicians in practice, and other health care professionals about issues relating to health, wellness, and disease prevention. It is crucial, given the changing health care needs of society, that these educational interventions be effective. How can we ensure effectiveness? By considering carefully not only what we teach but also how we teach.

THE GOAL OF EDUCATION

What elements are important to consider in designing an educational intervention? What pedagogical philosophies, strategies, and learning settings are most likely to produce effective learning? What are the roles of the teacher and the student? To answer these questions, it is critical first to define the learning outcomes we seek.

Numerous educators, researchers, and philosophers have proposed definitions for the ultimate goal of education. More than half a century ago, Alfred North Whitehead defined the goal of education as wisdom. He stated, "You cannot be wise without some basis of knowledge, but you may easily acquire knowledge and remain bare of wisdom." Whitehead saw wisdom as the mastery of knowledge and education as the acquisition of the art of the utilization of knowledge.[4] More recently, Paul Ramsden has referred to the goal of education as understanding not just the acquisition of facts but rather "the ability to use these facts to solve real problems."[5]

Benjamin S. Bloom and a group of cognitive psychologists have classified educational outcomes, with the result that the lowest cognitive level is acquisition of knowledge. Higher levels include application, analysis, synthesis, and evaluation. The mission of education from the standpoint of cognitive psychology is thus to help students move from memorization of discrete facts to more complex and more difficult cognitive levels.[6]

For the most thoughtful description of the goal of education, we return to Whitehead. He viewed the mission of education as the imaginative acquisition of knowledge: "The university imparts information but it imparts it imaginatively. . . . A university which fails in this respect has no reason for existence. This atmosphere of excitement, arising from imaginative consideration, transforms knowledge. A fact is no longer a bare fact: it is invested with all its possibilities. It is no longer a burden on the memory; it is energizing as the poet of our dreams and as the architect of our purposes."[4] Unfortunately, in many medical schools in the United States, little imagination is evident in the curriculum, and the students show little excitement about what they are learning. Excessive attention is paid to the acquisition of "bare facts," and little attention is paid to the development of wisdom or understanding. However, new alternatives to the traditional fact-based, lecture-based education of medical students are beginning to emerge and spread.

PRINCIPLES OF TEACHING AND LEARNING

How then do we help students to gain wisdom, to understand, and to function at higher cognitive levels? A number of principles need to be considered in the design and implementation of effective educational interventions.

Teaching methods should focus less on the transfer of information and more on the development of higher cognitive skills. Lecturing remains the dominant method of teaching at most American medical schools.

This approach to teaching is often effective and efficient as a means of transferring information, but often no deeper understanding of the material results from it. As Ramsden points out, "Research indicates that, at least for a short period, students retain vast quantities of information. On the other hand, many of them soon seem to forget much of it, and they appear not to make good use of what they do remember." In fact, medical educators have recognized this problem for many years. In 1932, the Association of American Medical Colleges (AAMC) Rappleye Commission stated, "The almost frantic attempt to put into the medical course teaching all phases of scientific and medical knowledge, and the tenacity with which traditional features of teaching are retained, have been responsible for great rigidity, overcrowding, and a lack of proper balance in the training." [7] More recently, the AAMC report on the General Professional Education of the Physician (GPEP) included in its first recommendation that "medical faculties must limit the amount of factual information that students are expected to memorize."

The acquisition and development of skills, values, and attitudes by students should be emphasized at least to the same extent as acquisition of knowledge. What are the skills, values, and attitudes that we want students to develop, and how can we help students develop them? The skills important in medical practice include the more difficult and complex tasks found in the higher cognitive domains, such as analysis, evaluation, critical thinking, and problem solving. Educators have also identified other important skills that students need to acquire. One is the skill of self-evaluation. It is crucial for students, particularly medical students, to have a sense of the limits of their knowledge—what they know and do not know. Svinicki believes that students also need to develop an awareness of "how their own biases and behaviors filter the information they receive." [8] Students also need to be able to communicate effectively with patients, families, and professional colleagues, and they need to be skilled in caring for people from diverse cultural backgrounds.

For physicians and other health care professionals, the acquisition of appropriate values and attitudes is as important as the acquisition of skills. Honesty, integrity, dedication, compassion, humanism, and an abiding concern for patients and colleagues are essential values that need to be fostered and nurtured.

Unfortunately, in traditional medical education, particularly in the first two preclinical years, little opportunity is provided for students to develop self-reflective skills, communication skills, and other appropriate values. The passive and impersonal experience of sitting in a lecture hall is unlikely to produce changes—at least positive ones—in skills and values. As an alternative to lecturing, small-group teaching has been used with success. In this teaching format, the focus is on understanding—through interaction and active participation—not just knowledge acquisition. Students take a more active role in learning. They discuss, analyze, evaluate, share perceptions of values, and reflect on gaps in knowledge or understanding. Students thus have the opportunity to practice some of the very skills we want them to develop.

A related approach to teaching in medical school that has received substantial attention and increased acceptance is problem-based learning (PBL), which is a systematic, structured approach to learning in which small groups of students work with faculty facilitators to solve clinical problems. Faculty have a very different role in PBL. Rather than serving as repositories of information that needs to be passed on to students, faculty act as guides to help direct student learning. The development and practice of higher-level cognitive skills is inherent in the process of problem-based learning. Students work through several steps to arrive at a solution:

1. Problem definition
2. Hypothesis generation
3. Data analysis
4. Identification of present knowledge and learning needs
5. Independent inquiry
6. Synthesis and reevaluation of problem
7. Problem resolution

Problem-based learning has been used extensively around the country in basic science teaching, but we believe that it is particularly well suited to teaching issues such as disease prevention, health promotion, and cross-cultural care.

To learn most effectively, students need to feel motivated. How are students motivated? One key factor is that learning should be engaging and enjoyable. The dominance of lecturing and the focus on the passive acquisition of vast quantities of information needed to pass the next series of exams can have a deadening and dispiriting effect on many students. There is strong evidence that students in small-group, problem-based curricula are happier and enjoy the learning experience more than their counterparts in traditional lecture-based curricula. For example, at Harvard Medical School, students in the PBL curriculum were more likely to describe their preclinical years as engaging and useful, while students in the conventional curriculum were more likely to describe these years as boring and passive.[9]

Another important factor in motivating students to learn is the bond between teacher and learner. In lecture-based courses, there is little opportunity for any meaningful connection between teachers and learners. The GPEP panel recognized this problem and recommended that "the practice of having a large number of faculty members, each of whom spends a relatively short period of time with medical students, should be examined critically and probably abandoned." They also stated that the "anonymous relationship between students and faculty is inconsistent with a general professional education directed toward the personal development of each student." [10] By contrast, in small-group settings, students have an opportunity for real dialogue with faculty. When faculty meet with students in small groups over the course of an academic year, meaningful interpersonal connections can be made.

Learning must be meaningful for the students. Learning can be made more meaningful for students in a number of ways:

1.   The content should be relevant and recognized as important by the students. The goal of medical education is to prepare future physicians for the practice of medicine. To be relevant, the content of the curriculum must therefore address important health needs in society and reflect the actual practice of medicine. Health care educators must thus help students recognize the importance of prevention in medical practice today.

2.   Teaching approaches should encourage easy retrieval of what has been learned. The traditional lecture-, discipline-, and fact-based curriculum does not encourage effective storage and future retrieval of information that has been learned by the student. Much of what is learned is soon forgotten, and that which is remembered cannot be easily utilized to solve clinical problems. By contrast, the educational strategies used in PBL courses facilitate this process of storage and retrieval. H. G. Schmidt termed the recall mechanism "encoding specificity." He hypothesized that retrieval of information is enhanced when the knowledge that is learned is acquired in a context that is similar to the future setting where it will be needed to solve a problem [11]—hence the theoretical strength of case- or problem-based learning: Knowledge begins to take on meaning when it is acquired in the appropriate context.

3.   Content should be developmentally sequenced, and planned repetition and opportunities for students to use knowledge in different contexts should be built into the curriculum. The meaning of what is learned
by third- and fourth-year medical students is very different from the
meaning of what is learned in the first year. By paying attention to the developmental level of medical students, learning opportunities can be constructed that provide deeper meaning by allowing students to build on
what they have learned and to make connections with other curricular
experiences. With planned repetition, students can use what they have
learned before to solve problems in new and somewhat different contexts.

A classic example of a case for developmental sequencing is the teaching
of medical ethics. Until recently, ethics at the University of California, Los
Angeles (UCLA), was taught in a brief course in the first eight weeks of
medical school and was never formally addressed again. Clearly, students
at this very early stage in their medical education have neither the prior
knowledge nor the clinical experience to develop a deep understanding
or appreciation of this important subject. Ethics (and other topics, such
as prevention) should be woven longitudinally throughout the curriculum. Students can then use the concepts they have learned in the first
years to solve new and more complex problems as they gain experience
and progress in their studies.

Students must be encouraged to develop independent learning skills.
There is simply no way that medical students can be provided with all
the information they will need to solve all the clinical problems they will
encounter in their careers. New knowledge about diagnostic techniques
and therapeutic approaches is constantly emerging and must be evaluated
by physicians. Also, clinical problems do not always fit classical or typical patterns, and physicians need to be able to recognize gaps in their
own understanding and know how to rectify these deficiencies.

In traditional medical education, students are not rewarded for independent inquiry and endeavor; in fact, these activities are often sup-
pressed and extinguished by the oppressive focus on specific knowledge
acquisition and the emphasis on learning what is needed to excel in the
next exam. In PBL courses, independent inquiry is an essential part of
the process for all students.

Student and faculty roles must change. This new paradigm for learning calls for a new partnership between students and faculty. Students
must take a more active role, assuming greater responsibility for their
own learning. They can no longer expect to sit passively and simply

absorb as much information as possible. For their part, faculty cannot serve as mere sources of information that must be passed on to the students. Rather, they need to facilitate and guide the process of learning by helping students ask the right questions, helping direct their inquiry, and providing appropriate and timely feedback, and they must be open to learning themselves.

CHANGING PHYSICIAN PRACTICE BEHAVIORS

The principles outlined here have proven helpful in designing effective undergraduate medical curricula. These and additional factors should also be considered, however, in designing better ways to change the behaviors of practicing physicians.

For some time the public has assumed that clinicians actively seek out new medical information and respond by changing their behaviors if they believe that the information will improve care for their patients. In this scenario, effective dissemination of new information is thought to be the key variable in changing physician behaviors. Dissemination is understood to involve the communication of information from one or more sources through various channels (journals, conferences, word of mouth, and popular press) to an audience of clinicians. Physicians are assumed to be active consumers of new information, eager to keep abreast of the latest developments and willing and able to devote the time necessary to ferret out sources of information for practical clinical pearls.

The task of changing clinicians' behaviors has traditionally been thought to be limited only by an inability to reach the practitioners with accurate, timely information. However, researchers have failed repeatedly to find much change in practitioner behaviors, even when all conditions for effective dissemination of information are ideal. Alternative views of clinician behavior have been suggested to explain this failure. It has been postulated that changing physicians' behaviors requires more than simply providing believable and relevant information; it requires a better understanding of the context in which clinical decisions are made.[12-14] Some educators have applied social psychology—specifically, concepts of social influence—to understand methods of behavioral change,[15-17] others have used cognitive psychology, and still others have invoked theories that derive from sociology. Whatever the explanation, rarely does dissemination alone change physician practice behaviors.

It could be argued that physicians will change a behavior if the information provided to them is accurate and well proven, such as findings from randomized controlled trials (RCTs). Despite the difficulty in discerning behavior changes, it is clear that physicians do not respond rapidly or in large numbers to newly published findings of RCTs. In many cases, little or no change in practice may occur, even after a considerable amount of time has elapsed.

Others might feel that physicians want their colleagues or groups of experts to endorse or recommend a given change in behavior before they incorporate it into their practice. The most extensive exercise of professional influence involves the dissemination of consensus recommendations. The dissemination strategies used by different consensus projects vary, but the dominant strategy has been publication of consensus statements both in booklet form and in medical journals. In surveys, however, only 25% to 60% of physicians in the United States report hearing about conference recommendations addressing their medical specialties.[18,19] Behavioral change is thus not ensured by practitioners' reading habits, a finding that is not encouraging to those who seek to affect physicians' behaviors by written interventions.[19]

Physicians also rank the importance of various information sources somewhat differently. For example, different publications may hold different credibility levels for practitioners. Ideally, we would like to know how influential different channels are in changing practice behaviors, but this turns out to be difficult to measure; most studies rely on providers' self-reports through questionnaires or interviews. Providers' ability to report accurately on what influences their decisions in such circumstances is open to question.

How, then, are physician behaviors determined? A host of different factors, including environmental, organizational, clinical, specialty, patient, and provider characteristics, affect behaviors. Environmental characteristics are external influences, such as laws and financial incentives. Organizational characteristics are determinants unique to a practice setting, such as a managed care organization or hospital. Clinical characteristics are determinants of behavior based on patient disease characteristics, such as those associated with HIV infection or substance abuse. Specialty determinants are related to specialty training and socialization. Patient characteristics are factors related to the patient (age, gender, race, affect, education, and values) that determine provider behavior. A number of provider characteristics (socioeconomic background, schooling, and gender) also contribute to determine behavior. Finally, information—the form that it takes and the way in which it is delivered to clinicians—has the potential to change behavior. In order to change physician behavior effectively, each of the previously mentioned determinants must be recognized, and those that pose barriers must be dealt with explicitly.

CONTINUING MEDICAL EDUCATION

Continuing medical education (CME) is the primary educational forum for the acquisition of knowledge by practicing physicians. Ninety-seven percent of a random sample of physicians reported that they had participated in continuing medical education activities in the last year, many because it is a state licensing requirement.[19] The purposes of CME vary. In some cases, CME results from a physician's self-recognized need for new knowledge in order to improve patient outcomes. Some courses, however, may be chosen mainly because of the attractiveness of the locale. In other cases, an organization (hospital, HMO, or state licensing board) may look to CME to increase the likelihood that physicians will implement an appropriate therapeutic or diagnostic approach under a given set of circumstances.

Continuing medical education seems to be an effective method of disseminating some types of simple factual knowledge but is not very effective in other respects, particularly in terms of influencing a behavioral change. To gain an understanding of the conditions under which CME is an effective intervention for disseminating information and thereby changing physicians' behavior, we should first recognize that there are several contextual issues. These include the characteristics and level of interest of those engaged in the CME activity, the requirement for attendance (state license, HMO mandate, or physician choice), the behavior targeted for change, and the methods of instruction employed. (As in undergraduate medical education, the standard approach of most CME courses has been to provide fact-laden lectures to the learners.)

Researchers have examined these issues and identified some attributes of successful education. For example, face-to-face contact is an especially effective way to achieve behavioral change.[20–23] This and other conclusions are suggested largely by considering the shared characteristics of interventions that have been successful. Unfortunately, randomized trials in which the same practice recommendations or guidelines are promulgated through more than one intervention are practically nonexistent, so far-reaching conclusions are not possible. However, based on a careful review of the literature, additional elements of continuing medical education that appear most likely to produce behavioral change include the following:

- Involving opinion leaders wherever possible
- Addressing real and perceived barriers to implementation of new practice behaviors
- Offering realistic alternatives to the practices being discouraged
- Repeating and reinforcing major points in the message
- Actively involving the learner, preferably with a chance to practice the behavior(s) or see others perform the behaviors
- Following the intervention with behavioral feedback to the learner
- Providing supportive materials for later use
- Using multiple teaching methods during the course of the intervention

Not surprisingly, the strategies listed here, which have been successful in changing practicing physicians' behaviors, are very similar to those that are beginning to be employed in medical schools.

THE UCLA DOCTORING CURRICULUM

A curriculum that incorporates these educational principles is Doctoring, a three-year, longitudinal program for medical students at the UCLA School of Medicine.[24,25] The overarching goal of Doctoring is to ensure competencies in areas that allow our graduates to care for patients, families, and communities in a compassionate, humanistic, and competent manner. Such a daunting educational mission could not be contained within a single course, a single semester, or even a single department or discipline. Thus, Doctoring was designed as a three-year sequence, emphasizing special areas in each year, but with a cascading approach to major goals. The curriculum is coordinated by faculty from the three generalist disciplines (i.e., internal medicine, pediatrics, and family medicine) with input from multiple expert working groups. Curricular time and content for Doctoring came from a merger of previously existing courses, such as behavioral sciences, medical ethics, clinical correlates, epidemiology, and clinical fundamentals. These orphan courses, each standing alone, had little status relative to the basic science courses, but together they formed nearly a fifth of total curricular time. In addition, topics such as violence, substance abuse, and AIDS, largely absent in the curriculum before, were incorporated into Doctoring.

A major concept of Doctoring is integration, which works at three levels. First, in each module we integrate material from a variety of subject areas (ethics, epidemiology, and behavioral medicine) needed to understand and provide care for the patient. The second level of integration is horizontal and is directed toward the basic science courses. During a module that focuses on elder abuse, for example, students simultaneously learn about health problems, psychopathology, and neurology in the elderly within their basic science courses. The third level of integration involves a vertical approach across the three years of the Doctoring sequence, ensuring that content areas such as ethics or interviewing are not limited to one semester but rather reappear on a regular basis. This allows students to build sequentially on their knowledge base by applying familiar content in new contexts. What students learn about confidentiality in the third year, for example, is built on the basic principles they learn in the first year.

In the first and second years, Doctoring combines an ambulatory patient care experience with a small-group, problem-based learning experience that stresses the development of communication skills and self-directed learning. Students work in groups of eight with two faculty tutors (one generalist and one mental health professional/social scientist). Learning in both years is organized into a series of four-week modules, each driven by a particular clinical problem. In week 1 of each module, the group is introduced to a problem using a standardized patient (an actor trained to portray a patient in a reproducible manner), a videotaped vignette, an iterative paper case, or a real patient. Using an inquiry approach, students seek to define the problem, identify and acquire relevant data, formulate explanatory models and hypotheses, and identify questions for independent learning. (Preliminary evaluation has shown that the vast majority of learning issues that the faculty have designated as key are also identified by the students as important areas of study.) A protected half day for independent study in week 2 of the module allows students to pursue their special interests, build on prior life experiences, and apply their preferred learning styles. Students research their learning issues in locations such as nontraditional health care facilities (jail clinics, hospices, and homeless shelters), a patient's home, religious centers, and community-based support groups. In addition, community experts are invited to the medical center at designated times so that students can easily contact them to ask specific questions.

During week 3, students visit a generalist preceptor in the community (someone working in private practice or at an HMO or county clinic) for a longitudinal clinical experience. During these sessions the emphasis is on perfecting interviewing and physical examination skills. Students also spend up to a half day working through a set of clinical epidemiology problems that relate to the case at hand.

In the fourth and final week of the module, students again meet in their Doctoring groups and discuss learning issues in a manner that allows the group to explore the topics in greater depth, focusing on how they relate to the care of the patient.

In Doctoring 1, the first year of the Doctoring Curriculum, major themes include eliciting a patient's experience of illness, taking a comprehensive psychosocial history, promoting health through nutrition, understanding ethical issues in the context of patient care, and understanding major health care issues at different stages of life.

The major foci for Doctoring 2 are the physical examination, basic clinical reasoning skills, population-based medicine, an approach to solving ethical dilemmas, counseling for promotion of health, and an awareness of cultural and social perspectives of illness and disease.

As with nearly all U.S. medical schools, once the clinical years begin at UCLA, students tend to consider a substantial part of the knowledge acquired in years 1 and 2 as nonessential to the actual practice of medicine. Without reinforcement, the skills, knowledge, and attitudes developed in Doctoring 1 and 2 might be quickly extinguished by the culture in the clerkships, which focuses on treatment of acute disease in hospitalized patients, mechanisms of disease, memorization of lists and facts, and professionalization through indoctrination. A major goal, then, of Doctoring 3 is to reinforce and preserve concepts acquired in Doctoring 1 and 2 while at the same time introducing important new content areas not covered elsewhere in the curriculum. Throughout the third year, students in their small groups are encouraged to discuss real and perceived barriers to practice. In Doctoring 3 we do not use a four-week module system; rather, each small group manages a fictitious panel of patients for the entire year.

Doctoring deals with a broad range of wellness and prevention issues over the three years of the curriculum. An example of a wellness issue of critical educational importance that Doctoring deals with is violence, particularly domestic violence.

Violence in the United States

Over the last decade, violence has been recognized as a major threat to the health, well-being, and safety of an increasing number of Americans.

The problem of violence crosses demographic and socioeconomic lines; it affects all ages, from children to the elderly. The magnitude of the problem is enormous, and the available statistics are staggering. Over 25,000 homicides occur each year in the United States, with murder being the leading cause of death for both Black men and Black women between 15 and 24 years of age. There are approximately 30,000 deaths from suicide each year, and the suicide rate among 15- to 24-year-olds has tripled in the past three decades.

Violence against women is endemic in the United States, and the greatest risk occurs in the home. It is estimated that between two and four million women are severely physically abused each year by their partners.[26] Even pregnancy offers no protection but actually appears to increase the risk of abuse: An estimated 4% to 8% of pregnant women are physically abused.[27] Sexual violence against women is also widespread. The incidence of date rape has been estimated to be as high as 20% for adolescent females.[28]

Another group at high risk for violence is children, 1.6 million of whom experience some form of nonfatal abuse or neglect each year.[29] One hundred and sixty thousand are seriously harmed, and between 1,200 and 5,000 children die each year as a result of injuries inflicted by an abusive relative.[29] The elderly are equally at risk: The prevalence of elder abuse is estimated to be between 4% and 10%, which translates to 1.5 to 3.2 million Americans.[30]

No single approach can address or combat the problem of violence; it would be naive to think so, given the prevalence and complexity of the problem. Nevertheless, it is clear that the medical profession and clinicians must play a far larger role in defining and implementing potential solutions. Health care professionals are the ones most likely to see victims of violence or those at risk for becoming victims. As such, the medical community constitutes a front line for identification, intervention, and prevention.

Unfortunately, substantial evidence suggests that health care professionals are not fulfilling this essential role. It has been reported that between 11.7% and 35% of women visiting emergency rooms are there because of symptoms of ongoing abuse, yet only 5% of victims of domestic violence are so identified.[26,31,32] In one study, 20% of domestic violence victims reported seeking medical care for injuries more than 10 times. Another 23% had seen a physician between 6 and 10 times for care of abuse-related injuries.[33]

In the area of domestic violence in particular, a number of barriers have been identified that may help to explain the general unresponsiveness of physicians in terms of recognition and intervention. Close identification with patients, fear of causing offense, feelings of powerlessness, an inability to control outcomes, and time constraints in practice have all been found to be significant factors.[34] One of the most important factors, however, is the lack of training that most physicians have received in this area. Physicians and other health professionals are ill prepared to help their patients largely because of the absence of violence-related education in undergraduate, graduate, and CME curricula. Numerous community and professional groups have called for increased attention to violence at all levels of medical education. Yet there has been little improvement to date. In 1994, over 50% of graduating medical students in the United States rated their instruction in family and domestic violence as inadequate.[35] Through the Doctoring course, UCLA was one of the first medical schools to institute an integrated substantive educational intervention relating to domestic violence.

Domestic Violence Module

The domestic violence module, which focuses primarily on partner abuse, is one of eight educational units in the second year of Doctoring. It is worth describing in detail since it employs many of the educational elements mentioned previously. Beyond the goal of developing a substantial knowledge base about the epidemiology of domestic violence, signs and symptoms of abuse, legal and ethical issues relating to violence, and resources and options for victims, the module is designed to help students develop the essential clinical skills (interviewing, counseling, and diagnosis) and values (empathy and trust) required to apply this knowledge in practice to provide sensitive care to patients.

The specific learning objectives are as follows:

Knowledge

K1. Define domestic violence (societal and legal definitions)

K2. Recognize the prevalence of domestic violence in the United States today; recognize how frequently women seek medical care for this problem and how frequently physicians miss this diagnosis

K3. Identify predisposing and predictive characteristics of both victims and abusers

K4. Recognize common presenting signs, symptoms, "stories," and red-flag indicators of abuse

K5. Describe reasons why a victim may not recognize a relationship as abusive

K6. Describe reasons why a victim may be reluctant to make disclosure of domestic violence or seek help

K7. Identify reasons why a victim may remain in an abusive relationship

K8. Identify questions with which physicians can encourage patients to talk about domestic violence

K9. Describe reasons why physicians may avoid inquiring about abuse or intervening when abuse is uncovered

K10. Identify local legal requirements regarding reporting domestic violence and potential limits of confidentiality

K11. List elements that should be included when documenting a case of abuse

K12. Identify community resources and legal recourse available to victims

K13. Identify steps that a victim may take to increase safety

Skills

S1. Conduct a sensitive, empathetic, detailed history when domestic violence is suspected

S2. Conduct a sensitive screening history for domestic violence when abuse is not suspected

Attitudes

A1. Appreciate the central roles that physicians may play in helping victims of domestic violence

A2. Feel a personal responsibility to identify domestic violence victims and intervene appropriately when domestic violence is identified

A3. Appreciate the need to screen all patients for the risk or presence of domestic violence

In the first week of the module, students and faculty meet in their small groups to view a videotape of a clinical encounter. A young man brings his girlfriend to the emergency room, saying that she has some kind of eating disorder. The man's approach toward the woman and the physician is aggressive and controlling. The physician pursues the boyfriend's agenda and begins to ask the patient questions about her diet and her weight. When the visit does not proceed as he wishes, however, the boyfriend is verbally and physically abusive to the patient and then storms out of the examining room. Despite these obvious signs of problems with the couple's interactions, the physician quietly returns to questioning the traumatized woman about her supposed eating disorder.

After viewing the videotape, students have the opportunity to discuss their perceptions and feelings about the encounter. What was really going on? Despite the fact that no obvious physical harm was inflicted, does this constitute abuse on the part of the boyfriend? Do our own ethnic or social backgrounds influence our perceptions and understanding of abuse? How did the doctor handle the situation? Should he have done anything differently? Why did he miss or ignore the signs of abuse? What might he have been feeling? Following this discussion, students participate in an "invent-an-interview" exercise. They explore what questions should be asked when someone is at risk for or a victim of abuse. After constructing their own list of questions, students compare their list with the recommended questions from the American Medical Association's Diagnostic Treatment Guidelines on Domestic Violence.

In the next segment of the session, students are told that they will interview a standardized patient (SP) using the skills that they have just discussed. They are then given Mrs. Rita Brown's medical records to examine prior to her arrival. The triage note states that Mrs. Brown is a "48-year-old female requesting pain medication for headaches following a car accident the day before." In fact, she is a victim of ongoing abuse at home. Mrs. Brown's medical record (physician notes, X-ray reports, and emergency room encounter forms) chronicles a long history of different types of injuries.

The SP is then brought in, and one student begins the interview in front of the group. Time-outs can be called by the interviewer or faculty when students need guidance from their peers or when the seminar leader feels a sufficient number of teaching points have been raised. During these time-outs, the action freezes and the SP goes into "suspended animation." The group can then assess what is transpiring. These discussions are particularly rich, as attention is paid both to what is being learned about the patient and to how it is being learned. Consideration is given to the most effective communication approach and the feelings that the interviewer experiences while talking to the patient. Finally, approaches and strategies for continuing the interview are explored and, after a "time-in," the same student resumes the interview.

When initially confronted about violence at home, Mrs. Brown is reticent to discuss her circumstances and denies any problem. With a supportive and compassionate approach to interviewing, however, she eventually admits that her husband has physically abused her.

After the completion of the interview, students identify learning issues that they will pursue to help them better understand and provide care for Mrs. Brown and other victims of domestic violence. These learning issues constitute many of the objectives outlined previously. For example, one student might choose to look into ethical and legal issues surrounding the reporting of domestic violence to law enforcement; another might research resources such as hotlines and shelters.

In the second week of the module, students are given protected time to pursue their learning issues. Expert resource persons from the faculty and the community (victims, victim advocates, shelter directors, physicians with expertise in domestic violence, police officers, assistant district attorneys, and social workers) meet with the students at prearranged times. The experts are told not to give a lecture but rather to respond to students' questions and needs. In addition, students are given required and optional readings on the problem of violence. Finally, students can research their learning issues in other ways. Some students, for example, may independently arrange to visit shelters and support groups for battered women.

In week 3 of the module, the entire second-year class attends a Doctoring forum in which several women talk about their own experiences with domestic violence and the response, or lack of response, of physicians in their cases. In addition, the male director of a residential counseling center for abusers shares his perspective. The forum gives students the opportunity to hear firsthand accounts, which has proved to be a very powerful and moving experience for them—and for the panelists. During this week the students also work through a problem set concerning the epidemiology of domestic violence. In this exercise, students evaluate the reliability of data from different sources, assess the quality of data on the incidence/prevalence of domestic violence arising from hospital emergency rooms, and identify approaches to improving surveillance for this problem. In the final week of the module, students return to their tutorial groups and discuss what they have learned in the context of Mrs. Brown's case and review what advice they might offer her.

The teaching approach used in this module affords students the opportunity to begin to develop a deeper understanding of the problem of domestic violence rather than just accumulating a group of facts and statistics that are not grounded in real experience. Students are actively engaged in the educational process and can tailor their learning by pursuing independent study. There is also a substantial focus on essential clinical skills, such as communication with patients and diagnostic reasoning. Finally, students have the opportunity to compare their values with those of other students and to consider some important questions for themselves: What is abuse? Where should the line be drawn? What has been accepted as appropriate behavior in different cultures?

CONCLUSION: IMPLICATIONS FOR THE EDUCATION OF HEALTH PROFESSIONALS

Just as it is increasingly important to teach medical students about the problem of domestic violence, many practicing physicians need to be trained in this area as well. Internists, family physicians, pediatricians, orthopedists, obstetricians, neurosurgeons, and ophthalmologists all encounter—and yet often fail to recognize—patients who suffer from injuries due to abuse. Other health care professionals, such as nurses, physical therapists, psychologists, and social workers, also need to receive formal and effective education on violence prevention and treatment. The same holds true for prevention and health promotion in such areas as smoking, drug and alcohol abuse, high-risk sexual activity, and depression.

In developing new and innovative curricula for these groups, the Doctoring Curriculum does not necessarily need to be replicated. Rather, the educational principles that underlie Doctoring should be taken and applied to the particular teaching setting. For example, in the typical CME course, the time is not available for longitudinal, PBL experiences. The teaching format could, however, make use of small groups and interactive learning techniques. A three-hour CME workshop on domestic violence could use activities similar to those of the first week of the domestic violence module: viewing a videotape of the clinical encounter with the abusive boyfriend, inventing a domestic violence interview, and interviewing a standardized patient. Instead of pursuing learning issues (as is done in a PBL approach), learners could attend a lecture that provides an overview of the key issues in providing appropriate care for the patient. Finally, for a CME workshop, it would be essential to address barriers to appropriate clinical responses to domestic violence.

Given the great need for more effective approaches to prevention and health promotion in our society, it is more important than ever that health care educators assume a key role in effecting change. Our hope is that this chapter will stimulate others to think creatively about teaching, particularly where behavioral change is the goal.

NOTE

We wish to thank the many faculty, staff, and students who helped in the creation of the Doctoring Curriculum at the UCLA School of Medicine. In particular, we appreciate the contributions of Richard Usatine, Marjorie Covey, Elizabeth O'Gara, LuAnn Wilkerson, David Schriger, and the Curricular Working Group on Violence. Brenda Hanning provided invaluable assistance in the editing and preparation of this manuscript.

REFERENCES

1. Rodgers, David. 1991. *Adapting Clinical Medical Education to the Needs of Today and Tomorrow*. Proceedings of the Josiah Macy, Jr. Foundation National Seminar on Medical Education, 1988.
2. Pew Health Professions Commission. 1991. Survey of practitioners' perceptions of their education.
3. Association of American Medical Colleges, Section for Educational Research. 1996. *Graduating Student Survey Results*. Washington, D.C.: AAMC.
4. Whitehead, A. N. 1967. *The Aims of Education and Other Essays*. New York: The Free Press.
5. Ramsden, P. 1992. *Learning to Teach in Higher Education*. New York: Routledge.
6. Bloom, B. S., Englehard, M. D., Furst, E. J., et al. 1956. *Taxonomy of Educational Objectives: Cognitive Domain*. New York: McKay.
7. Rappleye, W. C. 1932. *Medical Education: Final Report of the Commission of Medical Education*. New York: Association of American Medical Colleges.
8. Svinicki, M. D. 1991. Practical implications of cognitive theories. *New Directions for Teaching and Learning* 45, 27–37.
9. Moore, G. T., Block, S. D., Briggs-Style, C., and Mitchell, R. 1994. The influence of the new pathway curriculum on Harvard medical students. *Academic Medicine* 69, 983–989.
10. Muller, S. 1984. Physicians for the twenty-first century: Report of the project panel on the general professional education of the physician and college preparation for medicine. *Journal of Medical Education* 59(2).

11. Schmidt, H. G. 1983. Problem-based learning: Rationale and description. *Medical Education* 17, 11–16.
12. Eisenberg, J. M. 1986. *Doctors' Decisions and the Cost of Medical Practice: The Reasons for Doctors' Practice Patterns and Ways to Change Them.* Ann Arbor, Mich.: Health Administration Press.
13. Kanouse, D. E., and Jacoby, I. 1988. When does information change practitioners' behavior? *International Journal of Technology Assessment in Health Care* 4, 27–33.
14. Lomas, J., and Haynes, R. B. 1988. A taxonomy and critical review of tested strategies for the application of clinical practice recommendations: From "official" to "individual" clinical policy. *American Journal of Preventive Medicine* 4(Suppl.), 77–94.
15. Deutsch, M., and Gerard, H. B. 1955. A study of normative and informational social influences upon individual judgment. *Journal of Abnormal and Social Psychology* 51, 629–636.
16. French, J. R. P., and Raven, B. 1959. The bases of social power. In *Studies in Social Power,* edited by D. Cartwright. Pp. 150–167. Ann Arbor, Mich.: Institute for Social Research.
17. Schopler, J. 1965. Social power. *Advances in Experimental Social Psychology* 2, 177–218.
18. Hill, M. N., Levine, D. M., and Whelton, P. K. 1988. Awareness, use, and impact of the 1984 Joint National Committee Consensus Report on High Blood Pressure. *American Journal of Public Health* 78, 1190–1194.
19. Kanouse, D. E., Winkler, J. D., Kosecoff, J., et al. 1989. *Changing Medical Practice through Technology Assessment: An Evaluation of the NIH Consensus Development Program.* Ann Arbor, Mich.: Health Administration Press.
20. Avorn, J., and Soumerai, S. B. 1983. Improving drug-therapy decisions through educational outreach: A randomized controlled trial of academically based "detailing." *New England Journal of Medicine* 308, 1457–1463.
21. Palmer, R. H., Louis, T. A., Hsu, L. N., et al. 1985. A randomized controlled trial of quality assurance in sixteen ambulatory care practices. *Medical Care* 23, 751–770.
22. Stross, J. K., and Bole, G. G. 1980. Evaluation of a continuing medical education program in arthritis. *Arthritis and Rheumatism* 23, 846–849.
23. Stross, J. K., Hiss, R. G., Watts, C. M., et al. 1983. Continuing education in pulmonary disease for primary-care physicians. *Annual Review of Respiratory Diseases* 127, 739–746.
24. Wilkes, M. S., Slavin, S. J., and Usatine, R. 1994. Doctoring: A longitudinal generalist curriculum. *Academic Medicine* 69(March), 191–193.
25. Slavin, S. J., Wilkes, M. S., and Usatine, R. 1995. Innovations in generalist education in the clinical years. *Academic Medicine* 70(12, December), 1091–1095.
26. Novello, A. C., Rosenberg, M., Saltzman, L., and Shosky, J. 1992. A medical response to domestic violence. *Journal of the American Medical Association* 267(23), 3132.
27. Council on Ethical and Judicial Affairs, American Medical Association.

1992. Physicians and domestic violence: Ethical considerations. *Journal of the American Medical Association* 276(23), 3190–3193.

28. Davis, T. C., Peck, G. Q., and Storment, J. M. 1993. Acquaintance rape and the high school student. *Journal of Adolescent Health* 14, 220–224.

29. Reiss, A. J., and Roth, J. A., eds. 1993. *Understanding and Preventing Violence*. Washington, D.C.: National Academy Press.

30. Council of Scientific Affairs, American Medical Association. 1987. Elder abuse and neglect. *Journal of the American Medical Association* 257(7), 966–971.

31. Randall, T. 1990. Domestic violence intervention calls for more than treating injuries. *Journal of the American Medical Association* 264, 939–940.

32. Abbott, J., Johnson, R., Koziol-McLain, J., and Lowenstein, S. R. 1995. Domestic violence against women: Incidence and prevalence in an emergency department population. Journal of the American Medical Association 273, 1763–1767.

33. Council on Scientific Affairs, American Medical Association. 1992. Violence against women: Relevance for medical practitioners. *Journal of the American Medical Association* 267(28), 3184.

34. Sugg, N. K., and Inue, T. 1992. Primary care physicians' response to domestic violence: Opening Pandora's box. *Journal of the American Medical Association* 267(27), 3157–3160.

35. Association of American Medical Colleges, Section for Educational Research. 1994. *Graduating Student Survey Results*. Washington, D.C.: AAMC.

18

■

Philip R. Nader

UNIVERSITY-COMMUNITY PARTNERSHIPS
TO PROMOTE WELLNESS IN CHILDREN,
YOUTH, AND FAMILIES

Wellness promotion can be defined as the enhancement of physical, mental, and social well-being and the prevention of disease and disability. Efforts to promote wellness are difficult because (1) wellness promotion does not have the "press appeal" of a dramatic cure or a high-technology advance, (2) the benefits of wellness promotion may be delayed (3) wellness promotion may encounter strong industry lobby interests (e.g., tobacco), and (4) the crisis of immediate unmet needs overshadows allocation of resources for prevention.

The enhancement of physical, mental, and social well-being and the prevention of disease and disability for all children and youth in our society will require new partnerships and collaboration among a broad range of public, private, and community organizations that interact with youth and families on a routine basis. These may be organizations that traditionally have not worked together very effectively. To form these new partnerships and collaborations, certain barriers will have to be overcome, including professional and turf issues, categorical funding, fragmentation, diverse institutional missions, bureaucracy, communication problems, and lack of involvement of the community as a source of power to solve problems (Morrill, 1992).

This chapter proposes that the university, and specifically the university medical school, along with other academic branches, become a leading force in forging the necessary collaborations and partnerships that will be required to promote wellness in a community (Nader, 1979).

Many universities are already involved with preventive medicine and public health. Wellness promotion includes, but is much broader than, what is already known in medicine as HPDP: health promotion, disease prevention, and health protection endeavors. An institutional emphasis on wellness promotion will place a higher value for HPDP endeavors as legitimate academic currency throughout the university. Thus, this chapter advocates an active application of the principles of social learning, family, and systems theories to practical and researchable population-based interventions designed to promote wellness. This chapter illustrates first a need for a broad-based approach to wellness promotion in San Diego, followed by a description of two examples of wellness promotion activities. The chapter concludes with a proposed model for institutionalization and dissemination of wellness promotion via university-community partnerships.

A COMMUNITY APPROACH
TO WELLNESS PROMOTION

Prevention sounds like a good idea, but it will take a great deal of effort to realize the benefits of an emphasis on prevention. It has been conceptualized as primary, secondary, and tertiary. What most of medicine does on a daily basis fits into tertiary (rehabilitation) or secondary (early detection and treatment) categories. In pediatrics, primary prevention of diseases for which active immunization is possible has now become routine. However, the promotion of wellness, which includes the availability of immunizations to each and every child in the community, obviously encompasses a great deal more than strictly biologically determined issues of susceptibility, host response, and reactions to immunization. Many much broader factors, including economics, delivery systems, and education, must be considered in implementing a community emphasis on immunizing all children. One quickly realizes the complexity of the problem if one includes these additional factors.

The problem is greatly magnified when attempting to consider primary prevention of the leading causes of mortality and morbidity. These include cardiovascular disease, cancer, accidents (including motor vehicle), morbidity and violence related to alcohol and substance abuse, and morbidity related to both premature and unprotected sexual activity. Therefore, while it is true that operationalizing wellness promotion requires specific activities with measurable outcomes, the approach must be very broad based in order to maintain effective, ongoing health promotion programs in a community. This is because many factors in a community affect the overall wellness of the population. Clusters of behaviors and factors often coincide. For example, we know that for young people the risks of school failure, smoking, involvement in gang violence, unprotected sexual behavior, and drug use experimentation tend to go together (Campanelli et al., 1987; Chassin et al., 1990; National Research Council, 1993). These behaviors are compounded by economic status, racial/ethnic bias, and unemployment of family members.

The school is a crucial site for wellness promotion for youth and a good place to gather information as well (Bruhn and Nader, 1982). The school tends to cut across many segments of society. Every school day, nearly 47 million students attend school in the United States; about six million certified and classified personnel staff these schools. Schools are the center of work activity for nearly one-fifth of the U.S. population (Green and Kreuter, 1991). While there are children who do not attend school, families with no school-age children, or newly emigrated families who may still not be comfortable with the school setting, the school does reach a large number of youth and their families at perhaps crucial times in their development of health habits and lifestyle choices. The school is also important because it offers educational resources that may be useful in planning interventions. In both projects described in this chapter, the school plays an important role.

Nationally, the leading causes of adult mortality and morbidity are cardiovascular disease and cancer. The roots of these diseases are often reflected by lifestyle habits that may be formed early, for example, diet habits, physical activity, and nonsmoking (World Health Organization, 1982). Risk-taking behaviors in youth are also directly related to morbidity and mortality in youth. Among persons ages 1 through 24, nearly 70% of all deaths are due to accidents (especially motor vehicle accidents), injuries, and violence (homicide and suicide) (Centers for Disease Control and Prevention, 1993). In addition, an estimated 2.5 million teenagers are infected with a sexually transmitted disease each year. About 20% of new AIDS diagnoses are in 20- to 25-year-olds. Given the relatively lengthy incubation period, many of these individuals become infected with HIV during adolescence.

In San Diego, the statistics are similar to national norms. In San Diego County, the big killers are heart disease, stroke, cancer, injury, and HIV (San Diego County Department of Health, 1991). Because of San Diego's proximity to Mexico and because immigration patterns may bring tropical diseases to the locale, residents must also be alert to infectious diseases thought to have been controlled years ago. For tuberculosis, for example, the case rate in the 0- to 13-year-old age range in 1991 was 9.6 per 100,000 (48 cases), with an overall case rate of 15.1 per 100,000 (390 cases) in 1991 (San Diego County Department of Health, 1991).

When examining demographic characteristics for San Diego County, some interesting trends for the future are revealed. The age-groups that increased the most in the decade 1980–1990 were the oldest and the very young. The 75-and-older age-group grew by 60.1%. Of tremendous impact for those interested in prevention among children, however, is that the 0- to 4-year-old age-group increased by 53.7%, adding more than 69,000 people (San Diego Association of Governments, 1990).

As this cohort ages, it will require more and more emphasis on education and prevention directed toward basic immunization, access to health care, and accident and violence prevention. We have other information on San Diego County that suggests that a broad-based approach to prevention is needed.

In 1990, there were three deaths and 985 cases due to measles in San Diego County; all of these could have been prevented with timely immunizations. Surveys in San Diego and California indicate that more than half of all preschool-age children are behind on their immunizations (San Diego County Department of Health, 1990). A recent grocery store/mall interview survey of parents was conducted by the Maternal and Child Health Section of the Health Department in selected San Diego County census tracts with predicted difficulty in accessing health care (American Academy of Pediatrics, 1992). The results suggested that 31% of children are not covered by either health insurance or Medi-Cal; 14% said they do not obtain well-child preventive care. These figures are probably underestimated since some San Diego areas with the highest levels of poverty and highest levels of immigrant residents were not surveyed. "Financial difficulty" was given as a major reason for not accessing health care. Forty-six percent of the respondents did not have dentists for their children.

In addition to difficulty in meeting basic physical health needs, a myriad of other issues and conditions work against the chances for a child or youth in San Diego to experience total wellness. For example, national surveys indicate that 20% to 25% of parents report that their children have had some school problems (Haggerty and Roghmann, 1993). There is no evidence to suggest that San Diego is different. The current predicted four-year dropout rate (as of 1991) (San Diego City Schools, 1991) for a class of ninth-graders is 27.6%, higher than the previous year's 26.9%. In other words, 276 of every 1,000 San Diego City School District ninth-graders are likely to drop out before high school graduation. Estimated rates for the major racial/ethnic groups are as follows:

Ethnicity	% Dropout
Hispanic	41.7
African American	29.2
Indochinese	23.4
White	23.0
Filipino	17.8
Asian	15.0

Most dropouts occur at age 16 or after eighth grade, but a disturbing number begin as early as seventh grade. Forty percent (1,022) of the 2,679 dropouts that occurred in 1989–1990 involved eighth- or ninth-graders. Dropouts are balanced between boys and girls. Having a health problem and being held back in school have been associated with dropping out (Grunbaum and Basen-Engquist, 1993).

Since there are increasing data linking poor health, risk-taking behaviors, and academic underachievement, there is interest in examining adolescents' own self-reported health habits and behaviors.

A recent survey of student (self-reported) health was conducted in the San Diego Unified School District under the auspices of the Centers for Disease Control (Campana, 1992). The results suggest that there is room for a great deal of improvement in health education efforts with youth. It is also likely, even though the surveys are anonymous, that the levels of risk-taking behaviors may be even higher, given the fact that the survey was available only in English and that only those present in school responded to it.

The survey results indicated that San Diego youth reported that 31% had been passengers in a car driven by someone who had been drinking, 26% said that there had been at least one instance in the past month in which they had consumed five or more drinks, and 11% said that they had driven a car while under the influence of alcohol. Twenty-three percent of students said that they had carried a weapon such as a knife, gun, or club in the month prior to the survey; 4% said that they had carried a gun. Thirty-six percent said that they had tried marijuana, 3% said that they had injected illegal drugs and used cocaine or heroin at least once. Thoughts of suicide and depression were not uncommon. About one-third had contemplated suicide in the past year. Six percent said that they had actually tried to kill themselves.

Slightly less than half the students reported that they had engaged in sex at least once. Sixteen percent said that they had had four or more partners ever, and 3% percent said that they had had that many partners in the past three months. Only 22% said that they or their partner had used a condom during their last sexual intercourse. However, this figure included all the respondents to the survey in the denominator. When considering only those who said that they were sexually active, 45% reported that they or their partner had used a condom during their last sexual intercourse. An interesting age-related trend emerged: Proportionately more sexually active ninth-graders (52%) reported condom use, while the proportion decreased each successive grade to only 34% of sexually active 12th-graders reporting condom use. Six percent said that they had been pregnant or had made someone else pregnant.

Fifty percent to 60% of the students reported frequently consuming high-fat foods, such as french fries, potato chips, cookies, and cake. Sixty percent reported engaging in regular vigorous exercise. Eighteen percent—lower than the national average of 36%—report smoking tobacco. This may reflect vigorous local educational programs, or it may reflect regional differences in smoking in the general population (San Diego City Schools, 1992).

All these data support the need for a broad-based approach to prevention and health promotion. Clearly, much more emphasis is required in order to improve the picture that emerges of a significant population at risk.

EXAMPLES OF A UNIVERSITY RESPONSE

In democratic countries the science of associations is the mother science; the progress of all the rest depends upon the progress it has made.
—Alexis de Tocqueville, originally published
in *Democracy in America* (1835)

A number of countywide effects involving the university and its community have been under way from the University of California, San Diego. Over 100 such initiatives were recently identified by a University K–12 Task Force (University of California, San Diego, 1997), and only a few that pertain to youth and schools are described here.

The San Diego Health Coalition
for Children and Youth

The San Diego Health Coalition for Children and Youth is an attempt to move from a situation in which many groups and agencies that impact and serve youth are frustrated that little is done for prevention to a situation in which an organized collaboration can actually begin to demonstrate the benefits of preventive programs.

However, there are many steps and barriers to overcome in moving from a stage of loose networks to coordination of efforts and, finally, to a real collaboration for this purpose. The process itself is worthy of study. "What we don't need is another meeting to attend." "Another coalition?" These are commonly heard complaints during days already filled with emergency meetings to deal with fiscal and other crises. Yet there is a growing awareness among all human services personnel of an increasing pressure to intervene earlier in the stream of life events. It is believed by many, with striking new evidence supporting the conclusion, that such preventive interventions will be much more cost-effective than treating problems later. For example, a home visitor program has been shown in several studies to markedly reduce the incidence of physical child abuses to improve both health and developmental outcomes of low-birth-weight infants and to improve pregnancy outcomes and prenatal care (Hawaii Healthy Start, 1991; Olds et al., 1986; Ramey et al., 1992). Another study estimated that merely by applying preventive health strategies known to be effective—such as car safety restraints, hot water heater temperature controls, and safety bars on windows—the morbidity/mortality due to childhood injuries could be reduced significantly (Rivera, 1985). As Liz Schorr (1988) has reminded us, goals for youth are within our reach. However, there is a striking lack of a broad-based constituency to support health promotion and disease prevention for youth and families.

The recognition of the need for such a constituency led several UCSD staff to enlist the support of others in the community to develop such a coalition. The first meeting, with 10 to 12 people attending, representing five agencies, occurred on January 26, 1990. At a retreat led by a volunteer professional facilitator on September 8, 1990, 50 attendees designed a mission/vision statement and established four working groups. The mission is to achieve optimal health and development of children and youth of the San Diego region. A data group was charged with conceptualizing a plan to develop a system for ongoing needs assessment and monitoring of child health and wellness data for the county. The other three groups were designed to respond to the outline of *Healthy People 2000*, with health promotion, protection, and disease prevention objectives (U.S. Department of Health and Human Services, 1990). Each group devised a pilot project proposal for the coalition as a whole to consider.

The pilot project selected was a measles immunization project, targeting selected neighborhoods with known low immunization rates. These neighborhoods were predominantly low income and Hispanic. While the project actually resulted in special immunization sessions at a community clinic on two weekend days with more than 100 children immunized, the real benefit of the project was the demonstration that multiple private and public agencies, as well as government and media, could work together. The County Health Department gave specialized training to members of a Latino health education group called Por La Vida, who canvassed the target area. The Children's Hospital Public Relations Department coordinated media coverage with local Spanish print and radio media. An exit interview held at the clinic site documented that children who were brought to the clinic were significantly behind in their immunizations and that the home visitor counselors, or "consejeras," as well as information from the school, were effective in informing the parents of the clinic. This pilot project was timely since immunizations were being targeted by national and local health officials in San Diego. As a result of Health Department initiatives and this pilot project, funding has been obtained for several additional projects that could significantly affect immunization levels in San Diego in the future.

The All Kids Count Project, which was initially a response to a Robert Wood Johnson Foundation request for proposal, fit nicely into the coalition's plans. An application was made by the Health Department with coalition support. Although not funded, its objective was the establishment of a computerized tracking system and database for immunizations for San Diego children. Once the computerized system was established, it was envisioned that a number of health and wellness indicators for youth could be continuously collected and made available to the community to serve as a status report and to serve as a database for future program evaluation. As of 1997, the All Kids Count Immunization Registry is in its final pilot phase, supported by grants from the State of California and the Anna B. Casey Foundation.

As of 1997, there are 50-plus individuals who are members of the San

Diego Health Coalition. In February 1997, a new work plan was laid out with major goals of broadening membership and pursuing existing projects (San Diego Health Coalition for Children and Youth, 1997).

University-community partnerships are also required to implement community-based research in health promotion and disease preventions. The Child and Adolescent Trial for Cardiovascular Health (CATCH) Project, funded by the National Institutes of Health, is a clinical trial of the efficacy of promoting healthy eating, physical activity, and nonsmoking by working with elementary school children and their parents via schools (Perry et al., 1990). This project is a national collaborative trial with sites in Minnesota, Texas, Louisiana, and California. The coordinating center is the New England Research Institute in Boston, Massachusetts. The University of California, San Diego, was selected as a study site in a competitive granting process. Part of the reason we were selected as a site was our previous work in the area of cardiovascular disease prevention with Mexican-American and Anglo families—Project SCAN (Study of Child Activity and Nutrition)—and our studies of the determinants of cardiovascular disease risk factor behaviors in children ages 4 to 6 and 9 to 14 years (Broyles et al., 1996; Elder et al., 1998; McKenzie et al., 1991, 1992; Nader et al., 1989a, 1995; Sallis et al., 1995b; Sallis et al., 1997; Zive et al., 1995, 1998).

There is good evidence that modifiable precursors of cardiovascular disease—namely, smoking, dietary habits, and sedentary lifestyle—lead to elevations of total and LDL cholesterol, which in turn promote premature cardiovascular disease morbidity and mortality (Luepker et al., 1996). There is also good evidence that preclinical disease processes can be detected in childhood and that, although not in every case, the various relative levels of physiologic risk factors (e.g., weight, blood pressure, and cholesterol) tend to persist through childhood, adolescence, and into adulthood (Fraser, 1986). It would seem logical, then, to attempt interventions that are not extreme, that do not label children or cause undue concern or worry, and that are hygienic from a public health perspective. As mentioned earlier, the school is an obvious site for such an intervention. The school has opportunities for adult and peer modeling of health habits and behaviors (Perry et al., 1990). The school potentially can exercise control over the environmental aspects of the school lunch program, physical education programs, and smoking policies. In addition, there are the usual opportunities to involve children and parents in curricular learning activities to reinforce healthful choices (Perry et al., 1990).

TABLE 18.1   CATCH PHASE II
RESEARCH DESIGN

96 Schools (24/Site)

Random Assignment

School Year	Grade	School-Based CATCH Program (n = 28)	School-Based Plus Family CATCH Program (n = 28)	Control Schools (Usual programs) (n = 40)
1991–1992	3	Baseline measurements; CATCH programs	Baseline measurements; CATCH programs	Baseline measurements; usual programs
1992–1993	4	CATCH programs	CATCH programs	Usual programs
1993–1994	5	CATCH programs; follow-up measurements	CATCH programs; follow-up; measurements	Usual programs; follow-up measurements

Reprinted with permission from Perry et al. (1990).

CATCH was evaluated in Austin, Minneapolis, New Orleans, and San Diego among public school populations of third- to fifth-grade students that include a range of socioeconomic groups and minority students (including Blacks and Hispanics) and that are representative of the larger U.S. school population (for the study design, see Table 18.1). The results were published in 1996 (Luepker et al., 1996) and presented the effects of the three-year intervention (grades 3 through 5) compared to control schools who received only their usual health education programs. In intervention school lunches, the percentage of energy intake from fat fell significantly more (from 38.7% to 31.9%) than in control lunches (from 38.9% to 36.2%) (P < .001). The intensity of physical activity in physical education classes during the CATCH intervention increased significantly in the intervention schools compared with the control schools (P < .02). Self-reported daily energy intake from fat among students in the intervention schools was significantly reduced (from 32.7% to 30.3%) compared with that among students in the control schools (from 32.6% to 32.2%) (P < .001). Intervention students reported significantly more daily vigorous activity than controls (58.6 minutes vs. 46.5 minutes; P < .003). Blood pressure, body size, and cholesterol measures did not differ significantly between treatment groups. No evidence of deleterious effects of this intervention on growth or development was observed (Luepker et al., 1996). In summary, the CATCH intervention was able to modify the fat content of school lunches, increase moderate to vigorous physical activity in physical education, and improve eating and physical activity behaviors in children during three school years. A recent follow-up, at eighth grade, shows persistence of these behavior changes among intervention students (Nader et al., 1999).

Why the University?

The mission of the university is to define and investigate new knowledge, to teach the applications of knowledge to its students and its faculty, and to provide a resource and service to the surrounding community. The third of this triad has received increasing attention as public support for higher education has become more precarious and as universities strive to enrich their faculties and student populations with more people of color.

Active collaboration with the community provides rich opportunities for the university to enhance its traditional missions as well as to respond to the community and recruit and attract students from varied ethnic backgrounds. The balance provided by in-the-field, real-life experiential learning combined with more didactic and contemplative approaches within the university classroom or seminar session is exciting for both teachers and students. In medicine, recent concern has been expressed over the lack of students entering the primary care fields. This has been attributed to lack of financial rewards. It has also been attributed to lack of exposure of medical students and doctors in training to real life, primary care, out-of-the-medical-center learning activities, and relatively more exposure to predominantly subspecialty research physicians in tertiary care centers.

At UCSD, there are a number of examples of involvement of university students and trainees in community sites and programs. The Independent Study Project (ISP) frequently involves community outreach. Several years ago, one UCSD medical student conducted an ISP examining San Diego youth's knowledge and attitudes about HIV/AIDS. He compared a group of gay youth and groups of urban and suburban high school students to a group of incarcerated youth. The incarcerated group demonstrated significantly poorer knowledge and lower agreement with health guidelines, a lower perceived personal threat of AIDS, a lower personal efficacy to prevent AIDS, and the lowest perceived norms of safe-sex practices (Nader et al., 1989b). Another student, who was president of the American Women's Medical Student Association, based one of her ISPs on initiating and conducting a program of volunteer medical student health education teachers for local high schools. Although initiated in San Diego, this program was replicated nationally in a number of other medical schools. The program is still active and has been incorporated formally into the medical school curriculum as an elective. Currently, 50 medical students per quarter discuss selected topics with adolescents in area schools, including mental health issues, HIV prevention and spread, drug and tobacco use, growth and development, human sexuality, diet and physical activity habits, and simple "Q&A" ask-the-doctor sessions. The sessions seem to be well received by young people, and medical students report learning a great deal about adolescent development and the concerns of youth.

At the postdoctoral level of medical education, we have incorporated community and school experiences for pediatric residents. In these activities, residents become familiar with community consultation activities of the pediatrician. The resident witnesses firsthand the numerous social and health concerns buffeting families and becomes aware of resources in the community to help children and families with a wide variety of physical health, learning, and behavioral problems of children. At times, residents have been able to provide a source of ongoing health care for a child identified by the school as having special needs. Both schools and residents indicate satisfaction with these educational experiences.

Data collected on similar resident training in Texas and other settings indicate that pediatricians in practice who had such training experiences continue to be more active in school and community consultations later when they enter their practices, compared to those without such community activities during their residency training (Black et al., 1991).

Currently, UCSD is examining its medical school curriculum and is likely to expand primary care and community-based education. The desire is not to diminish the contribution and importance of basic biomedical research and teaching but rather to complement it with the richness and breadth of application of advances in the biomedical sciences using behavioral sciences and epidemiology, thereby exposing medical students to the challenge of delivering quality primary care medical services in the community.

Interaction with the community in service and educational areas leads naturally to collaboration and mutual pursuit of research projects. This fits well with the primary mission of the university. Unfortunately, too often the university is perceived by the community as coming in, doing its research, and then leaving without even sharing the results of the study with community participants. We utilize the following guidelines in approaching schools with ideas for research: (1) What benefit will the school or participants in the study derive from the research? (2) Does the project require minimal interruption of classroom instructional or teacher time? (3) What will happen when the research is completed?

INSTITUTIONALIZATION AND REPLICATION: A MODEL

In 1990, a project was initiated at the Harvard School of Public Health. This project undertook a nationwide examination and policy analysis of the potential contributions made by university and public K–12 schools in health promotion efforts. A first step was the review and synthesis of 25 selected panel expert group reports, including reports by the American Medical Association, the Carnegie Council, the Center for the Study of Social Policy, the Children's Defense Fund, the Congress of the United States Office of Technology Assessment, the Council Chief of State School Offices, the National Commission on Children, the National School Boards Association, the U.S. Department of Education, and the U.S. Department of Health and Human Services. Five common themes emerged:

Theme 1: Education and health are interrelated. It is accepted and well demonstrated that knowledge and skills learned by individuals can assist them in improving their health. Similarly, health influences education. Recent research documents the role of potentially preventable conditions in the development of learning impairments from birth to age five, including low birth weight, prenatal exposure to alcohol, parental smoking, prenatal drug exposure, lead poisoning, child abuse and neglect, and malnutrition. In addition, direct morbidity and mental deficits can occur if children are not immunized in a timely manner. The interrelation between academic failure and health risk behaviors has already been noted.

Theme 2: The biggest threats to health are "social" morbidities. The American Medical Association defines social morbidities as those that are primarily the result of behavior and the social environment. This is evident in the current burden on the health care system of low-birth-weight infants, alcohol-related birth impairments, drug use during pregnancy, and physical and sexual abuse. Add accidents, homicide, suicide, and the additional impact of alcohol on these morbidities, and the need for a broad-based approach to prevention is evident.

Theme 3: There is a clear need for a more comprehensive, integrated approach. Many of the reports reviewed examples of effective interventions that can be made, but all reports called attention to the fact that there is no consistent effort to apply effective interventions to the general population. The major reason for this is fragmentation of programs and services. There is a major need for more comprehensive and coordinated programs and services. This will require system changes. Changes are required in the way health and education programs are funded, how professionals are trained, and how each system relates to the other. The university will need to play an important role in defining and experimenting with these changes.

Theme 4: Health promotion and education efforts should be centered in and around schools. We have long attempted as a society to solve many problems by placing the brunt of the responsibility for change on the schools. At the same time, we have been unable to provide increasing resources or support from other institutions and government (or the private sector) to enable schools to respond effectively. The difference in the call today for school-centered health promotion is the realization that the school cannot, and should not, be expected to do this job alone. The stakes are high for everyone, and all must contribute. Efforts will be needed from all sectors of society—public and private.

Theme 5: Prevention efforts are cost-effective. The social and economic costs of inaction are too high and still escalating. The Children's Defense Fund estimates that every dollar spent on prenatal care saves $3 in the child's first year of life by reducing the need for remedial medical care. Every dollar spent in immunizing a child saves $10 by reducing death and disease. The costs of preventable problems are also documented by the Carnegie Council, which concluded that a year's class of dropouts would cost the nation $260 million in lost earnings and forgone taxes. Each added year of secondary education reduces the probability of public welfare dependency by 35%. Alcohol and drug abuse in the United States cost more than $136 billion in 1980 in reduced productivity, treatment, crime, and related costs.

It behooves the university to take an active role in increasing savings and decreasing costs to society by facilitating health promotion and wellness promotion programs. The university is an educational institution, and so are community schools. It makes sense to have a structure within the university that will facilitate the types of community interactions with schools that have been described. A university-wide committee with membership of departments, divisions, and colleges that could interact beneficially with K–12 schools in the area, along with school leaders as consultants to the committee, could be one mechanism for institutionalizing a university's commitment to wellness promotion for a community. The University of Texas Medical Branch at Galveston established such a committee, the Dean's School Health Committee, in 1974. The committee is still active in 1997 despite the fact that the dean and many members of the original committee have since departed. Representatives from local school districts, as well as all medical school departments that interact with public and parochial schools in the Galveston area, are members of the committee. The committee regularly publishes a newsletter on child health and education issues that is distributed to many teachers. The committee also sponsors minority student summer research and academic year fellowships and conducts an annual continuing education program for school nurses and teachers on health issues. I recently had the pleasure of addressing the gathering of the 15th annual conference, attended by more than 200 school health and education personnel. The committee has also been helpful to university teachers and researchers in implementing community-based training and research activities in area schools. Thus, the committee has successfully institutionalized a community-school-university collaboration of 15 years' duration. The committee has not yet tackled the issue of a broad-based effort in health promotion, although there are many examples of health promotion activities that have emerged over the years.

CONCLUSION

This chapter has described examples of how a university can promote wellness for children, youth, and families. There are many other examples that could have been described. The particular emphasis that the university brings to wellness promotion is on education and on researching the best and most effective methods of promoting wellness. Both of these contributions are important to the advancement of knowledge and practice of health promotion and disease prevention. The benefits to the university include improved responsiveness to the needs of the community surrounding the university while at the same time furthering the traditional missions of the university. The university can become an important catalyst in a community without diluting or detracting from traditional academic pursuits. The eventual bottom line should be a significant increase in investment in our nation's families and youth—an investment in time, cooperation, collaboration, and resources that will result in enhanced physical, emotional, and social well-being for all of our society.

NOTE

This chapter was initially prepared for the 1992 University of California/Health Net Wellness Lecture Series under a grant from Health Net.

REFERENCES

American Academy of Pediatrics, San Diego County Chapter, Community Access to Child Health Care Committee. (1992, July). *Access to Health Care for Children in San Diego County.* San Diego: Division of Maternal and Child Health, CHDP Program, San Diego County Department of Health Services.

Black, J. L., Nader, P. R., Broyles, S. L., and Nelson, J. A. (1991). Pediatric training and activities in school health: A national survey. *Journal of School Health* 61(6), 245–248.

Broyles, S. L., Nader, P. R., Sallis, J. F., et al. (1996). Cardiovascular disease risk factors in Anglo- and Mexican-American children and their mothers. *Family Community Health* 19(3), 57–72.

Bruhn, J. G., and Nader, P. R. (1982). The school as setting for health education, health promotion, and health care. *Family Community Health* 4, 57–69.

Campana, J. (1992, February). *Report to the San Diego City Schools Board of Education.* San Diego: Student Services Division, San Diego City Schools.

Campanelli, P. C., Dielman, T. E., Shope, J. T., et al. (1987) Pretest and treatment effects in an elementary school-based alcohol misuse prevention program. *Health Education Quarterly* 16(1), 113–130.

Centers for Disease Control and Prevention. (1993). *Youth Risk Behavior Summaries.* Atlanta: Division of Adolescent and School Health.

Chassin, L., Presson, C. C., Rose, J. S., and Sherman, S. J. (1996). The natural history of cigarette smoking from adolescence to adulthood: Demographic predictors of continuity and change. *Health Psychology* N15(6), 478–484.

Elder, J., Broyles, S., McKenzie, T., et al. (1998). Direct home observations of the prompting of physical activity in sedentary and active Mexican- and Anglo-American children. *Journal of Developmental and Behavioral Pediatrics* 19, 26–30.

Fraser, G. (1986). *Preventive Cardiology.* New York: Oxford University Press.

Green, L. W., and Kreuter, M. W. (1991). *Health Promotion Planning: An Educational and Environmental Approach.* New York: Mayfield Publishing, 350.

Grunbaum, J. A., and Basen-Engquist, K. (1993). Comparison of health risk behaviors between students in a regular high school and students in an alternative high school. *Journal of School Health* 63(10), 421–428.

Haggerty, R. J., and Roghmann, K. J. (1993). *Child Health and the Community.* 2nd ed. New Brunswick, N.J.: Transaction Publishers.

Hawaii Healthy Start. (1991). *Study of Reduction of Child Abuse.* Honolulu: Department of Health, National Child Health Bureau.

Luepker, R. V., Perry, C. L., McKinlay, S. M., et al. (1996). Outcomes of a field trial to improve children's dietary patterns and physical activity. *Journal of the American Medical Association* 275(10), 768–776.

McKenzie, T. L., Sallis, J. F., Nader, P. R., et al. (1991). BEACHES: An observational system for assessing children's eating and physical activity behaviors and associated events. *Journal of Applied Behavioral Analysis, 24(1),* 141–151.

McKenzie, T. L., Sallis, J. F., Nader, P. R., et al. (1992). Anglo- and Mexican-American preschoolers at home and at recess: Activity patterns and environmental influences. *Journal of Development and Behavioral Pediatrics* 13(3), 173.

Morrill, W. A. (1992). Overview of service delivery to children. In R. E. Behram, ed., *The Future of Children, School Linked Services.* 2nd ed. Pp. 32–43. Center for the Future of Children, The David and Lucille Packard Foundation.

Nader, P. R. (1979). The university medical center and school health. *Texas Report of Biology and Medicine* 38, 169–179.

Nader, P. R., Sallis, J. F., Patterson, T. L., et al. (1989a). A family approach to cardiovascular risk reduction: Results from the San Diego Family Health Project. *Health Education Quarterly* 16(2), 229–244.

Nader, P. R., Wexler, D. B., Patterson, T. L., et al. (1989b). Comparison of beliefs about AIDS among urban, suburban, incarcerated, and gay adolescents. *Journal of Adolescent Health Care* 10(5, September), 413–418.

Nader, P. R., Sallis, J. F., Broyles, S. L., et al. (1995). Ethnic and gender trends for cardiovascular risk behaviors in Anglo- and Mexican-American children, ages four–seven. *Journal of Health Education* 26(2, Suppl.), S27–S35.

Nader, P. R., Stone, L. J., and Lytle, L. A. (1999). Three-year maintenance of improved diet and physical activity: The CATCH cohort. *Archives of Pediatric and Adolescent Medicine* 153(July), 695–704.

National Research Council. (1993). *Losing Generations: Adolescents in High Risk Setting.* Washington, D.C.: National Academy Press.

Olds, D. L., Henderson, C. R., Tatelbaum, R., and Chamberlin, R. (1986). Improving the delivery of prenatal care and outcome of pregnancy: A randomized trial of nurse home visitation. *Pediatrics* 77(1), 16–28.

Perry, C. L., Stone, E. J., Parcel, G. S., et al. (1990). School-based cardiovascular health promotion: The Child and Adolescent Trial for Cardiovascular Health (CATCH). *Journal of School Health* 60(8), 406–413.

Ramey, C. T., Bryant, D., Wasek, B., et al. (1992). Infant and development program for low birth weight premature infants: Program elements, family participation, and child intelligence. *Pediatrics* 89, 454–465.

Rivera, F. P. (1985). Traumatic deaths of children in the United States: Currently available prevention strategies. *Pediatrics* 75, 456–462.

Sallis, J. F., Broyles, S. L., Frank-Spohrer, G., et al. (1995b). Child's home environment in relation to the mother's adiposity. *International Journal of Obesity* 19, 190–197.

Sallis, J. F., McKenzie, T. L., Elder, J. P., et al. (1997). Factors parents use in selecting play spaces for young children. *Archives of Pediatrics and Adolescent Medicine* 151, 414–417.

San Diego Association of Governments. (1990). *Population Projections.* San Diego: SANDAG.

San Diego City Schools. (1991, March). *Report to the Board of Education on Grades 8–12 Dropouts during 1989–90.* San Diego: San Diego City Schools, Planning, Research, and Evaluation Division, Research Department.

———. (1992). *Report on Youth Risk Behaviors Survey to the School Board.* San Diego: San Diego City Schools, Planning, Research, and Evaluation Division, Research Department.

San Diego County Department of Health. (1990). *Morbidity Reports.* San Diego: SDDH.

———. (1991). *Morbidity Reports.* San Diego: SDDH.

San Diego Health Coalition for Children and Youth. (1997). *Newsletter,* March.

Schorr, L. B. (1988). *Within Our Reach: Breaking the Cycle of Disadvantage.* New York: Anchor Press, Doubleday.

University of California, San Diego. (1997). *Outreach Task Force Report.* San Diego: UCSD.

U.S. Department of Health and Human Services. (1990). *Healthy People 2000. National Health Promotion and Disease Prevention Objectives.* DHHS Publication PHS91–50213. Washington, D.C.: U.S. Government Printing Office.

World Health Organization. (1982). *Prevention of Coronary Artery Disease.* WHO Technical Report (Series 678). Geneva: WHO.

Zive, M. M., Frank-Spohrer, G. C., Sallis, J. F., et al. (1998). Direct home observations of the prompting of physical activity in sedentary and active Mexican- and Anglo-American children. *Journal of Developmental and Behavioral Pediatrics* 19, 26–30.

Zive, M. M., Taras, H. L., Broyles, S. L., et al. (1995). Vitamin and mineral intakes of Anglo- and Mexican-American preschoolers. *Journal of American Dietetic Association* 95(3), 329–335.

PART FOUR

WELLNESS PROMOTION POLICY: TOWARD A MORE EXPLICIT CONSIDERATION OF THE POLITICAL CONTEXT

The chapters in part 4 are grouped together because each addresses the role of the political context as an influence on wellness promotion, whether as impediment or facilitator. As an impediment, the political context has stalled wellness promotion efforts in the areas of adolescent sexuality, safety in the agricultural workplace, women's health, and HIV/AIDS. Hofmann (chapter 20) addresses the first of these topics in a detailed analysis of the data relating to adolescent reproductive health and pregnancy. Noting the combination of biological, social, cognitive, developmental, and cultural factors that confound teens' best intentions with respect to sexual activity, she points out the insufficiency of the abstinence-only approach currently favored by the political climate. Similarly, Schenker (chapter 21) argues that a widely held perception of agricultural employment as salutagenic interferes with the establishment of effective legislation to protect farmworkers' health. Stanton, Danoff-Burg, and Gallant (chapter 22) and Villablanca (chapter 23) discuss ways in which the political/cultural climate has stunted progress in women's health. Specifically, the historical bias toward conducting research with male subjects and the general absence of women within the circles of power have served to delay significant advances in promoting wellness among women. With respect to HIV/AIDS, Waldo and Coates (chapter 24) relate the failure of HIV/AIDS prevention to live up to its promise to political and cultural biases that have thwarted the translation of scientific knowledge into effective intervention (e.g., the current legislation forbidding needle exchange programs despite their established efficacy). In contrast to the other chapters in part 4, Wallack (chapter 19) gives an overview of a wellness program that was explicitly designed to work within the political structure to bring about change. The Violence Prevention Initiative has worked with the media and the community to leverage scientific knowledge to bring about political and legislative changes that reduce the threat to public health posed by firearms. Thus, as a whole, this part paints a picture of the power of the political context as an influence on wellness promotion efforts.

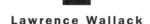
Lawrence Wallack

STRATEGIES FOR REDUCING
YOUTH VIOLENCE

Media, Community, and Policy

INTRODUCTION

Violence scars the contemporary American landscape. There are more
guns, more violent crimes, and more murders per capita in the United
States than in any other industrialized country.[1] Violence is like a virus
that infects and weakens the essential relationships and structures that
bind our society. Individuals, families, schools, work sites, and entire
communities are devolving toward a state of *dis-ease* as their basic sense
of security and well-being is undermined. Fear, mistrust, hopelessness,
and social isolation spread with this violence virus and perpetuate some
of the very conditions that create and feed the epidemic. Donna Shalala,
secretary of the Department of Health and Human Services, notes, "Of
all the health and human service challenges we face, perhaps one of the
most devastating and, ironically, the most preventable is the epidemic of
violence sweeping across this nation."[2]

Youth-related violence, in particular, is a reflection of the tensions,
conflicts, hopes, and fears pervasive in our society. That so many youth
are injured or killed by their peers and by adults signals a tragic crisis of
morality and justice. It forces us, as individuals and as a society, to reflect on how we value children and youth; to consider how we allocate
resources and assign priorities; to ponder racial, ethnic, and cultural factors; to confront basic constitutional issues such as the presumed right
to carry firearms; and to search our souls about what is right and just.

In California, violence prevention efforts have increasingly focused on
reducing the widespread and easy availability of handguns—an essential

first step in making the problem of violence less lethal. New laws being passed at the local and state levels in California are designed to make handguns more difficult for youth to obtain. Passing such laws was not politically feasible a few years ago; however, the Violence Prevention Initiative (VPI) of The California Wellness Foundation has helped to create a new environment for handgun policy and given rise to a movement that has important lessons for others working on this issue. This chapter explores some important characteristics of the VPI and describes some of the progress that has been made. It is based on interviews with key informants, reviews of VPI documents, and personal observations on the design and implementation of the project. Although the VPI has a much broader focus than handguns, this chapter addresses only those activities related to the goal of reducing the availability of handguns to youth. The VPI includes an extensive evaluation being conducted by RAND and the Stanford Center for Research in Disease Prevention. This detailed evaluation will address all components of the VPI. Also, the limited scope of this chapter does not allow for a full critical analysis of the VPI. Indeed, I have elected to focus on the fruits of the progress and have slighted the pain of the struggle. My intent is to be observational rather than evaluative. As with any new, large undertaking, the VPI has had its share of growing pains and may have suffered from some false starts or missed opportunities. Nonetheless, there is much to be learned from the VPI, and I hope that this chapter is a useful beginning in highlighting some of the lessons.

A PRIMARY INDICATOR OF VIOLENCE

There are many indicators of violence, but perhaps none conveys a greater sense of urgency than homicide rates. In 1995 there were 21,597 homicides in the United States, or roughly 59 people murdered every day.[3] Homicide accounted for 2,555 deaths of those under age 18 in 1994 and was one of the top two causes of death for children and young people aged 5 to 24.[4]

In California, there were 3,699 homicides in 1994. Homicide was the leading cause of death for males aged 15 to 24 and the second-leading cause of death for those in the 10- to 14-year age-group. For females, homicide was the second-leading cause of death in the 15- to 24-year age-group and the third-leading cause of death for girls aged 10 to 14. In 1995, there were 1,565 homicide deaths in California for those under the age of 25.[5]

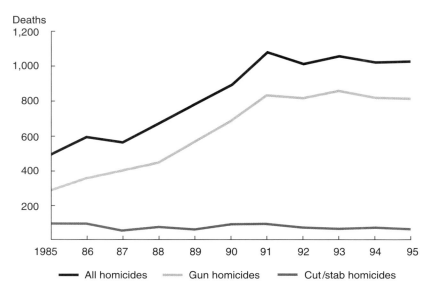

Figure 19.1. Homicides for youth under 21 years of age, California (1985–1995). Source: California Department Of Health Services.

Figure 19.1 shows that from 1985 to 1995, the overall number of youth homicides increased 106%, slightly down from peaks in 1991 and 1993. During that same period, deaths due to cutting/piercing declined 28%, while firearm-related homicides increased 189%.[6] Overall, 76% of homicides involved firearms; of those, 88% were handgun deaths.[7,8]

The increase in youth homicide is especially alarming because overall homicide rates have been declining.[9] A violence expert has noted, "Youth are now killing youth at rates far higher than any other time this century,"[10] and it is widely accepted that the increase in deaths is attributable to guns.[11–14] Overall, the United States has the highest rate of firearm death for children aged 1 to 14 in the industrialized world—a rate almost 12 times higher than that for children in the other 25 countries combined.[15] In 1995, 35,957 people died from firearm injuries in the United States, with suicides accounting for 51% of these deaths and homicides for 44%.[16] Firearm deaths for youth, however, are much more likely to be linked to homicide than suicide.

Research indicates that ownership of a gun is more likely to put individuals and their families at risk for violence than it is to provide protection from it.[17–19] When guns are primarily in the hands of youth who live in a hostile environment, who lack restraint, and who participate in a subculture that accepts violence as a basic means for resolving conflict, the risk will be substantially higher. Blumstein has calculated an estimate of "excess" murders for the period 1985–1992 based on what the number of homicides would have been if the homicide rate had remained at the average for the period 1970–1985. He found an "excess" of 18,600 murders for 15- to 21-year-olds, most of those attributable to guns.[20] As Cook explains, "When guns are the instrument for conducting violent encounters, the likelihood that someone will die is multiplied."[10]

HANDGUN POLICY AS PREVENTION STRATEGY

There are an estimated 192 million to 216 million firearms in the United States.[21,22] Handguns are the firearm of choice for homicide: "While handguns make up only about one-third of all firearms owned in the United States, they account for 80 percent of the homicides committed with a firearm."[22] Handguns are relatively cheap and easy for youth to obtain, and their availability increases the risk of homicide and suicide for urban youth.[23] Guns may not cause violence, but they do make violence more lethal and allow traditionally nonfatal incidents to become fatal. Further, these incidents can set into motion a cascade of negative effects across the community by creating a spiral of revenge and retribution. Removing guns from the violence equation may not reduce the frequency of violence, but it will reduce the mortality from violent encounters.

It is widely accepted that violence is an enormously complex issue with many causes and potential solutions.[24–26] (Accordingly, the VPI has developed a broad policy agenda that includes other approaches, such as increasing social and educational resources for youth.)[27] Nonetheless, taking handguns out of violence is a significant step to creating a more supportive environment in which other prevention programs have a better chance of success. Also, getting handguns that are killing youth out of the picture is an important way to get people involved in the larger issue of violence prevention. In California, this strategy is working.

June 4, 1997, was a historic day for California. A front-page story the next day in the *Los Angeles Times* reported, "In what would be landmark legislation, the Senate and Assembly approved separate bills Wednesday to ban the manufacture and sale of cheap handguns known as Saturday night specials and junk guns."[28] The two bills were later reconciled, and a new bill was passed by both bodies of the state legislature. This new bill was sent to the governor for his signature. Sometimes referred to as "starter guns"—in part because their low cost and concealability make them accessible to youth—Saturday night specials are usually defined as short-barreled, inexpensive, poor-quality handguns that lack even basic safety features. The quality of these guns is so poor that under federal regulations they would not be able to be imported into the United States. Because they are made here, however, they are exempt from these regulations. They are disproportionately involved in violent crime and account for the great majority of guns confiscated in California. What made this proposed legislation even more significant was the fact that approximately 80% of the Saturday night specials manufactured in the United States are produced by just six companies located in southern California. Noting that these are "weapons of choice among young criminals," an editorial in the *Los Angeles Times* went on to observe that "[the ban] assuredly would save lives of an untold number of innocent Californians, including children and police officers." [29]

One day prior to the votes on the junk-gun ban in the state legislature, the voters of Livermore, a suburban community in the San Francisco Bay Area, passed Measure H, banning the sale of junk guns in that city. In fact, the state assembly approved the junk-gun ban at 11:30 P.M. on the night of the Livermore vote. The senate passed its version the following day. Some advocates thought that the Livermore victory influenced the vote in the state legislature. The referendum, the first public vote in California on junk guns, was called to ratify the decision of the city council, which had passed the ordinance on a 3-to-2 vote.

The passage of a proposed statewide ban on junk guns and the victory in Livermore marked the culmination of an intense period of handgun policy activity in California that has continued to spark the introduction of local ordinances. This period of dramatic action began in January 1996, when the city council of West Hollywood proposed an ordinance banning the sale of Saturday night specials. The ordinance passed in May and went into effect in July. On November 15, 1996, the Los Angeles Superior Court upheld West Hollywood's ban. This success opened the door for many other communities; by the summer of 1997, 52 cities and six counties had passed local ordinances placing limits or additional requirements on firearm sales. [30] Thirty-four of these were bans on Saturday night specials.

Passing local ordinances to limit the availability of handguns had thus become a trend when five years earlier it had seemed an unlikely possibility. No one at that time would have suggested that a handgun ban of any kind might pass the state legislature. The transformation from the impractical to the pragmatic, from the improbable to the common-place, was largely due to the VPI and other related projects funded by The California Wellness Foundation. Virtually all the ordinances have some imprint of the educational and policy materials from the VPI. The influence of the VPI has been pervasive; many of its themes, messages, and data have become part of the public conversation and are routinely used by public officials who, according to one advocate, "now own this language."

THE CALIFORNIA VIOLENCE PREVENTION INITIATIVE

The VPI was introduced in the spring of 1993. Conceived by The California Wellness Foundation (TCWF), the VPI is a five-year, $35 million grant-making program designed to reduce violence among youth up to age 24. The VPI includes multiple components, including policy development, community action programs, leadership development, public education, and research.[31]

Interestingly, the VPI was conceived in a challenging environment in which the supports for those most at risk for violence were eroding, in part because of a stagnant California economy and an increasing public fear of crime, violence, and immigration. April 1992 had witnessed civil unrest in Los Angeles following the Rodney King verdict, the state budget was tight, and crime and violence were framed primarily as criminal justice problems that should be addressed by harsher penalties, especially for youth. The seeds of a growing social conservatism would soon sprout in the form of ballot initiatives and public policies limiting health and social services for undocumented immigrants, requiring 25-year to life terms for three-time offenders, and eliminating affirmative action. In an ironic reversal, the prison budget briefly exceeded the budget for higher education.

Despite this adverse political climate, TCWF decided to make a significant commitment to violence prevention, including the development of controversial policies to limit the availability of handguns. This commitment was, in part, a response to the rising trend of death and injury from violence in California (gunshot homicides had increased sharply since 1985 and were on their way to a 204% increase by 1993),[6] wide-spread public concern about violence, and the increasing acceptance of a public health approach to violence prevention. The commitment also reflected the assertiveness of a new, large foundation with a desire to get on the map and address leadership gaps in the philanthropic world. No other foundation had supported a broad-based public health approach to violence prevention.[27]

In considering its first grant-making initiative, TCWF commissioned five white papers on topics identified by a series of community focus groups conducted around the state in the spring of 1992. Violence prevention was one of the top concerns expressed, and the violence prevention white paper became the basis for a national advisory committee meeting in August 1992.[27] This meeting brought together a diverse group of 40 individuals, including former gang members, law enforcement officials, clergy, trauma physicians, community activists, policy advocates, and researchers. Together this group crafted the essential elements that became the Violence Prevention Initiative.[27] The diversity at this first meeting became a hallmark of the VPI. The initiative continues to build and support broad-based coalitions that "include unexpected allies and speak with many voices from many perspectives."

In October 1992, TCWF's board approved the VPI and committed $25 million for an initial five-year effort. Within a few months, a public education campaign and new community program sites were added, increasing TCWF commitment to $30 million. Eventually, through the added support of several other California foundations, the VPI became a $35 million project. The structure of the VPI includes several components designed to work together to reduce youth-related violence in California. Some of the major components are discussed in the following.

The Policy Program

The VPI has three ambitious policy goals designed to promote a favorable environment for all violence prevention activities:

Goal 1: Shift society's definition of youth violence from a law-enforcement-only perspective to include a public health perspective that addresses societal and environmental influences contributing to youth violence.

Goal 2: Advocate for public policies that reduce access to alcohol and other drugs that contribute to youth violence.

Goal 3: Advocate for public policies that reduce firearm injury and death among youth.

The Pacific Center for Violence Prevention (PCVP), established by a TCWF grant to the Trauma Foundation located at San Francisco General Hospital, has the primary responsibility of coordinating activity toward the policy goals, particularly on the issue of handguns. It also serves as the information and strategic policy center of the VPI. In this capacity, the PCVP provides other VPI components with a range of support activities, including policy and media advocacy training and consultation, an electronic communication network, market research, monitoring of news media presentations of violence, an information resource center, technical assistance for community collaboratives, gathering of expert opinion, legal advice and assistance on crime and violence policy, publication of position papers, education of policy makers, and organization of an annual meeting for all VPI participants. The PCVP also coordinates the Academic Fellows Program, which seeks to increase the number of public health professionals committed to working on violence prevention.

A grant to conduct the public education campaign was awarded to Martin & Glantz, a national consulting firm located in northern California and specializing in grassroots organizing and communications strategies involving public policy issues. Martin & Glantz has developed two major public education campaigns: "Prevent Handgun Violence Against Kids" and "Resources for Youth: An Honest Dialogue About Strategies to Prevent Youth Violence." The firm also developed "Youth Want You to Know," an innovative effort to facilitate the involvement of young people in the policy debate. The primary emphasis of the public education program is to develop an infrastructure of opinion leaders throughout California that will actively support policies to reduce youth violence.

Community Action Programs

The California Wellness Foundation also awarded grants for community action programs (CAPs) serving diverse populations in communities extending from Mendocino to San Diego (Figure 19.2). Compared to the rest of California, the areas served by CAPs are much more likely to include census tracts with African-American, Latino, and Asian/Pacific Islander populations. Also, these communities are marked by greater population density, higher school dropout rates, more people below the poverty level, and higher levels of unemployment.[32] The 16 (originally 18) CAPs provide youth-related program services, such as conflict resolution and peer mediation training, leadership and self-esteem development, cultural awareness, recreation, and education.[27] More generally,

1. Asian Resources
2. Barrios Unidos
3. Bayview Hunter's Point Foundation
4. Boys' and Girls' Club of Stockton
5. EYE Counseling and Crisis Service
6. First Presbyterian Church
7. International Mutual Assistance
8. Inland Agency
9. La Familia Counseling Center
10. Los Angeles Commission on Assaults
11. Mendocino Family and Youth Services
12. Neighborhood House of North Richmond
13. Proyecto Pastoral at Dolores Mission
14. Real Alternatives Program
15. West Oakland Health Council
16. Southern California Youth and Family Services

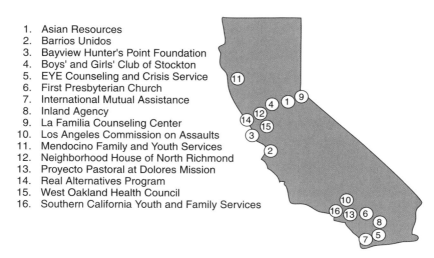

Figure 19.2.   Community action programs funded by The California Wellness Foundation.

they mobilize the broader community on violence prevention issues and apply policy and media advocacy toward this end.

The Leadership Program

The Leadership Program is designed to recognize community leadership, provide resources for leaders and youths, and support professional training in three ways. First, the Community Leader Fellowship Program gives annual awards to 10 individuals, each with an established track record in violence prevention. These remarkably diverse and highly experienced community fellows receive opportunities to increase their advocacy skills; in addition, each fellow is required to identify and mentor two youth leaders. Second, the Academic Fellows Program seeks to increase the number of health professionals committed to violence prevention and provides opportunities for fellows to develop new research, advocacy, clinical, and policy development skills. Third, each year the California Peace Prize honors three outstanding individuals to provide public recognition of the highest level of achievement in the prevention of youth-related violence.

The Research Program

The California Wellness Foundation recognized that there were significant gaps in our knowledge of violence that needed to be filled by scientific inquiry. Grants were thus funded to support research consistent with each of the three VPI policy goals. For example, one project examined the relationship between socioeconomic status, immigrant status, ethnicity, other public health problems, and youth violence. This research developed new information consistent with goal 1, concerning societal and environmental influences contributing to youth violence. Two other studies explored ways to reduce youth access to alcohol (goal 2). The first of these assessed the relationship between retail alcohol outlet density and violence among Mexican-American youth. The second explored legal strategies for reforming alcohol policies to promote prevention efforts at the local level. Research directed toward goal 3 of reducing firearm injury and death among youth applied an epidemiological framework to determine the source of handguns that appeared to be most frequently implicated in youth violence.

A PUBLIC HEALTH APPROACH TO SOCIAL CHANGE

The conception of violence as a public health issue put forth by the Centers for Disease Control and Prevention provided a way for TCWF to justify its significant involvement in this potentially controversial and contentious area of public policy.[33] The adoption of a public health approach provides the VPI with a general framework for engaging the issue of violence. This includes (1) a strong commitment to values based on social justice concepts, (2) advocacy of public policy solutions, (3) use of a scientific and applied research base, (4) mobilization of a broad range of constituencies, and (5) strategic use of the mass media. These were key ingredients in the VPI recipe for successful social change.

Pursuing Social Justice

Public health is the blending of science, advocacy, and politics in the context of community values to improve health.[34] The mission of public health is to "fulfill society's interest in assuring conditions in which people can be healthy."[35] This means placing a primary focus on prevention rather than treatment and on education rather than punishment. The public health approach to violence uses epidemiological methods to assess the distribution of the problem as it varies geographically and within populations in order to identify risk factors, it applies social and behavioral science research to design and assess interventions and inform policy development,[36] and it mobilizes communities to participate in the definition and solution of violence problems through community organizing, coalition building, and policy advocacy.[37]

Inherent in the public health model is a clear commitment to a set of values linked to fairness, equity, participation, and social justice.[38] Virtually every public health problem varies according to social class—the less well-off a group is, the fewer its social and physical resources, the poorer its health status.[39-41] Violence is no different. The primary risk factor for violence is poverty. In an extensive review on violence and youth, the American Psychological Association concluded, "[I]t is the condition of social and economic inequality in which many ethnic minority youth live—and not their ethnicity—that places them at increased risk of becoming victims of violence."[24]

Another characteristic of the public health approach is that it addresses the multiple layers of causality of social and health problems. The model not only calls for efforts to strengthen the ability of individuals to make good health choices but also advocates policies to address the social inequalities that put people at risk. Individuals and their behavior are seen as inextricably linked to a broader social and physical environment; ignoring these environments and focusing exclusively on personal behavior inevitably creates inadequate approaches to public health problems.[42] In terms of violence, the public health approach suggests (1) a wide range of education and training programs aimed at strengthening individual and community resources; (2) specific policies to reduce economic inequality, reduce discrimination, and improve life circumstances for those most at risk; and (3) limits on the availability and design of guns and limits on the availability of alcohol—two major contributors to the frequency and lethality of violence.[36,43-47]

Addressing the adverse social conditions that contribute to violence requires a progressive view of society that links group disadvantage to social factors. This very link separates basic conservative punishment-oriented policy positions from more liberal prevention-oriented policy positions. As Lakoff explains, "The logic of conservatism locates so-called 'social' problems within people, not within society."[48] In the conservative view, programs that try to change social conditions in order to limit crime and violence are fundamentally misguided because they do not focus on the "real" problem—a moral failing of the individual. Building more prisons and instituting tougher penalties to punish criminals is, from a conservative point of view, the appropriate place to focus.

By contrast, the VPI's basic concept of shifting our societal understanding of youth-related violence away from a primarily criminal justice orientation toward a public health focus entails an explicit recognition of a social justice perspective. This is not a complete rejection of punishment; indeed, the public health model recognizes the role of criminal justice in controlling violence.[33] However, in the criminal justice view, "prevention" is believed to occur by threatening punishment (deterrence); in the public health model, prevention is believed to occur by strengthening the personal and social resources for the groups most affected.

Setting Clear, Specific Policy Goals

Public health approaches often begin from the perspective that it is not possible to be healthy in an unhealthy environment.[49,50] Public policy is a means of creating healthy environments. Clear policy goals also allow people to have a shared understanding of what they are trying to achieve, and they provide a basis for evaluating activities and resource allocations. The essential question is, How will this action help advance our policy goal?

Growing out of the firearm policy goal were the following objectives:

· Banning Saturday night specials (also referred to as "junk guns")
· Promoting local authority for firearm policy
· Establishing regulatory authority for the manufacture of firearms under the federal Bureau of Alcohol, Tobacco, and Firearms
· Making the carrying of a concealed firearm a felony rather than a misdemeanor, to be consistent with penalties for concealing other weapons, such as knives

Each of the firearm objectives was strategically determined. Banning Saturday night specials capitalized on a popular issue with broad support in public opinion polls that cut across liberal-conservative lines. Even gun owners supported limits on these handguns, which were seen to be of poor quality with little legitimate use for legal purposes.[51] Promoting local authority was part of a strategy borrowed from the tobacco control movement in California. Because of the difficulty in getting any state legislative activity on the issue of secondhand smoke, these groups had taken the issue to the local level, passing ordinances in more than

100 counties and municipalities; as a result, they had virtually eliminated smoking in enclosed public places. In terms of firearms, it had
been widely accepted that any authority to regulate the availability of
guns resided at the state rather than the local level. Such a situation—in
which the state maintains an authority to regulate that supersedes that
of the locality—is known as preemption. Breaking the hold of preemption was seen as a way to bring the battle to the local level, where communities potentially had more power than pro-gun lobbies. Once the
barrier of preemption was overcome, there were a number of other local
legislative options that could be pursued. These included requiring
ammunition registration, requiring trigger-locking devices, prohibiting
firearm dealers in residential neighborhoods, and imposing a "gross re-
ceipts tax."

The policy objective to establish a federal regulatory authority for the
manufacture of firearms was a way to link the California handgun policy agenda to a national issue. The final policy objective, to make carrying a concealed weapon a felony, built a bridge to the law enforcement
community, which strongly supported this policy.

Translating and Applying Research

Advocacy is inevitably based on the conviction that a significant wrong
must be righted and is often propelled by a sense of moral outrage. The
gun death of one parent's child may be enough to transform that parent
into a tireless gun-control advocate for a lifetime. However, scientific research can help to establish the broader scope of the problem and inform possible solutions. Research is equally important in communicating with policy makers. And because crime, violence, and gun policy are
controversial public issues with powerful advocacy groups promoting
different solutions, it is particularly important to be able to marshal research to counter the claims of the opposing side.

The California Wellness Foundation was influenced from the outset
by research highlighting the problem of youth violence and the role of
guns as a major cause of death. There was a strong epidemiological
knowledge base about the level of youth violence. The research clearly
showed that youth violence had increased in recent years, that the violence had become more deadly, and that the reason for the increased
lethality was guns. State and federal data sources, as well as specific research studies, provided compelling evidence from which TCWF could

confidently justify its involvement in this controversial area. Over the course of the VPI, various types of research were instrumental in advancing the handgun policy issue.

Literature and Database Reviews The strategic use of existing research by the PCVP, complemented by specific compilations from raw data, provided important legitimacy and credibility to the focus on handguns as an important issue in the prevention of youth violence. It also allowed others working on the issue to have access to key findings. The policy papers and fact sheets were based on a large scientific literature that was often difficult to access. This information was effectively "translated" for popular use by VPI grantees and later disseminated through the public education campaign to opinion leaders, policy makers, and the general population as well.

Literature and database reviews provided an early empirical foundation for the significant educational effort that was to unfold. One PCVP policy paper, for example, presented the public health approach to violence and reviewed studies on firearm-related suicide and homicide.[52] The paper discussed legal and regulatory issues at both the state and the federal level, reported findings regarding the cost of firearm injuries, reviewed a range of policy issues, and put forth specific policy recommendations. This policy paper and two others on related topics were widely circulated within the VPI and more broadly to opinion leaders statewide.

One of the most important "data bites" emerged from an analysis of California records by the PCVP. Although it was clear from the start that firearms were *a* leading cause of death for youth in the state, a review of basic data indicated that handguns were *the* leading cause of death for those up to age 19, greater than motor vehicle crashes, drugs, or disease. This important piece of information would become the linchpin of public education efforts and a significant tool in shaping the public conversation about violence.

Another product of PCVP literature and database reviews was a series of well-documented fact sheets that could be used by advocates and journalists. For example, one fact sheet that was part of a "local action kit" provided concise statements and scientific documentation supporting the idea that a gun in the house actually increased rather than decreased the likelihood of becoming a victim of gun violence. Other fact sheets focused on the enormous hospital costs associated with firearm injuries and the effectiveness of gun safety features that could be required by law.

Market Research Market research techniques, like focus groups and public opinion polls, were used to assess public views on violence. Basic ideas were first tested in a series of small focus groups and then further assessed in statewide surveys. This type of research served three functions: (1) It provided a "hook" for gaining media attention and thus contributed to public education, particularly for opinion leaders attending to the news media; (2) it provided intelligence for strategic planning; and (3) it provided local advocates with site-specific data regarding local attitudes on various handgun policy options.

The initial announcement of the VPI was accompanied by the release of a statewide poll on perceptions of violence and approaches to prevention in California. The public opinion poll was explicitly used to enhance the newsworthiness of the announcement on the initiative. This strategy for using polling data was repeated several times and successfully generated news coverage, thus helping to create a supportive information environment for the VPI.

Focus group and public opinion data also provided critical strategic insights for planning public education efforts and identifying policy options. For example, the data showed that people were not aware that handguns were the leading cause of death for children in California. Furthermore, when people became aware of this fact, their level of support for policies to limit handgun availability increased. Also, the data showed that people differentiated between long guns—and firearms in general—and handguns relative to policy options. Thus, policy options needed to be worded accordingly. Other important information on likely supporters of various policies was used to tailor paid advertising buys to reach those most likely to respond to the educational messages.

Polling data for specific communities allowed local groups to provide policy makers with highly relevant information. This information proved interesting and useful to policy makers and opinion leaders and increased the credibility and legitimacy of those providing it. One person noted, "Access to local data gave people the courage to argue more strongly for what they needed in their communities. Polls alone are not enough—it takes a constituency to really use this information." Also, community advocates were linked through the data with the broader statewide effort. One local advocate explained, "We used the poll data. We could talk about guns, but it was really the statistics and information that came from places like the PCVP that impressed people."

Epidemiological and Legal Research Other research was funded to provide information that could help advance the firearm policy goal. The most important research was that of Garen Wintemute, a physician/ epidemiologist at the University of California, Davis. Wintemute had been applying an epidemiological approach to violence for years and had focused on the loading docks of the gun manufacturers as a source of the problem. In other words, Wintemute traced a large part of lethal violence to guns and then sought to find out which manufacturers were producing the guns that caused the deaths. Wintemute wanted to track the problem back to its source and close down the loading dock. His approach was reminiscent of that of John Snow, the father of epidemiology, who, more than a hundred years earlier, stopped a cholera epidemic by ripping the handle off the Broad Street pump that was supplying contaminated water.

Wintemute found that in 1992 six companies, all located within a small radius in Southern California, produced 685,934 handguns, or 34% of all handguns made in the United States. These companies, dubbed the "ring of fire" by Wintemute, produced 80% of all Saturday night specials.[53]

Wintemute's research had a profound effect on highlighting the importance of handgun policy as an essential strategy and on engaging local groups. The *Ring of Fire* report was a significant event in the VPI because it helped people understand guns as a local issue. Everyone already knew that there were far too many guns in the community and that they were too easy to get, but the report made people wonder whether guns were being "dumped" into poor communities of color. If that were the case, it was now clearer where the guns might be coming from. One person explained, "People began to see a tangible enemy instead of constantly feeling surrounded by a vague sense of faceless danger." *Ring of Fire* provided an opponent that might be profiting from the flood of guns and death that was plaguing these communities. The message found an even broader audience when the Public Broadcasting System's television program *Frontline* used Wintemute's research as the basis for "Hot Guns," a one-hour documentary that was partly supported by TCWF.

Another important study was done by Eric Gorovitz, legal director of the Trauma Foundation. Gorovitz reviewed the issue of whether local communities could legally regulate firearms. His law review article indicated that total state preemption of local authority was a myth that was not substantiated by the legal codes. Although local governments were indeed prohibited from regulating in some areas, such as licensing and registration of firearms, they could regulate in a number of other areas, such as banning sales, limiting where guns could be sold, regulating ammunition, and taxing firearm dealers.[54] This research opened the door for people around the state to exercise their power to control guns in their own community, an option that prior to Gorovitz's work was not thought to be possible. "Now," a legal expert noted, "community groups could go to their city attorney with documents in hand that explained how an ordinance could be enacted and who to go talk with to learn more."

Gorovitz's research was not funded by TCWF. It is, nevertheless, a powerful example of how VPI resources leveraged other efforts. Much work that might not have been done, or that would have found little or no audience had it been done, had an impact because of the supportive context provided by the VPI. This principle of leverage would play out many times over on many different levels during the course of the VPI.

Organizing, Supporting, and Expanding the Constituency

Implicit in the VPI's far-ranging policy goals was the mission to develop a statewide network of advocates that could be mobilized to advance violence prevention policy related to youth. This was particularly important for handgun issues, which are emotionally charged and highly controversial. Also, the opposition is well funded, politically sophisticated, and well organized, and refining their arguments and strategies over many years has made the pro-gun groups effective in achieving their legislative goals. Therefore, building a strong violence prevention movement required engaging the CAPs and other VPI grantees, coordinating the existing as well as the new gun control groups emerging around the state, and expanding the constituency by mobilizing additional opinion leaders. It also required ensuring that all grantees had access to a wide range of support materials on policy and media advocacy; legal, epidemiological, and public opinion research; and model local ordinances.

Engaging the Broader VPI The funding of CAPs as part of larger community collaboratives with broad representation provided the basis for a statewide network of advocates. Also, community fellows and academic fellows were situated around the state. However, the handgun policy agenda was not necessarily shared by the other components of the VPI.

The focus on reducing youth access to handguns had been developed independently by TCWF and approved by their board prior to funding the initiative. The broad policy goals had been given to the PCVP as their main charge, but the rest of the VPI was not required to participate in pursuing these goals. Opinion on the policies varied throughout the VPI groups: Some just did not agree with the firearm focus, some were simply too busy providing services and did not have time to get involved in policy issues, some felt that they had had no say in developing the goal and so felt no ownership or commitment to it, and still others felt that they wanted to maintain their autonomy and independence. Thus, building trust with the other components of the VPI and engaging their support became a key concern for the PCVP. In the beginning it was, as one person noted, "like a bad blind date."

Building trust took many forms, including education through the wide range of materials that were available from the PCVP and the "Prevent Handgun Violence Against Kids" (PHVAK) campaign. Fact sheets and policy papers provided a basic understanding of the issues, and events such as annual meetings for all VPI grantees, special meetings for the CAPs, and policy and media advocacy training sessions provided opportunities for building personal relationships and developing new advocacy skills.

Engaging the broader VPI in handgun issues proved a difficult task, but an intensive effort was made to gain support. The PCVP and the public education campaign presented the important research in this area and highlighted the links between handgun availability and local concerns. The PCVP also provided extensive informational materials through its quickly expanding resource center, Web site, and technical assistance. Youth involvement was a primary concern for the CAPs, and PHVAK provided materials such as the "Youth Want You to Know" packets, which provided opportunities for youth to get involved in the policy debate through circulating petitions and writing letters about gun violence to legislators and newspapers. A 1995 statewide video conference was a seminal event in this process, creating an opportunity for VPI grantees to participate in the handgun policy debate with other important leaders in their communities.

In August 1996, the CAPs attended a retreat and agreed to work as an integrated group over the short term to support banning the manufacture and sale of handguns while also working on the longer-term goal of increasing violence prevention resources for youth. This was a significant shift in the support of the CAPs, and it occurred for several reasons. First, PHVAK had increased the visibility and credibility of the issue by effectively using the mass media and providing opportunities for CAPs to participate in the policy education process. Second, the video conference on gun policy had connected local policy makers and opinion leaders with violence prevention professionals and local activists. Third, the *Ring of Fire* report and a resulting perception that companies might be dumping guns in communities of color created an understanding of a common "enemy." Fourth, the PCVP's new policy director had extensive experience developing local gun ordinances in Contra Costa County and had worked closely with the CAPs. As a person of color, he was sensitive to underlying cultural issues attached to this topic and was effective in communicating the importance of the issue to the CAPs. Also, the relationships with the CAPs that the PCVP had cultivated over time had increased trust. Finally, things were changing in the handgun policy environment. In 1995, for the first time, a ban had passed one house of the state legislature before failing in the other, and local ordinances were being introduced around the state. There was a sense that victories could be won, and there were opportunities to participate in the process. Ultimately, interest in the issue of youth access to handguns increased, and various CAPs, as well as community and academic fellows, played significant roles in educating policy makers on both the state and the local level.

Creating a Firearm-Strategy Network While many of those in the VPI had no strong initial commitment to gun policy, there were groups around the state, including new groups funded by TCWF, whose primary concern was the easy availability of handguns. Shortly after the VPI was launched, and as a result of the firearm murders of eight people at a law office in San Francisco in July 1993, the Legal Community Against Violence was founded. This group provided pro bono legal assistance to local governments who were interested in passing ordinances and produced a handbook on developing such local ordinances.[55] In addition, the California Police Chiefs Association, another key group linking law enforcement with some of the VPI objectives, published a position paper supporting limits on firearms.[56]

The League of Women Voters, the Parent Teacher Association, Women Against Gun Violence, and Orange County Citizens Against Gun Violence were among the other groups now getting active in the effort to educate policy makers about the problems associated with cheap, easily available handguns. These groups had lots of information, lots of ideas, and lots of contacts through their political, community, and professional networks.

A new network formed to capture the energy, experience, and expertise of those concerned about handgun availability. Existing groups and the new organizations that were popping up in different parts of the state joined together as a firearm-strategy network to air issues and pursue common goals. The network shared intelligence, monitored the latest developments, kept everyone updated, and used its expanding connections to participate in the policy process. The network agreed on priorities, identified specific policy makers as targets for change, divided up workloads, and followed up on assignments. It also linked up with local efforts, such as the Measure H campaign in Livermore, and, when possible, provided expertise and resources.

The leadership skillfully created an environment in which competitiveness and egos were put aside in the interest of the larger goal of saving lives. Prior to the VPI, few organizations had existed to inform and educate California policy makers about the role of handguns in violence, and the ones that did exist, while on the same side, were often in a competitive relationship. As one advocate put it, "In the past we talked, but didn't share." Now there were many voices united to provide the same message.

The network included gun policy experts from both northern and southern California. One expert explained that "there were many important pieces in the gun control puzzle, but the network was probably the most important piece." Various groups participated, some of whom had no desire to be publicly identified with each other. Some of the groups carried considerable political clout, and other groups were developing important legislative relationships so that "when things came up, people knew who to call."

The network was initially coordinated by the PCVP as a means for sharing the increasing body of information regarding handgun violence, but it soon became apparent that the network could be moving into policy areas that might cross the line of what constituted appropriate participation by nonprofits whose sole funding came from private foundations. At that point, the PCVP representatives no longer participated as part of their PCVP jobs but shifted to other funding sources where there would be no conflict. This approach reflected a growing sophistication within the movement, as groups that might have forgone participation in policy efforts in the past now created alternative structures so they could continue their involvement.

While TCWF did not fund the network, it did, as one person explained, "construct the table around which people sat." The VPI public education campaign and other policy development activities had increased the visibility and urgency of this issue. The California Wellness Foundation helped create a climate in which the goal of reducing handgun availability to youth—a goal supported by those in the network and opinion leaders around the state—could better resonate with policy makers. While the activities of the network were mostly carried on behind the scenes, the impact appears to have been significant. Just a few years ago, advocates had worked largely in isolation, and now they were part of a broader statewide social movement at the core of which was the network. One advocate noted, "As the size of the network grew, so did the movement."

Mobilizing Opinion Leaders Another key part of "growing and feeding" the constituency was the opinion-leader communication program, which was part of the PHVAK public education campaign. This campaign was a sophisticated effort designed to "develop and implement a multimedia public education campaign focused on voters and opinion leaders with the goal of reducing the availability of and access to firearms by youth." In addition to the development of a statewide infrastructure of opinion leaders, it involved extensive message development and testing through focus groups and public opinion polls, strategies to enhance the visibility and importance of handgun violence through the news media, and a video conference to link various parts of the state to the campaign. Each aspect of PHVAK relied on careful research to develop strategy and provide assessment of the value of different tactics.

The opinion-leader effort created a statewide infrastructure for advancing policy for reducing youth access to handguns. The purpose was to increase the capacity of opinion leaders to communicate on violence prevention and handgun policy and hence increase their comfort with these issues. The opinion-leader strategy involved identifying an audience who was supportive of the VPI policy positions but who might not have the knowledge, tools, or confidence to participate in the public debate and then providing those leaders with the necessary information to make it easier to participate in the violence prevention discussion. Many of these opinion leaders have the ear of policy makers, other opinion leaders, or members in organizations to which they belong. They are potential "champions" who can influence members in their groups, introduce resolutions in their organizations, communicate with policy makers, and add their voice to the public debate. One community leader explained that people believed "they should take a stand against guns but had no way to express it. Now people are able to speak out, there is sentiment for gun control, and people feel safer joining in." An opinion leader who received mailings as a result of her position with the Parent Teacher Association (PTA) requested additional material to distribute to the membership. Soon she had organized a task force within the PTA on gun violence. The statewide PTA convention, consisting of 4,000 local presidents, eventually passed a resolution supporting a ban on Saturday night specials.

The cultivation of the opinion-leader group included disseminating policy updates on issues related to handgun violence. "Communities on the Move," developed with the Legal Community Against Violence as part of PHVAK, surveyed cities and counties in California to determine the extent of local ordinances to limit access to guns. Information primarily developed by the PCVP was sent out in a PHVAK mailing that provided survey results and updates on banning Saturday night specials and on other policy options. This was the kind of educational information that opinion leaders could give to others in their organizations and also provide to policy makers and friends.

The opinion-leader database proved to be an especially important tool for organizing supporters. It includes approximately 12,000 people who receive mailings that provide a wealth of information, encourage networking, and encourage opinion leaders to increase their participation on issues central to prevention. This database includes 20 categories of opinion-leader types (e.g., business, education, health, and law enforcement) and approximately 7,000 "prime" records. This separate "prime group" within the database represents an important opinion-leader constituency made up of people who responded to previous mailings or attended a video conference.

Developing Media Strategies to Set the Agenda and Shape the Debate

The mass media set the agenda and shape the public discussion regarding potential solutions to social problems.[57,58] The media tell people not only what issues to think about but also *how* to think about those issues.[59] Youth violence is a highly visible issue and commands extensive coverage in the news media. Unfortunately, this coverage tends to sensationalize the problem and reinforce incarceration and punishment approaches rather than broader public health approaches emphasizing prevention.[60] Solutions, if they are presented, focus on instituting tougher penalties, treating youth as adults in the criminal justice system, and building more prisons.

Importantly, information in the media is disseminated via a two-step model in which information moves from the media to opinion leaders to the broader public.[61] Advocates' media strategies, then, seek not to reach all people but rather to increase the saliency and legitimacy of an issue, to inform and reinforce opinion leaders on that issue, and to directly reach the policy makers. Because these two groups pay special attention to the news media, it is important to augment a public education campaign with various events, direct-mail communication, and news coverage of the issue (earned media).

Paid Television Commercials The first task of PHVAK was to focus the youth violence debate on youth as victims rather than just as perpetrators and to educate people that handguns are the leading cause of death for youth in California. From this core position, a "reframing" of the problem could begin, and PHVAK could move into the need for policy options to limit handgun availability. A key component of the reframing process was the use of paid television commercials.

Public education campaigns usually have limited resources to accomplish substantial goals and thus must be very strategic in their planning. Although PHVAK could not reach every person in California, it sought to mobilize a critical mass of supportive people to become more involved. In addition, a highly visible media campaign would reinforce the efforts of the opinion leaders and create a more favorable public climate in which it was easier for them and others to speak out. Paid media served several purposes: They provided credibility for the broader educational campaign among the media, supported and punctuated key periods of campaign activity, and, in the markets where the ads ran, increased public awareness that handguns were the leading cause of death for youth, that there were too many handguns, and that something must be done. After extensive message development, three spots were created for the first year. One spot explained that a handgun was produced every 20 seconds and that they were being used to kill kids, while a second stressed that handguns were the leading cause of death for youth. A third spot provided a plea from two mothers who had lost children to handgun violence. Subsequent ads addressed the potential for communities to reduce the number of gun dealers through local ordinances and the need to maintain limits on the ability to carry concealed firearms.

Television time for the ads was purchased in Los Angeles and Sacramento and placed to reach populations identified through polling as being most likely to support policies to limit handgun availability. The first six-week buy cost $1 million and reached 85% of television households in the market. Each spot had a toll-free number (800-222-MANY), and people who called received a Citizen Involvement Kit, which included fact sheets about guns and postcards to be sent to policy makers that asked them, "What are you doing to prevent handgun violence against kids?" Evaluation results indicated that there was a significant increase in the number of people identifying handguns as the leading killer of kids, and more than 10,000 Citizen Involvement Kits were distributed. Overall, 62% of those calling the 800 number said that they supported stricter laws, and 19% sent postcards. This indicated that the campaign was successful in reaching the anticipated audience and accomplishing the behavioral objective.[62]

The Video Conference A defining event of the public education campaign to energize people about the handgun issue was a video conference held in February 1995. This event brought diverse elements of the community together around the single issue of the availability of handguns to youth. Community organizers were hired to ensure that a broad spectrum of the community would be represented, and the video conference was downlinked to all the sites where CAPs were located. Panels to discuss next steps in each location immediately followed the video conference and included policy makers, violence prevention professionals, members of law enforcement, and health care workers. This was followed by regional meetings four months later to build on the new relationships that had been established.

In the southern California city of Pomona, for example, the police chief, mayor, leaders from the business and education communities, and the local CAP all attended the video conference. It was here that the idea for a local junk-gun ban was conceived. The police department later requested information from the 800 number. By May 1997, with a lot of community support, Pomona had a junk-gun-ban ordinance as well as an ammunition registration law. Others attending the video conference included aides of those city council members who would later introduce the critically important Saturday night specials ban in West Hollywood and more than 1,500 other key people in 18 cities around California.

Though the video conference was not without its critics, it was a turning point. It successfully brought together key people and gave participants a sense that they were part of a larger movement. Later, when ordinances were being considered, many local people had easier access to their policy makers because they had met them at the video conference. The event was also crucial in framing limits on handgun availability to youth as a mainstream, inclusive issue. Now people were talking not just about the problem but about solutions as well. One southern Californian said, "[Gun control] was not on the agenda before the video conference. It made it real, it made it immediate, it made it important, it made it a battle."

Media Advocacy Another element of working through the mass media to shape the debate and advance handgun ordinances was the use of media advocacy.[37] The Berkeley Media Studies Group, as a subcontractor to the PCVP, trained most VPI grantees in media advocacy and worked with many on an ongoing basis. The media advocacy training complemented the public health focus and helped groups and individuals to frame their violence issues from the policy rather than the personal perspective. In addition, it helped build the capacity in groups to maintain a media presence and advance their policy goals over time.

Media advocacy training presented media strategy as part of overall policy advocacy and explained the role of the news media in setting the agenda, framing the issue, and advancing policy goals. Participants developed skills in gaining access to the news media, talking about violence prevention from a policy perspective, writing letters to the editor, producing op-ed pieces, and developing counterarguments to those of the opposition. Basic tips on the logistics of holding news conferences, developing media lists, and appearing on talk radio were provided. In some cases, on-camera training was used to help advocates prepare for interviews.

The VPI media approach illustrates that media must be combined with other activities and integrated with a broader strategy. It needs to support community action, not substitute for it. Gina Glantz, senior partner in the firm that developed the public education campaign, explained, "Using media without doing constituency building doesn't work. Real community voices need to be carrying the same messages that appear in the media. The combination is what policy makers respond to."

CONNECTING THE DOTS

In the last week of May 1997, the state legislature was considering the ban on the sale and manufacture of Saturday night specials. The makings of a milestone were at hand, and gun control advocates, violence prevention professionals, concerned citizens, and opinion leaders newly versed in the debate came together to secure the victory. One advocate suggested a "Caravan for the Junk-Gun Ban": People would travel from San Diego to Sacramento and rally on the capitol steps to focus attention on the deliberations of the state legislature. The caravan quickly gathered several sponsors, and planning for the trip began.

The mission of the caravan was to educate opinion leaders and policy makers about the problem of youth access to handguns. The group planned the trip strategically, choosing to hold rallies in the districts of key undecided legislators in order to highlight the issue. The firearm-strategy network provided intelligence on where the votes were. Research and education materials from PHVAK and PCVP provided necessary background on the facts of handgun violence and its toll on youth. The Trauma Foundation, parent of the PCVP, coordinated strategy for the planning process, while VPI grantees along the route provided logistical support. Media advocacy skills from previous trainings were put to use in conferences in key legislative districts; in some communities, events were held at trauma centers to emphasize the health perspective.

Media coverage of the caravan was extensive in print and on television, and in nearly every case the coverage reflected the advocates' frame: Personal stories of tragedy were used to highlight the call for a junk-gun ban. Statistics and media bites from the caravanners appeared in the coverage, while the opposition perspective was virtually absent. Copies of the newspaper stories were sent to the legislators. In addition, Handgun Control Inc. aired radio spots in Sacramento, and PHVAK purchased $200,000 in placements in Los Angeles and Sacramento for two commercials emphasizing that there were too many guns and referring viewers to an 800 number for further action. The PHVAK placements were mostly around the evening news shows (excellent opinion-leader time), which were carrying stories about the caravan. As a result, requests to the 800 number shot up from an average of 13 calls per day for the four days preceding the caravan to an average of more than 200 calls a day for the four days of the caravan. Overall, the television commercials contributed to a positive backdrop for the caravan's message to limit handgun availability to youth.

Many letters and phone calls had gone to the legislature. They came from youth in the VPI communities, opinion leaders, and probably some people who had read the news or seen the television commercials in the days leading up to the passage of the ban. In the final rally on the steps of the state capitol, "parents held a 75-foot quilt memorializing the 75 victims of handgun violence in Santa Ana two years ago."[63] This was the same quilt that had draped the dais in the city council chambers in West Hollywood when it became the first city to ban junk guns.

Many people had spoken in many ways to the legislature. Voices were raised on the radio, on television, in print, and in rallies the length of the state. People spoke from the research, and they spoke from their own personal tragedies. The legislators listened because they knew that when they returned to their districts, they would be held accountable for their votes. In the final days, key votes fell into place. Where a few years earlier there had been no voice about limiting handgun availability, now there was an uproar. More than noise, there was now political power and sophistication. One advocate, noting the role of the emerging firearm-strategy network, said, "In the hours that led up to the final vote [in the assembly], you could identify whose vote you needed and who had the clout to get the vote."

The opposition spoke too, but this time it did not prevail. In California, there was now a powerful network of people united on the broad issue of violence prevention and committed to reducing the number of cheap handguns that were available to kill youth.

CONCLUSION

The Violence Prevention Initiative has been a catalyst for transforming the nature of the discussion about handgun policies in California. Just a few years ago, there was no organized constituency supporting limits on the availability of handguns. There was no loud, clear statewide voice linking guns, violence, and youth in a way that called people to action and provided a means to participate. Also, there was no shared long-term vision from which a strategy for change could evolve. If constituencies, voices, and vision did exist, they were isolated and struggling.

Within four years after the start of the VPI, 28 municipalities and six counties had passed junk-gun bans, and a bill banning the statewide manufacture and sale of junk guns was awaiting the governor's signature (see the next section). The community of Livermore had passed a ban through their city council, but before they had a chance to celebrate, it was turned into a referendum—and for the first time in California, a community voted to ban the sale of junk guns.

We are still a great distance from having policies that can reduce the almost 36,000 firearm deaths that we can expect this year in the United States. In California, the dramatic changes in the handgun environment may not produce quick changes in gun fatalities among youth. However, doing nothing to stem the widespread and easy availability of guns could hardly make the problem better. A large footprint has been left in the legislative landscape, and this will lead to more policy options that were not part of the pre-VPI environment.

The VPI set out to mobilize the state to prevent violence, not to pass a specific law or set of laws. Such a mobilization has occurred, but how did it happen? Some of the effect can be attributed to a unique blending of science, advocacy, and politics with a level of resources that were adequate to implement a sophisticated strategy. The VPI provided vision, commitment, and an opportunity for broad participation, creating a synergy that allowed the effect of each single effort to be magnified through the action of many others.

Vision. The VPI was based on a vision of what was possible in the long term rather than what was necessary in the short term. Service providers and advocates often lack even the limited resources necessary to meet the pressing needs of the day, much less the energy to take on a major public policy issue with strong opposition from well-funded groups. Yet in the planning and construction of the VPI, there was always someone looking beyond the horizon. As Andrew McGuire, PCVP director, explained, "The VPI provided the vision that allowed people to believe that the deadly role of handguns in youth violence could be reduced by changing policy."

Commitment. The VPI comprised an extremely diverse group of people, many of whom had been touched personally by violence. During the project, some of those working on this issue in their community were injured and even killed as a result of violence. In these communities, people are committed to change as a matter of survival, and they teamed up with advocates who have a long history of working to make things better. Even the researchers in the VPI, through the topics that they chose to study, evidenced the same kind of commitment to change.

Participation. The extensive constituency-building effort was designed both to create an expanded base of opinion leaders with access to the debate about handgun policies and to provide those leaders with the knowledge, language, and tools to participate. Law enforcement, business, education, and health professionals joined with violence prevention specialists and others in their communities to create change. In addition, the extensive firearm-strategy network that evolved over the course of the project focused in a more concentrated way on those legislators who had the direct power to effect policy change. Where a few years ago legislators might have heard primarily from the pro-gun groups, by 1996 they were hearing from many diverse voices concerned about the devastating effects of handguns and committed to supporting limits on their availability.

Synergy. Many voices with one message about limiting handgun availability created a drumbeat for change. However, the power of those voices was their credibility and the implicit threat in their message. The credibility came from three sources: (1) the scientific research documenting the terrible toll of gun violence among youth and supporting the importance of limiting handgun availability, (2) the market research that provided local data, and (3) the connection of individual voices to a larger movement. The threat was clear, and it was reinforced by the results of the 1996 elections in California: Gun control was a voting issue, as it always had been, but now the votes were in favor of limiting handgun availability rather than against it.

The struggles over public policy are contentious because there is so much at stake. Public policy is the way that we, as a society, allocate risks and benefits to the population and establish norms for personal behavior and social intercourse. Public health, because of its focus on prevention, is inevitably about politics and policy. The VPI was drawn into the political process because that is one of the key arenas in which the struggle for change is waged. Importantly, TCWF and the VPI grantees have a keen understanding of how to educate policy makers within the context of Internal Revenue Service regulations limiting the activities of nonprofits. When they thought that these limits were being reached, they found alternative structures that allowed them the kind of participation they needed to make a difference. While it is too soon to say if the VPI has succeeded in its larger task of reducing violence, it can reasonably be said that a foundation has been laid that makes further progress inevitable.

POSTSCRIPT

On September 26, 1997, Governor Wilson vetoed the proposed legislation that would have banned the manufacture and sale of Saturday night specials in California.[64] However, almost two years later, on August 27, 1999, Governor Gray Davis signed a bill to ban the manufacture and sale of Saturday night specials in California as of January 1, 2000. What was thought virtually impossible at the beginning of the VPI was now the law of the state.[65]

NOTE

Prepared for the 1997 California Wellness Foundation / University of California Wellness Lecture Series under a grant from The California Wellness Foundation. I wish to thank The California Wellness Foundation/UC Wellness Lectures Steering Committee for selecting me as a Distinguished Wellness Lecturer for 1997. I want to express my great appreciation to the following people for their contribution to various aspects of this chapter: Frank Acosta, Michael Balaoing, Mary Leigh Blek, Ralph Catalano, Carole Ching, Iris Diaz, Lori Dorfman, Tracy Fried, Gina Glantz, Eric Gorovitz, Jennifer Logan, Andrew McGuire, Kae McGuire, Meredith Minkler, Holly Potter, Bernardo Rosa, Susan Shaw, Andres Soto, Stephen Teret, Esther Thorson, Luis Tolley, Robin Tremblay-McGaw, Jan Vernick, Elaine Villamin, Liana Winett, Katie Woodruff, and Gary Yates. I am especially grateful to Linda Nettekoven and Kathryn Chetkovich for their extensive editing contributions. Also, I want to express my appreciation to, and admiration for, all those working on the Violence Prevention Initiative of The California Wellness Foundation. Their efforts will mean safer communities for all people in California. Finally, in the interest of disclosure, please note that I have worked for several years on the Violence Prevention Initiative and have received compensation for that work.

REFERENCES

1. Hubner, J., and Wolfson, J. 1997. *Somebody Else's Children*. New York: Random House.
2. Shalala, D. E. 1993. Addressing the crisis of violence. *Health Affairs* (winter), 30–33.

3. Federal Bureau of Investigation. 1995. *Crime in the United States 1995, Uniform Crime Reports.* Washington, D.C.: Federal Bureau of Investigation, 14.

4. U.S. Department of Health and Human Services, National Center for Health Statistics, National Vital Statistics System. 1995. *Health United States, 1995.* Washington, D.C.: U.S. Department of Health and Human Services, 117.

5. California Department of Health Services. 1997, May 22. *Injury Deaths for Homicides by Age and Cause, California 1995.* Sacramento: California Department of Health Services.

6. California Department of Health Services, Emergency Preparedness and Injury Control Branch. 1996. *Epic Proportions: Violent Injuries to California Youth.* Sacramento: California Department of Health Services, 7.

7. California Department of Justice, Division of Law Enforcement, Bureau of Criminal Information and Analysis. 1996. *Homicide in California, 1994.* Sacramento: California Department of Justice.

8. California Department of Justice, Division of Law Enforcement, Bureau of Criminal Information and Analysis. 1995. *Crime and Delinquency in California, 1994.* Sacramento: California Department of Justice.

9. Wilkinson, D. L., and Fagan, J. 1996. The role of firearms in violence "scripts": The dynamics of gun events among adolescent males. *Law and Contemporary Problems* 59, 55–89.

10. Cook, P. J. 1996. Foreword. *Law and Contemporary Problems* 59, 1–4.

11. Hemenway, D., Prothrow-Stith, D., Bergstein, J. M., et al. 1996. Gun carrying among adolescents. *Law and Contemporary Problems* 59, 39–53.

12. Zimring, F. E. 1996. Kids, guns, and homicide: Policy notes on an age-specific epidemic. *Law and Contemporary Problems* 59, 25–37.

13. Kennedy, D. M., Piehl, A. M., and Braga, A. A. 1996. Youth violence in Boston: Gun markets, serious youth offenders, and a use-reduction strategy. *Law and Contemporary Problems* 59, 147–196.

14. Blumstein, A., and Cork, D. 1996. Linking gun availability to youth gun violence. *Law and Contemporary Problems* 59, 5–24.

15. Rates of homicide, suicide, and firearm-related death among children— 26 industrialized countries. 1997. *Morbidity and Mortality Weekly Report* 46(5), 101–106.

16. Anderson, R. N., Kochanek, K. D., and Murphy, S. L. 1997. Report of final mortality statistics, 1995. *Monthly Vital Statistics Report* 45(11, Suppl. 2), 1–5.

17. Kellermann, A. L., Rivara, F. P., Rushforth, N. B., et al. 1993. Gun ownership as a risk factor for homicide in the home. *New England Journal of Medicine* 329, 1984–1991.

18. Kellermann, A. L., Rivara, F. P., Sommes, G., et al. 1992. Suicide in the home in relation to gun ownership. *New England Journal of Medicine* 327, 467–472.

19. Cummings, P., Koepsell, T. D., Grossman, D. C., et al. 1997. The association between the purchase of a handgun and homicide or suicide. *American Journal of Public Health* 87, 974–978.

20. Blumstein, A. 1995. Violence by young people: Why the deadly nexus? *National Institute of Justice Journal* 229, 2–9.

21. Cook, P. J., and Ludwig, J. 1997, May. *Guns in America: National Survey on Private Ownership and Use of Firearms.* Research in Brief. Washington, D.C.: National Institute of Justice.

22. Nieto, M., Dunstan, R., and Koehler, G. 1994, October. *Firearm-Related Violence in California: Incidence and Economic Costs.* California Research Bureau.

23. Elliott, D. S. 1994. *Youth Violence: An Overview.* Boulder, Colo.: Center for the Study and Prevention of Violence, Institute for Behavioral Sciences, University of Colorado, F-693.

24. American Psychological Association, Commission on Violence and Youth. 1993. *Violence and Youth: Psychology's Response.* Vol. 1. Washington, D.C. American Psychological Association.

25. Reiss, A. J., and Roth, J. A., eds. 1993. *Understanding and Preventing Violence.* Washington, D.C.: National Academy Press.

26. Rosenberg, M. L., and Fenley, M. A., eds. 1991. *Violence in America: A Public Health Approach.* New York: Oxford University Press.

27. RAND and Stanford Center for Research in Disease Prevention. 1997, June. The California Wellness Foundation Violence Prevention Initiative Mid-Initiative Assessment. Vol. 1. Santa Monica, California.

28. Morain, D. 1997. Assembly, Senate approve curbs on cheap handguns. *Los Angeles Times,* June 5, A1.

29. Editorial. 1997. This could be the year for killing off junk guns. *Los Angeles Times,* August 1, B8.

30. Wilgoren, J. 1997. Gun control backers set sights on bullets. *Los Angeles Times,* May 27, B1.

31. The California Wellness Foundation. 1994. *The California Wellness Foundation Violence Prevention Initiative: A New Direction for Improving Health and Well-Being in California.* Woodland Hills, Calif.: The California Wellness Foundation.

32. Stanford Center for Research in Disease Prevention. 1996, June. *Violence Prevention Initiative Community Action Grantee Program, Mid-Initiative Report.* Palo Alto, Calif.: Stanford Center for Research in Disease Prevention.

33. Rosenberg, M., O'Carroll, P., and Powell, K. 1992. Let's be clear—Violence is a public health problem. *Journal of the American Medical Association* 267, 3071–3072.

34. Wallack, L., and Dorfman, L. 1996. Media advocacy: A strategy for advancing policy and promoting public health. *Health Education Quarterly* 23, 293–317.

35. Institute of Medicine. 1988. *The Future of Public Health.* Washington, D.C.: National Academy Press.

36. Mercy, J. A., Rosenberg, M. L., Powell, K. E., et al. Public health policy for preventing violence. *Health Affairs* (winter), 7–29.

37. Wallack, L., Dorfman, L., Jernigan, D., and Themba, M. 1993. *Media Advocacy and Public Health.* Newbury Park, Calif.: Sage Publications.

38. Beauchamp, D. 1976. Public health as social justice. *Inquiry* 12, 3–14.

39. Wilkinson, R. G. 1992. National mortality rates: The impact of inequality. *American Journal of Public Health* 82, 1082–1084.

40. Adler, N., Boyce, T., Chesney, M., et al. 1993. Socioeconomic inequalities in health. *Journal of the American Medical Association* 269(24), 3140–3145.
41. Kaplan, G., Pamuk, E., Lynch, J., et al. 1996. Inequality in income and mortality in the United States: Analysis of mortality and potential pathways. *British Medical Journal* 312, 999–1003.
42. Wallack, L., and Winkleby, M. 1987. Primary prevention: A new look at basic concepts. *Social Science in Medicine* 25, 923–930.
43. Cohen, L., and Swift, S. 1993. A public health approach to the violence epidemic in the United States. *Environment and Urbanization* 5, 50–66.
44. Robinson, K., Teret, S., Vernick, J., and Webster, D. 1996, September. *Personalized Guns: Reducing Gun Deaths through Design Changes*. Baltimore: The Johns Hopkins Center for Gun Policy and Research.
45. Wintemute, G. 1996. The relationship between firearm design and firearm violence. *Journal of the American Medical Association* 275, 1749–1753.
46. McLoughlin, E., and Wang, C. 1990. Alcohol, tobacco, and firearms—Filling or spilling the National Treasury. *Problems in General Surgery* 7, 306–320.
47. Parker, R. 1993. The effects of context on alcohol and violence. *Alcohol Health and Research World* 17, 117–122.
48. Lakoff, G. 1996. *Moral Politics*. Chicago: University of Chicago Press.
49. Wallack, L. 1992. What is public health? *Propaganda Review* 9, 4–6.
50. Labonte, R. 1986. Social inequality and healthy public policy. *Health Promotion* 1, 341–351.
51. EDK Associates. 1994. *Handguns and Violence: A Survey of California Public Attitudes*. New York: EDK Associates.
52. Pacific Center for Violence Prevention. 1994. *Preventing Youth Violence: Reducing Access to Firearms*. San Francisco: Pacific Center for Violence Prevention.
53. Wintemute, G. 1994. *Ring of Fire—The Handgun Makers of Southern California*. Davis: Violence Prevention Program, University of California, Davis.
54. Gorovitz, E. 1996. California dreamin': The myth of state preemption of local firearm regulation. *University of San Francisco Law Review* 30(2), 395–426.
55. Legal Community Against Violence. 1995. *Addressing Gun Violence through Local Ordinances: A Legal Resource Manual for California Cities and Counties*. San Francisco: Legal Community Against Violence.
56. California Police Chiefs Association. 1995. *Confronting the American Tragedy: The Need to Better Regulate Firearms*. Vol. 95-1. California Police Chiefs Association.
57. Lippmann, W. 1965. *Public Opinion*. Reprint, New York: The Free Press.
58. Dearing, J. W., and Rogers, E. M. 1996. *Agenda-Setting*. Newbury Park, Calif.: Sage Publications.
59. Iyengar, S. 1991. *Is Anyone Responsible? How Television Frames Political Issues*. Chicago: University of Chicago Press.
60. Dorfman, L., Woodruff, K., Chavez, V., and Wallack, L. 1997. Youth and violence on local television news. *American Journal of Public Health* 87(8), 1311–1316.

61. Katz, E. 1975. The two-step flow of communication. In W. Schramm, ed., *Mass Communication.* Pp. 346–366. Urbana: University of Illinois Press.

62. Martin & Glantz. *The Campaign to Prevent Handgun Violence Against Kids: A Report on the February 22, 1995, Statewide Video Conference.* San Rafael, Calif.: Martin & Glantz. 1995.

63. Bancroft, A. 1997. Grieving parents back ban on cheap handguns. *West County Times,* May 30, A12.

64. Gunnison, R. 1997. Governor vetoes bill banning cheap guns. *San Francisco Chronicle,* September 27, A1.

65. Wallack, L. 1999. The California Violence Prevention Initiative: Advancing policy to ban Saturday night specials. *Health Education and Behavior* 26(5, December), 841–857.

ADOLESCENT SEXUALITY
AND HEALTH CARE REFORM

More than half of all adolescents are sexually experienced well before the end of their second decade, leading to such serious consequences as unintended pregnancies, sexually transmitted diseases, and acquired immunodeficiency disease (AIDS/HIV).[1] Yet we, as a nation, have not given a high priority to the primary prevention of these outcomes among sexually active youth in terms of either health education or health care itself. Public policy too often has swept teen pregnancy under the rug until after conception has occurred or has limited preventive concerns to seeking universal teen abstinence—an unrealistic goal at best. As a result, we have one million teenagers becoming pregnant each year, equivalent to one out of every nine 15- to 19-year-old girls, or one out of five among those who are sexually active.[2] Some 600,000 give birth, becoming parents far too soon and curtailing their future potentials. Rates of gonorrhea, chlamydia, and syphilis among sexually active youth today are higher than among sexually active persons of any other age. While the number of cases of clinical AIDS remains low in the adolescent years, the incidence of HIV seropositivity is rising exponentially and is particularly high among inner-city, homeless, and runaway teens. It also is true that those who manifest AIDS between ages 20 and 26 in all probability become infected as adolescents. The costs to all these young people and to the nation are incalculable.[3]

Answers are far more complicated than simply telling adolescents to be abstinent until marriage and hoping that will happen—as has been our policy to date. Young people today are faced with an exceptionally difficult and ambiguous situation in which both developmental and societal factors combine to confound their best intentions. First is the dichotomy between biological maturity and societal adulthood. Most young people are biologically prepared for procreation, with all the associated instinctive drives, some 10 years or more before society condones activation of these drives in wedlock. Girls are capable of reproduction at an average age of $12\frac{1}{2}$ years, and boys are capable of fathering a child at age 13. At the same time, the typical young woman in the United States today marries at age 24 and the average young man at age 26.[2]

Cognitive and psychosocial developmental factors also come into play. Younger teens, in particular, are still concrete in their thought processes. It is not until midway in the second decade that they will gain the ability to think in an abstract manner. Concrete thinkers are existential, focused on the here-and-now. They cannot fully appreciate the future consequences of their current acts. At the same time, adolescents are defining their identities and seeking emancipation, processes that, by nature, involve a good bit of experimentation and at least some denial of associated risks.[4]

Societally, while our basic moral message continues to be one of no premarital sex, we do everything possible to promote it in an exceptionally provocative environment. In 1988, American television viewers were exposed to some 14,000 instances of sexual material, of which more than 9,000 were scenes suggestive of sexual intercourse with varying degrees of explicitness.[5] Most such scenes were highly romanticized. Only 1% addressed sex education, sexually transmitted diseases (STDs), birth control, or abortion. In an even more recent study of televised sexual material conducted in the fall of 1996 during the prime-time family hour,[6] three out of four programs (75%) on the major networks contained sexual content; 61% showed some degree of sexual behavior (up from 48% in 1986 and 26% in 1976), with 30% featuring scenes with a primary emphasis on sex (up from 23% in 1986 and 9% in 1976.) Further, during the three-week sample period, 15 cases of sexual intercourse were either depicted or clearly implied. Here again, only a handful (6%) had an overall emphasis on sexual risks and responsibilities, such as waiting until a relationship matures before having sex or pursuing efforts to prevent STDs or unwanted pregnancy when sexually active. Further, many MTV rock videos give messages that encourage not only sexual activity but also sexual exploitation—particularly in "heavy metal."

The clothing industry seems equally bent on turning juniors into young Lolitas. Take a look at the junior department displays in any clothing store. Also take a look at such teen-oriented magazines as *Seventeen*. Although most commonly read by 12- to 13-year-old girls, advertisements, in particular, regularly depict overt flirting behavior, seductive cosmetic use, and provocative clothing styles. "Adult" magazines also are readily available to teens. Youths with even a modicum of curiosity can easily purchase a copy of *Playboy, Playgirl,* or *Penthouse* at the nearest magazine store.

These images create an environment in which there is an extraordinary degree of pressure to be sexually active, to "make out" in the pursuit of autonomy and identity, especially among males. In many respects, we continue to maintain the double standard of old in valuing and encouraging boys to press on and be sexually aggressive while valuing girls who can resist. But major societal changes have occurred in the female role. Prohibitions against sexual activity among unmarried women today are considerably less than in the past. Pregnancy and childbearing no longer need be an invariable outcome—contraception and abortion have changed the odds greatly. Further, single parenthood no longer results in social ostracism.

For many youths, sexual intimacy is something more than an impulsive response to pheromones, passion, or curious experimentation. Teens have a difficult and ambiguous status in our society. We call them "transitional," which implies that they are neither here nor there but in transit between one place and another—in limbo. They have no significant role or place other than as students. They are not needed either to support the concept of the family, as are little children, or to contribute to society, as are adults. They are segregated away from the societal mainstream in schools and stratified in the classroom according to age. As a result, adolescents today comprise a distinct and separate subculture with powerful peer-group influences and few external ameliorating forces. Sexual activity frequently is perceived as an important marker of this subculture and something that "all kids do."

Many adolescents who have a negative view of the world are chronically depressed with poor self-esteem and believe that sexual intimacy will provide the love and closeness that they so urgently want. As an added bonus for those teen girls who also are drifting with no sense of the future or personal goals and are doing poorly in school, having a baby often is perceived as providing someone to love and to love them unconditionally, as bestowing instant adulthood, and as ending their "in limbo" status. In a national longitudinal survey of eighth-grade students, more than half of all dropouts had at least one child before the time they normally would have graduated as compared to only 9% of those who did graduate.[7] Low socioeconomic status was a particular predictor of both dropping out and parenthood, and, in many cases, the birth of a child was the particular event that precipitated leaving school.

Other youths are angry and feel deprived, both of which can lead to sexual acting out. Some teens have a self-interested, hedonistic view of life and a belief that they are personally entitled to get their due, including sexual gratification. The new phenomenon of the shrinking "American Dream," in which young people rightly perceive that they will have less economic opportunity than their parents, may well promote a sense of disappointment and of being cheated by life with little point in delaying sexual activity.

All these societal and developmental factors combine to make it very difficult for adolescents to be fully responsible for their sexual behavior and create a situation that forces intimacy to be clandestine, unintended, and unplanned. Sexual risks tend to be denied by teens who often are both ambivalent about being sexually active and not cognitively mature enough to appreciate the potential risks. Powerful environmental and biological forces often overwhelm even the best of abstinence intentions. Once abstinence intentions give way to action, far less anxiety, fear, blame, and guilt are experienced if the adolescent allows himself or herself to be just swept away by overwhelming emotion, without conscious planning and in denial of risks in the mistaken belief that pregnancy or AIDS "can't happen to me."

In countering these pressures, parents continue to find it difficult to give guidance to their young about sex beyond prohibition. Few mothers or fathers have open discussions about sexual decision making or sexual responsibility.[8,9] Few even know whether their offspring are sexually active or even make such an inquiry. Many parents unwittingly even facilitate sexual activity. It is they who pay the bills for bikini bathing suits and miniskirts. It is they who no longer insist on adult chaperones at teen get-togethers. It is they who are very free with the keys to the family car or even buy their 16-year-old a car of his or her own as a rite of passage. And it is they who often are so self-preoccupied that they demand little accountability from their adolescent.

From another perspective, parental discord and divorce, together with the associated family chaos surrounding such an event, is a major contributor to adolescent health-risk behaviors, including sexual activity.[10] The rate of divorce over the past decade has escalated to such a degree that 26% of all children under 18 now live with a divorced parent, a separated parent, or a stepparent[11] and are subjected to all the emotional distress of the process of marital dissolution.

A number of recent popular movies, humorous and good-natured in tone, provide clear models for adolescent sexual freedom by portraying young heroes who monumentally exceed the boundaries of parental permission—and get away with it—while their parents are not at home. In *Risky Business,* for example, Tom Cruise sets up his home as a bordello for his high school classmates as an entrepreneurial fund-raiser and barely returns the house to normal as his parents walk up the front walk. He does not get caught or suffer any penalty. This is a far different message from teen cult movies of the past, such as James Dean's *Rebel without a Cause,* so full of anguish and painful consequences for defiant behavior, or the resentful attitudes toward adult authority and adult limit setting expressed by adolescents in *The Breakfast Club.*

Schools do little better than parents at promoting responsible adolescent sexual behavior. While AIDS education has now been introduced into most secondary school classrooms, relatively few programs employ an approach based on combining social learning, social inoculation, and cognitive-behavioral learning theories, now recognized as the most effective method for modifying behavior (see the section "Modifying Adolescent Sexual Risk Taking"). The vast majority simply provide young people with information about the risks of sexual intimacy and advocate abstinence, an approach that has been found to have only a small effect. Few students are provided answers to all their questions in an honest, straightforward manner; nor are they equipped with the skills and support systems that they need to deal with our highly sexualized society. Moreover, none of these courses reaches the large number of sexually active young people who have dropped out of school. Current conservative political forces also seek to severely restrict sex education to teens. In 1966, the federal legislature appropriated $50 million annually for abstinence-only education in schools, mandating that "sexual activity outside of the context of marriage is likely to have harmful psychological and physical effects" be the only message taught and banning inclusion of any information about other means of pregnancy, AIDS, or STD prevention.[12] Such actions totally ignore the fact that abstinence-only education is not very effective for the large numbers of young people who already are sexually experienced.

As far as the health care sector is concerned, with the exception of such specialized programs as family planning and adolescent medicine clinics, there has been widespread abdication of professional responsibility for providing preventive sexuality health care to youth. Strong forces promote sexual activity among our adolescents while, at the same time, we tell them not to respond to such temptations. We then go one step further and punish those who do become sexually active by not providing them with readily available and appropriate health care services that will promote responsible sexual behavior and prevent its adverse consequences.

THE STATISTICS

Sexual Activity

In 1995, the Centers for Disease Control's (CDC's) national school-based Youth Risk Behavior Survey (YRBS)[13] found that 53% of students in all grades reported being sexually experienced, with 17% having been involved with four or more lifetime partners. By the end of their senior year, nearly three out of every four male students (70%) and two-thirds of all female students (66%) had experienced sexual intercourse at least once, and 7% reported that they either had been pregnant or had impregnated a partner. Nine percent had even initiated sexual intercourse before they were age 13. African-American students (73%) were significantly more likely than White and Hispanic students (49% and 58%, respectively) to have ever had sexual intercourse (Table 20.1). These data were not singularly different from those found in the 1993 YRBS.[14]

The proportion of adolescent females who report being premaritally sexually experienced not only has increased dramatically over the past two decades but is the culmination of a trend that began at the turn of the 20th century and clearly suggests a fundamental and permanent societal change in teenage girls' sexual behavior. Despite their many statistical flaws and dominantly Caucasian subjects, Kinsey's surveys in the 1940s still provide significant information.[15,16] Kinsey found that among women born before 1900, only 3% were premaritally sexually experienced by age 18—and this usually during the period of engagement with their fiancé. But for those born just a few years later, or after 1900, the number increased sixfold to 18%, again primarily with a fiancé. The incidence of sexual activity among adolescent boys, however, has not changed a great deal. In Kinsey's time, 40% of men reported that they were experienced by age 15 and 60% by age 17. The cardinal difference between past and present patterns of adolescent male sexual activity is

TABLE 20.1   PERCENTAGE OF HIGH SCHOOL
STUDENTS WHO REPORTED ENGAGING
IN SEXUAL INTERCOURSE BY ETHNICITY/
RACE, GRADE, AND HAVING FOUR
OR MORE LIFETIME PARTNERS —
UNITED STATES, 1993 AND 1995

	1993			1995		
	Female	*Male*	*Total*	*Female*	*Male*	*Total*
Ethnicity/race						
White	47.4	49.8	48.4	49.0	48.9	48.9
Black	70.4	89.2	79.7	67.0	81.0	78.4
Hispanic	48.3	63.5	56.0	53.3	62.0	57.6
Grade						
9th	31.6	43.5	37.7	32.1	40.6	36.9
10th	44.9	47.4	46.1	46.0	50.0	48.0
11th	55.1	59.5	57.5	60.2	57.1	58.6
12th	66.3	70.2	68.3	66.0	67.1	66.4
Four+ partners	15.0	22.3	18.8	14.4	20.9	17.8
Total	50.2	55.6	53.0	52.1	54.0	53.1

SOURCES: Centers for Disease Control (1995 [14], 1996 [13]).

that much of the earlier cohort's experience was with prostitutes in contrast to the dating partner of today. Among women born somewhat later (between 1938 and 1940), approximately one in four was sexually experienced by age 18. There was a modest increase of 25% for the 1947–1949 birth cohort but a 100% increase among those born between 1956 and 1958 (Figure 20.1).[17] In subsequent years there again has been a further doubling in the prevalence of sexual activity with approximately twice as many 15- to 19-year-old young women (53%) being sexually experienced in 1995 as were experienced in 1970 (28%) (Figure 20.2).[18,19]

There has, however, been a recent modest drop in the proportion of both teens who are sexually active, as evidenced in the CDC's series of high school youth surveys,[13,14,19] and females, as seen in the 1995 National Survey of Family Growth (NSFG).[20] In the 1990 YRBS, 59% of all students reported that they were sexually experienced as compared to 55% in 1991 and 53% in 1995. Over the same period, there was a drop of 3%, from 40% to 37%, in the number of students reporting two or more lifetime partners and a decrease of 6% for four or more partners.

In the 1995 NSFG, the percentage of teenage females aged 15 to 19 years declined to a slightly greater degree (Figure 20.2), with only

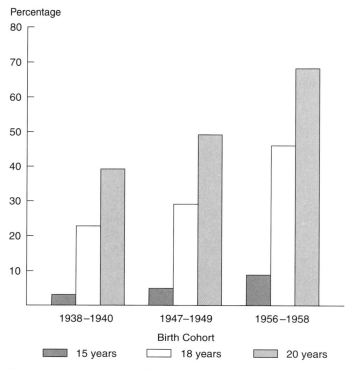

Figure 20.1. Percentage of women aged 15, 18, and 20 who had premarital sexual intercourse by birth cohort. Source: Cates (1990 [17]).

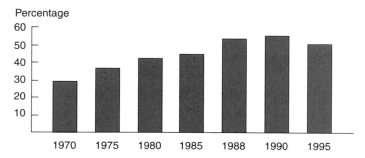

Figure 20.2. Percentage of women aged 15 to 19 years who reported having had premarital sexual intercourse—United States, 1970–1995. Source: Abma et al. (1997 [20]).

50% reporting that they ever had sexual intercourse as compared to a peak of 55% found in 1990. According to a series of surveys conducted by the Urban Institute for the National Institute of Child Health and Development, a similar reversal in trends has been reported for teenage males, with a decline in the number of males who report that they are sexually active declining from 60% in 1988 to 55% in 1995.[21]

Despite the overall drop in the percentage of sexually active youth found in these surveys, a return to universal teen abstinence is highly unlikely. First, taking an overall figure is misleading in not considering the data by both ethnicity and age (Table 20.1). A closer examination of YRBS findings reveals that three-quarters of all Black adolescents continue to be sexually active, that rates among Hispanic girls are increasing, that more 11th-grade females of all ethnicities were sexually active in 1995 than in 1993, and that the percentage of sexually active 12th-grade females has not changed. Second, the trend toward an increasing incidence of premarital sexual intercourse, particularly among teenage girls, has taken place over a span of nearly nine decades and can only be seen as reflecting a major and persistent societal change in normative adolescent behavior. It is clear that a substantial number of teenagers will continue to be at risk from sexual activity and that initiatives promoting abstinence alone will be far from sufficient to meet the task of protecting our adolescents from serious health harm.

The initiation of sexual activity appears to be determined by the interaction of a number of biological, psychological, cultural, and social factors, either singly or severally, including early pubertal onset (particularly in girls), cognitive immaturity, ethnicity, dysfunctional home situations, past physical or sexual abuse, chronic depression, poor self-esteem, absence of future plans, poor schooling, and economic disadvantage.[22-33] Most of these studies also show a significant association of an early coital debut, multiple partners, choice of a high-risk partner, and nonuse of protection with a wide range of other problem behaviors, such as alcohol use, marijuana use, school problems, minor delinquent acts, depression, and suicide attempts. Only Stanton[34] showed no such relationship in a survey of African-American youths in a public housing project. These adolescents perceived sex as being in a very different domain.

None of these studies, however, assess the degree to which these other associated risk behaviors are within the experimental or committed range and the degree to which they can be considered truly dysfunctional and deviant. Further, all persons are sexual beings from the time of birth, and the exploration of intimacy in general is a normal behavior for ado-

lescents as well as adults. It is the progression of intimacy to sexual intercourse prior to marriage that violates conservative moral values. But
when the increase in the incidence of adolescent female sexual intercourse
has taken place over the course of many decades and when half of all
teenagers are sexually experienced, this behavior can well be interpreted
as reflecting fundamental cultural change and as now being within the
range of normal behavior for older teens. The risk is not so much in the
fact of being sexually active, provided that the couple are relatively mature, no exploitation is involved, and the choice has been willingly, ratio-
nally, and responsibly made as it is in the adverse consequences when
protection is not used. Younger adolescents who are cognitively immature and have not yet established effective decision-making skills are quite
another matter and do cause developmental concern; they are far less
likely to be discriminating in their partner choice or to use consistent
protection and much more likely to be coerced into sexual intercourse
against their will or otherwise exploited.

Pregnancy

As previously noted, about one million teenagers become pregnant each
year.[2] In 1990, 11% of all adolescent girls became pregnant, 5% gave
birth, 3.3% had an out-of-wedlock birth (although many in-wedlock
births were premaritally conceived), 4.6% had an abortion, 1.5% experienced a miscarriage, and only 0.13% gave up their baby for adoption.[35] Another way of looking at this epidemic is to state that 43% of
the approximately 17 million teen females in the United States will become pregnant at least once before they reach their 20th birthday.[36] Further, the vast majority of current teen births are out of wedlock. In 1960,
only 15% of all adolescent births were to single mothers, but by 1993
this figure had increased nearly fivefold to 72% (Figure 20.3).[37] Rates
are highest among teenagers of Mexican, Puerto Rican, and African-
American ethnicity, as they are for Mexican, Puerto Rican, and African-
American women of all age-groups.[38]

There has, however, been a recent reversal in the birth rate to teens
(Figure 20.3). Although the rate among 15- to 19-year-olds rose by
nearly 10% from 53.0 births per 1,000 in 1980 to a high of 62.1 per
1,000 in 1991, the subsequent three years saw a drop of 3% to a rate
of 58.9 per 1,000 in 1994.[37] This drop, however, was considerably less
(only 1%) when 18- to 19-year-olds were excluded, with rates for 1980,
1991, and 1994 among 15- to 17-year-olds being 32.5%, 38.7%, and

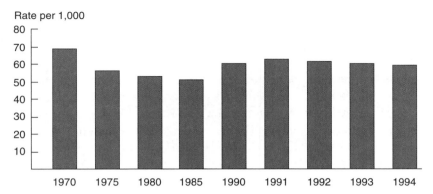

Figure 20.3. Birth rates for women aged 15 to 19 years—United States, 1970–1994. Source: National Center for Health Statistics (1996 [37]).

37.6%, respectively. It is apparent that efforts to reduce the pregnancy rate among younger high school girls have been limited at best.

Whatever decrease in adolescent birth rates has occurred is almost exclusively due to more effective contraception (particularly among older teens), not a higher incidence of abortions—which actually has declined—or a reduction in the percentage of sexually active youths, which has only modestly changed. Further, despite this recent decline, the 1994 teen pregnancy rate is still higher than in any year prior to 1990.

California is no exception to high teen birth rates and, in fact, has a substantially higher 15- to 19-year-old rate (68 per 1,000) than the national average (58.9 per 1,000).[39] Here too, however, there has been a significant drop of 5.5% from 69.9 births per 1,000 population in 1993 to 64.4 per 1,000 in 1995. These statistics, however, do not reflect the wide geographic variation within the state with singularly high teen birth rates ranging from 92 to 100 per 1,000 15- to 19-year-olds and comprising 18% to 20% of all births reported in Fresno, Kern, Kings, Madera, Merced, and Tulare, all agricultural counties, with the largest number of births (both adolescent and adult) being to mothers of Hispanic ethnicity.[40] Nor do these figures represent the true scope of the problem, as California has an even higher adolescent pregnancy rate than reflected in teen birth statistics alone. In 1992, this state had both the highest total number of estimated abortions (338,700) and the highest abortion ratio (564 abortions per 1,000 live births) of any state in the United States.[41] As approximately one in five of all abortions are in teenage girls, it can be concluded that California has one of the highest, if not the highest, teen pregnancy rate in the nation.

The cost of births to adolescents alone argues for a greatly expanded program of contraception. Few teen mothers place their babies for adoption (only 2%), and most establish families of their own, often as single parents. In a 1989 study by the Center for Population Options, it cost $21.55 billion to support these young families, or 53% of the public funding spent for Aid to Families with Dependent Children (AFDC), food stamps, and Medicaid (Medi-Cal in California).[42] By 1992, this figure had risen to $34 billion,[43] with the typical AFDC household receiving $1,426 per month in benefits, or $17,112 per year.[44] Effective contraceptive programs could result in substantial savings, particularly in California, where teen births impose a singularly high toll on our financial resources. For every $1 spent on family planning services in this state, $7.70 is saved by averting an unintended birth and its attendant health and welfare costs as compared to an average national savings of $4.40.[45] These costs are but the tip of the iceberg when one considers all that is required to support teenage families. In 1992, for example, more than 1,900 kindergarten classes were needed in California to serve just the children born to teen mothers five years earlier and cost the state almost $262 million.[46]

The United States fares poorly when measured against teen pregnancy and pregnancy outcomes in other developed countries. Rates in this country for 15- to 19-year-olds are twice as high as in England, New Zealand, or Canada; three times as high as in Sweden; and nine times as high as in the Netherlands.[2,47] In a detailed comparative study conducted in 1981,[48] the average pregnancy rate in selected European countries was 36 per 1,000 adolescent girls, with one-third terminating in abortion and two-thirds resulting in a live birth. In the United States, there were three times as many conceptions, or 98 per 1,000 (Figure 20.4). Moreover, the adolescent abortion rate in the United States alone exceeded the total conception rate of any of the comparison countries. Somewhat more recent data reveal even more dire findings, with 1989 teen pregnancy rates having substantially declined throughout Europe to 13% in Germany, 8.6% in the United Kingdom, and 0.9% in the Netherlands and Denmark[49] at a time when the teen pregnancy rate in this country was at a high of 38.7%.[19] The primary difference in both studies was not in the incidence of sexual activity—it was similar in all countries—but rather in public policy. The European countries had adopted a vigorous primary prevention approach and provided comprehensive sex education and readily available contraception to all adolescents in need. The United States, on the other hand, approached the issue by promoting abstinence

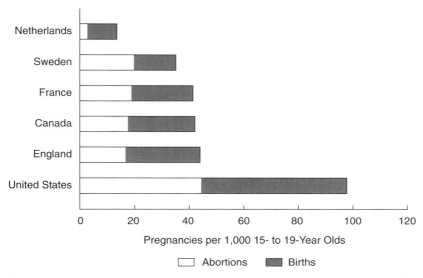

Figure 20.4.   Pregnancy rates and outcomes among adolescent women aged 15 to 19 years in selected western European countries and the United States. Source: Jones et al. (1985 [48]).

at one end of the sexuality spectrum and dealt with the problem of pregnancy only once it had occurred at the other end, giving scant attention to protecting sexually active youth before the pregnancy occurred.

Abortion

Between 1980 and 1990, the annual ratio of legal abortions to live births for all age-groups in the United States remained relatively constant at approximately 350 per 1,000. Since 1990, however, this ratio has gradually declined to 321 per 1,000, as has the total number of abortions (from a high of 1,429,577 in 1990 to 1,267,415 in 1994).[50] The proportion of all abortions occurring in adolescents 19 years of age or less has decreased from a high of 32.6% in 1972 to 20.2% in 1994, although this latter figure has decreased less than 1% since 1991 (21%) and reflects a lesser effect of prevention efforts in this age-group than in others (Table 20.2). Adolescents aged 15 to 19 years are 1.5 times more likely than adults to terminate a pregnancy, with an abortion ratio of 440 per 1,000. When broken down for each year of age, the ratios for younger adolescents are even higher. In 1992 (the latest date for which detailed data are available), the abortion ratio was 790 per 1,000 for those 14 years of

TABLE 20.2   SELECTED DATA ON REPORTED LEGALLY INDUCED ABORTIONS
IN ADOLESCENT FEMALES—UNITED STATES, 1972–1994

Year	All abortions in 10- to 19-year-olds[a] (%)	Total no. of abortions in 10- to 19-year-olds (in 1,000s)[a]	Abortion ratio in 10- to 14-year-olds[b]	Abortion ratio in 15- to 19-year-olds[b]	Abortion rate in sexually active 10- to 14-year-olds[c]	Abortion rate in sexually active 15- to 19-year-olds[c]
1994	20.2	256.0	—	—	—	—
1993	20.0	266.0	—	—	—	—
1992	20.1	273.2	—	—	—	—
1991	21.0	291.7	502	379	—	—
1990	22.4	320.2	515	403	41.7	55.5
1985	26.3	349.4	624	462	48.0	73.7
1980	29.2	378.9	—	—	41.2	78.3
1976	32.1	317.2	—	—	—	—
1972	32.6	191.3	—	—	—	—

[a] From Centers for Disease Control, Abortion surveillance: Preliminary data—United States, 1994, *Morbidity and Mortality Weekly Report* 45(1997), 1123.
[b] Number of legally induced abortion per 1,000 live births in age-group (from S. K. Henshaw and J. Van Vort, Abortion services in the United States, 1991 and 1992, *Family Planning Perspectives* 26 [1994], 100).
[c] Number of legally induced abortions per 1,000 sexually active females in age-group (from A. M. Spitz, P. Velabil, L. M. Koonin, et al., Pregnancy, abortion and birth rates among US adolescents—1980, 1985, and 1990, *Journal of the American Medical Association* 275[13, 1975], 989).

age or less, 553 per 1,000 for 15-year-olds, and 477 per 1,000 for 16-year-olds.[44]

Sexually Transmitted Diseases

The prevalence of STDs among adolescents at risk from sexual activity is higher than among at-risk individuals of any other age. In 1995, the rate of gonorrhea among 15- to 19-year-olds was 665 per 100,000, with rates of 840 per 100,000 for teen females and 498 per 100,000 for teen males (Table 20.3).[51] There were striking differences, however, when race and ethnicity was taken into account. Rates in African-American adolescents were more than 20 times those who were White or Hispanic. Teen females led all age-groups in reported prevalence; teen males were second only to 20- to 24-year-olds. If these data were modified to include only those individuals who were sexually active and at actual risk, the teenage rate would be even higher; considerably fewer adolescents are sexually active (50%–55%) as compared to older populations (80%–90%).[52] It is true, however, that there has been a significant drop in reported gonorrhea rates since 1992 for all age-groups, including adolescents, with a greater decline in males than females.[51,53] Nonetheless, inter-age-group gonorrhea ratios remain the same, and teen females continue to have the highest prevalence of this disease even when not factored for at-risk status.

The gonorrhea data parallels the high prevalence of other common STDs in adolescents and often is a comorbid infection. Cervical and vaginal cultures of various sexually active female adolescent populations find an average of 11% (range: 3%–18.3%) positive for gonorrhea, 22% (range: 15%–37%) for chlamydia, 21% (range: 6%–48%) for trichomonas, and 39% (range: 32%–46%) for human papilloma virus as detected by positive cervical cytology or DNA probe. Among urethral cultures in sexually active adolescent males, an average of 6% (range: 3%–9%) are positive for gonorrhea and, in one study, 3% for chlamydia.[35]

The greater incidence of STDs in sexually active adolescents as compared to older sexually active populations is attributed to a combination of an early coital debut, exposure to a greater number of partners, and a less frequent use of the condom. The highest STD rates are seen in disadvantaged inner-city teens, for whom these behaviors are even more prevalent than in advantaged youths.[35] The primary exception is human papilloma virus infection, which has been found to be as frequent in college-age females as in female juvenile detainees.[54]

Pelvic inflammatory disease (PID) is one of the most serious com-

TABLE 20.3   REPORTED RATES OF
GONORRHEA PER 100,000 ADOLESCENTS
AGES 15 TO 19 YEARS BY GENDER
AND RACE/ETHNICITY—
UNITED STATES, 1992–1995

	1992	1993	1994	1995
All races/ethnicities				
Total	869	733	739	665
Male	770	616	590	498
Female	974	857	897	840
White, non-Hispanic				
Total	166	137	151	143
Male	72	49	50	45
Female	264	230	258	246
Black, non-Hispanic				
Total	4,979	4,333	4,328	3,843
Male	4,888	4,062	3,893	3,267
Female	5,073	4,611	4,772	4,433
Hispanic				
Total	279	280	257	NA
Male	209	207	180	NA
Female	359	361	343	NA

SOURCE: U.S. Department of Health and Human Services, Public Health Service, Division of STD Prevention, *Sexually Transmitted Disease Surveillance, 1995* (Atlanta: Centers for Disease Control, 1996).

plications of infection, with gonorrhea and chlamydia and the leading cause of ectopic pregnancy and infertility. When factored for sexual activity, African-American 15- to 19-year-olds have the highest PID rate of all races and all age-groups; White teen women have the same rate as their African-American 20- to 24-year-old counterparts.[55,56]

From 1981 through 1991, syphilis rates among both male and female 15- to 19-year-olds accounted for 10% to 12% of all primary and secondary cases, with a 1991 rate of 18 cases per 100,000 males and 35 cases per 100,000 females.[57] Although rates were highest among 20- to 29-year-olds of both sexes throughout this period, between 1987 and 1990 rates for adolescents rose by 41% among 15- to 19-year-old males and by 112% for 15- to 19-year-old females, contributing significantly to the overall 21% increase in the prevalence of primary and secondary syphilis that occurred during this time. By 1991, the rate for 15- to 19-year-old females (35 per 100,000) was almost twice that of males, reflecting a dramatic increase among women of all ages in the latter half of the 1980s.

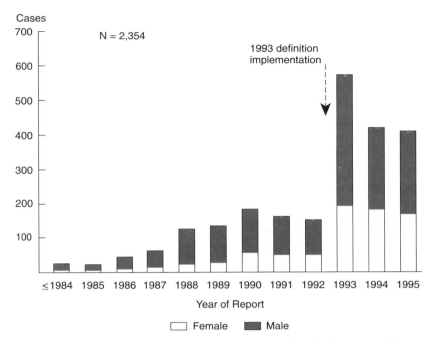

Figure 20.5. Annual number of AIDS cases reported in adolescents aged 13 to 19 years by sex—United States, 1984–1996. Source: Centers for Disease Control (1997 [58]).

Acquired Immunodeficiency Disease (AIDS/HIV)

As of December 1996,[58] a cumulative total of 2,754 cases of clinical AIDS had been reported in 13- to 19-year-old adolescents; 63% of these cases occurred in males and 37% in females (Figure 20.5). Among 20- to 24-year-olds, who most likely became infected as adolescents, there was a cumulative total of 21,097 cases with a male-to-female ratio of three to one. This represents a dramatic increase in total AIDS cases since just 1993, when only 157 cases among 13- to 19-year-olds were reported.[59] Data about AIDS cases prior to this time are difficult to interpret, as the diagnostic criteria were greatly expanded in 1993, admitting a far greater number of cases than before. Cumulative 1996 data for HIV seropositivity revealed a total of 3,193 cases in 13- to 19-year-olds for nearly a one-to-one male-to-female ratio, with females predominating (1,563 and 1,630 cases, respectively).

The adolescent age-group is the only one to demonstrate such a high proportion of HIV/AIDS cases occurring in females. All other groups

TABLE 20.4   CUMULATIVE REPORTED
AIDS CASES IN ADOLESCENTS AND YOUNG
ADULTS THROUGH DECEMBER 1995
BY EXPOSURE CATEGORY

	13–19 years		20–24 years	
Exposure Category	N	(%)	N	(%)
Males				
Men who have sex with men	501	(33)	9,084	(63)
Injecting drug use	97	(6)	1,803	(13)
Men who have sex with men and inject drugs	77	(5)	1,562	(11)
Heterosexual contact	646	(42)	539	(4)
Hemophilia/coagulation disorder	38	(2)	505	(4)
Recipient of blood transfusion, blood components, or tissue	66	(4)	101	(1)
Other/undetermined [a]	109	(7)	802	(6)
Total	1,534	(100)	14,396	(100)
Females				
Injecting drug use	132	(16)	1,430	(31)
Coagulation disorder	9	(1)	12	(<1)
Heterosexual contact	440	(54)	2,338	(51)
Recipient of blood transfusion, blood components, or tissue	60	(7)	105	(2)
Other/undetermined [a]	179	(22)	674	(15)
Total	820	(100)	4,559	(100)

[a] Includes patients pending medical record review; patients who died, were lost to follow-up, or declined interview; and patients whose mode of exposure to HIV remains undetermined.

SOURCE: Centers for Disease Control, U.S. HIV and AIDS cases reported through December 1995, *HIV/AIDS Surveillance Report* 7(2, 1996), 1.

show a three-to-one male-to-female ratio or greater. This discrepancy is probably best accounted for by the growing prevalence of HIV/AIDS in females in general. At the same time, homosexual transmission is a significant cause of teenage male AIDS/HIV, as it is among adults, although transfusions necessitated by hemophilia or other coagulation disorders remain the most common source of infection among male adolescents and young adults (Table 20.4). Among teen females, transmission is primarily through heterosexual contact.[60]

While the incidence of HIV/AIDS infection in adolescents is low compared to older individuals, certain youth populations show an alarmingly high prevalence of HIV infection (Table 20.5). For comparison, the

TABLE 20.5   PREVALENCE OF HUMAN
IMMUNODEFICIENCY VIRUS INFECTION
IN DIFFERENT ADOLESCENT POPULATIONS

Group	Age (Years)	% HIV Positive
Military active duty five-year conversions	17–19	0.01
Military applicants	17–19	0.03
College youth	College age	0.2
Juvenile detainees	16–17	0.2
Job Corps enrollees	16–21	0.4
Youths seen in an inner-city adolescent clinic	15–18	0.7
Adolescents attending an STD clinic	15–19— males	2.0
	15–19— females	2.5
Runaway and homeless youth	15–18	3.0

SOURCE: U.S. Congress, Office of Technology Assessment, *Adolescent Health—Volume 2* (Washington, D.C.: U.S. Government Printing Office, 1991).

lowest seropositivity rate has been found in 17- to 19-year-olds on active military duty.[61] Higher rates have been reported among adolescents known to engage in high-risk behaviors. This includes inner-city adolescents attending an adolescent medical clinic, juvenile detainees, 16- to 21-year-old Job Corps enrollees, 15- to 19-year-olds attending STD treatment clinics, and runaway and homeless youth.[62–64] The wide demographic variability in HIV seropositivity is documented in a study of 16- to 21-year-old Job Corps enrollees.[65] HIV testing on entry into the program is mandatory. The highest seropositivity rates were found in African-American and Hispanic adolescents (5.3 per 1,000), inner-city youths from large urban areas in the Northeast (5.5 per 1,000), and a surprisingly disproportionate number from rural areas and small towns in the Southeast (4.2 per 1,000). For African-American and Hispanic youths from large northeastern cities, seroprevalence increased by 4.3 per 1,000 at each year of age to a high of 24.8 at age 21. Males and females had similar rates of 3.7 and 3.2 per 1,000, respectively.

Risk Taking: Contraceptive and Condom Use

Risks of pregnancy, STDs, and HIV seropositivity are all greater in those sexually active youth who fail to use protection and in those who use protection, but inconsistently. In the CDC's 1995 YRBS,[13] slightly more than half of all sexually active high school students (54%) used a condom at their last sexual encounter with 49% of females and 61% of males reporting this behavior. Use was highest for 9th- and 10th-graders (63% and 60%, respectively) and lowest for 11th- and 12th- graders (52% and 50%). African-American students (61%) were more likely to use condoms than Caucasian (53%) or Hispanic students (44%). These condom use rates were only slightly higher than the rates reported in 1993, when use at the last sexual encounter was reported by 53% of all students, again with the highest percentage of use being among younger youths and those of African-American ethnicity.[14] Both the 1993 and the 1995 surveys found significantly higher condom use than in 1990, when condom use at the last sexual encounter among all students was only 45%.[19] Birth control pill use was much lower than use of condoms. In 1995, pill use at the last encounter was only reported by one in five high school girls (20%). The frequency of use among different class and ethnic groups, however, was the reciprocal of condom use, with senior girls (29%) and Caucasian females (25%) reporting being on the pill at the last sexual encounter more frequently than others. Pill use in 1995 was up only 2% from use in 1993 (18%).

Data from the 1995 NSFG shows a similar trend employing somewhat different questions.[20] Among 16-year-old females, 57% had used some method of protection at their first coital episode, with 15% relying on the pill and 32% on the condom. For teen women less than 20 years of age, use of any method was lowest among Hispanics (53%) and highest among non-Hispanic Whites and non-Hispanic Blacks (83% and 72%, respectively).

Other studies support a picture of wide variability in contraceptive and condom practices depending on the population studied. Different surveys have found that anywhere from 31% to 80% report that they always use a method, and from 16% to 58% state that they never use one.[21–24,66–69] When adolescents themselves are asked why they do not use protection, two-thirds (65%) state that sex was unexpected, one in four (25%) do not know how to obtain protection or where to go, one in four (24%) fear parental discovery or method side effects or are too embarrassed to seek out services, and one in six (15%) believe that they are safe without birth control and will not get pregnant.[70] Although condom and pill use appears to be slowly increasing among sexually active adolescents as a class, a significant number continue to remain unprotected at least some if not all of the time.

Not all teenagers seek to avoid pregnancy, as much as one might think to the contrary. Any efforts to promote contraceptive use among these young women only fall on deaf ears. Several surveys of teen girls have shown that poor contraceptive use may well be associated with a definite intent to become pregnant or at least the absence of any objection.[71,72] Such intents often remain unspoken while the unknowing clinician diligently provides careful but unavailing contraceptive instruction. Adolescents in this group perceive pregnancy and parenthood as a desirable state and as providing answers to some other dilemma, such as having no future goals other than parenthood and drifting aimlessly in the interim.

Factors that have been found to support contraceptive and condom use include the following:[20,24–28,61,63,73,74]

- Having educational goals
- Doing well at school
- Ability to pay
- Married parents
- An older partner
- Fewer other risk behaviors
- A belief in the efficacy of condom use against HIV infection

- Suburban residence
- Cognitive maturity, older age
- Prior satisfactory contraceptive use
- Higher parental educational level
- Fewer life-time partners
- Friends who use condoms
- A low perception of undesirable aspects of condom use

It is significant to note that HIV knowledge, fear and anxiety about HIV infection, or intentions toward avoiding other risk behaviors were not found to have any substantial effect on sexual risk taking or on contraceptive and condom use.[24,25,63,65]

MODIFYING ADOLESCENT SEXUAL RISK TAKING

Educational Interventions

Evaluations of educational intervention strategies all show that knowledge alone has little effect on modifying behavior. Simply telling adolescents not to have sex, providing them with information about associated risks, or informing them about protective measures through passive learning methods neither increases nor decreases the age of coital debut, the frequency of sexual intercourse, the number of partners, or the use of protective methods.[72,75,76] Even those educational programs that are interactive and focus on building skills only delay the onset of the coital debut and have little effect on modifying the frequency of coitus once sexual activity has begun.[66,77]

The health belief model offers an explanation of the complexities of health behavior modification as well as direction for developing effective intervention strategies.[27,78] This theory holds that an adolescent will modify his or her behavior only when he or she perceives a clear and personal benefit in doing so. Three separate but interactive elements collectively determine this perception. First, a youth must perceive that his or her sexual risk taking poses an immediate and serious personal threat. Second, the youth must have appropriate knowledge about the benefits of behavior modification (e.g., being abstinent, using effective contraception). That is, he or she must believe in the new behavior's effectiveness, know how to implement it (e.g., resist sexual pressures, obtain and use protection), and have positive attitudes about it. The last element consists of a number of variables that support or undermine these perceptions and beliefs, including sociodemographics, cognitive maturity, motivation, self-esteem, the presence or absence of other risk-taking behaviors, emotional risks, and health-seeking and compliance behaviors. An external catalyst that brings the matter close to home often is required to move intention into actual practice, such as a friend's becoming pregnant or the promptings of a meaningful and supportive person in the adolescent's life.

This health belief model, together with social learning theory, social inoculation theory, and cognitive/behavioral learning theory, has served as the basis for new and innovative sex education programs with the goal of delaying the coital debut and enhancing contraceptive use in cognitively immature adolescents.[75,76,79-82] Curricula are narrowly focused on program goals and are participatory in nature. The prediction is that successful enactment of a desired behavior will encourage that behavior in the future (e.g., convincing a partner to delay having sex though rehearsal will lead to delaying in actuality). Course activities closely look at social and media influences and pressures to have sex as well as provide the modeling and practicing of communication and negotiation skills. Abstinence as a positive behavior is strongly supported, as is effective protection for those who are sexually active. Students who participate in these courses are significantly more likely to continue to delay their coital debut for at least 18 months. In one such program, given over 10 sessions to eighth-grade students in Atlanta, only 24% of inexperienced students had become sexually active at the end of the following year as compared to 39% of students in schools that did not offer the program.[78] Although these programs have only a limited effect in either promoting a return to abstinence or decreasing coital frequency among those who already are sexually active, there is a significant decrease in the number of partners and an increase in the frequency of condom use.

Health Care Interventions

Over the past few decades, an increasing number of health programs specifically targeted at adolescents have emerged. The vast majority are school-linked, hospital-based, or community-based clinics.[83] All are comprehensive in that they address biological, psychological, and social needs; seek to provide an optimal adolescent health care environment; and offer preventive and early intervention services for health risk behaviors. Many family planning programs also have special programs for adolescents' reproductive health care needs.

Most attention and interest has been given to school-based and school-linked clinics (SBSLCs), which provide a wide range of health services, particularly to disadvantaged and uninsured youth.[84–90] The impetus for what has been a rapid expansion of SBSLCs, particularly in relation to a belief in their effectiveness in pregnancy prevention, comes from the initial evaluation of the first such program, which was initiated in St. Paul–Minneapolis in 1977.[91] Originally, there appeared to be both a significant increase in contraceptive use with a 93% 12-month continuation rate and a reduction in schoolwide births from 79 to 35 per 1,000 students over the first three years. Subsequent reevaluation of the St. Paul data, however, uncovered significant problems with the first analysis, suggesting that the initial findings were more artifact than real.[92] A broader look at longitudinal data, both before and after program implementation, found wide fluctuations in schoolwide birth rates from one year to the next that originally had not been taken into account. When these variations were included in the statistical analysis, there was no significant difference in overall schoolwide birth rates in the postprogram years from those that preceded it.

The reproductive health programs of six SBSLCs in different parts of the country also have been evaluated.[93,94] While these clinics demonstrate modest effects on diminishing sexual risk taking, at the same time it is important to note that they did not promote sexual activity in any way, neither hastening the onset of sexual activity nor increasing its frequency. Effects on contraceptive use were varied. Simply providing birth control pills or condoms on site was not enough by itself to significantly increase use. Use did increase, however, when other factors were brought to bear. Condom use was enhanced in three different SBSLCs, each of which included one of the following in addition to adolescent-oriented health care:

- A strong school AIDS education program in a community where AIDS was a significant issue
- A school policy and educational program that placed pregnancy prevention as a matter of high priority
- Identification of and focusing on high-risk youth with a strong emphasis on pregnancy prevention

While these strategies definitely increased contraceptive use in those SBSLCs that dispensed them, use remained inconsistent, and none of the six clinics demonstrated a statistically significant effect on school-wide pregnancy rates, although a small number of conceptions may have been averted.

One SBSLC that has shown dramatic results (not included in the previous study) is linked to a Baltimore school.[66,95,96] In the three years following inception of the clinic, there was a 30% drop in the pregnancy rate compared to a 57% pregnancy rate increase in regional schools without SBSLCs during the same time. Factors contributing to this success were thought to be the high priority given to pregnancy prevention as a matter of school policy and curricular objectives; the fact that the clinic was located near but not on the school campus, affording greater privacy; and the fact that the clinic was open during after-school hours, affording greater accessibility.

Community-based programs aimed at adolescent pregnancy prevention also have had mixed success as measured by teen fertility rates.[66] One such program, the Multimodal School/Community Program for Sexual Risk Reduction Among Teens, implemented in rural South Carolina, was a comprehensive coordinated approach involving schools, churches, homes, community agencies, and public media. The message to youth was to postpone the onset of sexual activity but, if they were sexually active, to use contraception consistently. A trained school nurse based in an SBSLC provided males with condoms and took females to a local family planning clinic. In the first year, pregnancy rates dropped from 61.7 to 25 per 1,000. A nearby county without such a program showed an increase of 8.5 per 1,000. Reduced rates persisted for three years but then rose to preprogram levels because of program erosion. The school nurse resigned, new state-mandated minimum competency requirements reduced teacher time for the program's educational component, the state legislature imposed a ban on condom distribution in all SBSLCs, and the nearest family planning clinic was nine miles away with poor public transportation.

Earls[97] compared the effectiveness of seven hospital-based adolescent medical clinics funded by the Robert Wood Johnson Foundation to provide comprehensive health care to high-risk adolescents with three similar but nonfunded clinics. Funded clinics detected and treated a substantially wider range of medical and behavioral problems than those that were not funded, but effectiveness was limited. Measures of improvements in lifestyle, risk-taking behaviors, and related medical outcomes showed minimal change.

Studies of family planning clinic effectiveness are mixed. Those clinics with special programs for or special emphasis on adolescents result in greater contraceptive use. Those with less emphasis conduct more teen abortions.[66] As a result, both demonstrate similar teen birth rates but, obviously, for very different reasons.

While the ability of special adolescent health care programs to reduce adolescent pregnancies appears to be limited, the model should not be discarded. Overriding factors must be taken into account.

First, given the high-risk nature of many of the adolescents seen in these programs (most are from low-income families and live in disadvantaged environments), any interventions, no matter how well conceived, are likely to be seriously compromised by such central issues as poverty, dysfunctional families, disrupted schools, neighborhood violence, and, for many, limited English proficiency. State and local restrictions on contraceptive and condom distribution in schools and community opposition to dealing openly with the reality of adolescent sexuality also impose substantial barriers.

Second, many young people attending teen clinics have no other source of health care and cannot afford it. Subsidized teen clinics often are the only place they can obtain attention for their health needs.

Third, the highly supportive and comprehensive orientation of SBSLCs, wherever based, and the delivery of care by professionals skilled in working with teens—as opposed to the orientation and care practices found in most private practice offices—are far more likely to promote disclosure of behavioral risks and psychosocial problems and to provide age-appropriate care and counseling to individual youths in need.

Lastly, the adolescent clinic model, wherever based, embodies many of the elements thought to be important for adolescent health care (as discussed in detail in the following) and can well serve as a springboard for further research.

ADOLESCENT HEALTH CARE RESOURCES
AND UTILIZATION BY ADOLESCENTS
Special Adolescent Clinics

A national survey of special adolescent clinics identified 664 such programs.[98] Nearly half (45%) were connected with schools (SBSLCs), and one-quarter (22%) were hospital based. One in five (20%) were community or neighborhood centers, and 8% were located in departments of health. More than 90% of these programs provided pregnancy testing, AIDS education, family planning counseling, and STD treatment. Three-quarters (76%) dispensed condoms and provided contraceptive services on site; the remainder had linkages with off-site resources. Confidentiality was regularly afforded, although many SBSLCs required parental permission for the adolescent to use the clinic at all. Young people who attended these clinics averaged 3.6 visits per year and expressed considerable satisfaction with care. Only 44% of the clinics collected patient fees, which were on a sliding scale based on the adolescent's ability to pay. Seventy-two percent received federal funding subsidization, and 75% received state and/or local support. Unfortunately, these special youth programs serve only 5.3% of all 15- to 19-year-olds, meeting the health care needs of only a very few.

Adolescents tend to use family planning clinics more often than private physicians for birth control. In the 1988 NSFG, 30% of all 15- to 19-year-old females reported at least one family planning clinic visit in the previous year. Attracting factors include low cost (private physician fees for similar services are four times as great) and confidentiality. Nearly 9 out of 10 (87%) family planning clinics provided birth control to minors without parental consent.[66]

The Private Sector

Data from the 1985 National Ambulatory Care Survey and the 1988 National Health Information Survey found that there were 50.216 million visits by 10- to 18-year-olds, an average of 1.6 visits per adolescent per year. This rate was significantly lower than for any other age-group and well below the national average of 2.7 visits per year. Thirty-five percent of these visits were to family medicine and general practitioners, 23% to pediatricians (largely limited to those under age 16), and only 5% to internists. The remainder was to various subspecialists with dermatology predominating.[99]

Leading reasons for these visits were general medical and routine physical examinations (10%), symptoms referable to the throat (7%), acne (4%), and routine prenatal care (6%).[100,101] The time spent during a physician visit averaged 14 minutes for adolescents compared to the national norm of 16.5 minutes. But nearly half of all visits (48%) were 10 minutes or less, and only 1 in 25 (4%) lasted 30 minutes or more. There is little to suggest that the length of such visits has increased in the intervening years, particularly in light of the expansion of managed care and its focus on lowering health care costs through increasing physician productivity (e.g., seeing more patients in less time).

Only a minority of visits to primary care physicians deal with sexuality issues. A recent survey of more than 1,000 primary care physicians, for example, found that only 40% of respondents routinely inquired about sexual activity among their adolescent patients, only 17% screened for the teenager's number of sexual partners, and only 9% ever provided condoms.[102] In a survey of youths themselves, fewer than two out of five (39%) had ever discussed how to avoid getting HIV or STDs with a physician, only 13% had received information about how to use condoms, and only 15% had been asked about their own personal sexual behaviors.[103] There does, however, appear to be a positive change in these data from those of the last decade, when a survey of college freshmen revealed that 81% had never received counseling about contraception from a physician, and 79% had never received counseling about STDs.[104]

Most adolescents (80%–90%) and parents (80%) see physicians as an important resource for discussions about sexuality.[103,105] Inquiries of teens themselves, however, find a wide disparity between what they would like to talk to a physician about and what actually does get talked about. In one survey of urban high school students, although the vast majority wanted information about STDs (80%), AIDS (85%), condoms (73%), and safe sex (80%), only 27% reported ever having discussed any of these subjects with their physicians.[106] Of particular interest is the finding in this and similar surveys that adolescents find it difficult to initiate a discussion about sexuality issues and look to the physician to do so. At the same time, physicians themselves find this difficult to do. Parents also have observed that physicians generally appear uncomfortable when discussing such personal issues as a teenager's sexuality.[107]

Confidentiality

Privacy surrounding sexuality issues is an essential ingredient of health care for adolescents.[108] There is considerable variation, however, in the degree to which teenagers trust their physicians to keep confidences, depending on the nature of the problem. In one survey,[109] most adolescents trusted that their physician would keep it secret if they asked questions about sex (75%), if they were having sex (65%), or if they were using contraception (68%). Only a minority, however, would trust their physician to keep secret the actual presence of an STD (44%) or pregnancy (44%). The level of trust rose among adolescents who knew that physicians in their state do not have to tell parents about either of these conditions, but only to 54%. In another report of 10th-grade students, more than half (58%) would not seek STD care for fear parents would find out, and three-quarters (78%) were afraid that friends would find out. Other perceived barriers were that they did not know where to go (38%), had no transportation (29%), did not think that they could afford care (48%), or were too embarrassed to talk to a doctor (43%).[66,108] Among a randomly selected group of adolescents residing in Massachusetts, more than half (58%) had health concerns they wished to keep private from their parents and were concerned about whether a physician would respect their confidences. Of those with a regular source of health care, four out of five (86%) would go to their physician for a physical illness, but only half (57%) would go if there was a question about pregnancy, AIDS, or substance abuse. Three out of every four (77.7%) felt that being sexually active should be kept confidential, 46% felt the same way for STD infection, 55% for pregnancy, and 35% for HIV seropositivity.[110]

Teenagers generally have poor information about their legal rights to confidential care and the fact that, in all jurisdictions, minors can consent on their own to care for STDs and, in many states, also can consent on their own to contraceptive services, pregnancy diagnosis, and prenatal care. In one study, two out of every three adolescents did not know that they had a legal right to consent to care for STDs. Three-quarters (75%) either believed that STD clinics would tell parents of their visit or did not know whether parents would be notified. Nearly four in five (79%) believed that STD treatment required parental consent.[66] Over half of another group of teenagers (54%) reported that no health provider had ever talked to them about privacy or provided time for confidential discussion.[107]

This lack of trust of the private sector is not entirely misguided. One national survey of general practitioners and family medicine practitioners—who account for the largest proportion of adolescent visits—found that only 59% were willing to provide contraception to minors without parental consent, and only 57% believed that minor adolescents should have this right.[105] An inquiry into physician attitudes about selected ethical dilemmas found that 61% of all respondents would tell a mother of her 15-year-old daughter's pregnancy even against the girl's strongly stated wishes to the contrary and even despite her legal right to confidential care.[107] A substantial majority of pediatricians, however, are accepting of the confidentiality option.[111] Further, the American Academy of Pediatrics has specifically adopted the position that confidentiality is an important ingredient in adolescent health care, enabling minor youths to seek out early and timely services for sensitive and personal health problems. While strongly encouraging parental participation, the Academy views that mandatory parental consent results only in adolescents maintaining silence about their medical need, unnecessarily delays treatment, and places them at greater risk of health harm.[112–114]

Competence and Interest
of Private-Sector Physicians

Surveys of physician attitudes toward adolescent patients find that general practitioners, family medicine practitioners, and internists have only a modest interest in this age-group, with only one in four expressing definite interest.[115] Even if interested, many are not skilled. Currently, there are insufficient primary care physicians in the United States with the type of training and experience required to provide the nation's 35 million adolescents with age-appropriate care.[115,116]

Most physicians and other health care providers have limited competence in identifying and treating the health problems of adolescence. Studies have shown that general and family practitioners, pediatricians, and internists all have difficulty identifying adolescents who have behavioral and emotional problems and consider themselves relatively untrained in managing adolescent sexuality, contraception, and psychosocial concerns. Further, only 30% of those who perceive themselves to have such deficiencies have any interest in increasing their competence.[115]

There may be change among future pediatricians and internists. All approved pediatric residency programs[117] now are required to have a full-time faculty member trained in adolescent medicine, and all residents must have at least a one-month rotation with teenage patients exclusively as well as additional experience with young people in ambulatory and inpatient settings. Internal medicine residency training requirements also call for specific experience in adolescent medicine, including health-risk behaviors, but without defining the length of time that must be devoted to this discipline.[118] Family medicine, on the other hand, has not yet incorporated specific adolescent medicine training requirements into its curriculum,[119] presumably because of the view that training residents to provide comprehensive care to families axiomatically includes adolescents as well. The incorporation of adolescent medicine experiences into the resident curricula of pediatrics and internal medicine, however, is a relatively recent event, and it will be many years before all practicing pediatricians and internists will be appropriately skilled.

Financing

Even if all physicians were both interested and trained, providing care to adolescents in a manner that promotes compliance and behavioral modification is time intensive. Public and private third-party reimbursement rates do not reflect this fact and, when adolescents are given the time they need for counseling and anticipatory guidance, do not even compensate for overhead costs. This problem is even further compounded by the increasing emphasis on "productivity" and efforts to decrease health care costs by increasing the volume of patients seen in a given span of time. No specific coverage yet exists for comprehensive adolescent preventive services (see the following discussion of Guidelines for Adolescent Preventive Services). Coverage for mental health and substance abuse problems, often associated with high levels of sexual risk taking, has been substantially cut back in recent years and also is highly limited in availability.

A lack of adequate financing deprives many poor youths of even the most basic services. Yet poor adolescents are the ones at greatest risk of unintended pregnancy, teen parenthood, STDs, and HIV seropositivity. One in every seven adolescents has no public or private health insurance.[120] Nearly one-third live in families with incomes at or below 150% of the federal poverty level, and one in three is not eligible for Medicaid/Medi-Cal. These data do not take into account the ever increasing number of undocumented poor young people in the southwestern United States and in southern California in particular.

Even when adolescents are insured, they often are reluctant to seek out care for confidential problems out of concern for discovery if payment is dependent on their parents' or family insurance plan. It is virtually impossible to make a private third-party payer claim for a minor without the signature of the insured adult and without the latter receiving notice of claims made and paid. Equal barriers exist in public payment programs (Medicaid, Medi-Cal); a sticker or eligibility card generally must be presented before services can be rendered. These items usually are in the possession of parents, and adolescents do not have independent access to them.

The recent expansion in managed care and health maintenance organizations (HMOs) poses both problems and solutions. In prepaid systems, it becomes possible for adolescents to gain independent access and see a provider without the need for parental payment authorization for each visit. Whether this actually does occur depends on the policies of the particular program in question, and this is a variable matter. Some programs do provide for adolescent confidential care, while others continue to require parental permission for each visit, even though time may be spent with the teenager alone and confidences respected. One of the disadvantages of prepaid and managed care systems is the requirement that all members of a subscribing family receive care at a single location with no reimbursement for services rendered elsewhere. Adolescents may well require services at several sites, such as regular care by their personal physician or HMO and confidential care from a school-based clinic or family planning program. Increasingly, however, public managed care programs for low-income teens are beginning to recognize the unique needs of this age-group and to establish payment linkages between these various types of services.

Summary of Adolescent Health Care Delivery Issues

All in all, the mainstream health care delivery system for adolescents, while making some headway, still has room for considerable improvement. Key issues include inadequate professional training, inadequate reimbursement rates, insufficient visit time allotments to properly evaluate and counsel teens, access difficulties for youths seeking confidential care, and a large segment of economically disadvantaged adolescents who are uninsured.

There is considerable resistance on all fronts to dealing openly with adolescent sexual activity and denial of the fact that sexual intercourse is now a normal behavior on the part of at least half our nation's adolescents today. Nor have we effectively addressed the many problems such as poverty, poor schooling, and community violence that underlie the motives of those teens who see parenthood as a desirable state. Communities tend to resist the overwhelming evidence showing that sex education programs and the availability of contraception to adolescents do not promote an earlier age of coital debut and do not promote greater sexual risk taking.[121,122] On the contrary, new sex education programs can, in fact, delay the initiation of sexual activity and, for those already involved, enhance contraceptive use and reduce the number of partners. In the past, policy makers have been all too reluctant to accept these facts and, instead, oppose the formation of services that will best assist adolescents in contending with their own sexuality and with the sexual pressures of the world around them in a responsible manner.

Fortunately, changes are being undertaken in federal administrative policy. In 1997, the U.S. Department of Health and Human Services established the National Strategy to Prevent Teenage Pregnancy and funded two new community grant programs at $1 million per year. The primary target group, however, is 9- to 14-year-olds, with a focus on helping communities to develop horizon-broadening opportunities for youth and experiences that they can say "yes" to. While such initiatives are critical to the solution of teen risk-taking behaviors, this still does not address the needs of those young people who remain at risk and need age-appropriate reproductive health services and effective sex education.

OPTIMAL ADOLESCENT HEALTH SERVICES

In 1992, 15% of the U.S. population (38.4 million) were 10- to 19-year-old youths. Of these, approximately 20% were living below the federal poverty line. Minority adolescents were disproportionately poor, with 43% of African-American teens and 38% of those of Hispanic ethnicity living in poverty as compared to only 15% of White adolescents.[123] By the year 2000, the total population of adolescents will have increased by an additional 15%, with more than one-third being members of racial or ethnic minorities.[124]

We certainly cannot turn back the clock to a time when abstinence among unmarried individuals was the expected norm and governmental policies kept contraceptives out of the hands of the poor, the unmarried, and the young, to a time before the U.S. Supreme Court clearly established the right of all women, including adolescents, to control their own reproductive fate,[125,126] but we still do not make it easy for teenagers to do so. Although most minor young people today have the right to consent on their own to contraceptive services, to the diagnosis and treatment of STD, and to confidential HIV testing, they continue to find access to such care difficult at best. American adolescents of the 1990s face a very different world than that of their parents, a world in which they have considerably greater autonomy than ever before and one in which they face a myriad of pressures with perplexing decisions to make. Systems must be developed to effectively meet these young people's comprehensive health needs in contemporary terms.

Goals

Realistic goals for managing adolescent sexuality are, first, to foster delay in the initiation of sexual activity, at least until the young person is sufficiently cognitively mature to handle this in a responsible manner; second, to ensure that, when adolescents are sexually active, such activity is consonant with their own personal value codes and is not exploitative of themselves or others; and, finally, to support the consistent use of protection by sexually active youth against the risks of pregnancy, STDs, and AIDS.

The U.S. Public Health Service has established the following specific 10-year objectives relative to adolescent sexuality in its *Healthy People: 2000* report:[127]

• Reduce the number of pregnancies among girls aged 17 and younger to no more than 50 per 1,000 adolescents. (Objective 5.1)
• Reduce the proportion of adolescents who have engaged in sexual intercourse to no more than 15% by age 15 and no more than 40% by age 17. (Objectives 5.4, 18.3,and 19.1)
• Increase to at least 90% the proportion of sexually active, unmarried adolescents aged 19 and younger who use contraception, especially combined-method contraception that both effectively prevents pregnancy and provides barrier protection against disease. (Objective 5.6)
• Increase to at least 60% the proportion of primary care providers who provide age-appropriate adolescent care and counseling aimed at primary unintended pregnancy prevention. (Objectives 5.10 and 14.12)

Optimal Adolescent Preventive Care

The American Medical Association has developed a set of specific guidelines as a standard for teenage preventive care (*Guidelines for Adolescent Preventive Services*) calling for annual visits by all adolescents.[128] The primary objective of these visits should be to identify both psychosocial and biomedical concerns and to provide anticipatory guidance. In the absence of specific complaints, physical examinations need be performed on only three occasions; once in early, middle, and late adolescence. Services should be age- and developmentally appropriate and sensitive to individual and sociocultural differences. Office policies should be established regarding confidential care and how parents will be involved in that care. Recommendations relating to sexuality include annual anticipatory guidance of all adolescents regarding responsible sexual behavior, including abstinence. All youths should be asked about their involvement in sexual risk-taking behaviors once a year. Those who are sexually active should be screened for STDs, should be given latex condoms for protection, and, if female, should be screened annually for cervical neoplasia. Appropriate methods of birth control also should be made available, as should instruction on how to use them. Adolescents at risk for HIV infection should be offered confidential HIV screening.

Optimal Adolescent Health Care Systems

The U.S. Congress Office of Technology Assessment,[31] the Study Group on Adolescent Health of the National Academy of Sciences,[129,130] the American Medical Association,[128] the National Association of State Boards of Education,[131] and the Carnegie Corporation[1] have all examined adolescents' health care needs in depth, are in agreement that these needs have been badly neglected, and call for essential change. Their recommendations have major implications for health care reform and include the following:

- All adolescents should be assured of access to services that provide affordable, accessible, and age-appropriate comprehensive care.
- These services should be located in schools and communities where adolescents live, should be easily reachable by walking or public transportation, should be available on a walk-in basis, and should be open during at least some evening and weekend hours.

• Young people should be able to go to these services by themselves. Confidential care should be provided when the nature of the adolescent's need is such that he or she would not seek out medical assistance otherwise. At the same time, parental involvement always should be encouraged.

• Health care providers who deliver care to adolescents should care about them, be effective in communicating with them, and be specifically trained in meeting young people's health care needs.

• High priority should be given to preventive and early intervention measures for health risk behaviors, including pregnancy, STDs, and AIDS.

• Close linkages and liaisons should exist with schools and other youth-serving resources in the community. Integrated multidisciplinary and multimodal programs are particularly important. Educational programs should include a combination of personal skill-building and life-option components and be interactive in nature.

• Health services should be free or based on a sliding fee scale according to the adolescent's own ability to pay.

• Those adolescents who are insured under a family policy should have the ability to secure reimbursement for confidential services without risking disclosure.

• Provider reimbursement rates must be appropriate to the type of specialized services that adolescents need, including preventive anticipatory guidance and intervention counseling.

CONCLUSIONS

Adolescent sexual activity, with its potential consequences of pregnancy, STDs, and HIV infection, is the single largest health problem in this age-group. Yet for many teenagers our current health care system does not address these problems very effectively, and our health care policies have not, until recently, held primary pregnancy and STD prevention in adolescents as a matter of high concern. Even though the nation is waking up to the problem, current policies primarily seek methods of promoting abstinence and still overlook the needs of the many youths who remain sexually active. Most adolescents are not provided affordable, accessible, and age-appropriate comprehensive care despite compelling arguments in support of this need and despite the recommendations of leading study groups.

Indeed, little attention has been given to adolescents by the health care sector except within the small group of specialized adolescent health care clinics that see only 5% of the nation's youth. The results are unacceptable costs both to the young person who must suffer the consequences of health care's neglect and to society, which must pay for it.

Current health care reform initiatives tend to make matters worse by limiting access to the health care system to a single point of entry where there would be no guarantee that the gatekeeping primary practitioner will have any competence in caring for youth or that confidential care will be an option. If managed care is to be the primary administrative structure for health care delivery in the future, adolescents should be able to choose their own managed care program or, minimally, have access to multiple health care sites. Their choices should include both office-based practices and alternative specialized adolescent health care programs, such as school-linked clinics, hospital-based and community-based adolescent medicine programs, and family planning clinics. All such special services should be covered and should not require referral from a primary care gatekeeper for reimbursement.

Further, there is a clear need for a substantial increase in effective sex education programs and in the number of school-based clinics; both are particularly necessary in reaching teenagers who so far have been underserved and comprise that portion of the adolescent population at greatest risk of pregnancy, STDs, and AIDS. There also is a need for both public and private third-party reimbursement systems that support the young people's comprehensive health care needs. We need to ensure that all primary health care providers are trained in adolescent health—particularly those who will be managed care's gatekeepers—and to develop resources to provide such training. We need to give as much time and concern to preventive interventions for adolescent sexual risk behaviors as we now do for younger children and their immunizations. And we need to establish specific objectives for preventive care interventions and ensure that they are met.

Admittedly, there is limited information about exactly what types of interventions are effective in modifying adolescent sexual risk-taking behaviors. We have some evidence that the initiation of sexual activity can be delayed by educational programs that are based on the health belief model and social inoculation theory and that employ an interactive learning approach. We also have some evidence that sexually active adolescents can be encouraged to be more effective users of protection against STDs and pregnancy when these matters are given high priority and backed by strong community support. Effective interventions for reducing pregnancy rates short of all-out integrated community efforts are less clear, although giving high priority to primary pregnancy prevention at home, in schools, and by the community is a requisite foundation.

Research is needed in many areas. First, we need to know much more about adolescent sexual activity, including those factors that contribute to its initiation and what factors can delay it. We also need to know much more about the determinants of condom and contraceptive use. Areas that require additional study include the influence of the media and other aspects of our highly sexualized environment, the role of cognitive maturation on decision making, the role of parents and the nature of parent-adolescent communications about sexuality (not simply whether adolescents have ever talked to their parents about sex), the role of adolescents' perception about power and powerlessness, and the role of negative societal attitudes toward adolescents. We need considerably more research on how the health care and educational systems can effectively reach youth not only to delay their coital debut but also to influence those who are already sexually active to take consistent protective measures. We need more research on how to provide young people with early intervention and prevention counseling in the most cost-effective manner possible. And we need to examine how we can help parents be better communicators with their adolescents about sex. We also need more information on why physicians do not address adolescents' sexuality needs and what it would take to have them provide such services and to feel more enthusiastic about caring for this age-group.

In conclusion, I propose that access to age-appropriate care be provided to all adolescents and that teenage sexuality issues be fully addressed in any health care reforms. In particular, I propose that primary pregnancy prevention become a matter of the highest priority both for those who have not yet engaged in coitus and for those who are already experienced. No adolescent should have to make the choice between having an unintended baby and terminating a pregnancy in abortion, and no adolescent should have to risk STD or HIV infection because of a health care system that fails to provide for these needs. I further propose the establishment of multidisciplinary adolescent health research and training centers to find effective ways of influencing adolescent health risk behaviors and to train primary health care providers in these methodologies.

These initiatives will take commitment and courage in braving the criticism of those who seek only universal teen abstinence and rigorously oppose any public support for educational and health services aimed at sexually active adolescents, even if targeted at preventing unintended pregnancy or disease. Providing our young with age-appropriate care also will take considerable financial resources, scarce enough in these times of the shrinking dollar. But the saving in both dollars and the wellness of our youth will be incalculable.

NOTE

Prepared for The University of California/Health Net Wellness Lecture Series, 1993.

REFERENCES

1. Hechinger, F. M. 1992. *Fateful Choices: Healthy Youth for the 21st Century.* New York: Carnegie Council on Adolescent Development, Carnegie Corporation of New York.
2. Alan Guttmacher Institute. 1994. *Teen Sex and Pregnancy.* New York: Alan Guttmacher Institute.
3. Brown, S. S., and Eisenberg, L., eds., Committee on Unintended Pregnancy, Institute of Medicine. 1995. *The Best Intentions: Unintended Pregnancy and the Well-Being of Children and Families.* Washington, D.C.: National Academy Press.
4. Hofmann, A. D. 1997. Adolescent growth and development. In *Adolescent Medicine,* 3rd ed., edited by A. D. Hofmann and D. E. Greydanus. Stamford, Conn.: Appleton & Lange.
5. Harris, L., and Associates. 1988. *Sexual Material on American Network Television During the 1987–88 Season.* New York: Planned Parenthood Federation of America.
6. Children Now and the Kaiser Family Foundation. 1997. *Sex, Kids and the Family Hour: Sexual Images on Television.* Sacramento: Children Now.
7. U.S. Department of Education, National Center for Education Statistics. 1994. National education longitudinal study of 1988, third follow-up survey (unpublished data).
8. Pick, S., and Palos, P. A. 1995. Impact of the family on the sex lives of adolescents. *Adolescence* 30(119), 667–675.
9. Jaccard, J., Dittus, P. J., and Gordon, V. V. 1996. Maternal correlates of adolescent sexual and contraceptive behavior. *Family Planning Perspectives* 28(4), 159–165.
10. King, C. A., Radpour, L., Naylor, M. W., et al. 1995. Parents' marital functioning and adolescent psychopathology. *Journal of Consulting and Clinical Psychology* 63(5), 749–753.
11. Behrman, R. E., and Quinn, L. S. 1994. Children and divorce: Overview and analysis. *The Future of Children* 4(1), 4–14.

12. Section 510, Title V of the 1996 Social Security Act (PL 104–193).
13. Centers for Disease Control. 1996. Youth risk behavior surveillance—United States, 1995. *MMWR* 45(SS-4), 1–83.
14. Centers for Disease Control. 1995. Youth risk behavior surveillance—United States, 1993. *MMWR* 44(SS-1), 1–55.
15. Kinsey, A. C., Pomeroy, W. B., Martin, C. E., et al. 1953. *Sexual Behavior in the Human Female*. Philadelphia: W. B. Saunders.
16. Kinsey, A. C., Pomeroy, W. B., and Martin, C. E. 1948. *Sexual Behavior in the Human Male*. Philadelphia: W. B. Saunders.
17. Cates, W. 1990. The epidemiology and control of sexually transmitted diseases in adolescents. *State of the Art Reviews: Adolescent Medicine* 1, 409–427.
18. Centers for Disease Control. 1991. Premarital sexual experience among adolescent women—United States, 1970–1988. *MMWR* 39, 929–931.
19. Centers for Disease Control. 1992. Sexual behavior among high school students—United States, 1990. *MMWR* 40, 885–887.
20. Abma, J. C., Chandra, A., Mosher, W. D., et al. 1997. Fertility, family planning, and women's health: New data from the 1995 National Survey of Family Growth. National Center for Health Statistics. *Vital Health Statistics* 23(19).
21. National Center for Health Statistics. 1997. Teen sex down, new study shows. NCHS press release, May 1. www.cdc.gov/nchswww/releases/97news/nsfgteen.htm.
22. Centers for Disease Control. 1992. HIV instruction and selected HIV-risk behaviors among high school students—United States, 1989–1991. *MMWR* 41, 866–868.
23. Joffe, A. 1993. Adolescents and condom use. *AJDC* 147, 746–754.
24. Kann, L., Anderson, J., Holtzman, D., et al. 1990. HIV-related knowledge, beliefs, and behaviors among a national sample of high school students in the United States. 1989 Internat Conf AIDS (abstract S.C.568), 6, 231.
25. Morris, N. M. 1992. Determinants of adolescent initiation of coitus. *State of the Art Reviews: Adolescent Medicine* 3, 165–180.
26. Orr, D. P., Beiter, M., and Ingersoll, G. 1991. Premature sexual activity as an indicator of psychosocial risk. *Pediatrics* 87, 141–147.
27. Orr, D. P., Langerfeld, C. D., Katz, B. P., et al. 1992. Factors associated with condom use among sexually active female adolescents. *Journal of Pediatrics* 120, 311–317.
28. Orr, D. P., and Langerfeld, C. D. 1993. Factors associated with condom use by sexually active male adolescents at risk for sexually transmitted disease. *Pediatrics* 91, 873–879.
29. Pendergrast, R. A., Jr., DuRant, R. H., and Gaillard, G. L. 1992. Attitudinal and behavioral correlates of condom use in urban adolescent males. *Journal of Adolescent Health Care* 13, 133–139.
30. Shafer, M., and Boyer, C. B. 1991. Psychosocial and behavioral factors associated with risk of sexually transmitted diseases, including human immunodeficiency virus infection, among urban high school students. *Journal of Pediatrics* 119, 826–833.
31. Stiffman, A. R., Dore, P., Earls, F., et al. 1992. The influence of mental health

problems on AIDS-related risk behaviors in young adults. *Journal of Nervous and Mental Disease* 180, 314–320.

32. Stiffman, A. R., and Earls, F. 1990. Behavioral risks for human immunodeficiency virus infection in adolescent medical patients. *Pediatrics* 85, 303–310.

33. Spingarn, R. W., and DuRant, R. H. 1996. Male adolescents involved in pregnancy: Associated health risk and problem behaviors. *Pediatrics* 98(2, pt. 1), 262–268.

34. Stanton, B., Romer, D., Ricardo, I., et al. 1993. Early initiation of sex and its lack of association with risk behaviors among adolescent African-Americans. *Pediatrics* 92, 13–19.

35. U.S. Congress Office of Technology Assessment. 1991. *Adolescent Health, Volume 1: Summary and Policy Options*. Publication OTA-H-468. Washington, D.C.: U.S. Government Printing Office.

36. National Center for Health Statistics. 1992. Trends in pregnancies and pregnancy rates, United States, 1980–88. *Monthly Vital Statistics Report* 41(6, Suppl.).

37. National Center for Health Statistics. 1996. Advance report of final natality statistics, 1994. *Monthly Vital Statistics Report* 44(11, Suppl.).

38. Centers for Disease Control. 1995. State-specific pregnancy and birth rates among teenagers—United States, 1991–1992. *MMWR* 44(37), 677–684.

39. Children Now. 1997. *California: The State of Our Children 1996*. Sacramento: Children Now.

40. California Center for Health Statistics. *Live Births and Birth Rates by Age of Mother—California 1993–1995*. Sacramento: California Department of Health Services.

41. Centers for Disease Control. 1996. Abortion surveillance—United States, 1992. *MMWR* 45(SS-3), 1–36.

42. Center for Population Options. 1992. *Teenage Pregnancy and Too-Early Childbearing: Public Costs, Personal Consequences*. 6th ed. Washington, D.C.: Center for Populations Options.

43. U.S. Government Accounting Office. 1995. *Welfare Dependency: Coordinated Community Efforts Can Better Serve Young At-Risk Teen Girls*. Publication RCED-95-108. Washington, D.C.: U.S. Government Printing Office.

44. Regional Economic Studies Program. 1994, September. Government means tested programs in Maryland FY 1992. University of Baltimore (http://www.cfoc.org).

45. Children Now. 1993. *California: The State of Our Children 1993*. Sacramento: Children Now.

46. California Department of Education, Special Programs Branch. 1991. *Children of Teen Parents: Fiscal Impact upon California Schools*. Sacramento: State of California.

47. Alan Guttmacher Institute. 1996. *Issues in Brief: Risks and Realities of Early Childbearing Worldwide*. Washington, D.C.: Alan Guttmacher Institute.

48. Jones, E. F., Forrest, J. D., Goldman, N., et al. 1985. Teenage pregnancy in developed countries: Determinants and policy implications. *Family Planning Perspectives* 17, 53–63.

49. Creatsas, G. C, 1995. Adolescent pregnancy in Europe. *International Journal of Fertil Menopaus Stud* 40(2, Suppl.), 80–84.
50. Centers for Disease Control. 1994. Abortion surveillance: Preliminary data —United States, 1994. *MMWR* 45(51, 52), 123–127.
51. Division of STD Prevention, Centers for Disease Control. 1996. *Sexually Transmitted Disease Surveillance, 1995*. Atlanta: Centers for Disease Control.
52. Biro, F. M. 1992. *Adolescents and Sexually Transmitted Diseases*. Maternal and Child Health Technical Information Bulletin. Washington, D.C.: Maternal and Child Health Bureau.
53. Division of STD Prevention, Centers for Disease Control. 1996. *Sexually Transmitted Disease Surveillance, 1995*. Atlanta: Centers for Disease Control.
54. Fisher, M., Rosenfeld, W. D., and Burk, R. D. 1991. Cervicovaginal human papillomavirus infection in suburban adolescents and young adults. *Journal of Pediatrics* 119, 821–825.
55. Shafer, M., and Sweet, R. L. 1990. Pelvic inflammatory disease in adolescent females. *State of the Art Reviews: Adolescent Medicine* 1, 545–564.
56. Spence, M. R., Adler, J., and McLellan, R. 1990. Pelvic inflammatory disease in the adolescent. *Journal of Adolescent Health Care* 11(4), 304–309.
57. Centers for Disease Control. 1993. Surveillance for gonorrhea and primary and secondary syphilis among adolescents, United States—1981–1991. *MMWR* 42(SS-3), 1.
58. Centers for Disease Control. 1997. US HIV and AIDS cases reported through December 1996. *HIV/AIDS Surveillance Report* 8(2), 1.
59. Centers for Disease Control. 1994. US HIV and AIDS cases reported through December 1993. *HIV/AIDS Surveillance Report* 5(4), 1.
60. Centers for Disease Control. 1996. US HIV and AIDS cases reported through December 1995. *HIV/AIDS Surveillance Report* 7(2), 1.
61. McNeil, J. G., Brundage, J. F., Gardner, L. I., et al. 1991. Trends of HIV seroconversion among young adults in the US army, 1985 to 1989. *Journal of the American Medical Association* 265, 1709–1714.
62. Bowler, S., Sheon, A. R., D'Angelo, L. J., et al. 1992. HIV and AIDS among adolescents in the United States: Increasing risk in the 1990s. *Journal of Adolescence* 15, 345–371.
63. Vermund, S. H., Hein, K., Gayle, H. D., et al. 1989. Acquired immunodeficiency syndrome among adolescents: Case surveillance profiles in New York City and the rest of the United States. *American Journal of Diseases of Children* 143, 1220–1225.
64. Centers for Disease Control. 1992. Selected behaviors that increase risk for HIV infection among high school students—United States, 1990. *MMWR* 41, 231–240.
65. St. Louis, M. E., Conway, G. A., Hayman, C. R., et al. 1991. Human immunodeficiency virus infection in disadvantaged adolescents: Findings from the US Job Corps. *Journal of the American Medical Association* 266, 2387–2391.
66. U.S. Congress Office of Technology Assessment. 1991. *Adolescent Health, Volume II: Background and Effectiveness of Selected Prevention and Treat-*

ment Services. Publication OTA-H-466. Washington, D.C.: U.S. Government Printing Office.

67. Emans, S. J., Grace, E., Woods, E. R., et al. 1987. Adolescents' compliance with the use of oral contraceptives. *Journal of the American Medical Association* 257, 3377–3381.

68. Baldwin, W. 1990. *Adolescent Pregnancy and Childbearing: Rates, Trends, and Research Findings from the Center for Population Research of the National Institute of Child Health and Human Development.* Washington, D.C.: U.S. Government Printing Office.

69. Brown, L. K., DiClemente, R. J., and Park, T. 1992. Predictors of condom use in sexually active adolescents. *Journal of Adolescent Health Care* 13, 651–657.

70. Louis Harris and Associates, Inc. 1986. *American Teens Speak: Sex, Myths, TV and Birth Control.* New York: Planned Parenthood Federation of America.

71. Gordon, C. P. 1996. Adolescent decision making: A broadly based theory and its application to the prevention of early pregnancy. *Adolescence* 31(123), 561–584.

72. Stevens-Simon, C., Kelly, L., Singer, D., et al. 1996. Why pregnant adolescents say they did not use contraceptives prior to conception. *Journal of Adolescent Health* 19(1), 48–53.

73. DiClemente, R. J., Durbin, M., Siegel, D., et al. 1992. Determinants of condom use among junior high school students in a minority, inner-city school district. *Pediatrics* 89, 197–202.

74. Stiffman, A. R., Earls, F., Dore, P., et al. 1992. Changes in acquired immunodeficiency syndrome-related risk behavior after adolescence: Relationships to knowledge and experience concerning human immunodeficiency virus infection. *Pediatrics* 89, 950–956.

75. Kirby, D. 1991. *Sexuality Education: An Evaluation of Programs and Their Effects.* Vol. 1. Atlanta: Centers for Disease Control.

76. Kirby, D., Barth, R. P., Leland, N., et al. 1991. Reducing the risk: Impact of a new curriculum on sexual risk-taking. *Family Planning Perspectives* 23, 253–263.

77. Weinman, M. L., Smith, P. B., and Mumford, D. M. 1992. A comparison between a 1986 and 1989 cohort of inner-city adolescent females on knowledge, beliefs, and risk factors for AIDS. *Journal of Adolescence* 15, 19–28.

78. Irwin, C. E., Jr. 1990. The theoretical concept of at-risk adolescents. *State of the Art Reviews: Adolescent Medicine* 1(1), 1–14.

79. Coyle, K., Kirby, D., Parcel, G., et al. 1996. Safer Choices: A multicomponent school-based HIV/STD and pregnancy prevention program for adolescents. *Journal of School Health* 66(3), 89–94.

80. Galbraith, J., Ricardo, I., Stanton, B., et al. 1996. Challenges and rewards of involving community in research: An overview of the "Focus on Kids" HIV Risk Reduction Program. *Health Education Quarterly* 23(3), 383–394.

81. Kipke, M. D., Boyer, C., and Hein, K. 1993. An evaluation of an AIDS risk reduction education and skills training (ARREST) program. *Journal of Adolescent Health* 14(7), 533–539.

82. Orr, D. P., Langerfeld, C. D., Katz, B. P., et al. 1996. Behavioral interven-

tions to increase condom use among high-risk female adolescents. *Journal of Pediatrics* 128(2), 288–295.

83. Klein, J. D., Starnes, S. A., Kotelchuck, M., et al. 1992. *Comprehensive Adolescent Health Services in the United States, 1990.* Carrboro, N.C.: Center for Early Adolescence.

84. Dryfoos, J. G. 1994. *Full-Service Schools: A Revolution in Health and Social Services for Children, Youth, and Families.* San Francisco: Jossey-Bass.

85. Dryfoos, J. G. 1994. Medical clinics in junior high school: Changing the model to meet demands. *Journal of Adolescent Health* 15(7), 549–557.

86. Hacker, K., Fried, L. E., Bablouzian, L., et al. 1994. A nationwide survey of school health services delivery in urban schools. *Journal of School Health* 64(7), 279–283.

87. Klein, J. D., and Cox, E. M. 1995. School-based health clinics in the mid-1990s. *Current Opinion in Pediatrics* 7(4), 353–359.

88. Peak, G. L., and McKinney, D. L. 1996. Reproductive and sexual health at the school-based/school-linked health center: An analysis of services provided by 180 clinics. *Journal of Adolescent Health* 19(4), 276–281.

89. American Medical Association, Council on Scientific Affairs. 1990. Providing services through school-based health programs. *Journal of School Health* 60(3), 87–91.

90. Society for Adolescent Medicine. 1988. School-based health clinics: A position paper. *Journal of Adolescent Health* 9(6), 526–530.

91. Edwards, L. E., Steinman, M. E., Arnold, K. A., et al. 1980. Adolescent pregnancy prevention services in high school clinics. *Family Planning Perspectives* 12, 6–14.

92. Kirby, D., Resnick, M. D., Downes, B., et al. 1993. The effects of school-based health clinics in St. Paul on school-wide birthrates. *Family Planning Perspectives* 25, 12–16.

93. Kirby, D., and DiClemente, R. J. 1993. School-based behavioral interventions to prevent unprotected sex and HIV among adolescents. In *Preventing AIDS: Theories and Methods of Behavioral Interventions,* edited by R. J. DiClemente and J. L. Petersen. New York: Plenum.

94. Kirby, D., Waszak, C., and Ziegler, J. 1991. Six school-based clinics: Their reproductive health services and impact on sexual behavior. *Family Planning Perspectives* 23, 6–16.

95. Santelli, J., Alexander, M., Farmer, M., et al. 1992. Bringing parents into school clinics: Parent attitudes toward school clinics and contraception. *Journal of Adolescent Health* 13(4), 269–274.

96. Beilenson, P. L., Miola, E. S., and Farmer, M. 1995. Politics and practice: Introducing Norplant into a school-based health center in Baltimore. *American Journal of Public Health* 85(3), 309–311.

97. Earls, F., Robins, L. N., Stiffman, A. R., et al. 1989. Comprehensive health care for high-risk adolescents: An evaluation study. *American Journal of Public Health* 79, 999–1005.

98. Klein, J. D., Starnes, S. A., Kotelchuck, M., et al. 1992. *Comprehensive Adolescent Health Services in the United States 1990.* Carrboro, N.C.: Center for Early Adolescence.

99. National Center for Health Statistics. 1991. Office visits by adolescents. *Advance Data* 196, 1–12.

100. U.S. Congress Office of Technology Assessment. 1991. *Adolescent Health, Volume III: Crosscutting Issues in the Delivery of Health and Related Services*. Publication OTA-H-467. Washington, D.C.: U.S. Government Printing Office.

101. National Center for Health Statistics. 1991. Office visits by adolescents. *Advance Data* 196, 1–12.

102. Millstein, S. G., Igra, V., and Gans, J. 1996. Delivery of STD/HIV preventive services to adolescents by primary care physicians. *Journal of Adolescent Health* 19(4), 249–257.

103. Shuster, M. A., Bell, R. M., Peterson, L. P., et al. 1996. Communication between adolescents and physicians about sexual behavior and risk prevention. *Archives of Pediatrics and Adolescent Medicine* 150(9), 906–913.

104. Joffe, A., Radius, S., and Gall, M. 1988. Health counseling for adolescents: What they want, what they get, and who gives it. *Pediatrics* 82, 481–485.

105. Croft, C. A., and Asmussen, L. 1993. A developmental approach to sexuality education: Implications for medical practice. *Journal of Adolescent Health* 14(2), 109–114.

106. Rawitscher, L. A., Saitz, R., and Friedman, L. S. 1995. Adolescents' preferences regarding human immunodeficiency virus (HIV)–related physician counseling and testing. *Pediatrics* 96(1, pt. 1), 52–58.

107. Novack, D., Detering, B., Arnold, R., et al. 1989. Physicians' attitudes toward using deception to resolve difficult ethical problems. *Journal of the American Medical Association* 55, 96–98.

108. Council on Scientific Affairs, American Medical Association. 1993. Confidential health services for adolescents. *Journal of the American Medical Association* 269(11), 1420–1424.

109. American School Health Association, Association for the Advancement of Health Education, and Society for Public Health Education, Inc. 1989. *The National Adolescent Student Health Survey: A Report on the Health of America's Youth*. Oakland, Calif.: American School Health Association.

110. Cheng, T. L., Savageau, J. A., Sattler, A. L., et al. 1993. Confidentiality in health care: A survey of knowledge, perceptions and attitudes among high school students. *Journal of the American Medical Association* 269, 1404–1407.

111. Fleming, G. V., O'Connor, K. G., and Sanders, J. M., Jr. 1994. Pediatricians' views of access to health services for adolescents. *Journal of Adolescent Health* 15(6), 473–478.

112. American Academy of Pediatrics, Committee on Adolescence. 1990. Contraception and adolescents. *Pediatrics* 86(1), 134–138.

113. American Academy of Pediatrics, Task Force on Pediatric AIDS. 1993. Adolescents and human immunodeficiency virus infection: The role of the pediatrician in prevention and intervention. *Pediatrics* 92(4), 626–630.

114. American Academy of Pediatrics, Committee on Adolescence. 1996. The adolescent's right to confidential care when considering abortion. *Pediatrics* 97(5), 746–751.

115. Blum, R. 1987. Physicians' assessments of deficiencies and desire for training in adolescent medicine. *Journal of Medical Education* 62, 401–407.

116. U.S. Bureau of the Census. 1993. *Population of the United States, 1992.* Washington, D.C.: U.S. Government Printing Office.

117. Accreditation Council for Graduate Medical Education. Program requirements for residency education in pediatrics (http://www.acgme.org/progreq/peds.htm).

118. Accreditation Council for Graduate Medical Education. Program requirements for residency education in internal medicine (http://www.acgme.org/progreq/im.htm).

119. Accreditation Council for Graduate Medical Education. Program requirements for residency education in family practice (http://www.acgme.org/progreq/fp.htm).

120. U.S. Bureau of the Census. Health insurance coverage for children in the United States, 1995 (http://www.census.gov/hhes/hlthins/childins).

121. Sellers, D. E., McGraw, S. A., and McKinlay, J. B. 1994. Does the promotion of condoms increase teen sexual activity? Evidence from an HIV prevention program for Latino youth. *American Journal of Public Health* 84(12), 1952–1959.

122. Wolk, L. I., and Rosenbaum, R. 1995. The benefits of school based condom availability: Cross-sectional analysis of a comprehensive high school-based program. *Journal of Adolescent Health* 17, 184–188.

123. U.S. Bureau of the Census. 1995. *Population Estimates and Projections, 1950–1992.* Current Population Reports, Series P-25.

124. U.S. Bureau of the Census. 1995. *Projections of the Population for the United States: 1992 to 2050.* Current Population Reports, Series P-25.

125. Hofmann, A. D. 1980. A rational policy toward consent and confidentiality in adolescent health care. *Journal of Adolescent Health* 1(1), 9–17.

126. Mauldon, J., and Luker, K. 1996. Does liberalism cause sex? *The American Prospect* 24, 80–85.

127. U.S. Public Health Service. 1991. *Healthy People 2000: National Health Promotion and Disease Prevention Objectives.* Publication 017-001-00474-0. Washington, D.C.: U.S. Government Printing Office.

128. American Medical Association. 1992. *Guidelines for Adolescent Preventive Services.* Chicago: American Medical Association.

129. National Academy of Science, Committee on Child Development Research and Public Policy, Panel on Adolescent Pregnancy and Childbearing, and Hayes, C. D., ed. 1987. *Risking the Future: Adolescent Sexuality, Pregnancy, and Childbearing.* Vol. 1. Washington, D.C.: National Academy Press.

130. Bearinger, L. H., and McAnarney, E. R. 1988. Integrated community health delivery programs for youth: Study Group report. *Journal of Adolescent Health* 9, 36S–40S.

131. The National Commission on the Role of the School and the Community in Improving Adolescent Health. 1990. *Code Blue: Uniting for Healthier Youth.* Alexandria, Va.: National Association of State Boards of Education.

IMPROVING HEALTH AND SAFETY
IN THE AGRICULTURAL WORKPLACE

THE HISTORY OF OCCUPATIONAL HEALTH
AS AN AGRICULTURAL CONCERN

In one of the earliest references to occupational disease, the Swedish archbishop Olaus Magnus warned in 1555 in his *Historia de Gentibus Septentrionalibus* (History of the Nordic peoples) about the "damage to the vital organs of threshers from inhaling grain dusts" (1). This respiratory hazard of farmwork was again noted 150 years later by the Italian physician Bernadino Ramazzini in his seminal work on occupational health hazards, *De Morbis Artificum* (The diseases of workers) (2). While these early observations called attention to occupational hazards in agriculture, the field of occupational health has been driven, since the late 18th century, by the urban engines and industries of the industrial revolution, and this focus on heavy industry has continued to the present time.

The industrial revolution in Great Britain was a direct cause of numerous occupational and nonoccupational health hazards in British cities. Charles Dickens's *Hard Times* paints a grim picture of the filth and pollution in his fictional but realistic Coketown:

> It was a town of red brick, or of brick that would have been red if the smoke and ashes had allowed it; but as matters stood it was a town of unnatural red and black like the painted face of a savage. It was a town of machinery and tall chimneys, out of which interminable serpents of smoke trailed themselves for ever and ever, and never got uncoiled. It had a black canal in it, and a river that ran purple with ill-smelling dye. (3)

Urban pollution and its associated public health hazards in Great Britain led to one of the earliest triumphs of epidemiology, the recognition by John Snow that cholera in London was spread by sewage-contaminated water (4). In addition to improved public sanitation, the 19th century saw many improvements in workplace conditions, but these efforts continued to focus on the heavy industries—the mines and mills—of the industrial revolution.

One English medical practitioner of note at that time was Charles Turner Thackrah (1795–1833). His seminal work, *The Effects of the Principal Arts, Trades and Professions, and of Civic States and Habits of Living, on Health and Longevity, with Suggestions for the Removal of Many of the Agents Which Produce Disease and Shorten the Duration of Life* (5), is particularly noteworthy because it focused on the prevention of disease by removal of workplace exposures. It was also prescient in its attention to bad occupational postures as a source of disability. But Thackrah's treatise failed to mention the hazards of agriculture except where those agricultural products, such as cotton, reached the urban mills and factories.

One can imagine that Thackrah and his contemporaries viewed the agricultural countryside as a healthy alternative to the filth and pollution of the industrializing cities and to the hazards of long work hours and terrible working conditions in the factories. This image of pastoral beauty, cleanliness, and health, reinforced by the artists of the time (6,7), supported the belief that agriculture itself was healthier, more wholesome, and more virtuous than urban industry. In the United States, this "agrarian myth" was embraced by Thomas Jefferson when he stated that "cultivators of the earth are the most valuable citizens. They are the most vigorous, the most independent, the most virtuous, and they are tied to their country and wedded to its liberty and interests by the most lasting bonds" (8).

These themes were echoed in the 19th century in the United States by Dr. Benjamin McCready, who noted in his treatise *On the Influence of Trades, Professions, and Occupations in the United States, in the Production of Disease* that "agriculture is the oldest, the healthiest, and the most natural of employments. The husbandman, in general, enjoys pure air, and varied and moderate exercise. In this country his diet is always abundant and nutritious, and his habits much more temperate than those of the manufacturing or laboring classes" (9).

The modern era of occupational health has also failed, until recently, to focus its efforts on the occupational hazards in agriculture. Dr. Alice Hamilton began her career by exploring the health hazards of lead and other heavy metals among working-class residents of Chicago (10).

While her efforts were instrumental in focusing public health efforts on occupational diseases in the United States, her work completely ignored the occupational hazards of agriculture (11).

One of the experiences that moved Dr. Hamilton from laboratory research to field studies was attending the International Congress on Occupational Accidents and Diseases in Brussels in 1915. At that meeting, Dr. Glibert of Belgium dismissed the subject of occupational health in the United States by stating, "It is well known that there is no industrial hygiene in the United States. Ça n'existe pas." During the first half of the 20th century, industrial hygiene and occupational health were indeed more advanced in Europe than they were in the United States. While since then that situation has been corrected for heavy industry, the United States has continued to lag behind Europe in many areas of agricultural health and safety.

Agriculture was further removed from modern occupational health efforts by the Occupational Safety and Health Act of 1970, which excluded the agricultural workplace from the jurisdiction of the new Occupational Safety and Health Administration (OSHA) and its research counterpart, the National Institute of Occupational Safety and Health (NIOSH). This exclusion contributed to a drastic disparity in federal funding levels for occupational safety: In 1985, federal spending for safety was $181 per miner but only 30 cents per agricultural worker, or over $350,000 per miner death but only $600 per agricultural worker death (12).

There was finally an effort to correct the discrepancy in the late 1980s. In 1987, an international conference in Iowa City focused attention on the tragically high rates of occupational injury and fatalities in agriculture and on the diminishing local and federal resources for addressing the problem (12). That conference and the resulting report were instrumental in passing federal legislation in 1989 supporting several broad initiatives in agricultural health and safety. The momentum from this effort was continued with the Surgeon General's Conference on Agricultural Safety and Health in 1991 (13). Since 1990, most of the increase in NIOSH's extramural funding has been to support its programs in agricultural health and safety, a step toward correcting the agency's neglect of this area in its first two decades. Nevertheless, the NIOSH effort and other federal programs are still much too little to address the magnitude of the problem.

THE AGRICULTURAL WORKFORCE

In addition to overlooking the hazards of agriculture in espousing the agrarian myth, Jefferson ignored much of the workforce doing the farmwork—the southern slave population (including his own slaves). When he spoke about the valuable citizens and virtuous employment of the cultivators of the earth, he was certainly ignoring the unpaid, noncitizen slaves. This neglect of a large portion of farm labor continues even today. The "farm family" may evoke the classic iconography of Grant Wood's painting *American Gothic,* but that image is not an accurate one for much of the country.

The number of hired farmworkers, including migrant and seasonal workers, in the United States is greater than the number of farmers and family workers (14). Further, the number of persons residing on farms has been declining for the past 50 years, while there has been an increase in hired labor (15). But even these data fail to illustrate the dependence of U.S. agriculture on hired workers, which varies with specific commodities and farm practices. For example, the average labor requirement for fruits and vegetables is 120 hours per acre, compared to only three hours per acre for grains, and these labor-intensive crops are farmed primarily by hired farm labor. Over 50% of hired farmworkers on farms employing more than 10 workers are located in California and Florida, two states with a predominance of high-value, labor-intensive crops. In California, there are 18 farmworkers for each farmer, and over 80% of farmwork is performed by hired labor.

Hired farmworkers are also demographically very different from family farmers (16). The population is young and predominantly male, foreign born, and Hispanic (Table 21.1). Almost half have less than eight years of education. This contrasts markedly with family farmers, who are an aging population, predominantly White male and U.S. born. The differences in income are also striking. One-half of migrant and seasonal farmworkers are below the poverty level, as defined by the U.S. Bureau of the Census, with a median family income of between $7,500 and $10,000 (16). Six of the 10 poorest Standard Metropolitan Statistical Areas in the United States are in California's Central Valley, and median family income is negatively correlated with employment in farmwork. In contrast, our study of California farm operators found that over 50% had a household income above $50,000 per

TABLE 21.1 DEMOGRAPHIC
CHARACTERISTICS OF U.S. FARMWORKERS
VERSUS FARM OPERATORS

Characteristic	Farm-workers	Farm Operators
Age		
Under 25 years	30%	2%
25–34 years	35%	9%
35–44 years	19%	20%
45–54 years	8%	22%
55–64 years	7%	22%
65+ years	1%	25%
Sex		
Male	71%	92%
Female	29%	8%
Ethnicity		
White (non-Hispanic)	23%	96%
Hispanic	72%	1%
African-American	2%	1%
Asian	2%	0.4%
Other	1%	1%
Education		
0–3 years	16%	na[a]
4–7 years	32%	na
8–11 years	27%	na
12+ years	25%	na
Place of birth		
U.S. born	38%	na
Foreign born	62%	na

[a]na = not available.
SOURCES: Farmworker data from U.S. Department of Labor (1991
[16]). Farm operators data from U.S. Census of Agriculture, 1992.

year and that over 25% had an annual income above $100,000 (un-published).

Globally, agriculture is even more dominant as a source of occupa-tional livelihood and potential health hazards, although a detailed dis-cussion of this topic is beyond the scope of this chapter (17). The size of the agricultural workforce relates inversely to level of development (17). In many developing countries, 70% or more of the economically active population are involved in agriculture (18).

OCCUPATIONAL FATALITIES AND INJURIES
IN AGRICULTURE

Jefferson may have ignored the occupational hazards of agriculture to the slaves who provided the labor for southern farms, but the facts amply demonstrate that the "agrarian myth" is just that—a myth. This myth was exploded by John Powers in a 1939 article in the *Journal of the American Medical Association,* in which he noted,

> During the past quarter century the hazards of industry, transportation, mining and construction have been recognized; the economic value of safety has become clearly apparent and measures have been adopted to insure its promotion. For agriculture, because of its primarily individualistic character, there has been no such recognition or supervision, and farming, though the oldest occupation in the world, remains the most hazardous. (19)

Powers went on to note in a 1950 article that 26.6% of the occupational fatalities in the United States were in agriculture, and this was approximately 70% more than in manufacturing or construction (20). He also reported that over a quarter of a million people annually were estimated to incur a disabling injury in agriculture, resulting in more than six million days of lost time.

Perhaps John Powers's most prophetic observation was that the rate of fatal injuries in construction and transportation was declining, while it was increasing in agriculture. Over the past 50 years, there has been a significant decline in the work-fatality rates in mining and construction, but a comparable decline has not occurred in agriculture (Figure 21.1). A similar discrepancy has occurred for occupational injuries and illness over the past 20 years, with significant declines occurring in mining and construction but not in agriculture (Figure 21.2). While there may be many contributing factors to this absence of significant improvement in agricultural fatality and injury rates, the limited occupational health and preventive medicine programs and the exclusion of many regulatory efforts are likely to be contributing factors.

How do occupational health indicators for agriculture compare to those of other major industries? One direct measure of occupational hazardousness is the rate of unintentional work fatalities. According to the National Safety Council, agriculture had the highest rate of unintentional fatalities in 1993, with 1,100 deaths, or 35 deaths per 100,000 workers (Figure 21.3, Table 21.2) (21). This is higher than the rates for mining or construction, and while the exact rates may vary depending

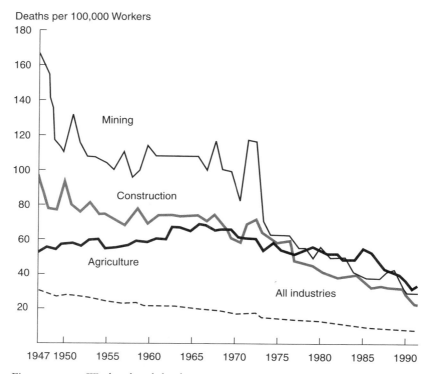

Figure 21.1. Work-related death rates in U.S. industries. Source: National Safety Council (1994 [21]).

on the method of ascertainment and population estimation, this indicator confirms that agriculture is clearly among the most hazardous occupations, with a death rate approximately four times that of all industries combined. Further, many studies have demonstrated that farming is underreported as an occupation in standard injury surveillance data, with actual mortality rates being 30% to 100% greater (22,23).

Consideration of farm residents paints an even worse picture, with 2,400 deaths in 1993, or 51 deaths per 100,000 farm residents (21). This reflects the hazards to farm family members, who are not counted among the agricultural worker totals. For example, there are nearly 300 deaths per year to children and adolescents from farm injuries, a particularly tragic statistic unique to agriculture, where the home and the workplace are the same (24).

Another perspective on agricultural fatalities is obtained from studies of cause-specific mortality in agricultural populations. The California Occupational Mortality Study found that the mortality rate for falls

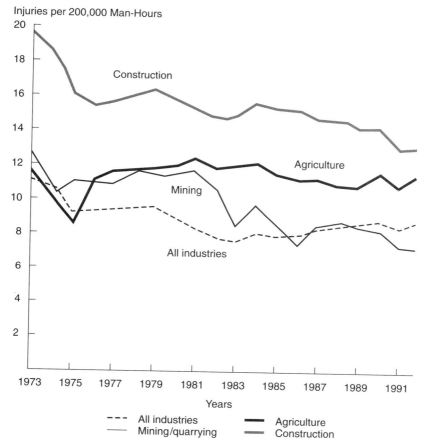

Figure 21.2.   Occupational injury and illness incidence rates by industry.
Source: National Safety Council (1994 [21]).

and machinery accidents among male farmworkers was 3.8 times the
age- and race-adjusted rates for men in all other occupations (25). Studies of mortality in other agricultural populations similarly have shown
deaths from injuries to be several times the rate in the general population (26).

Farm machinery is an obvious work hazard in agriculture and has repeatedly been shown to be the major cause of fatal work injuries. Farm
vehicles account for approximately half the fatal farm injuries, and the
majority of these deaths are due to tractors (21,27). Farm equipment,
and specifically tractors, are also the predominant cause of fatal injuries
to children in agriculture, accounting for approximately half the deaths

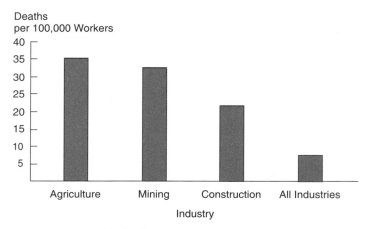

Figure 21.3. Work death rates by industry, 1993. Source: National Safety Council (1994 [21]).

TABLE 21.2   UNINTENTIONAL WORK-RELATED
DEATHS AND DISABLING INJURIES IN THE
UNITED STATES, 1993

Industry	Workers (1000s)	Deaths	Death Rates[a]	Disabling Injuries
Agriculture	3,100	1,100	35	130,000
Mining, quarrying	600	200	33	20,000
Construction	5,900	1,300	22	280,000
All industries	118,700	9,100	8	3,200,000

[a]Deaths per 100,000 workers in each group.
SOURCE: National Safety Council (1994 [21]).

of children (24,28). In our study of agricultural fatalities to children in California, deaths of children due to machinery were 80 times more likely to occur in a farm setting (29).

Data on occupational injuries and illnesses show similarly increased rates in agriculture. Agriculture consistently ranks with construction and manufacturing in having the highest incidence rates for occupational injuries and illnesses, based on Bureau of Labor Statistics data (21). Since these data exclude workplaces with fewer than 11 employees—a category that includes 95% of U.S. farms—the actual rates in agriculture may be much higher. Underreporting of injuries among migrant and seasonal farmworkers may also contribute to the underestimate of agricultural injuries. It is likely that this total is one-half or less of the actual rate (30). Nevertheless, in California alone, there are over

20,000 reported disabling injuries annually among agricultural workers. In Iowa, hospital admissions for traumatic injuries among farmers are more than three times the rate for nonfarmers (31).

CHRONIC ILLNESSES AMONG FARMERS

While traumatic injuries are the most obvious cause of death and disability among agricultural populations, a wide range of chronic illnesses are also more prevalent in agriculture, putting another nail in the coffin of the "agrarian myth." Chronic diseases also may be made worse for farmers and farmworkers because of barriers to health care in rural locations (32).

The National Health Interview Survey (NHIS) provides some perspective on chronic diseases and impairments among U.S. farmers (33). An analysis of health outcomes among 2,681 White male farmers found significantly increased age-adjusted prevalences of amputations, arthritis, cardiovascular disease, and hypertension among farmers compared to blue- or white-collar workers (Table 21.3). Although hearing loss was not more prevalent among farmers as a whole, it was significantly more prevalent in farmers over 65 years of age. Both asthma and chronic respiratory diseases were increased (70% and 30%, respectively), although not quite achieving statistical significance. Many of these findings are even more remarkable because cigarette smoking prevalence is lower among farmer populations, thus reducing the impact of one of the major preventable causes of chronic disease in society (34).

Mortality of farmers in California was significantly increased for many chronic illnesses, including cerebrovascular disease, chronic obstructive pulmonary disease, and cirrhosis (27). Studies of cause-specific mortality also have found increased suicide deaths among farmers, often attributed to the economic stresses of farming (35).

Finally, analysis of cause-specific mortality in 23 states found excess mortality among farmers from vascular lesions of the central nervous system, asthma, and several cancers, in addition to several types of fatal injuries (36).

CHRONIC ILLNESSES AND MORTALITY
AMONG FARMWORKERS

Data on chronic diseases and mortality among migrant and seasonal farmworkers are more difficult to obtain because of the lack of separate

TABLE 21.3   AGE-ADJUSTED PREVALENCE FOR
SELECTED CHRONIC CONDITIONS
BY OCCUPATIONAL GROUP

			Age-Adjusted Prevalence (%)[a]			
			Blue-Collar		White-Collar	
Condition	Farmers	95% CI[b]	Workers	95% CI	Workers	95% CI
Amputations	3.1	1.3–4.9	1.4	1.0–1.8	0.8	0.6–0.9
Arthritis	11.7	8.8–14.6	9.7	8.7–10.7	6.8	6.0–7.6
Cardiovascular diseases	18.7	14.4–23.0	14.9	13.3–16.4	13.4	12.4–14.4
Ischemic heart disease	2.9	1.5–4.3	2.2	1.2–3.2	2.4	2.0–2.8
Hypertension	15.5	11.8–19.2	12.3	11.1–13.5	10.8	9.8–11.8
Hearing loss	11.6	8.5–14.7	13.0	11.8–14.2	10.2	9.2–11.2
Skin cancer	1.4	0.4–2.4	0.9	0.5–1.2	1.2	0.8–1.6
Chronic respiratory diseases	6.7	3.4–10.0	5.2	4.4–6.0	5.3	4.5–6.1
Asthma	5.2	2.7–7.8	2.8	2.2–3.3	3.5	2.9–4.1
Back pain	7.8	4.9–10.7	6.9	6.1–7.7	6.0	5.2–6.8
All selected conditions	76.0	66.0–86.0	68.1	64.1–71.9	56.9	55.0–59.9

[a] Indirectly age-adjusted using the employed population as the standard.
[b] Confidence interval.
SOURCE: National Health Interviews Survey, 1986–1990. Reprinted from Brackbill et al. (1994 [33]).

enumeration in most surveillance data sets, missing or inaccurate denominator data, and numerous difficulties in conducting epidemiologic
investigations in this population (37,38). A comprehensive assessment
of the health status of farmworker families in McFarland, California,
confirmed the poor health status and inadequate health care in this population (38). Forty percent of families reported barriers to medical care,
the greatest of which was cost (39). In a screening of almost all (92%)
of the children 1 to 12 years of age in the town, 71% were found to have
one or more medical problems requiring referral. Forty percent of the
children were referred for vision problems, 37% for dental care, and
22% for anemia. This study and others emphasize the lack of preventive
health services in this population (40). A Michigan study found that less
than 1% of office visits for 1- to 4-year-old children of migrants were for
preventive care, compared to 34% of visits by nonmigrants (41).

Clinic-based surveys of farmworkers show that proportionately more
health care is provided for acute, infectious disease problems and less
for chronic diseases, such as hypertension (42). Among farmworkers,
health problems are exacerbated by poverty, lack of access to health

care, lack of workers' compensation coverage in many states, migratory or seasonal work patterns, and legal or regulatory impediments to health care access (37,43,44).

Limited mortality studies among farmworkers provide evidence of increased mortality from infectious and parasitic diseases (45). Increased tuberculosis mortality has been specifically identified among farmworkers and farmers (28), consistent with recent data indicating an increased prevalence of tuberculosis among farmworkers in some parts of the United States (46).

SPECIFIC CHRONIC ILLNESSES AND HAZARDOUS EXPOSURES IN AGRICULTURE

Respiratory Disease

A wide range of respiratory hazards exists within the agricultural workplace, often in concentrations much higher than in other industries (Table 21.4) (47–50). Most studies of respiratory hazards have focused on organic dust hazards, such as those that exist in hay barns, grain silos, and animal confinement units. These complex, antigenic exposures are associated with acute and chronic respiratory disease, including bronchitis, asthma, organic dust toxic syndrome, and hypersensitivity pneumonitis. Acute gaseous exposures to nitrogen oxides can occur in confinement situations and result in "silo-filler's disease," which may range clinically from transient respiratory symptoms to acute pulmonary edema and death. In New York State, deaths occur from this exposure every year, with an estimated annual incidence rate of 5 deaths per 100,000 silo-exposed farmers (51). Respiratory morbidity and mortality are also common from exposure to animal confinement–generated gases, such as ammonia, chlorine, and hydrogen sulfide (50).

Chemical exposures cause respiratory disease, either directly affecting the respiratory tract or causing systemic illness via respiratory absorption. Paraquat is an herbicide that causes death from respiratory failure following ingestion and may result in respiratory morbidity from occupational exposures (52). Examples of agricultural chemicals absorbed through the lungs that cause significant morbidity and mortality include the fumigants phosalone and methyl bromide (53,54).

Recent studies have focused on inorganic dust exposures in agriculture, particularly in dry climates such as California and other western states (55). Exposures to dusts in agriculture may be substantially

TABLE 21.4   RESPIRATORY HAZARDS IN AGRICULTURE

Agent	Examples	Sources	Diseases
Dusts			
Organic	Grain, cotton, hay, endotoxin, vegetable fiber, sugarcane	Barns, silos, storage facilities, harvesting operations	Asthma, hypersensitivity pneumonitis, organic dust toxic syndrome (ODTS), byssinosis, chronic bronchitis
Inorganic	Silica (quartz), silicates	Soil-disturbing operations	Pulmonary fibrosis, chronic bronchitis
Gases	NH_3, H_2S, NO_2, CH_4, CO, CO_2	Silos, animal confinement facilities	Silo-filler's disease, acute tracheobronchitis, pulmonary edema, asphyxiation
Chemicals			
Herbicides	Paraquat	Applicators, storage	Pulmonary fibrosis
Fertilizers	NH_3	Storage containers	Mucous membrane irritation, tracheobronchitis
Miscellaneous			
Solvents, fuels	Diesel fuel	Storage containers	Mucous membrane irritation
Welding fumes	NO_x, O_3, phosgene, metals	Welding operations	Bronchitis, emphysema

greater than levels for nuisance dusts in general industry. Further, toxic components in inorganic agricultural dusts, such as the fibrogenic agent crystalline silica, may be present at levels above the allowable industry standard in a majority of samples (55). We have recently demonstrated an independent association of wheezing and chronic bronchitis with agricultural dust exposure among California farmers (56), and our earlier work found reduced vital capacity of the lungs among grape workers (57), a crop with higher exposure to dust and silica (55). Earlier studies have shown fibrotic dust diseases of the lungs of agricultural workers in California and elsewhere (50,58), and recent work has also identified increased prevalence of interstitial or fibrogenic disease of the lungs among farmers, although the extent of these disorders is largely unknown.

Pesticide Illnesses

While most popular impressions of agricultural health hazards immediately focus on pesticides and other agrochemicals, these toxic agents actually account for only a small proportion of known disease and illness in the agricultural workplace in the United States and other developed countries. Conversely, pesticides account for a disproportionate share of the agricultural morbidity and mortality in developing countries (59). Nevertheless, many pesticides are potent systemic toxins and neurotoxins that result in acute illnesses and deaths each year, and the long-term effects of exposures are largely unknown. In California, where pesticide illness is reportable, there are over 1,000 acute illnesses among agricultural workers reported annually (60). The spectrum of acute effects, or "toxidromes," from pesticides ranges from eye and skin toxicity to several systemic manifestations, including respiratory, gastrointestinal, central, and peripheral neurologic impairments (61).

Many chronic illnesses have also been associated with pesticide exposure, including cancer (62), respiratory insufficiency, chronic neurologic disorders (63,64), and miscarriage and other reproductive toxicity (33). While most of these findings have not achieved a scientific consensus as to causality, others have shown consistent, biologically plausible associations in several studies. An example of this latter situation is the association of lymphoma with exposure to the phenoxy herbicides (62,65,66). For other health outcomes, such as Parkinson's disease (64) and neurobehavioral impairment (63), provocative hypothesis-generating studies exist that require further investigation before any causal linkage can be confirmed. The possibility exists that cumulative low-level exposures or acute high-dose exposures may result in delayed adverse health effects (63). Surveillance of acute illnesses will not detect these effects, which occur years after the exposure.

Musculoskeletal Trauma

Many characteristics of farmwork typify ergonomic factors associated with an increased risk for musculoskeletal trauma and degenerative disorders. Farmwork often requires heavy lifting, commonly in abnormal postures. This situation exists for the farmer loading hay into a barn as well as for the farmworker harvesting fruit into bags while balancing on a ladder. Incorrect postures and whole-body vibration are associated with driving tractors and other farm equipment, and these factors increase the risk of low-back pain (67). This exposure may be further exacerbated by the very long hours of tractor driving required in agriculture. Many harvesting tasks require farmworkers to perform rapid, repetitive motions of the upper extremities, factors known to cause or exacerbate ergonomic stress and cumulative trauma injuries.

Is there evidence of increased musculoskeletal trauma and degenerative disease in agriculture? Poor ergonomic design is associated with increased traumatic injury, which is well established in agriculture, as noted previously. The NHIS found a significantly increased age-adjusted prevalence of arthritis among male farmers compared to other currently employed males (36). An analysis of U.S. workers' compensation injury data for agriculture showed that over one-third of claims were for strains/sprains, and one-half of these were for back injuries (68). Farmwork in the fruit and nut tree industry was specifically identified as having increased sprain and strain injuries, and the highest percentage of these were from back injuries caused by lifting. Other analyses of farmwork have identified manual lifting in the field by farmers as the greatest risk for low-back pain.

An Italian study of tractor drivers found significant reduction in spine mobility compared to a control population, a likely result of the ergonomic stresses of tractor driving (69). Other degenerative joint diseases are also more common in agriculture. For example, two studies of hip joint degeneration have found it to be significantly more common among farmers than among control groups (70,71). In one study, hip osteoarthritis was almost 10 times more common in those who had farmed for more than 10 years and was not associated with any single type of farming (70). There are little or no data on degenerative joint disease among hired farmworkers, although the nature of the work would suggest that these late-onset outcomes would be increased in frequency.

Noise-Induced Hearing Loss

Ample literature has demonstrated that excessive noise exposure is associated with high-frequency sensorineural hearing loss. Noise and vibration are integral parts of many agricultural operations. In one study, 75% of tractors without cabs had noise levels in excess of 90 decibels, the occupational standard and a level associated with increased hearing loss (72).

The NHIS found significantly increased hearing loss among farmers over age 65 (36). In a study of New York dairy farmers, 65% had high-frequency hearing loss, which was significantly greater than the rate among control subjects (73). Other studies have confirmed the association of noise exposure in farming with increased hearing loss (74). Of even greater concern is a Wisconsin study finding an increased prevalence of hearing loss among teenage children who did farmwork compared to those who did not (75).

Cancer

Agricultural workers are exposed to a wide variety of potential carcinogens, including chemicals and physical and biologic agents (76). Potentially carcinogenic chemicals include not just herbicides and pesticides but also solvents, oils, welding fumes, wood preservatives, and other chemicals used on the farm. Ultraviolet radiation from sunlight is a physical factor directly associated with skin cancer, and biologic agents of particular concern in agriculture are viruses associated with farm animals.

Analysis of U.S. mortality data and numerous other data sources indicates that male farmers have excess mortality from cancers of the lymphatic and hematopoietic systems, lip, eye, brain, and prostate (39,65). Other cancers are increased among farmers, including cancers of the pancreas, kidney, and bone, but with less consistency. Farmers have decreased mortality from cancers of the lung and bladder, in large part because of their lower prevalence of cigarette smoking.

Most etiologic studies have focused on chemical agents, particularly pesticides. The data are consistent for an association of phenoxyacetic acid herbicides—in particular, 2,4-dichlorophenoxyacetic acid (2,4-D) —with a two- to eightfold increase of non-Hodgkin's lymphoma in studies conducted in Sweden, Kansas, Nebraska, Canada, and elsewhere (66).

Skin cancer is increased among farmers, and exposure to sunlight, a known risk factor, during work is the likely etiologic factor (77). For other cancers, a consistent increase is observed among farmers, but specific etiologic agents have not been identified; for example, many studies have documented an increase in prostate cancer among farmers (78–80).

Stress

An often overlooked health problem in farming is stress. The numerous sources of stress on the contemporary farm include financial uncertainty and losses, intense time pressures, drought and other natural disasters, intergenerational conflicts, and health and safety concerns (81). Manifestations of this stress may include causation or exacerbation of relationship problems, substance abuse, increased home violence, suicide, and several chronic diseases. While farm stress has been the subject of much speculation and many popular novels, few studies have looked at stress in farming populations. Surveys of urban versus rural populations have generally shown no differences in levels of overall stress or psychologic distress, but several specific factors in farm populations suggest that stress may be an important risk factor for disease. Suicides are increased among male farmers in the Midwest (82,83), although not in California (25). There are little data on stress among migrant and seasonal farmworkers, but poverty, job uncertainty, poor housing conditions, and family separations may all contribute to stress-related health outcomes (84).

Other Chronic Diseases

Many other chronic health conditions may be increased in agricultural populations, although specific etiologic factors often have not been identified. Dermatitis is increased in agriculture and may significantly contribute to workplace morbidity, although it is rarely a cause of death (85). Numerous agricultural exposures may result in adverse reproductive outcomes, including miscarriage, infertility, and birth defects (33). A few specific risk factors have been identified, such as the permanent infertility associated with DBCP (a nematocide) manufacturing (86), but most studies have observed ecologic associations and require further investigation (87) or require confirmation in different settings and investigation of specific mechanisms (88). Other chronic diseases that are increased in agricultural populations and that deserve further investigation and preventive efforts include cardiovascular and infectious diseases (26,36,39).

RECOMMENDATIONS FOR DISEASE PREVENTION AND HEALTH PROMOTION

While occupational health and preventive medicine have only recently focused much attention on the agricultural workplace, these recent efforts and increased resources suggest that progress can be made in reducing illness and injury among farmers and farmworkers. The first step, recognition of the problem, was greatly advanced with the Surgeon

General's Conference on Agricultural Safety and Health in 1991 (12). There is also evidence that farmers are concerned with occupational health and safety. A survey of approximately 1,500 farmers in the Midwest and East found a high level of concern about farm health and safety, with the major areas of concern being stress, trauma, and respiratory problems (89). In a recent survey of California farmers, we also found a high level of concern about health and safety, with injuries, pesticides/farm chemicals, and respiratory problems ranking highest (90). However, unlike their midwestern and eastern counterparts, over two-thirds of the California farmers stated that farming was less hazardous than other occupations, and only 9% correctly recognized that it was a more hazardous occupation than others.

The classic approach to occupational disease prevention involves a combination of the triad of engineering, education, and enforcement. I believe that each of these has a role to play in preventing illness and injury in agriculture, and I will highlight a few examples. It is important to note that approaches to this problem are complex and multidisciplinary, and solutions must be sensitive to the unique needs and requirements of farm families. Approaches to some of these problems may require the input of epidemiologists, occupational health specialists, pediatricians, behavioral scientists, sociologists and anthropologists, agricultural engineers, media experts, public health officials, educators, regulators, and farm family members and farmworkers themselves.

Engineering

One of the most dramatic engineering solutions to an agricultural health problem is the rollover protective structure (ROPS) for tractors. Tractors are the most common cause of fatal farm injuries, and tractor overturns are the single most important cause of tractor-associated fatalities, accounting for over 50% of fatalities (27,91). The rate of tractor-associated fatalities has not changed in the United States for the past 15 years. In Sweden, the annual fatality rate from tractors overturning was reduced from 12 per 100,000 farmers in 1961 to 1 per 100,000 farmers, or virtual elimination, in 1981 (92). This dramatic reduction was achieved by a 1959 law mandating ROPS on all new tractors, followed by a 1978 law prohibiting the use of tractors without ROPS. In Iowa, of 90 tractor overturns analyzed, there were no fatalities involving tractors with ROPS (93). The persistence of traumatic fatalities in the United States from tractor rollovers, when an engineering solution exists and has been demonstrated to be effective, has been termed an "occupational obscenity" (13).

Many other agricultural hazards exist for which engineering solutions can and should be the first approach to exposure or injury prevention. For example, power takeoffs (PTOs) account for approximately 7% of tractor-related fatalities. Designing a simple, effective, and inexpensive guard for PTOs should be a high priority for reducing the morbidity and mortality associated with this piece of farm equipment.

Engineering solutions should also be developed to detect hazardous situations or to reduce the levels of exposure to toxins. For example, inexpensive monitors could be developed to detect excessive levels of endotoxin or toxic gases in enclosed farm environments. Farm equipment could be designed to be quieter, and monitors could signal excessive noise levels. Chemical exposures could be reduced by further development of enclosed systems for pesticide mixing and use and improved personal protection against agrochemicals in various climates. In general, the design and development of farm equipment should include consideration of potentially hazardous exposures in addition to improved production efficiency.

Education

Education is a fundamental element of any strategy to address agricultural health and safety issues. To be most effective, this effort should be directed to several audiences. These include the following:

• Farmers and farm family members, to increase their awareness of hazardous farm conditions and their knowledge of hazard reduction, proper equipment usage, and the proper emergency response to acute injuries and illnesses. Parents should also understand the importance of adequate supervision on the farm and the need for children to have age-appropriate tasks.
• Farm children, to increase their knowledge of farm safety and their ability to recognize hazardous situations.
• Rural residents, to promote general awareness of these issues and knowledge of first aid procedures.
• Primary care physicians and health care providers, who are often the only medical contacts for farmers and farmworkers.
• Hired farmworker populations, to educate this population by in-

creasing awareness of agricultural health hazards. An education must be culturally and linguistically appropriate.
• Agricultural extension agents.

Many potential avenues exist for these educational efforts, including schools in rural areas; volunteer organizations such as 4-H, FFA, and Farm Safety for Just Kids; and the popular media.

Educational efforts to promote farm safety have existed for decades, but there has been little improvement in agricultural injury or fatality rates. This does not mean that education should be abandoned but rather that it should be done more selectively and effectively. Educational efforts should be formally evaluated to determine their effects on knowledge, behavior, and, ultimately, health outcomes. It is no longer adequate to simply print up a poster or a brochure and expect that its existence or distribution will address the problem. Modern media and the behavioral sciences have developed powerful tools for affecting behaviors in the marketplace, and these can be applied to health and safety in agriculture and other work locations. These tools have been applied effectively, for example, to reducing cigarette smoking and other cardiopulmonary risk factors for disease. The marked decline of cigarette smoking in California, home to an aggressive antismoking campaign, provides dramatic evidence of the effectiveness of these methods. A review of the medical literature identifies hundreds of articles on strategies for reducing cardiopulmonary risk factors, including effective approaches with minorities and other special populations (94). In dramatic contrast, a search of the literature for behavioral interventions in agriculture turns up only a handful of articles.

Enforcement

Regulation has a role to play as one approach to improving farm health and safety, but its role must be both realistic and appropriate. The large number of small farms spread across the country means that most regulations would have little or no chance for enforcement. Small family farms also have few resources for additional regulatory burdens, such as record keeping, industrial hygiene assessments, or complex engineering changes. For large corporate farms, where resources do exist for the implementation of appropriate health and safety regulations, a more traditional industrial approach to health and safety may be possible. Some regulatory approaches are both logical and have proven effective. For example, banning of the most hazardous pesticides in California is a direct contributing factor in the reduction of agriculturally related pesticide illnesses (60). Mandated educational programs for pest-control operators in California also may have contributed to a reduction in acute pesticide illnesses in the state. Mandated safety changes in agricultural equipment should also be required as they are in the automotive industry.

Enforcement efforts should also focus on labor regulations for hired farmworkers as has recently been done in California with the joint CAL/OSHA and U.S. Department of Labor Targeted Industries Partnership Program (TIPP) (95). This novel program developed the first comprehensive electronic database of farm labor contractors and crew leaders who operate in California. This merged file made it possible for all agencies to cross-verify registration and license records, utilize the files for outreach to local employers, and develop strategies for education and enforcement. Subsequent work included adding compliance history information concerning specific labor contractors. Compliance records are utilized to schedule inspections, particularly involving contractors with a history of repeated citations.

Research

It is critical that research be done to identify the specific health hazards in agriculture, the factors that cause or contribute to those hazards, individuals at increased risk of disease or injury, and the effectiveness of proposed or attempted interventions. The Surgeon General's Conference noted several priorities for research to reduce agricultural injury and illness (13). These include the following:

• Better characterization of risk factors and specific physical, chemical, and biologic health hazards
• Research to address the effects on chronic diseases of combined exposures and repeated acute exposures
• Epidemiologic investigation of the safety and health problems of special populations (e.g., migrant workers, children, and women) and of regional patterns of injury and disease
• Research on intervention strategy alternatives (e.g., education, regulation, and engineering controls), protective technology, the efficacy of standards, and the role of personal actions

The Conference also identified the need for more surveillance of agricultural injuries and illnesses and for interventions in the areas of hazard elimination, passive controls, and behavioral changes. These intervention efforts must include appropriate evaluation of their effectiveness in reducing agricultural injuries and illnesses.

Recent work at the University of California, Davis, has identified risk factors for increased agricultural disease. In a study of agricultural dust exposure, a cause of adverse respiratory symptoms, specific factors associated with increased (and decreased) dust exposure were identified (96). An investigation using statewide pesticide illness surveillance and use data identified high risk factors for pesticide illness among agricultural workers in California (97). These studies are important for the prevention of respiratory disease and pesticide illnesses because they identify high-risk groups for whom educational efforts and engineering interventions will have the greatest benefit.

Other research by Davis investigators has focused on improving the standard cholinesterase assay used to measure pesticide exposure (98). With regard to California clinical testing of cholinesterase, they have found that systematic errors in the testing of blood enzymes, especially the cholinesterase of the red blood cells, introduced errors of at least 40% in the values. The application of these findings involves development and dissemination of new, more accurate methods of cholinesterase testing for medical surveillance of agricultural workers and for use in clinical research. This work is an example of agricultural health research, moving from fundamental mechanisms to application, outreach, and intervention.

THE FUTURE

Agriculture is an occupation whose hazards have historically been ignored in the United States. Other occupations thought to be "inherently" hazardous, such as mining, have seen dramatic reductions in injuries and illnesses at the same time as more productive technologies have been instituted. Unlike mining, agriculture has not suffered the sort of mass disasters that catalyze action and resources to address a problem; nevertheless, there is now increased recognition of the hazardous nature of agriculture, and the situation is changing.

Approaches to injury and illness prevention in agriculture must use modern techniques of disease prevention and health promotion. They also must take into account the changing nature of the agricultural workplace and of health care delivery, particularly in the rural setting. Agriculture is a very diverse industry, and solutions must be appropriate to the local political, geographic, and cultural factors and to the farm practices of the region. Farming is the oldest occupation and was one of the first in which it was recognized that work could be hazardous as well as rewarding; it deserves our best efforts and the necessary resources to make it as safe, and its workers as healthy, as possible.

NOTE

This work was supported by the National Institute for Occupational Safety and Health (NIOSH) cooperative agreement (U07-05) and by an award from The California Wellness Foundation and the University of California Wellness Lectures Award Program.

REFERENCES

1. Magnus, O. 1909. *In Historica om de Nordiska Folken* (History of the Nordic peoples). Uppsala, Sweden: Almquist & Wiksell, 13–41.
2. Ramazzini, B. 1940. *De Morbis Artificum Bernardini Ramazzini Diatriba* (The diseases of workers). The Latin text of 1713 revised, with translation and notes by Wilmer Cave Wright. The History of Medicine Series, Vol. 7. Chicago: University of Chicago Press, issued under the auspices of the Library of the New York Academy of Medicine.
3. Dickens, C. 1990. *Hard Times: An Authoritative Text, Backgrounds, Sources, and Contemporary Reactions, Criticism,* 2nd ed., edited by S. M. George Ford. New York: W. W. Norton.
4. Snow, J. 1936. *Snow on Cholera.* New York: The Commonwealth Fund.
5. Thackrah, C. T. 1832. *The Effects of Arts, Trades, and Professions, and of Civic States and Habits of Living, on Health and Longevity, With Suggestions for the Removal of Many of the Agents Which Produce Disease, and Shorten the Duration of Life.* 2nd ed. London: Longman, Rees, Orme, Brown, Green, & Longman.
6. Schenker, H. 1994. "Picturing the Central Valley." *Landscape* 32(2), 1–11.
7. Bermingham, A. 1986. *Landscape and Ideology: The English Rustic Tradition, 1740–1860.* Berkeley and Los Angeles: University of California Press.
8. Kelsey, T. W. 1994. "The Agrarian Myth and Policy Responses to Farm Safety." *American Journal of Public Health* 84(7), 1171–1177.
9. McCready, B. W. 1943. *On the Influence of Trades, Professions, and Occupations in the United States, in the Production of Disease.* Baltimore: The Johns Hopkins University Press.

10. Hamilton, A. 1943. *Exploring the Dangerous Trades: The Autobiography of Alice Hamilton, M.D.* With illustrations by Norah Hamilton. Boston: Little, Brown.

11. Hamilton, A. 1934. *Industrial Toxicology.* Harper's Medical Monographs. New York: Harper & Brothers.

12. Merchant, J., Kross, B., Donham, K., and Pratt, D. 1989. *Agriculture at Risk: A Report to the Nation.* Oakdale, Ia.: University of Iowa, National Coalition for Agricultural Safety and Health.

13. Meyers, M., Herrick, R., and Olenchock, S., et al., eds. 1992. *Papers and Proceedings of the Surgeon General's Conference on Agricultural Safety and Health.* DHHS (NIOSH) Publication 92-105. Washington, D.C.: U.S. Government Printing Office.

14. Schenker, M. B., and McCurdy, S. A. 1990. "Occupational Health among Migrant and Seasonal Farmworkers: The Specific Case of Dermatitis." *American Journal of Industrial Medicine* 18(3), 345–351.

15. Dacquel, L. T., and Dahmann, D. C. 1993. *Residents of Farms and Rural Areas: 1991.* Current Population Reports, U.S. Bureau of the Census. Washington, D.C.: U.S. Government Printing Office.

16. U.S. Department of Labor, National Agricultural Workers Survey. 1991. *A Demographic and Employment Profile of Perishable Crop Farm Workers.* Washington, D.C.: Office of Program Economics.

17. Schenker, M. 1996. "International Issues in Agricultural Health." *Sacramento Medicine,* May, 11–12.

18. Sekimpi, D. K. 1992. "Occupational Health Services For Agricultural Workers." In *Occupational Health in Developing Countries,* edited by J. Jeyaratnam. New York: Oxford University Press, 31–61.

19. Powers, J. H. 1939. "The Hazards of Farming." *Journal of the American Medical Association* 113(15), 1375–1379.

20. Powers, J. H. 1950. "Farm Injuries." *New England Journal of Medicine* 243(25), 979–983.

21. National Safety Council. 1994. *Accident Facts.* Itasca, Ill.: National Safety Council.

22. Murphy, D. J., Seltzer, B. L., and Yesalis, C. E. 1990. "Comparison of Two Methodologies to Measure Agricultural Occupational Fatalities." *American Journal of Public Health* 80(2), 198–200.

23. Russell, J., and Conroy, C. 1991. "Representativeness of Deaths Identified through the Injury-at-Work Item on the Death Certificate: Implications for Surveillance." *American Journal of Public Health* 81(12), 1613–1618.

24. Rivara, F. P. 1985. "Fatal and Nonfatal Farm Injuries to Children and Adolescents in the United States." *Pediatrics* 76(4), 567–573.

25. Health Data and Statistics Branch, Health Demographics Section, California Department of Health Services. 1987. *California Occupational Mortality, 1979–1981.* Sacramento: California Department of Health Services.

26. Delzell, E., and Grufferman, S. 1985. "Mortality among White and Nonwhite Farmers in North Carolina, 1976–1978." *American Journal of Epidemiology* 121(3), 391–402.

27. Etherton, J. R., Myers, J. R., Jensen, R. C., et al. 1991. "Agricultural

Machine-Related Deaths." *American Journal of Public Health* 81(6), 766–768.

28. Salmi, L. R., Weiss, H. B., Peterson, P. L., et al. 1989. Fatal Farm Injuries among Young Children." *Pediatrics* 83(2), 267–271.

29. Schenker, M. B., Lopez, R., and Wintemute, G. 1995. "Farm-Related Fatalities among Children in California, 1980 to 1989." *American Journal of Public Health* 85(1), 89–92.

30. Gunderson, P., Gerberich, S., Gibson, R., et al. 1990. "Injury Surveillance in Agriculture." *American Journal of Industrial Medicine* 18(2), 169–78.

31. Fuortes, L. J., Merchant, J. A., Van, L. S., et al. 1990. "1983 Occupational Injury Hospital Admissions in Iowa: A Comparison of the Agricultural and Non-Agricultural Sectors." *American Journal of Industrial Medicine* 18(2), 211–222.

32. Emanuel, D. A., Draves, D. L., and Nycz, G. R. 1990. "Occupational Health Services for Farmers." *American Journal of Industrial Medicine* 18(2), 149–162.

33. Brackbill, R. M., Cameron, L. L., and Behrens, V. 1994. "Prevalence of Chronic Diseases and Impairments among U.S. Farmers, 1986–1990." *American Journal of Epidemiology* 139(11), 1055–1065.

34. Nelson, D. E., Emont, S. L., Brackbill, R. M., et al. 1994. "Cigarette Smoking Prevalence by Occupation in the United States: A comparison between 1978 to 1980 and 1987 to 1990." *Journal of Occupational Medicine* 36(5), 516–525.

35. Gunderson, P. D. 1995. "An Analysis of Suicides on the Farm or Ranch within Five North Central United States, 1980 to 1988." In *Agricultural Health and Safety: Workplace, Environment, Sustainability*. Edited by H. M. McDuffie, J. A. Dosman, K. M. Semchuk, et al. Pp. 465–467. New York: CRC Lewis Publishers.

36. Blair, A., Dosemeci, M., and Heineman, E. F. 1993. "Cancer and Other Causes of Death among Male and Female Farmers from Twenty-Three States." *American Journal of Industrial Medicine* 23(5), 729–742.

37. Mobed, K., Gold, E., and Schenker, M. B. 1992. "Occupational Health Problems among Migrant and Seasonal Farmworkers." *Western Journal of Medicine* 157, 367–373.

38. Schenker, M. B. 1995. "General Health Status and Epidemiologic Considerations in Studying Migrant and Seasonal Farmworkers." In *Agricultural Health and Safety: Workplace, Environment, Sustainability*. Edited by H. M. McDuffie, J. A. Dosman, K. M. Semchuk, et al. Pp. 471–478. New York: CRC Lewis Publishers.

39. Coye, M., and Goldman, L. 1991. "Summary of Environmental Data: McFarland Childhood Cancer Cluster Investigation, Phase III Report." In *California Department of Health Services Environmental Epidemiology and Toxicology Program*. Sacramento: California Department of Health Services.

40. Schlesinger, D. P., and Cautley, E. 1981. "Medical Utilization Patterns of Hispanic Migrant Farmworkers in Wisconsin." *Public Health Reports* 96(3), 255–263.

41. Wilk, V. A. 1986. *The Occupational Health of Migrant and Seasonal Farmworkers in the United States.* 2nd ed. Washington, D.C.: Farmworker Justice Fund, Inc.

42. Bleiweis, P. R., Reynolds, R. C., Cohen, L. D., and Butler, N. A. 1977. "Health Care Characteristics of Migrant Agricultural Workers in Three North Florida Counties." *Journal of Community Health* 3(1), 32–43.

43. Coye, M. J. 1985. "The Health Effects of Agricultural Production: I. The Health of Agricultural Workers." *Journal of Public Health Policy,* 349–370.

44. U.S. General Accounting Office. 1992. *Hired Farmworkers, Health and Well-Being at Risk.* Report to Congressional Requesters. Publication GAO/ HRD-92-46. Washington, D.C.: U.S. Government Printing Office.

45. Stubbs, H. A., Harris, J., and Spear, R. C. 1984. "A Proportionate Mortality Analysis of California Agricultural Workers, 1978–1979." *American Journal of Industrial Medicine* 6(4), 305–320.

46. Ciesielski, S. D., Seed, J. R., Esposito, D. H., and Hunter, N. 1991. The Epidemiology of Tuberculosis among North Carolina Migrant Farm Workers." *Journal of the American Medical Association* 265(13), 1715–1719 (published erratum appears in *JAMA* 266(1), 66).

47. Schenker, M., Ferguson, T., and Gamsky, T. 1991. "Respiratory Risks Associated with Agriculture." *Occupational Medicine* 6(3), 415–428.

48. Zejda, J. E., and Dosman, J. A. 1993. "Respiratory Disorders in Agriculture." *Tubercle and Lung Disease* 74, 74–86.

49. May, J. J., and Pratt, D. S. 1993. "Occupational Lung Disease in Agriculture." In *Seminars in Respiratory Medicine,* vol. 14, no. 1, edited by T. L. Petty and R. M. Cherniack. New York: Thieme Medical Publishers.

50. May, J. J., and Schenker, M. B. 1995. "Agriculture." In *Occupational and Environmental Respiratory Disease.* Edited by P. Harber, M. B. Schenker, and J. R. Balmes. Pp. 617–636. St. Louis: C V Mosby.

51. Zwemer, F., Jr., Pratt, D. S., and May, J. J. 1992. "Silo Filler's Disease in New York State." *American Review of Respiratory Disease* 146(3), 650–653.

52. Weinbaum, Z., Samuels, S. J., and Schenker, M. B. 1995. "Risk Factors for Occupational Illnesses Associated with the Use of Paraquat (1,1'-Dimethyl-4,4'-Bipyridylium Dichloride)." *Archives of Environmental Health* 50(5), 341–348.

53. O'Malley, M. A., and McCurdy, S. A. 1990. "Subacute Poisoning with Phosalone, an Organophosphate Insecticide." *Western Journal of Medicine* 153(6), 619–624.

54. Herzstein, J., and Cullen, M. R. 1990. Methyl Bromide Intoxication in Four Field-Workers during Removal of Soil Fumigation Sheets." *American Journal of Industrial Medicine* 17(3), 321–326.

55. Popendorf, W. J. 1982. "Mineral Dust in Manual Harvest Operations." In *Agricultural Respiratory Hazards,* vol. 2, edited by W. D. Kelley. Pp. 101–116. Cincinnati: American Conference of Governmental Industrial Hygienists.

56. Schenker, M. B., Farrar, J. A., Green, R. S., et al. 1994. "Persistent Wheeze and Dust Exposure among California Farm Operators." *American Journal of Respiratory and Critical Care Medicine* 149(4), A400.

57. Gamsky, T. E., McCurdy, S. A., Samuels, S. J., and Schenker, M. B. 1992. "Reduced FVC among California Grape Workers." *American Review of Respiratory Disease* 145, 257–262.

58. Sherwin, R. P., Barman, M. L., and Abraham, J. L. 1979. "Silicate Pneumoconiosis of Farm Workers." *Laboratory Investigation* 40(5), 576–582.

59. Jeyaratnam, J. 1990. "Acute Pesticide Poisoning: A Major Global Health Problem." *World Health Statistics Quarterly* 43(3), 139–144.

60. Mehler, L. N., O'Malley, M. A., and Krieger, R. I. 1992. "Acute Pesticide Morbidity and Mortality: California." *Rev. Environ. Contam. Toxicol.* 129(51), 51–66.

61. Schenker, M., Albertson, T., and Saiki, C. 1992. "Pesticides." In Environmental and Occupational Medicine, 2nd ed., edited by R. Rom. Pp. 887–902. Boston: Little, Brown.

62. Morrison, H. I., Wilkins, K., Semenciw, R., et al. 1992. "Herbicides and Cancer." *Journal of the National Cancer Institute* 84(24), 1866–1874.

63. Steenland, K., Jenkins, B., Ames, R. G., et al. 1994. "Chronic Neurological Sequelae to Organophosphate Pesticide Poisoning." *American Journal of Public Health* 84(5), 731–736.

64. Goldsmith, J. R., Herishanu, Y., Abarbanel, J. M., and Weinbaum, Z. 1990. "Clustering of Parkinson's Disease Points to Environmental Etiology." *Archives of Environmental Health* 45(2), 88–94.

65. Pearce, N., and Reif, J. S. 1990. "Epidemiologic Studies of Cancer in Agricultural Workers." *American Journal of Industrial Medicine* 18(2), 133–148.

66. Zahm, S. H., and Blair, A. 1992. "Pesticides and Non-Hodgkin's Lymphoma." *Cancer Research* 52(19, Suppl.), 5485S–5488S.

67. Andersson, G. B. J. 1981. "Epidemiologic Aspects on Low-Back Pain in Industry." *Spine* 6, 53–60.

68. Bobick, T. G., and Myers, J. R. 1995. "Back Injuries in Agriculture: Occupations Affected." In *Agricultural Health and Safety: Workplace, Environment, Sustainability.* Edited by H. H. McDuffie, J. A. Dosman, K. M. Semchuk, et al. Pp. 325–332. New York: CRC Lewis Publishers.

69. Barbieri, G., Mattioli, S., Grillo, S., et al. 1995. "Spinal Diseases in an Italian Tractor Drivers Group." In *Agricultural Health and Safety: Workplace, Environment, Sustainability.* Edited by H. H. McDuffie, J. A. Dosman, K. M. Semchuk, et al. Pp. 319–323. New York: CRC Lewis Publishers.

70. Croft, P., Coggon, D., Cruddas, M., and Cooper, C. 1992. "Osteoarthritis of the Hip: An Occupational Disease in Farmers." *British Medical Journal* 304(6837), 1269–1272.

71. Thelin, A. 1990. "Hip Joint Arthrosis: An Occupational Disorder among Farmers." *American Journal of Industrial Medicine* 18, 339–343.

72. Holt, J. J., Broste, S. K., and Hansen, D. A. 1993. "Noise Exposure in the Rural Setting." *Laryngoscope* 103(3), 258–262.

73. Marvel, M. E., Pratt, D. S., Marvel, L. H., et al. 1991. "Occupational Hearing Loss in New York Dairy Farmers." *American Journal of Industrial Medicine* 20(4), 517–531.

74. Plakke, B. L., and Dare, E. 1992. "Occupational Hearing Loss in Farmers." *Public Health Reports* 107(2), 188–192.

75. Broste, S. K., Hansen, D. A., Strand, R. L., and Stueland, D. T. 1989. "Hearing Loss among High School Farm Students." *American Journal of Public Health* 79(5), 619–622.

76. Schenker, M., and McCurdy, S. 1986. "Pesticides, Viruses, and Sunlight in the Etiology of Cancer among Agricultural Workers." In *Cancer Prevention — Strategies in the Workplace.* Edited by C. Becker and M. Coye. Pp. 29–37. Washington, D.C.: Hemisphere Publishing.

77. Blair, A., Malker, H., Cantor, K. P., et al. 1985. "Cancer among Farmers: A Review." *Scandinavian Journal of Work, Environment, and Health* 11(6), 397–407.

78. Dosemeci, M., Hoover, R. N., Blair, A., et al. 1994. Farming and Prostate Cancer among African-Americans in the Southeastern United States." *Journal of the National Cancer Institute* 86(22), 1718–1719.

79. Brownson, R. C., Chang, J. C., Davis, J. R., and Bagby, J. J. 1988. "Occupational Risk of Prostate Cancer: A Cancer Registry-Based Study." *Journal of Occupational Medicine* 30(6), 523–526.

80. Morrison, H., Savitz, D., Semenciw, R., et al. 1993. "Farming and Prostate Cancer Mortality." *American Journal of Epidemiology* 137, 270–280.

81. Gerrard, N. 1995. "Farm Stress: A Community Development Approach to Mental Health Service Delivery." In *Agricultural Health and Safety: Workplace, Environment, Sustainability.* Edited by H. H. McDuffie, J. A. Dosman, K. M. Semchuk, et al. Pp. 433–444. New York: CRC Lewis Publishers.

82. Liu, T., and Waterbor, J. W. 1994. "Comparison of Suicide Rates among Industrial Groups." *American Journal of Industrial Medicine* 25(2), 197–203.

83. Stallones, L. 1990. "Suicide Mortality among Kentucky Farmers, 1979–1985." *Suicide* and *Life-Threatening Behavior* 20(2), 156–163.

84. Wiggins, N., and Castañares, T. 1995. "Mental and Psychosocial Health Issues among Migrant and Seasonal Farmworkers in Oregon: Preliminary Research with Intervention Applications." In *Agricultural Health and Safety: Workplace, Environment, Sustainability.* Edited by H. H. McDuffie, J. A. Dosman, K. M. Semchuk, et al. Pp. 503–510. New York: CRC Lewis Publishers.

85. Gamsky, T. E., McCurdy, S. A., Wiggins, P., et al. 1992. "Epidemiology of Dermatitis among California Farm Workers." *Journal of Occupational Medicine* 34(3), 304–310.

86. Eaton, M., Schenker, M. B., Whorton, D., et al. 1986. "Seven-Year Follow-Up of Workers Exposed to 1,2-Dibromo-3-Chloropropane." *Journal of Occupational Medicine* 28(11), 1145–1150.

87. McDonald, A. D., McDonald, J. C., Armstrong, B., et al. 1988. "Fetal Death and Work in Pregnancy." *British Journal of Industrial Medicine* 45, 148–157.

88. Nurminen, T., Rantala, K., Kurppa, K., and Holmberg, P. C. 1995. "Agricultural Work during Pregnancy and Selected Structural Malformations in Finland." *Epidemiology* 6(1), 23–30.

89. Thu, K., Donham, K. J., Yoder, D., and Ogilvie, L. 1990. "The Farm Family Perception of Occupational Health: A Multistate Survey of Knowledge, Attitudes, Behaviors, and Ideas." *American Journal of Industrial Medicine* 18(4), 427–431.

90. Farrar, J. A., Schenker, M. B., McCurdy, S. A., and Morrin, L. A. 1995.

"Hazard Perceptions of California Farm Operators." *Journal of Agromedicine* 2(2), 27–40.

91. "Use of Rollover Protective Structures—Iowa, Kentucky, and Ohio, 1992–1997." 1997. *Mortality and Morbidity Weekly Report* 46, 842–845.

92. Thelin, A. 1990. "Epilogue: Agricultural, Occupational and Environmental Health Policy Strategies for the Future." *American Journal of Industrial Medicine* 18(4), 523–526.

93. Lehtola, C. J., Donham, K. J., and Marley, S. J. 1995. "Tractor Risk Abatement and Control: A Community-Based Intervention for Reducing Agricultural Tractor-Related Fatalities and Injuries." In *Agricultural Health and Safety: Workplace, Environment, Sustainability.* Edited by H. H. McDuffie, J. A. Dosman, K. M. Semchuk, et al. Pp. 385–389. New York: CRC Lewis Publishers.

94. Marin, B. V., Perez, S. E., Marin, G., and Hauck, W. W. 1994. "Effects of a Community Intervention to Change Smoking Behavior among Hispanics," *American Journal of Preventive Medicine* 10(6), 340–347.

95. U.S. Department of Labor, Wage and Hour Division; California Employment Development Department; California Division of Occupational Safety and Health; California Division of Labor Standards Enforcement. 1996. *Targeted Industries Partnership Program: A Joint Enforcement and Educational Effort in the Agricultural and Garment Industries. Fourth Annual Report.* Sacramento, Calif.: U.S. Department of Labor.

96. Nieuwenhuijsen, M. J., Schenker, M. B., S. S, Farrar, J., and Green, S. 1996. "Exposure to Dust, Noise and Pesticides, Their Determinants and the Use of Protective Equipment among California Farm Operators." *Applied Occupational and Environmental Hygiene* 11(10), 1217–1225.

97. Weinbaum, Z., Schenker, M. B., Gold, E. B., et al. 1997. "Risk Factors for Systemic Illnesses Following Agricultural Exposures to Restricted Organophosphates in California, 1984–1988." *American Journal of Industrial Medicine* 31, 572–579.

98. Wilson, B. W., Sanborn, J. R., O'Malley, M. A., et al. 1997. "Monitoring the Pesticide-Exposed Worker." *Occupational Medicine: State of the Art Reviews* 12, 347–363.

22

Annette L. Stanton,
Sharon Danoff-Burg, and
Sheryle J. Gallant

ENHANCING WOMEN'S HEALTH

*Current Status and Directions
in Research and Practice*

Attending a university reception with a colleague some years ago, I (A.L.S.) reacted strongly when he referred to a study regarding the link between caffeine consumption and heart disease, which had just received considerable media attention (Grobbee et al., 1990). "I guess our hearts are safe if we have a cup of coffee," he said. "*Your* heart may be safe; I have no idea about the safety of *my* heart! That study was conducted on over 45,000 men," came my retort. Thus began a discussion of how little the scientific community knew, from either a psychological or a biomedical perspective, concerning many facets of women's physical health. Indeed, had this chapter been written only a decade ago, we would have had much less to say. Today, owing to the realization by researchers and practitioners that to understand women's health we need to study women and to include gender in conceptualizations of health and illness, the knowledge base in women's health is evolving rapidly. Rather than providing a review of the content of this large literature in this chapter (for comprehensive treatments, see e.g., Blechman and Brownell, 1998; Gallant et al., 1997; Stanton and Gallant, 1995), we first highlight historical and recent developments in the area. Specifically, it is important to understand the criticisms that have been leveled against the traditional body of thought regarding women's health and to be aware of the exciting initiatives designed to redress some of the deficiencies in earlier models and policies. We then provide recommendations for continuing to enhance our understanding and promotion of women's health.

WHAT IS A HEALTHY WOMAN? THE SOCIAL CONSTRUCTION OF WOMEN'S HEALTH

Observers of the literature on women's health have pointed out that health itself, and women's health in particular, are socially constructed phenomena (e.g., Corea, 1985; Ehrenreich and English, 1978; Travis, 1988). These writers argue that conceptualizations of women's health reflect prevailing sociocultural standards concerning women's proper place in the world. Lawrence and Bendixen (1992) illustrated this point through their analysis of depictions of male and female anatomy in medical texts. They first outlined two historical approaches to conceptualizing female and male anatomy: hierarchy and difference. Dominant from the time of the classical Greeks through the mid-17th century, the hierarchical approach framed women and men as sharing similar basic biological structures, albeit in imperfect form in women. They quoted Aristotle—"For the female is, as it were, a mutilated male" (p. 926)—to exemplify this understanding of female anatomy.

By contrast, post-17th-century writers began to present women's anatomy as quite distinct from that of men's. To illustrate the concept of difference, Lawrence and Bendixen (1992) quoted Sachs, a German physician, writing in 1830: "The male body expresses positive strength, sharpening male understanding and independence, and equipping men for life in the State, in the arts and sciences. The female body expresses womanly softness and feeling. The roomy pelvis determines women for motherhood. The weak, soft members and delicate skin are witness of woman's narrower sphere of activity, of home-bodiness, and peaceful family life" (p. 926). Other writers have pointed out that the scientists and physicians of the late 1800s used accepted scientific theories to promote the primacy of the maternal role for women (Travis, 1988). For example, Helmholtz's principle of energy conservation was used to support the proposition that because women's most important function was reproduction, it followed logically that other biological structures, especially those involved in intellectual pursuits and physical activities, could not and should not function at maximum capacities in women (Travis, 1988). Further, the purported primacy of cyclic biology and hormonal function in women is illustrated by one physician's (Virchow, cited in Fausto-Sterling, 1985) statement in the late 1800s that "woman is a pair of ovaries with a human being attached, whereas man is a human being furnished with a pair of testes" (p. 90). In addition, the exigencies of being a woman were used as a justification for female infirmity and for invalidism as an accepted role (Ehrenreich and English, 1978; Travis, 1988). Woven throughout is the notion of woman and female qualities as not merely different but inferior.

Returning to the present day, Lawrence and Bendixen (1992) found in their analysis of medical texts between 1890 and 1989 that although 63% of anatomy illustrations in medical texts they reviewed were not gender specific and that text space devoted specifically to males had declined over the century, medical texts in 1989 still evidenced a disproportionate use of male-specific figures and descriptions. Further, male structures often were presented as the norm with female as the variation, and female-specific content was at times vague or inaccurate.

These findings illustrate two primary contentions of social constructionists—that scientific and professional treatments of women's health have served (1) to perpetuate the view of male as normative and female as deviation from the norm and (2) to promote a focus on women's reproductive function to the exclusion of other aspects of health. Recent evidence also suggests that the social construction of women's health is apparent in researchers' selection of topics for study and in their interpretation of data (e.g., Meyerowitz and Hart, 1995; Stanton and Danoff-Burg, 1995). Fortunately, today many researchers are investigating women's health concerns in their own right, are broadening their focus to encompass a host of areas in addition to reproductive health, and are framing answers to the question "What is a healthy woman?" in terms of women's own experience.

HOW SHOULD WOMEN BE TREATED? DIFFERENTIAL TREATMENT OF WOMEN'S HEALTH CONCERNS

According to a number of writers, medical treatment for women in the United States is a reflection of women's subordinate status, and many point out that differences exist in health care for women and men that cannot be explained completely by differences in morbidity or illness behaviors (e.g., Ehrenreich and English, 1978; Travis, 1988). Differential treatment of women's health concerns is illustrated in a report of the Council on Ethical and Judicial Affairs of the American Medical Association (1991). The council cited gender disparities in access to kidney transplantation, diagnosis and treatment of cardiac disease, and diagnosis of lung cancer. Specifically, research was reviewed suggesting that (1) when age is controlled statistically, women are 25% to 30% less likely to receive cadaver kidney transplants than are men; (2) women are less likely to be referred for diagnostic testing for lung cancer than men, even when smoking status is taken into account; and (3) women are 6.5 times less likely to be referred for cardiac catheterization than are men, even when their radionuclide scans are abnormal. Further, physicians are more likely to attribute women's, as opposed to men's, cardiac-related symptoms to psychosomatic or noncardiac factors. The report's authors suggested that biological differences, such as women's greater longevity and accompanying higher disease rate, may in part account for the gender disparities. However, they also posited that gender stereotypic attitudes may affect medical decision making. Gender stereotypes may result in physicians' propensity to attribute women's health complaints to emotional rather than physical causes and to view women's societal contributions as relatively unimportant and therefore their health concerns as less deserving of serious attention.

The disadvantaged status of women, and particularly older women and women of color, also is reflected in their being more likely to live in poverty and to be unemployed than men. A result is that women are less likely to have adequate health insurance and access to health care. Given the consistent finding that lower socioeconomic status predicts less positive health outcomes even when controlling for access to health care (Adler et al., 1994), the disadvantaged status of women is of particular importance.

Another consequence of gender inequality has been the historical lack of participation of women in the upper echelons of the medical profession and the behavioral sciences. Indeed, the American Medical Association elected its first female president in 1997. Although women now are entering medical training in record numbers, women's relative nonparticipation is important because it may account in part for the lack of attention to women's health concerns and for less adequate treatment of women. For example, Lurie et al. (1993) found that male physicians were less likely than female physicians to refer their female patients for cancer screening (i.e., Pap smears, mammograms) or to perform such tests. Increased entry of women into important roles as researchers, practitioners, and policy makers may serve to improve attention to and increase effectiveness interventions for women's health concerns.

Many questions remain regarding differential treatment of women's health concerns, including the following:

• To what extent are gender disparities in specific medical diagnostic and treatment procedures accounted for by biomedical versus psychosocial factors?
• How often and in what contexts does a gender disparity reflect underattention to women's health or unnecessarily excessive attention to men's?
• Is it important to tailor medical and behavioral treatment strategies specifically for women, such as gender-sensitive interventions for alcohol abuse or smoking?
• Should research and practice in women's health be established as a distinct specialty within medicine and health psychology, should such activity be integrated into already existing structures, or should both integration and specialization be encouraged (Angell, 1993; Harrison, 1992; Rosser, 1993; Wallis, 1993)?

It is through addressing such questions that we will be able to facilitate optimal health care for women.

WHERE ARE THE WOMEN? THE EXCLUSION OF WOMEN AS PARTICIPANTS IN RESEARCH

Perhaps more than any other limitation, exclusion of women as research participants (Bennett, 1993; Johnson, 1992; Travis, 1988; U.S. General Accounting Office, 1990) has constrained progress in the area of women's health. This is most apparent in large clinical trials conducted solely on men, including those on the prophylactic effects of aspirin for cardiovascular disease, performed with more than 22,000 men (Steering Committee of the Physicians' Health Study Research Group, 1988), and on the identification of risk factors for coronary heart disease, in which more than 300,000 men were screened and more than 10,000 included in the clinical trial (Multiple Risk Factor Intervention Trial [MRFIT]; e.g., Ockene et al., 1990). Examples from the psychosocial literature also exist, including the relative absence of research on Type A behavior, hostility, and other psychosocial risk factors for heart disease in women (Baker et al., 1984; Shumaker and Smith, 1995; Wenger et al., 1993). Further, some have argued that the experience of and treatment for some female-prevalent health conditions, such as osteoporosis and systemic lupus erythematosus, have been understudied (U.S. Public Health Service [USPHS], 1985).

Several purported barriers to inclusion of women in clinical studies have been identified (Bennett, 1993; USPHS, 1985). These include (1) the responsibility to protect the reproductive capacity of women in their childbearing years and to protect the fetuses of pregnant women; (2) the need for convenient recruitment of participants and for easily identifiable cohorts (e.g., the Physicians' Health Study participants, who were recruited via the American Medical Association roster); (3) the potentially higher costs resulting from inclusion of women, given that women have lower mortality rates than men, and mortality often is the end point studied; (4) the need to recruit participants at high risk for the disease end points being examined (e.g., men's higher mortality rates for heart disease among particular age cohorts); (5) the goal of achieving homogeneity in study samples, thus not having to consider women's hormonal variation; and (6) the assumption that women are less likely than men to participate in clinical trials, to adhere to prescribed medical regimens, or to agree to random assignment (note that there is no empirical evidence for this assumption).

Specific neglect of poor, ethnic minority, and older women is apparent in the literature on women's physical health (Gatz et al., 1995; USPHS, 1985) and on aspects of women's psychological adjustment (Reid, 1993; Yoder and Kahn, 1993). This is of particular concern in light of the evidence that poor and ethnic minority women in general are at risk for greater morbidity and mortality than are their more affluent and White counterparts (USPHS, 1985). Moreover, older women are at risk for contracting multiple chronic conditions (i.e., comorbidities), may take multiple prescription medications, and, because of their greater likelihood of living in poverty than men, often are subject to inadequate health care (USPHS, 1985).

Consequences arising from the exclusion of women as research participants are profound. We know less about biological and psychosocial risk and protective factors for diseases in women than in men, and often the generalization of findings from studies on men's health and disease has occurred in the absence of knowledge of their applicability to women. Insufficient information exists regarding how endogenous and exogenous (e.g., oral contraceptives) hormones may interact with medications to affect the potency of medical treatments. Women (and sometimes fetuses in utero) are subject to pharmaceutical agents, medical treatments, and diagnostic procedures that are of undocumented safety and efficacy for them.

Fortunately, recent investigations suggest that the barriers to inclusion of women in health research are crumbling. Positive modifications in institutional and government policies will create pathways to knowledge about women's health and will diminish the necessity for the question "Where are the women?"

THE GOOD NEWS: NEW DIRECTIONS
IN ATTENTION TO WOMEN'S HEALTH

In 1985, documented recognition that the health concerns of women require substantial empirical attention occurred at the federal level. In that year, a report was released on the health status of American women by the Public Health Service Task Force on Women's Health Issues (USPHS, 1985). The following year, the National Institutes of Health (NIH) announced that all researchers applying for NIH funding should consider the inclusion of women in clinical trials or provide a clear rationale when women are excluded. However, in 1990 the U.S. General Accounting Office (GAO), the investigative arm of Congress, reported that few researchers were aware of this policy and that some scientific review panels had been instructed not to consider the inclusion of female participants as a criterion for evaluating the merit of a research proposal.

Along with other catalysts, the GAO report spurred the introduction in Congress of the Women's Health Equity Act of 1990. This act, developed by the Congressional Caucus on Women's Issues and introduced by Representatives Patricia Schroeder and Olympia Snowe, was designed to address deficiencies in women's health care in the areas of research, treatment, and prevention. Composed of 20 separate provisions, the bill proposed mechanisms for ensuring inclusion of women in study populations and bolstering empirical attention to women's health. Also proposed was authorization of funding for research, treatment, and prevention initiatives in women's health, including cancer, osteoporosis, reproductive health, AIDS, and sexually transmitted diseases. Many of these provisions saw favorable action in Congress, and others were introduced under the Women's Health Equity Act of 1993. A critical feature of this initiative's impact is that annual federal funding for breast cancer programs has increased from less than $100 million in 1990 to more than $600 million by 1997 (Blumenthal and Wood, 1997).

The establishment of the Office of Research on Women's Health represents another encouraging step in addressing a broad range of women's health concerns. This office, proposed in Congress and founded by the NIH in 1990, is charged with the coordination and oversight of efforts to enhance women's health research at the NIH. Its mission encompasses specifying pertinent research needs, supplementing extant funds for research on women's health, coordinating efforts among the various institutes, and promoting women's entry into and advancement in scientific careers. The office also monitors the inclusion of women in study populations, which now is mandated by the NIH unless a clear and compelling rationale for their exclusion is provided (NIH, 1994). Yet another stimulus for women's health research is the revision by the Food and Drug Administration (FDA) of a 16-year-old policy that excluded most women of reproductive age from the initial phases of clinical trials. The FDA's formal statement to drug developers that women should be represented sufficiently in drug studies and that appropriate statistical analyses for sex-related effects should be undertaken also is encouraging (Merkatz et al., 1993).

Federal attention to women's health set the stage for the development of the Women's Health Initiative, the largest clinical trial ever conducted in the United States. Following women aged 55 to 79 for up to 12 years, the initiative will investigate contributors to and treatments for important causes of death and disability among women, including cardiovascular disease, breast and colorectal cancer, and osteoporosis. An observational component is included; a randomized, controlled trial will test the efficacy of hormone replacement therapy and nutritional interventions in preventing major diseases; and psychosocial and behavioral factors will be investigated. Important implications for promotion of women's health and prevention of disease may be anticipated as findings from this large-scale study emerge.

DIRECTIONS IN RESEARCH, PRACTICE, AND POLICY IN WOMEN'S HEALTH

Promising developments at the federal policy level and in the empirical knowledge base provide encouragement to researchers and practitioners interested in women's health. A growing awareness exists among scientists that women's health concerns represent a crucial area for intensive study. However, progress is uneven, and many questions remain. In this section, we delineate themes that cut across substantive areas and identify challenges for future research and application in the psychology of women's health. The discussion is divided into three areas of emphasis: (1) conceptual frameworks in women's health, (2) methodological considerations, and (3) issues in application and policy.

CONCEPTUAL FRAMEWORKS IN WOMEN'S HEALTH

Research and practice in women's health will benefit from: (1) applying biopsychosocial models to the study and promotion of women's health; (2) promoting an expanded definition of health that includes psychological, functional, and social status as well as biological end points; (3) focusing increasingly on positive health outcomes in addition to morbidity and mortality; (4) incorporating established theories and considering multiple contextual determinants of health outcomes; and (5) considering women's diversity.

The Need for Biopsychosocial Models

In contrast to adhering strictly to a traditional biomedical model, the advantages of exploring interactions among biological, psychological, and social factors in order to understand health and disease have been documented for some time (Engel, 1977, 1980; Schwartz, 1982). The importance of assuming a biopsychosocial approach to research in women's health is highlighted by Hamilton's (1993) contention that "the social construction of gender implies that women's health can be understood only by a better appreciation of psychosocial aspects of women's lives, along with more integrative biological research. Indeed, every health discipline, with the notable exception of medicine, recognizes that psychology and the social sciences must be central to and at the very core of a woman-centered women's health movement" (p. 51). Several lines of evidence converge to suggest that psychological and social factors are prominent determinants of the health of women.

One such line of evidence comes from research exploring explanations for sex-related differences in mortality and morbidity. Echoing the observations of many researchers (e.g., Rodin and Ickovics, 1990; Strickland, 1988; Verbrugge, 1990), Riley (1990) cited a "familiar but still puzzling paradox: in the United States today, on the average, at every age women report more illness and health care utilization than men, yet life expectancy is consistently higher for women than for men" (p. vii). Indeed, in all economically developed countries, females' mortality advantage increased during the 20th century, particularly from 1930 to 1970, in large part owing to males' increase in deaths from lung cancer and ischemic heart disease (Waldron, 1993). Although a decline in the mortality advantage for females in most age-groups has been apparent since the 1970s, females currently outlive males by an average of seven years (Nathanson, 1990). In this context of greater longevity, women nevertheless appear to have higher rates of physical illness overall, especially acute illnesses and nonfatal chronic conditions; have more disability days and physician visits; and use more prescription and non-prescription medication than do men (Rodin and Ickovics, 1990; Verbrugge, 1990; Verbrugge and Wingard, 1987). Exceptions to women's greater morbidity are men's greater rates of sensory/structural impairments, life-threatening chronic diseases, and major disabilities due to chronic conditions (Verbrugge, 1990). These exceptions are consistent with men's higher death rates.

Certainly, sex differences in mortality and morbidity are accounted for in part by biological influences. These include such factors as the lack of genetic redundancy on the Y chromosome and other chromosomal influences (e.g., Smith and Warner, 1990; Travis, 1988), the protective effect of estrogen with regard to heart disease (e.g., Hazzard, 1990), and sex-related differences in neuroendocrine and cardiovascular response to stressors (e.g., Matthews, 1989; Polefrone and Manuck 1987). Psychological and social influences also play an important role. Health-related behaviors constitute one category of contributors. Changing sex differences in mortality, for example, can be attributed in part to changes in the behavior of cigarette smoking (Waldron, 1993). Although perhaps of lesser impact than smoking (Nathanson, 1990), other behaviors that confer health risk, including dietary practices, alcohol use, hazardous employment, unsafe sexual practices, lack of physical activity, reckless driving, and violent acts, also may produce differential impact on female and male morbidity and mortality (Verbrugge, 1990; Verbrugge and Wingard, 1987). Gender differences in illness and prevention orientation, including perception of symptoms, readiness to take preventive and curative actions, and health-reporting behaviors, also may contribute to morbidity and mortality differences (Verbrugge and Wingard, 1987). Furthermore, biological, behavioral, and social characteristics may interact to predict health risk in women and men (Matthews, 1989; Ory and Warner, 1990).

Other areas of inquiry also have illuminated the critical role of behavioral and psychosocial influences on women's health. For example, research has revealed the impact of sociodemographic transitions on health, such as the rapidly declining fertility rates in developing countries and the consequent decrease in maternal morbidity and mortality (Leslie, 1992). Also, although they reveal complex moderating and mediating factors, studies of women's social roles have demonstrated the relation of participation in multiple valued roles (e.g., worker, spouse, mother) to enhanced physical and psychological health and have suggested that paid employment may have particularly salutory effects (LaCroix and Haynes, 1987; Repetti et al., 1989; Rodin and Ickovics, 1990; Waldron and Jacobs, 1989). Certainly, women's experiences of poverty and victimization also carry health consequences (Koss et al., 1990; Plichta, 1992; USPHS, 1985). It is clear that most major causes of morbidity and mortality are multifactorial and involve biological, psychological, and social contributors.

Studying psychosocial, biological, and behavioral factors in isolation has contributed to fragmentation in research and health care. Rather, examining links among these factors may better serve to advance research and application in women's health. For example, depression may be associated with such health behaviors and outcomes as smoking maintenance (Mermelstein and Borrelli, 1995), diabetes (Butler and Wing, 1995), and cardiovascular disease (Shumaker and Smith, 1995). Marcus et al. (1995) cited research suggesting that participation in exercise may help women quit smoking. Conversely, the traditional biomedical model also may promote the treatment of isolated organ systems rather than the whole woman with complex and interacting health care needs. How is a woman to decide on electing exogenous hormone administration when it may confer benefit with regard to preventing heart disease but risk with regard to developing cancer (Barrett-Connor, 1994; Hulka, 1994; Lobo and Speroff, 1994)? Is women's optimal health promoted when researchers construct protocols that provide incentives to women for attending cancer screening but do not offer simple blood pressure checks at the same appointment? Research that prevents such fragmentation through examination of multiple determinants of multifaceted health outcomes is clearly indicated.

The Need for an Expanded Definition of Health

Not only are psychosocial factors significant contributors to health status, they also represent important end points in health research. Calls for increased empirical and applied attention to health-related quality of life have been issued in many arenas (e.g., Moinpour et al., 1989; Taylor and Aspinwall, 1990). Quality of life is a multidimensional construct that includes physical, psychological, and social functioning. As Gatz et al. (1995) have documented, older women, who are likely to have multiple chronic conditions, perceive themselves as healthier than their physical status would predict, suggesting that functional, social, and psychological status are important contributors to health perceptions.

The Need for a Focus on Positive Health Processes and Outcomes

We propose that the adequate conceptualization of multifaceted health outcomes implies examination not only of pathological psychosocial and biological processes but also of salutory health effects. A traditional biomedical approach often promotes a focus on pathology rather than health, and women's biology and health often have been viewed through a lens of difference and deficiency. Although it surely is important to explore what leads to disease in women, it is equally crucial to acknowledge women's health-related strengths and to examine factors that promote their optimal health and well-being. O'Leary and Ickovics (1995) have advanced a model of resilience as applied to women's health, and other researchers have developed psychological constructs shown to be related to positive psychological and physical health outcomes in both women and men, such as optimism (Scheier and Carver, 1992) and hope (Snyder et al., 1991). It is important to develop biopsychosocial models that focus on women's resilience and health to offset what traditionally has been a pervasive focus on distress and disease.

The Need for Theoretically Grounded Research

Researchers also should be aware that maintaining a narrow focus on a specific disease or behavior may prove limiting with regard to theory testing and development. For example, much of the research on postpartum depression failed to benefit from established theories regarding depression in general (Stanton and Danoff-Burg, 1995). As Marcus and colleagues (1995) suggested, general theories of behavior change can serve as a foundation for understanding and promoting physical activity in women. Theoretically grounded work will advance the study of specific diseases, and focusing on psychosocial constructs and theories that cut across health outcomes and behaviors may prove even more beneficial.

The Need for Attention to Contextual Determinants of Health

We observe that many of the theories and constructs applied to the psychology of women's health to date have centered on explanatory variables residing within the individual rather than in the sociocultural context of women's and men's lives. Women's reluctance to encourage condom use by their partners, for example, has been assumed to reflect women's health beliefs or lack of assertiveness rather than power differentials in intimate relationships (Morokoff et al., 1995). Depression following childbearing often has been assumed to be a result of biological upheaval rather than the demands that accompany assumption of the role of primary caretaker (Stanton and Danoff-Burg, 1995). Programs designed to promote exercise participation have focused on enhancing self-regulatory or other individual skills rather than addressing such barriers to activity as women's caretaking responsibilities or lack of convenient access to safe exercise facilities (Marcus et al., 1995).

A conceptual focus on intraindividual factors certainly is useful in accounting for some of the variance in health-related variables and in developing interventions to foster individuals' control over their health. However, narrow concentration on the individual woman and her internal attributes may result in misplaced blame for negative health behaviors and outcomes as well as in limited conceptual models and applications (see Bohan, 1993; Hare-Mustin and Marecek, 1990; Kahn and Yoder, 1989; Mednick, 1989; Prillentensky, 1989). Viewing a woman's "failure" to obtain a mammogram as reflecting her lack of interest in her own health, as opposed to attributing it to her physician's lack of referral or to her desire to devote all extra funds to her children's education, provides a considerably different conceptual picture and carries very different implications for maximally effective interventions. Contextual factors such as socioeconomic conditions, exposure to violence, ethnic and cultural norms, organizational (e.g., workplace) involvement, physical environments and hazards, and the sociopolitical milieu warrant far more theoretical and empirical attention (see Revenson, 1990, for other recommendations regarding conceptualizing contexts). The myriad positive and negative influences of interpersonal relationships on women's health also warrant continued attention. For example, interpersonal factors are potentially important determinants of women's drinking (Wilsnack, 1995), smoking (Mermelstein and Borrelli, 1995), exercise (Marcus et al., 1995), and sexual behaviors (Morokoff et al.,

1995). Women's roles as caretakers across the life span carry consequences for their own health as well as that of family members (Gatz et al., 1995). Health care providers' attitudes toward women translate into potentially differential treatment of women and men. Thus, the influences of relational contexts deserve increased consideration in conceptualizations of women's health. To conceptualize women's health without regard for the contexts of women's lives will result in a partial and potentially distorted picture.

The Need for Considering Women's Diversity

The recognition of contextual and individual differences among women highlights the need for considering issues of diversity in our conceptual models for women's health. Traditional disease-based approaches often have concentrated on the disease process itself, with minimal consideration of factors promoting vulnerability or resilience within the host or within the host's environment. Up to this point, we have addressed questions pertinent to conceptualizing "women's health." However, this is not meant to imply that women comprise a homogeneous group. Indeed, many researchers have pointed out the likelihood that within-group differences among women are greater in many domains than are average differences between women and men (e.g., Hyde, 1994; Worell and Etaugh, 1994). Thus, when one asks how best to conceptualize women's health, perhaps the question "Which women with which characteristics in what contexts?" would provide a useful frame. To date, much of the documented psychology of women's health in the United States must be classified as the study of White, relatively affluent women. Inclusion in conceptual models of sociodemographic and lifestyle characteristics, such as age, ethnicity, socioeconomic status, sexual orientation, and family structure, may serve as a starting point for capturing women's heterogeneity. However, like gender, these characteristics may act only as proxy variables for a host of other psychological and social mechanisms, and fine-grained analyses of these mechanisms are necessary.

Summary

In advocating a biopsychosocial model, we are not recommending that discrete disease-focused research be stopped. Indeed, we believe that ample room exists for both keen empirical concentration on specific diseases or behaviors and integration across health and psychosocial domains. Our view is that the most useful conceptual models for women's health (and humans' health in general) will be those that (1) take into account potential interactions among biological, psychological, and social factors in determining women's health; (2) include multifaceted outcomes, including both pathological and optimal indicators of health in multiple realms (e.g., physical, psychological, social); and (3) are grounded in carefully developed theories that account for the diverse contexts of women's lives. Of course, we do not expect that one comprehensive biopsychosocial theory will capture adequately the domain of women's health (see also Chesney and Ozer, 1995). Rather, we hope that researchers will meet the challenge of developing and testing conceptual frameworks in their specific areas of interest, as well as those that cut across health behaviors or outcomes, with the goal of adequately characterizing and promoting health for all women across the life span.

METHODOLOGICAL CONSIDERATIONS IN WOMEN'S HEALTH RESEARCH

What considerations merit attention in designing research to examine women's health issues? Of course, a first step is to devise questions that carry the potential to advance our understanding and promotion of women's health. In doing so, researchers must examine their assumptions regarding women and the topic of interest and ask what conceptual frameworks will be most useful, as discussed previously. Meyerowitz and Hart (1995) argued, with regard to psychosocial research on women and cancer, that gender-biased assumptions may have influenced the nature of the questions and hypotheses advanced. In addition to questioning our own assumptions, involving our colleagues and our potential research participants in the initial stage of research conceptualization may prove beneficial. Several other sources also provide suggestions for examining these assumptions and decreasing biases in conducting research, such as avoiding sexism (e.g., Denmark et al., 1988; McHugh et al., 1986), heterosexism (e.g., Herek et al., 1991), ageism (e.g., Schaie, 1993), and ethnocentricism (e.g., Betancourt and Lopez, 1993; Graham, 1992; Zuckerman, 1990).

Another crucial step in study conceptualization is selecting the unit of analysis. As previously noted, selection of the individual as the unit of analysis has been most typical in women's health research and in much psychological and biomedical research in general. For example, Felton and Shinn (1992; Shinn, 1989) have suggested that even in research on social support, the individual most often has been the focus of study.

Greater attention to the relational and larger environmental context is necessary. The relatively small bodies of work on couples coping with health threats (see Revenson, 1994, for a review) and women's daily transitions from paid employment to home contexts (e.g., Frankenhauser, 1991) provide examples of research that transcends the individual level of analysis or examines multiple contexts. Characteristics of the sociocultural, interpersonal, situational, and temporal contexts (Revenson, 1990) merit consideration as important influences on women's health. Even when the investigator studies individuals in a single setting, considering the larger contextual picture is important.

A number of different methodologies have been useful in advancing women's health research. Qualitative strategies such as intensive interviews and focus groups exploring women's experience regarding a particular issue may be especially helpful at the stage of hypothesis generation. Careful descriptive research is necessary in many areas, and longitudinal studies have the advantage of allowing researchers to gauge effects over time in natural settings and to assess the interplay of etiological factors as well as the long-term effects of interventions. Experimental investigations to explore causal relationships and to devise health-promoting interventions that subsequently can be tested in natural settings also are warranted. Feminist analyses have provided trenchant criticisms of the positivist, empirical tradition in science (e.g., Gergen, 1988; Harding, 1986; Keller, 1985; Riger, 1992), such as its assumption that science is value neutral and its emphasis on experimental control over external validity and the consequent tendency to decontextualize women's experience. We agree with Riger (1992) that no method is free of limitations, but given an awareness on the part of researchers of the value assumptions inherent in a research approach, a variety of methods can be of value in enhancing understanding and improvement of women's lives (see also Peplau and Conrad, 1989).

How should researchers in women's health construct their samples? Cogent arguments regarding the advantages and drawbacks of studying and reporting sex-related differences have been offered over the past several years (e.g., Baumeister, 1988; Eagly, 1990; Hare-Mustin and Marecek, 1990; McHugh et al., 1986). We suggest that the researcher's choice of study participants, whether females and males, females (or males) only, or a specific subgroup of females (e.g., reservation-dwelling Native American women), be guided by the questions and conceptual frameworks of interest. Certainly, study of underserved groups, such as poor women, older women, and women of color, is essential, as is inclusion of women participants in sufficient numbers for reliable analysis in research in which they have been underrepresented (e.g., psychosocial issues in cardiovascular disease). Of course, in research intended to reveal group differences, whether between women and men or African-American and White women, for example, we should not confuse description with explanation. That is, sex or other immutable group characteristics should not be viewed as explanatory variables, but rather the finding of a group difference should be further explored to illuminate the mechanisms for the difference. In addition, effect sizes should be included in reports of group differences to indicate their magnitude. Furthermore, the history of applying the results of studies on men to women illuminates the dangers of assumed generalization from any group to humans in general; careful description of our samples and specification of limitations on generalizability are critical.

Development of reliable and valid measures is crucial for women's health research. Consideration of the appropriateness of measures for women in particular contexts is essential. It is important to establish the validity of measures of such constructs as Type A behavior and quality of life (Shumaker and Smith, 1995), alcohol use (Wilsnack, 1995), exercise behaviors (Marcus et al., 1995) and pregnancy-related adjustment (Stanton and Danoff-Burg, 1995) in women. It is vital to ensure that researchers not overestimate pathology in women by including as indicators of maladjustment those items that characterize women's normative experiences (e.g., weight changes in pregnancy mistakenly counted as a symptom of depression). In addition, development of measures of positive health indicators is warranted, as is greater attention to measurement of dependent variables reflecting health outcomes more likely to affect women, such as specific morbidities and comorbidity (Gatz et al., 1995; Verbrugge and Jette, 1994). Researchers in women's health need to investigate links between psychosocial and physical health variables on the basis of careful conceptualization and measurement of several sorts of indicators. This will require the researcher to cultivate knowledge in a number of realms or to initiate involvement in interdisciplinary research teams possessing expertise in psychological, social, and biological health domains.

APPLICATIONS IN WOMEN'S HEALTH

How should research be translated into interventions that will promote optimal health for women? A first question regards the targets at which interventions should be directed. This question echoes themes of previous sections regarding appropriate units of analysis and consideration of context. Should interventions be designed to engender positive change in individual women, relationships, communities, or the larger sociopolitical context? Our answer is "yes" to all of these. Certainly, removing structural barriers to and expanding resources for women's optimal health are important goals. As suggested by Travis et al. (1995), greater access to such resources as adequate income and education, a safe physical environment, and effective health care is needed. Many psychologists have been involved in research translating health care policy into action, and lessons learned from effective community action groups (e.g., Boston Women's Health Collective, advocacy groups for women with breast cancer and people with AIDS) can be used to mobilize social change. In addition, it is essential to be cognizant of such structural impediments as lack of child care or transportation and to provide resources in order to promote women's participation in health-enhancing programs (e.g., Marcus et al., 1995; Morokoff et al., 1995; Wilsnack, 1995).

The stakes are high for women with regard to how American health care is delivered and financed, for the economic and social circumstances that determine access to health care are less stable for women than for men (UCLA Center for Health Policy Research, 1996; Wunsch, 1997). Women are more likely than men to utilize the health care system and to be responsible for coordinating the care of others. They also are more likely to live in poverty, head single-parent households, and work in uninsured occupations.

According to the UCLA Center for Health Policy Research (1996), 20% of the female population aged 18 to 64 in California (two million women) were uninsured in 1993, compared with the national rate for women of 16%. Seventy-five percent of these uninsured women were of reproductive age. The majority had family incomes below 200% of the poverty level, even though 80% were employed or in families with at least one employed adult. However, lack of health insurance coverage is not limited to poor women; 20% of these women had family incomes over 300% of the poverty level.

For those who do have health insurance, managed care plans, particularly health maintenance organizations (HMOs), are serving a growing number of Americans. At present, approximately 20% of Americans receive medical care through a managed care plan, and this figure is expected to increase (Group Health Association of America, 1995).

Among Californians, 75% of insured individuals are enrolled in managed care plans (Wunsch, 1997).

The majority of those enrolled in HMOs are female (Bernstein, 1996). Historically, HMOs have provided more generous coverage of women's health services (e.g., reproductive care) and preventive services (e.g., cancer screening) than have traditional insurance plans (Bernstein, 1996). However, women enrolled in HMOs report that they are less likely to receive needed medical services, less able to reach their physicians when needed, and less satisfied with their physicians than women with other types of insurance coverage; however, these experiences vary by type of plan and geographic location (Collins and Simon, 1996).

Although managed care plans have the potential to provide comprehensive health care for women, they also present many challenges. Such challenges include making a full range of reproductive health services available; providing screening and treatment for problems such as depression, domestic violence, and substance abuse; attending to issues of confidentiality (e.g., health care for sexually active adolescents); defining appropriate primary care for women; giving women adequate consultation time with health care providers; and identifying and addressing risks posed by incentives to underserve (e.g., "drive-by" deliveries and mastectomies) (Weisman, 1996; Wunsch, 1997).

Considerably more research directed toward improving treatment of women in the health care system is warranted. Shumaker and Smith (1995) cited research that suggested that health care providers manage heart disease in women less aggressively than in men, and women are less likely to attend rehabilitation programs after a cardiac event. Wilsnack (1995) indicated that physicians are less likely to identify problem drinking in women than men. Roter and Hall (1997) reviewed evidence suggesting that female physicians conduct medical appointments differently than males, in a manner more facilitative of a biopsychosocial approach. Determinants of differential treatment require study, and interventions are needed to enhance health care providers' provision of effective treatment to women. In addition, physician training in psychosocial and behavioral aspects of women's health is required to optimize their care of women.

Strategies designed to support change in health behaviors of individual women and men also are necessary, although they may not reach maximal success without attention to structural or relational barriers to change. Targeting men's behaviors, including drug use, smoking, condom use, and violence, will improve not only the health of men but also that of the women with whom they live. Programs to engender positive health behavior change in women, as well as their abilities to be informed and active consumers of health care, are necessary and require continued study. Rather than focusing solely on treatment of problematic behaviors or conditions after they have developed, proactive approaches are essential. Research designed to identify contextual and individual attributes that place girls and women at risk for unfavorable health outcomes and to specify effective methods for preventing those outcomes is merited (see e.g., Derby et al., 1997). In general, illness prevention and health promotion for women merit attention across the life span and at multiple levels of intervention.

In addition to considering appropriate targets for intervention, researchers must attend to the nature of the interventions. A primary challenge is to determine the varieties of content, format, and structure that will be most useful. One vital question regards the differential effectiveness of medical and psychosocial interventions for women and men. Although gender-related differences in treatment efficacy have not been tested in many realms, Butler and Wing (1995) demonstrated that women with diabetes may lose weight more successfully when treated with their partners and that men may be more successful when treated alone. Mermelstein and Borrelli (1995) found that women who smoke may prefer more formal smoking cessation programs and group treatment than do men. Identifying the mechanisms by which some interventions may be more effective for women than for men provides a fertile area for research. The question of what specific characteristics of health-promoting interventions render them most effective for which women (e.g., older women, women with young children) in which contexts is just beginning to be addressed. Again, meeting the diversity of women's health needs constitutes a central research challenge.

Researchers and practitioners also must be concerned with the consequences of interventions. We strongly advocate the inclusion of measurable outcomes so that the efficacy of interventions can be evaluated adequately. Both short- and long-range outcomes for individuals and larger social systems require scrutiny. Anticipating and attempting to minimize potential unintended, negative consequences of experimental interventions are critical to the research enterprise. For example, does instructing women in assertiveness with the aim of promoting condom use inadvertently misplace responsibility on women? Does encouraging the use of advanced reproductive technologies contribute to delayed resolution or option seeking in women with fertility problems?

The current impetus toward initiatives designed to promote women's health is exciting; it is important that this momentum not outstrip empirical support for the approaches being advocated. Careful evaluation of intervention outcomes is essential.

Increasingly, those implementing interventions will be called on to demonstrate their cost-effectiveness. Butler and Wing (1995) cited evidence that preconception health care for diabetic women is cost-effective, and Sobel (1994) provided evidence that an array of psychosocial and educational interventions can lower health care costs. Such documentation will provide strong argument for changes in health care policy and practice to promote women's health. Finally, dissemination of interventions that are shown to be effective is an important goal. Use of the media and other sources to communicate information regarding research and application in women's health to women themselves, as well as to the community of researchers and practitioners, is a responsibility of those working in this area.

CONCLUSIONS

Considerable progress has been made toward building a solid knowledge base in psychosocial aspects of women's health. Several issues require attention if that progress is to continue. No single encompassing biopsychosocial paradigm emerges to characterize women's health; rather, the challenge is to scrutinize and build on existing theories where possible and to revise and reframe the body of knowledge, research methods, and application where needed to reflect more fully women's experience of health and well-being.

It is clear that health is not a univariate phenomenon; rather, it is a function of the complex interplay of economic, sociopolitical, environmental, psychological, and biological determinants, the formula for which varies over the life course and across diverse groups of women. This complexity underscores the need for multivariate models and methods as well as broadened interdisciplinary collaboration in research and application. It also highlights the need for continued intensive study of women's diversity and their commonalities with regard to health. While recognizing that a range of important issues remain to be addressed, there is cause for optimism about the pace at which our understanding is increasing. We are confident that current lines of investigation will inspire a future generation of researchers and practitioners and will pave the way for achievement of optimal health in women's lives.

NOTE

This chapter was adapted and expanded from A. L. Stanton, Psychology of women's health: Barriers and pathways to knowledge (pp. 3–21), and A. L. Stanton and S. J. Gallant, Psychology of women's health: Challenges for the future (pp. 567–582), in A. L. Stanton and S. J. Gallant eds., *The psychology of women's health: Progress and challenges in research and application* (Washington, D.C.: American Psychological Association, 1995).

REFERENCES

Adler, N. E., Boyce, T., Chesney, M. A., et al. (1994). Socioeconomic status and health: The challenge of the gradient. *American Psychologist, 49,* 15–24.

Angell, M. (1993). Caring for women's health—What is the problem? *Journal of the American Medical Association, 329,* 271–272.

Baker, L. J., Dearborn, M., Hastings, J. E., and Hamberger, K. (1984). Type A behavior in women: A review. *Health Psychology, 3,* 477–498.

Barrett-Connor, E. (1994). Heart disease in women. *Fertility and Sterility,* 62(Suppl. 2), 127S–132S.

Baumeister, R. F. (1988). Should we stop studying sex differences altogether? *American Psychologist, 43,* 1092–1095.

Bennett, J. C., for the Board on Health Sciences Policy of the Institute of Medicine. (1993). Inclusion of women in clinical trials—Policies for population subgroups. *New England Journal of Medicine, 329,* 288–292.

Bernstein, A. B. (1996). Women's health in HMOs: What we know and what we need to find out. *Women's Health Issues, 6,* 51–59.

Betancourt, H., and Lopez, S. R. (1993). The study of culture, ethnicity, and race in American psychology. *American Psychologist, 48,* 629–637.

Blechman, E. A., and Brownell, K. D., eds. (1998). *Behavioral medicine and women: A comprehensive handbook.* New York: Guilford.

Blumenthal, S. J., and Wood, S. F. (1997). Women's health care: Federal initiatives, policies, and directions. In S. J. Gallant, G. P. Keita, and R. Royak-Schaler, eds., *Health care for women: Psychological, social, and behavioral influences.* Pp. 3–10. Washington, D.C.: American Psychological Association.

Bohan, J. S. (1993). Regarding gender: Essentialism, constructionism, and feminist psychology. *Psychology of Women Quarterly, 17,* 5–22.

Butler, B. A., and Wing, R. R. (1995). Women with diabetes: A lifestyle perspective focusing on eating disorders, pregnancy, and weight control. In A. L. Stanton and S. J. Gallant, eds., *The psychology of women's health: Progress and challenges in research and application.* Pp. 85–116. Washington, D.C.: American Psychological Association.

Chesney, M. A., and Ozer, E. M. (1995). Women and health: In search of a paradigm. *Women's Health: Research on Gender, Behavior, and Policy, 1*, 3–26.

Collins, K. S., and Simon, L. J. (1996). Women's health and managed care: Promises and challenges. *Women's Health Issues, 6*, 39–44.

Corea, G. (1985). *The hidden malpractice: How American medicine mistreats women.* New York: Harper Colophon Books.

Council on Ethical and Judicial Affairs, American Medical Association. (1991). Gender disparities in clinical decision making. *Journal of the American Medical Association, 266*, 559–562.

Denmark, F., Russo, N. F., Frieze, I. H., and Sechzer, J. A. (1988). Guidelines for avoiding sexism in psychological research: A report of the Ad Hoc Committee on Nonsexist Research. *American Psychologist, 43*, 582–585.

Derby, C. A., Winkleby, M. A., Lapane, K. L., and Stone, E. A. (1997). Community-based prevention studies: Intervention lessons for women. In S. J. Gallant, G. P. Keita, and R. Royak-Schaler, eds., *Health care for women: Psychological, social, and behavioral influences.* Pp. 405–424. Washington, D.C.: American Psychological Association.

Eagly, A. H. (1990). On the advantages of reporting sex comparisons. *American Psychologist, 45*, 560–562.

Ehrenreich, B., and English, D. (1978). *For her own good: 150 years of the experts' advice to women.* Garden City, N.Y.: Anchor Press/Doubleday.

Engel, G. L. (1977). The need for a new medical model: A challenge for biomedicine. *Science, 196*, 129–136.

———. (1980). The clinical application of the biopsychosocial model. *American Journal of Psychiatry, 137*, 535–544.

Fausto-Sterling, A. (1985). *Myths of gender: Biological theories about women and men.* New York: Basic Books.

Felton, B. J., and Shinn, M. (1992). Social integration and social support: Moving "social support" beyond the individual level. *Journal of Community Psychology, 20*, 103–115.

Frankenhaeuser, M. (1991). The psychophysiology of sex differences as related to occupational status. In M. Frankenhaeuser, U. Lundberg, and M. Chesney, eds., *Women, work, and health: Stress and opportunities.* Pp. 39–61. New York: Plenum.

Gallant, S. J., Keita, G. P., and Royak-Schaler, R., eds. (1997). *Health care for women: Psychological, social, and behavioral influences.* Washington, D.C.: American Psychological Association.

Gatz, M., Harris, J. R., and Turk-Charles, S. (1995). The meaning of health for older women. In A. L. Stanton and S. J. Gallant, eds., *The psychology of women's health: Progress and challenges in research and application.* Pp. 491–529. Washington, D.C.: American Psychological Association.

Gergen, M. M. (1988). Building a feminist methodology. *Contemporary Social Psychology, 13*, 47–53.

Graham, S. (1992). "Most of the subjects were white and middle class": Trends in published research on African Americans in selected APA journals, 1970–1989. *American Psychologist, 47*, 629–639.

Grobbee, D. E., Rimm, E. B., Giovannucci, E., et al. (1990). Coffee, caffeine, and cardiovascular disease in men. *New England Journal of Medicine, 323,* 1026–1032.

Group Health Association of America. (1995). *Patterns in HMO enrollment.* Washington, D.C.: Author.

Hamilton, J. A. (1993). Feminist theory and health psychology: Tools for an egalitarian, woman-centered approach to women's health. *Journal of Women's Health, 2,* 49–54.

Harding, S. (1986). *The science question in feminism.* Ithaca, N.Y.: Cornell University Press.

Hare-Mustin, R. T., and Marecek, J., eds. (1990). *Making a difference: Psychology and the construction of gender.* New Haven, Conn.: Yale University Press.

Harrison, M. (1992). Women's health as a specialty: A deceptive solution. *Journal of Women's Health, 1,* 101–106.

Hazzard, W. R. (1990). A central role of sex hormones in the sex differential in lipoprotein metabolism, atherosclerosis, and longevity. In M. G. Ory and H. R. Warner, eds., *Gender, health, and longevity: Multidisciplinary perspectives.* Pp. 87–108. New York: Springer.

Herek, G. M., Kimmel, D. C., Amaro, H., and Melton, G. B. (1991). Avoiding heterosexist bias in psychological research. *American Psychologist, 46,* 957–963.

Hulka, B. S. (1994). Links between hormone replacement therapy and neoplasia. *Fertility and Sterility, 62*(Suppl. 2), 168S–175S.

Hyde, J. S. (1994). Can meta-analysis make feminist transformations in psychology? *Psychology of Women Quarterly, 18,* 451–462.

Johnson, K. (1992). Women's health: Developing a new interdisciplinary specialty. *Journal of Women's Health, 1,* 95–99.

Kahn, A. S., and Yoder, J. D. (1989). The psychology of women and conservatism: Rediscovering social change. *Psychology of Women Quarterly, 13,* 417–432.

Keller, E. F. (1985). *Reflections on gender and science.* New Haven, Conn.: Yale University Press.

Koss, M. P., Woodruff, W. J., and Koss, P. G. (1990). Relation of criminal victimization to health perceptions among women medical patients. *Journal of Consulting and Clinical Psychology, 58,* 147–152.

LaCroix, A. Z., and Haynes, S. G. (1987). Gender differences in the health effects of the workplace. In R. C. Barnett, L. Biener, and G. K. Baruch, eds., *Gender and stress.* Pp. 96–121. New York: The Free Press.

Lawrence, S. C., and Bendixen, K. (1992). His and hers: Male and female anatomy in anatomy texts for U.S. medical students, 1890–1989. *Social Science and Medicine, 35,* 925–934.

Lobo, R. A., and Speroff, L. (1994). International consensus conference on postmenopausal hormone therapy and the cardiovascular system. *Fertility and Sterility, 62*(Suppl. 2), 176S–179S.

Lurie, N., Slater, J., McGovern, P., et al. (1993). Preventive care for women: Does the sex of the physician matter? *New England Journal of Medicine, 329,* 478–482.

Marcus, B. H., Dubbert, P. M., King, A. C., and Pinto, B. M. (1995). Physical activity in women: Current status and future directions. In A. L. Stanton and S. J. Gallant, eds., *The psychology of women's health: Progress and challenges in research and application*. Pp. 349–379. Washington, D.C.: American Psychological Association.

Matthews, K. A. (1989). Interactive effects of behavior and reproductive hormones on sex differences in risk for coronary heart disease. *Health Psychology, 8*, 373–387.

McHugh, M. C., Koeske, R. D., and Frieze, I. H. (1986). Issues to consider in conducting nonsexist psychological research: A guide for researchers. *American Psychologist, 41*, 879–890.

Mednick, M. T. (1989). On the politics of psychological constructs: Stop the bandwagon, I want to get off. *American Psychologist, 44*, 1118–1123.

Merkatz, R. B., Temple, R., Sobel, S., Feiden, K., Kessler, P. A., and the Working Group on Women in Clinical Trials. (1993). Women in clinical trials of new drugs: A change in Food and Drug Administration policy. *New England Journal of Medicine, 329*, 292–296.

Mermelstein, R. J., and Borrelli, B. (1995). Women and smoking. In A. L. Stanton and S. J. Gallant, eds., *The psychology of women's health: Progress and challenges in research and application*. Pp. 309–348. Washington, D.C.: American Psychological Association.

Meyerowitz, B. E., and Hart, S. (1995). Women and cancer: Have assumptions about women limited our research agenda? In A. L. Stanton and S. J. Gallant, eds., *The psychology of women's health: Progress and challenges in research and application*. Pp. 51–84. Washington, D.C.: American Psychological Association.

Moinpour, C. M., Feigl, P. Metch, B., et al. (1989). Quality of life end points in cancer clinical trials: Review and recommendations. *Journal of the National Cancer Institute, 81*, 485–492.

Morokoff, P. J., Harlow, L. L., and Quina, K. (1995). Women and AIDS. In A. L. Stanton and S. J. Gallant, eds., *The psychology of women's health: Progress and challenges in research and application*. Pp. 117–169. Washington, D.C.: American Psychological Association.

Nathanson, C. A. (1990). The gender-mortality differential in developed countries: Demographic and sociocultural dimensions. In M. G. Ory and H. R. Warner, eds., *Gender, health, and longevity: Multidisciplinary perspectives*. Pp. 3–23. New York: Springer.

National Institutes of Health. (1994). NIH guidelines on the inclusion of women and minorities as subjects in clinical research. *NIH Guide for Grants and Contracts, 23*(11), 2–10.

Ockene, J. K., Kuller, L. H., Svendsen, K. H., and Meilahn, E. (1990). The relationship of smoking cessation to coronary heart disease and lung cancer in the Multiple Risk Factor Intervention Trial (MRFIT). *American Journal of Public Health, 80*, 954–958.

O'Leary, V. E., and Ickovics, J. R. (1995). Resilience and thriving in response to challenge: An opportunity for a paradigm shift in women's health. *Women's Health: Research on Gender, Behavior, and Policy, 1*, 121–142.

Ory, M. G., and Warner, H. R., eds. (1990). *Gender, health, and longevity: Multidisciplinary perspectives.* New York: Springer.

Peplau, L. A., and Conrad, E. (1989). Beyond nonsexist research: The perils of feminist methods in psychology. *Psychology of Women Quarterly, 13,* 379–400.

Plichta, S. (1992). The effects of woman abuse on health care utilization and health status: A literature review. *Women's Health Issues, 2,* 154–163.

Polefrone, J. M., and Manuck, S. B. (1987). Gender differences in cardiovascular and neuroendocrine response to stressors. In R. C. Barnett, L. Biener, and G. K. Baruch, eds., *Gender and stress.* Pp. 13–38. New York: The Free Press.

Prilleltensky, I. (1989). Psychology and the status quo. *American Psychologist, 44,* 795–802.

Reid, P. T. (1993). Poor women in psychological research: Shut up and shut out. *Psychology of Women Quarterly, 17,* 133–150.

Repetti, R. L., Matthews, K. A., and Waldron, I. (1989). Employment and women's health: Effects of paid employment on women's mental and physical health. *American Psychologist, 44,* 1394–1401.

Revenson, T. A. (1990). All other things are not equal: An ecological approach to personality and disease. In H. S. Friedman, ed., *Personality and disease.* Pp. 65–94. New York: Wiley.

———. (1994). Social support and marital coping with chronic illness. *Annals of Behavioral Medicine, 16,* 122–130.

Riger, S. (1992). Epistemological debates, feminist voices: Science, social values, and the study of women. *American Psychologist, 47,* 730–740.

Riley, M. R. (1990). Foreword: The gender paradox. In M. G. Ory and H. R. Warner, eds., *Gender, health, and longevity: Multidisciplinary perspectives.* Pp. vii–xiii. New York: Springer.

Rodin, J., and Ickovics, J. R. (1990). Women's health: Review and research agenda as we approach the 21st century. *American Psychologist, 45,* 1018–1034.

Rosser, S. V. (1993). A model for a specialty in women's health. *Journal of Women's Health, 2,* 99–104.

Roter, D. L., and Hall, J. A. (1997). Gender differences in patient-physician communication. In S. J. Gallant, G. P. Keita, and R. Royak-Schaler, eds., *Health care for women: Psychological, social, and behavioral influences.* Pp. 57–71. Washington, D.C.: American Psychological Association.

Schaie, K. W. (1993). Ageist language in psychological research. *American Psychologist, 48,* 49–51.

Scheier, M. F., and Carver, C. S. (1992). Effects of optimism on psychological and physical well-being: Theoretical overview and empirical update. *Cognitive Therapy and Research, 16,* 201–228.

Schwartz, G. E. (1982). Testing the biopsychosocial model: The ultimate challenge facing behavioral medicine? *Journal of Consulting and Clinical Psychology, 50,* 1040–1053.

Shinn, M. (1989). Crossing substantive domains. *American Journal of Community Psychology, 17,* 565–570.

Shumaker, S. A., and Smith, T. R. (1995). Women and coronary heart disease:

A psychological perspective. In A. L. Stanton and S. J. Gallant, eds., *The psychology of women's health: Progress and challenges in research and application.* Pp. 25–49. Washington, D.C.: American Psychological Association.

Smith, D. W. E., and Warner, H. R. (1990). Overview of biomedical perspectives: Possible relationships between genes on the sex chromosomes and longevity. In M. G. Ory and H. R. Warner, eds., *Gender, health, and longevity: Multidisciplinary perspectives.* Pp. 41–55. New York: Springer.

Snyder, C. R., Harris, C., Anderson, J. R., et al. (1991). The will and the ways: Development and validation of an individuals-differences measure of hope. *Journal of Personality and Social Psychology, 60,* 570–585.

Sobel, D. S. (1994). Mind matters, money matters: The cost-effectiveness of clinical behavioral medicine. In S. J. Blumenthal, K. Matthews, and S. M. Weiss, eds., *New frontiers in behavioral medicine: Proceedings of the national conference.* Pp. 25–36. NIH Publication 94-3772. Washington, D.C.: U.S. Government Printing Office.

Stanton, A. L., and Danoff-Burg, S. (1995). Selected issues in women's reproductive health: Psychological perspectives. In A. L. Stanton and S. J. Gallant, eds., *The psychology of women's health: Progress and challenges in research and application.* Pp. 261–305. Washington, D.C.: American Psychological Association.

Stanton, A. L., and Gallant, S. J., eds. (1995). *The psychology of women's health: Progress and challenges in research and application.* Washington, D.C.: American Psychological Association.

Steering Committee of the Physicians' Health Study Research Group. (1988). Preliminary report: Findings from the aspirin component of the ongoing Physicians' Health Study. *New England Journal of Medicine, 318,* 262–264.

Strickland, B. R. (1988). Sex-related differences in health and illness. *Psychology of Women Quarterly, 12,* 381–399.

Taylor, S. E., and Aspinwall, L. G. (1990). Psychological aspects of chronic illness. In G. R. VandenBos and P. T. Costa, Jr., eds., *Psychological aspects of serious illness.* Washington, D.C.: American Psychological Association.

Travis, C. B. (1988). *Women and health psychology: Biomedical issues.* Hillsdale, N.J.: Lawrence Erlbaum Associates.

Travis, C. B., Gressley, D. L., and Adams, P. L. (1995). Health care policy and practice for women's health. In A. L. Stanton and S. J. Gallant, eds., *The psychology of women's health: Progress and challenges in research and application.* Pp. 531–565. Washington, D.C.: American Psychological Association.

UCLA Center for Health Policy Research. (1996). *Health insurance coverage of women in California.* PB 96-1. Los Angeles: Regents of the University of California.

U.S. General Accounting Office, Statement of Mark Nadel. (1990, June). *NIH: Problems in implementing policy on women in study populations.* Bethesda, Md.: National Institutes of Health.

U.S. Public Health Service, Task Force on Women's Health Issues. (1985). *Women's health: Report of the Public Health Service Task Force on Women's Health Issues.* Washington, D.C.: U.S. Government Printing Office.

Verbrugge, L. M. (1990). The twain meet: Empirical explanations of sex differences in health and mortality. In M. G. Ory and H. R. Warner, eds., *Gender, health, and longevity: Multidisciplinary perspectives.* Pp. 137–156. New York: Springer.

Verbrugge, L. M., and Jette, A. M. (1994). The disablement process. *Social Science and Medicine, 38,* 1–14.

Verbrugge, L. M., and Wingard, D. L. (1987). Sex differentials in health and mortality. *Women and Health, 12*(2), 103–145.

Waldron, I. (1993). Recent trends in sex mortality ratios for adults in developed countries. *Social Science and Medicine, 36,* 451–462.

Waldron, I., and Jacobs, J. A. (1989). Effects of multiple roles on women's health: Evidence from a national longitudinal study. *Women and Health, 15*(1), 3–20.

Wallis, L. A. (1993). Why a curriculum in women's health? *Journal of Women's Health, 2,* 55–60.

Weisman, C. S. (1996). Conference proceedings of Women's health and managed care: Balancing cost, access, and quality: Introduction to the proceedings. *Women's Health Issues, 6,* 1–4.

Wenger, N. K., Speroff, L., and Packard, B. (1993). Cardiovascular health and disease in women. *New England Journal of Medicine, 329,* 247–256.

Wilsnack, S. C. (1995). Alcohol use and alcohol problems in women. In A. L. Stanton and S. J. Gallant, eds., *The psychology of women's health: Progress and challenges in research and application.* Pp. 381–443. Washington, D.C.: American Psychological Association.

Worell, J., and Etaugh, C. (1994). Transforming theory and research with women: Themes and variations. *Psychology of Women Quarterly, 18,* 443–450.

Wunsch, B. (1997). Women's health and managed care. Paper presented at the Los Angeles County Women's Health Policy Summit, Los Angeles, April.

Yoder, J. D., and Kahn, A. S. (1993). Working toward an inclusive psychology of women. *American Psychologist, 48,* 846–850.

Zuckerman, M. (1990). Some dubious premises in research and theory on racial differences: Scientific, social, and ethical issues. *American Psychologist, 45,* 1297–1303.

23

Amparo C. Villablanca

CARDIOVASCULAR DISEASE IN WOMEN

Exploring Myths and Controversies

INTRODUCTION

Heart disease, a largely preventable disease, is the leading cause of death for women. Nonetheless, awareness of this epidemic by health professionals and the public is lagging. Total mortality from cardiovascular disease in women nearly equals that in men (approximately 500,000 deaths annually) and is nearly double the female mortality from breast, lung, uterine, cervical, and ovarian cancers combined. Yet women overwhelmingly perceive cancer, particularly breast cancer, and stress-related conditions as their two major health threats. The myth that coronary heart disease (CHD) is not a health threat for women continues despite more than 15 years of epidemiologic data to the contrary.

Recent interest in women who are at risk or have established heart disease has been accentuated by recognition of existing gaps in our knowledge of the impact of gender on a variety of variables, including the pathophysiology of atherosclerosis, its clinical manifestations, CHD risk factors, efficacy of conventional treatments and interventions, and the role of hormonal replacement therapy on risk factor modification. Currently available data point to several important gender differences in heart disease. A great deal of additional scientific study is needed to elucidate the optimal treatment and prevention of CHD in women. Similarly, equally concerted educational efforts for patients and health care providers will be needed to permit successful risk factor intervention and treatment implementation.

A variety of controversies exist. Is there gender bias in the current approach of the health care community toward the evaluation and management of heart disease in women? Should efforts be increased to augment use of hormone replacement therapy for cardiovascular risk reduction? Should scarce research funds be expended to study heart disease in women, or are male models of disease adequate? It is suggested that changes need to occur in our approach to the prevention and management of women with heart disease. Continuing along current trends may significantly and adversely impact present and future health care costs and delivery for men and women with cardiovascular disease.

BACKGROUND

In 1987 and 1992, the National Heart, Lung, and Blood Institute of the National Institutes of Health (NIH) convened task force conferences on cardiovascular health and disease in women. More recently, while under the directorship of Bernadine Healy, the NIH established a national Office of Research on Women's Health. These events have focused the national spotlight onto women's health issues. The task the nation has been charged with on the recommendation of the proceedings[1] from these national agencies is ambitious indeed: to direct health care resources toward improving all aspects of women's health and cardiovascular health to include clinical services, education, and research. This mandate will do much to help dispel the myths and address the controversies that have surrounded women's health issues and contributed to relative past inaction.

Although a number of health problems are unique to women or affect them disproportionately (e.g., pregnancy, breast and uterine cancer, and osteoporosis) this chapter focuses on cardiovascular disease in women and, in particular, CHD because of its overwhelming, though underrecognized, importance to the health of American women. Within this context, a number of significant myths and controversies have been identified and are highlighted here.

Myths surrounding the available medical and epidemiologic knowledge and its application are as follows:

• Coronary heart disease is a disease that affects primarily men, whereas breast cancer is the major health threat for women.
• Women appear to be at less risk for CHD than their male counterparts.

• Changing hormonal status and menopause confound our understanding of the impact of heart disease in women.
• No gender differences exist in therapeutic treatment approaches and applications for men and women with CHD.

Controversies in heart disease in women relate to the following:

• Perceptions of heart disease risk and cardiovascular disease outcomes by both patients and health care providers
• Differences in, and the role of, psychosocial perspectives and attitudes in clinical decision making
• Controversies in management decisions and treatment applications amid a gender gap in medical research

By understanding which factors are critical in the epidemiology, pathogenesis, treatment, and outcome for women with CHD, health care consumers, providers, educators, and policy makers can collectively become more informed partners and make a significant impact in a disease process that still remains largely undertreated and underdiagnosed in women.

MYTHS

Myth #1: Coronary Heart Disease Is a Disease That Affects Primarily Men

Coronary Heart Disease Coronary heart disease constitutes a major public health concern and has a substantial impact on utilization of U.S. health care resources (see Table 23.1). Coronary heart disease continues to be the leading cause of death for men and women in the United States. Age-adjusted death rates in the United States for men and women with cardiovascular disease (i.e., CHD and stroke) are similar and far outnumber deaths from all the other major causes (see Figure 23.1). In addition, cardiovascular disease deaths are more than double the combined total number of deaths from other major causes of mortality in women (including maternal mortality and uterine, ovarian, cervical, breast, and lung cancers). As demonstrated in Table 23.2, CHD is the leading cause of death for women over the age of 65 and the second-leading cause of death for perimenopausal women. This is in contradistinction to the pattern seen for men, where heart disease is the leading cause of death from middle age on. Therefore, CHD is significantly more age dependent in

TABLE 23.1   CORONARY HEART DISEASE:
MORBIDITY AND MORTALITY—
UNITED STATES, 1987

	Women	Men
Population	125 million	118 million
Deaths	244,000	268,000
Hospitalizations	0.9 million	1.3 million
Physician office visits	4.4 million	5.8 million
Prevalence	3.0 million	4.2 million
Health expenditures	$6 billion	$9 billion

SOURCE: Wenger et al., eds., *Cardiovascular Health and Disease in Women*. Greenwich, Conn: LeJacq Communications, 1987.

TABLE 23.2   LEADING CAUSES OF DEATH
BY AGE AND GENDER, 1989

	Age		
	25–44	*45–64*	*65+*
Women			
1	Cancer	Cancer	Heart disease
2	Accidents	Heart disease	Cancer
3	Heart disease	Stroke	Stroke
Men			
1	Accidents	Heart disease	Heart disease
2	HIV infection	Cancer	Cancer
3	Heart disease	Accidents	Stroke

SOURCE: National Center for Health Statistics.

women, with a 10-year lag seen in the age at which CHD becomes the leading cause of death in women compared to male counterparts. Although death rates for CHD have been declining nationally for the past 40 years, because of a combination of advances in medical and surgical treatments as well as an increased emphasis in prevention, the declines have not been at as rapid a rate for women as for men.

Myocardial Infarction Epidemiologic data for myocardial infarction (MI) show striking gender-related differences. Perhaps the most extensive data available come from 26 years of observation in the Framingham Heart Study.[2] For example, the mean age at presentation of MI was greater for women than for men (see Figure 23.2). Interestingly, of the three major presentations of CHD (sudden death, MI, and angina), the first two are significantly more common in men, whereas angina was

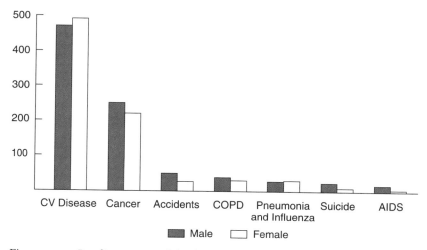

Figure 23.1. Leading causes of death in men and women in the United States (in thousands), 1987. Abbreviations: CV, cardiovascular; COPD, chronic obstructive pulmonary disease; AIDS, acquired immune deficiency syndrome.

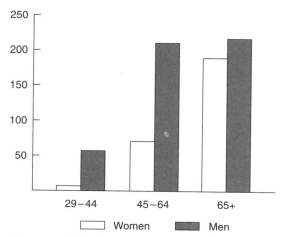

Figure 23.2. Heart attacks in the United States (in thousands). Adapted from American Heart Association, based on the Framingham Heart Study.

found to be the initial presentation for CHD in 50% to 60% of women. However, MI is the leading killer for women with cardiovascular disease (see Figure 23.3). In addition, MI in women was associated with higher case fatality rates (39% in women vs. 31% in men), and a higher percentage of all coronary deaths in women occurred as the initial manifestation of MI (68% in women vs. 49% in men). Therefore, in women MI

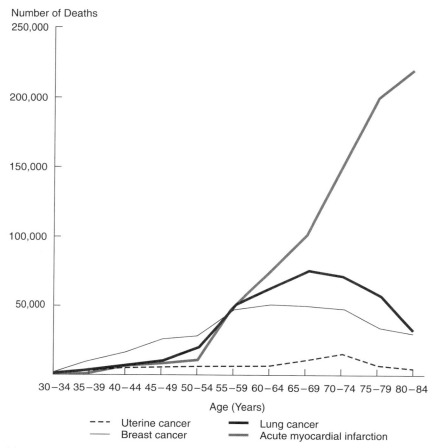

Figure 23.3. Number of deaths by cause and age in U.S. women (all races), 1988. Source: National Center for Health Statistics, *Vital Statistics of the United States, Vol. II, Mortality, Part A* (Washington, D.C.: U.S. Public Health Service, 1991).

was associated with greater morbidity and mortality than in men. Factors contributing to these differences in MI outcome may include women's older age at presentation, more advanced disease state, and greater likelihood of comorbid conditions. As a consequence of the progressive aging of the U.S. population and the predominance of women among the elderly, the number of women with CHD and MIs can be expected to continue to increase. Women in the Framingham Study were also more likely to have unrecognized silent MIs (35% in women vs. 27% in men). These infarcts were associated with an increased likelihood of subsequent stroke, heart failure, or death.

Postinfarction outcomes have been investigated by a number of studies[3-5] and demonstrate higher initial and long-term mortality for women as opposed to men, higher complication rates, and higher re-infarction rates. The role of ethnicity in mortality outcome from MI was highlighted by data from the Multicentre International Survival and Limitation of Infarct Size (MILIS) Trial,[6] which demonstrated that whereas combined mortality 48 months postinfarction was higher for women than for men (36% vs. 21%), African-American women had the highest postinfarction mortality, 48%. The reasons for the differences observed in the MILIS trial are incompletely understood but may relate to ethnic differences associated with cardiac risk factor prevalence, socioeconomic factors, and genetic predisposition.

Stroke In part because of the rapid decline in stroke rates in the United States in the last 40 years,[7-9] cerebrovascular accident (CVA) in women has received less attention than CHD. Yet CVA is an important entity in cardiovascular disease in women and, like MI, demonstrates significant gender and ethnic differences.[10] In general, stroke rates are uniformly higher among African-American men and women than they are for Caucasian men and women. Although deaths from CVA in men outnumber those for women by 30%,[9] women are more likely to have fatal strokes than men.[7,10] Furthermore, stroke mortality among African-American women is nearly two times that of Caucasian women until age 85, at which point the ethnic and gender trends for stroke are reversed, with Caucasian women having the highest mortality.[11] Gender differences in the association between stroke and blood pressure, the strongest and most consistent risk factor for CVA, have not been reported. Like for CHD, the economic and social impact of CVA is immense. The highest percentage of nursing home admissions in the elderly (age > 65) are due to disability from stroke; women comprise 76% of this group.[12] In addition, current epidemiologic studies appear to indicate a trend toward reversal of the decline in CVA morbidity and mortality observed in prior years, with stroke incidence rates rising in the past 10 to 15 years, particularly in older women.[13]

Myth #2: Women Appear to Be at Less Risk for CHD Than Their Male Counterparts

In order to gain a better understanding of the factors responsible for gender differences in cardiovascular disease as discussed previously, gen-

TABLE 23.3   MAJOR RISK FACTORS
FOR CORONARY HEART DISEASE

Positive risk factors for CHD other than LDL cholesterol
Age: males ≥45 years, females ≥55 years or premature menopause without
    estrogen therapy
Family history of premature CHD (≤55 years in male parent or sibling or
    ≤65 years in female parent or sibling)
Current cigarette smoking
Hypertension
Low HDL cholesterol (≤35 mg/dl)
Diabetes mellitus

Negative risk factor for CHD
High HDL cholesterol (≥60 mg/dl)

NOTE: LDL, low-density lipoprotein; HDL, high-density lipoprotein.
SOURCE: C. T. Sempos et al., Prevalence of high blood cholesterol among US adults: An update based on guidelines from the second report of the National Cholesterol Education Program Adult Treatment Panel, *Journal of the American Medical Association* 269, no. 23(1993), 3009–3014. Division of Health Examination Statistics, Centers for Disease Control and Prevention, Hyattsville, Maryland.

der differences in cardiovascular disease risk factors are outlined here. In addition to hyperlipidemia, the major well-established risk factors for CHD are listed in Table 23.3.[14] Although an exhaustive review of all major risk factors is not attempted here, the most significant risk factors for women[15] are highlighted, including age, diabetes mellitus, and hypertension.

Age   As the epidemiologic data on MI and CVA indicates, risk for cardiovascular disease in women is very importantly affected by aging. There is a 10-year lag between men and women in age as a risk factor for CHD (age > 45 for men, age > 55 for women) and in family history of premature CHD as a risk factor for CHD (male relative with CHD prior to age 55, female relative with CHD prior to age 65). The more advanced age of women at the time of CHD diagnosis coincides with a greater prevalence of other age-dependent risk factors, such as hypertension, diabetes, and hyperlipidemia. In addition, age contributes significantly to the higher complication rate, increased functional disability, and greater sense of social isolation that confronts women with CHD.[16] Social isolation (i.e., the absence of a spouse, significant other, or meaningful social contacts), an independent variable, has been identified to be the most important prognostic socioeconomic factor in patients with CHD.[17] The impact of social isolation becomes increasingly important in light of recognition that the average life span of U.S. women continues to exceed that of men, such that greater than 50% of women over the age of 65 are widowed.

Diabetes Mellitus A second important risk factor for CHD in women is diabetes mellitus (DM). Women with DM have a substantially higher relative risk of CHD and higher total CHD and congestive heart failure mortality as compared with diabetic men,[18,19] even after adjusting for other associated cardiovascular risk factors. The prevalence of DM is greater in African-American men and women than in Caucasian men and women. In women, the prevalence of DM is slightly lower than it is in men prior to age 65 but thereafter exceeds the prevalence in men.[20] The interrelationships between cardiovascular risk and DM are complex, such that the reasons for the increased risk conferred by DM in women are not entirely understood. Risk appears to be related to a variety of factors associated with DM, including obesity, hyperinsulinemia, and peripheral insulin resistance;[21] hyperestrogenemia;[22] and hyperlipidemia with resultant lipid profile abnormalities that are particularly unfavorable and atherogenic for women (i.e., small dense low-density lipoprotein [LDL], hypertriglyceridemia, and low levels of high-density lipoprotein [HDL] cholesterol).[23]

Hypertension Hypertension is an important risk factor for stroke and cardiovascular disease. Figure 23.4A and B demonstrates changes in mean systolic and diastolic blood pressures as a function of age in African-American and Caucasian men and women.[24] As can be observed from the figures, mean systolic blood pressure rises with age in African-American and Caucasian men and women. After age 54, mean systolic blood pressures are higher in women than in men.[25–28] In contrast, mean diastolic blood pressures also increase with age but decrease slightly at the older age-groups. At all ages, mean diastolic blood pressure levels are higher in men than in women. Although hypertension is a significant risk factor for excess mortality in both genders, hypertension appears to confer greater relative risk for women as compared to men. Specifically, systolic hypertension appears to be a more important predictor of mortality in both African-American and Caucasian women, whereas diastolic hypertension appears to have a much greater impact on mortality in African-American women.[29] Furthermore, hypertension has been demonstrated to be second only to age as the most important predictor of CHD in women.[15] As compared to endogenous hypertension, hypertension associated with oral contraceptive use, or with pregnancy, has not been demonstrated to be associated with an increased risk for CHD or an increased risk of developing hypertension later in life.

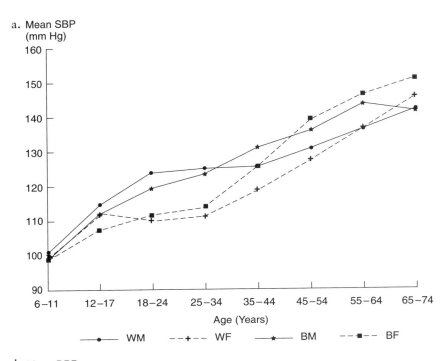

a. Mean SBP
(mm Hg)

Age (Years)

WM   ---+--- WF   —★— BM   --■-- BF

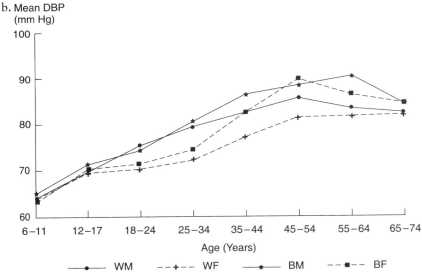

b. Mean DBP
(mm Hg)

Age (Years)

WM   ---+--- WF   —★— BM   --■-- BF

Figure 23.4 (A) Systolic blood pressure (SBP) by age, gender, and ethnicity. Adapted from Pyörälä et al. (1987 [23]). Abbreviations: WM, White male; WF, White female; BM, Black male; BF, Black female. (B) Diastolic blood pressure (DBP) by age, gender, and ethnicity. Adapted from Rowland and Roberts (1982 [24]). Abbreviations: WM, White male; WF, White female; BM, Black male; BF, Black female.

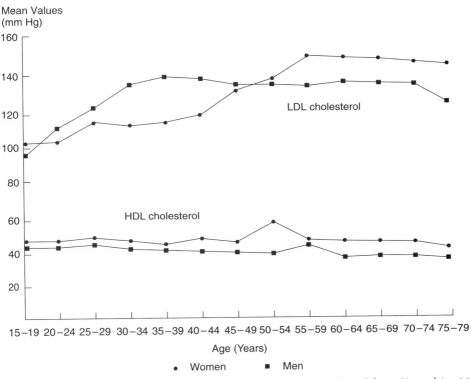

Figure 23.5. Age trends in lipoprotein-cholesterol fractions. Adapted from Kannel (1988 [33]). Abbreviations: LDL, low-density lipoprotein; HDL, high-density lipoprotein.

Hyperlipidemia Previous epidemiologic data have demonstrated a nonlinear relationship between serum cholesterol and cardiovascular risk: a 2% increase in cardiovascular risk for every 1% increase in serum total cholesterol above 200 mg/dl.[30] The components of total cholesterol are subfractionated on the basis of density ultracentrifugation and confer differing degrees of cardiovascular risk. In men and women, LDL is directly correlated with risk, whereas HDL inversely correlates with risk.[31,32] In addition, lipid levels change in men and women as a function of age. In premenopausal women, serum total and LDL cholesterol levels are generally lower than in men. Levels of HDL cholesterol are uniformly higher in women than in men at all ages. However, following menopause, and beginning in the premenopausal years, LDL cholesterol levels in women rise to higher levels than do men's (see Figure 23.5).[33] Levels of HDL in women fall slightly in postmenopause. Low HDL levels (<40–45 mg/dl) in women appear to confer greater increased risk than low HDL levels (<30–35 mg/dl) do for men,[32] underscoring the importance of low HDL cholesterol in cardiovascular risk in women. Levels of HDL cholesterol greater than 60 mg/dl are associated with significant cardioprotective effects and thereby constitute a negative cardiovascular risk factor. Elevations of HDL cholesterol of this magnitude are more commonly seen in women, particularly premenopausal women. Finally, elevations of lipoprotein(a) have been reported to be associated with increased cardiovascular risk in both men and women[34] and may be an additional factor associated with cardiovascular risk in women postmenopause, as lipoprotein(a) levels are higher in postmenopausal women than in premenopausal women.[34,35]

In general, hypertriglyceridemia and elevations in very low density lipoprotein (VLDL) cholesterol have not been clearly demonstrated to be associated with equivalent relative cardiovascular risk in men and women.[36-38] Elevations of VLDL triglycerides confer greater relative risk in women as compared to men.[39] The reasons for these differences are not presently clear but may in part relate to resultant interactions with other parameters associated with hypertriglyceridemia, including low HDL cholesterol, obesity, and low levels of exercise. In addition, hypertriglyceridemia in women may be less amenable to modification. For example, aerobic exercise training has been demonstrated to affect blood lipids differently and less favorably in women compared to men.[40]

Myth #3: Changing Hormonal Status and Menopause Confound Our Understanding of the Impact of Heart Disease in Women

Menopause An important physical and emotional transition in the lives of women is menopause, which is associated with a dramatic alteration in the vascular hormonal milieu, including a fall in estrogen levels. The sheer number of CHD risk parameters that are affected when a woman attains menopause, or age greater than 55 (the age by which most women are postmenopausal), strongly implies a role for menopause as an independent risk factor for CHD.[41] Menopause, whether natural or surgical, is associated with a two- to fourfold increase in CHD risk[41,42] (see Figure 23.6). A proportionately greater risk increase is seen the younger a woman is at the time of menopause.[43,44] As current life expectancy for women is greater than 80 years, many women will spend

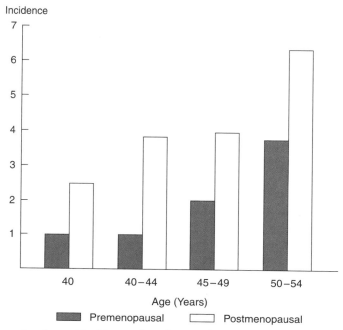

Figure 23.6. Annual incidence of cardiovascular disease per 1,000 women (by menopause status). Adapted from Department of Health, Education, and Welfare Publication 74, 1974, Framingham Study.

more than one-third of their lives in the postmenopausal state. Although aging is inextricably associated with menopause, it is a determinant of cardiovascular risk even in premenopausal women. Therefore, premenopausal women are relatively, but not absolutely, protected against CHD. Postmenopausal women have a greater risk of CHD than premenopausal women, even at comparable ages. Therefore, the interrelationship of menopausal state, age, and perhaps other cardiac risk factors are important determinants of the overall cardiovascular risk profile for women.

It is of interest that hysterectomy, perhaps the most frequently performed surgery on women, has also been postulated to be associated with an increase in CHD risk. The mechanism of risk enhancement may be associated with loss of uterine prostacyclin, a potent vascular vasodilator and inhibitor of platelet aggregation.[44] Keen interest also currently exists in evaluating the perimenopausal period, a period characterized by a changing hormonal status, as a time of accelerating CHD risk in women.

Myth #4: No Gender Differences Exist in Therapeutic Treatment Approaches and Their Applications for Men and Women with CHD

The health care costs associated with treatment for CHD are staggering[45] and highlight the need for judicious utilization of currently available management options. Yet there is little information regarding the benefits and efficacy of treatment and management options for women with CHD. The lack of information stems partly from past exclusion of women in clinical studies due to fear of pregnancy during an investigative trial and from concerns that fluctuations in hormone status in women would be a confounding variable in data interpretation. As a result, much of the available information on cardiovascular therapeutic interventions comes from studies done primarily in men. The relevance and appropriateness of applying the results of studies in men to women has been questioned. Currently, conventional medical and surgical treatment for women with CHD is not associated with similar benefits as for men. Women with CHD are underdiagnosed and undertreated when compared to male counterparts, resulting in delay in diagnosis and possible adverse outcomes. This section evaluates gender differences in the management of CHD.

Diagnostic Studies Chest pain, the most common presenting symptom of CHD in women, is often dismissed as a symptom of CHD. This stems in part from lack of physician awareness of women's risks for CHD, such as premenopausal women with a significant number of additional risk factors,[46,47] and discomfort with limitations of diagnostic modalities in women. Other factors contributing to the underdiagnosis of CHD in women include women's misperceptions of CHD as a health threat and the consequent dismissal, denial, or minimizing of symptoms; a higher frequency of noncardiac conditions associated with chest pain syndromes in women (e.g., mitral valve prolapse and anxiety disorders); a lower prevalence of CHD in women when compared to men of similar age; and exaggerated concerns of limitations of diagnostic testing in women. Although exercise treadmill testing is associated with a higher false-positive rate in women[47,48] and the interpretation of nuclear medicine scans can be hampered by breast artifact and breast attenuation,[48] both of these diagnostic studies remain useful in the evaluation of chest pain and ischemia in women.

Invasive Procedures and Revascularization Gender differences have been reported in utilization rates of invasive cardiovascular procedures for men and women, with women undergoing significantly fewer invasive procedures.[49] Specifically, women are referred for coronary arteriography, coronary angioplasty, and coronary artery bypass surgery at nearly half the rate as men,[50-53] even after the diagnosis of CHD has been established. The differences observed have been attributed to a variety of factors, including possible referral bias, inadequate access to care, more advanced age and overall poorer health status of elderly women, and anatomic considerations. Support for these postulates is provided by data from the Coronary Artery Surgery Study (CASS),[54] which indicated that women who undergo bypass surgery are typically sicker, more often require emergency surgery, and are referred for revascularization at a later and more symptomatic stage of their illness than men. In addition, the CASS study demonstrated that women undergoing bypass grafting had mortality rates two times greater than those for men, less initial and later symptomatic relief from angina, and shorter long-term graft patency rates. Therefore, bypass surgery may carry greater risks and be less efficacious in women as compared to men. Similarly, women have excess mortality after percutaneous transluminal coronary angioplasty.[55] Therefore, women may experience greater risks than men do with reperfusion and revascularization. The reasons for these differences are unclear but may in part relate to some of the factors mentioned previously and to anatomic variables, including smaller caliber coronary vessels and greater vessel friability as a direct result of hormonal vascular effects.

Medical Treatment Gender differences in response to pharmacologic management of CHD may be anticipated because of differences in body size, fat distribution, protein binding, and drug-drug interactions. The Nurses's Health Initiative Study[56] is the largest trial to date to include an investigation of the benefits of aspirin in women. This study found that aspirin use by women led to a 37% reduction in cardiovascular risk. The risk benefit was of similar magnitude to that previously established for men by the British Doctor's Study and other studies in men. Unfortunately, little comparable data are available regarding benefits to women who have been prescribed calcium channel blockers or beta blockers, other than the well-established benefits of beta blockers post-MI. Angiotensin converting enzyme inhibitors, used extensively for management

TABLE 23.4   HYPERTENSION TRIALS
AND OUTCOME

Study	Subjects	Outcome
Hypertension Detection and Follow-Up Program (1979)[a]	10,940 (46% female)	Female (Black)—28% reduction in mortality Male (Black)—19% reduction in mortality Male (White)—15% reduction in mortality Female (White)—3% reduction in mortality
Australian Therapeutic Trial (1980)[b]	3,427 (37% female)	Male—26% reduction total end points $p < .05$ Female—26% reduction in end points p = not significant
Medical Research Council Trial of Treatment of Mild Hypertension (1985)[c]	17,534 (48% female)	Female—26% INCREASE in all cause mortality Male—15% decrease in all cause mortality
European Working Party on High Blood Pressure in the Elderly (1985)[d]	840 (70% female)	Female—18% decrease in cardiovascular mortality Male—47% decrease in cardiovascular mortality

[a] From *Journal of the American Medical Association* 242(23), 2572–2577.
[b] From *The Lancet* 1(8181): 1261–1267.
[c] From the *British Medical Journal* 291(6488), 97–104.
[d] From *The Lancet* 1(8442): 1349–1354.

of hypertension and congestive heart failure, are associated with a greater incidence of cough in women. The benefits of antihypertensive therapy in women have been demonstrated by several studies (see Table 23.4), albeit with somewhat mixed results. Thrombolytic therapy for acute MI does not appear to be associated with similar benefits in men and women (see Table 23.5).

Hormone Use, Hormone Replacement Therapy, and CHD Risk Past use of oral contraceptives has not been linked to increased risk of cardiovascular disease,[57–59] with the well-recognized exception of enhanced thrombotic potential in women who are smokers, over the age of 35, and on oral contraceptives.[60] In addition, most epidemiologic studies of

TABLE 23.5 GENDER DIFFERENCES
IN THROMBOLYTIC THERAPY

Study	Subjects	Outcome
European Trial (SK, heparin)	730 (133 females)	Males—30% reduction mortality Females—24% reduction mortality
GISSI (SK)	11,806 (1,157 females)	Males—8.8% mortality Females—18.5% mortality
ISIS II (SK, ASA)	17,000 (4,000 females)	Males—44% reduction mortality Females—30% reduction mortality
ASSET (TPA, heparin)	5,000 (1,151 females)	Males—28% reduction mortality Females—21% reduction mortality
MILIS (hyaluronidase and propanolol)	816 (226 females)	Males—21% cumulative mortality Females—36% cumulative mortality

NOTE: SK, streptokinase; ASA, aspirin; TPA, tissue plasminogen activator. European, European Trial (*American Journal of Cardiology* 63[17], 1185–1192, 1989); GISSI, Gruppo Italiano per lo Studio della Streptochinasi nell Infarto Miocardico (*The Lancet* 2[8564], 871–874, 1987); ISIS II, Second International Study of Infarct Survival (*The Lancet* 2[8607], 349–360, 1988); ASSET, Anglo-Scandinavian Study of Early Thrombolysis (*The Lancet* 2[8610], 525–530, 1988); MILIS, Multi-Centre Investigation of the Limitation of Infarct Size (*Journal of the American College of Cardiology* 9[3], 473–482, 1987).

cardiovascular disease in postmenopausal women suggest that estrogen replacement therapy has a protective effect. The epidemiologic evidence for a protective effect of hormone replacement therapy (HRT) is compelling, such that HRT is a potent treatment option available to women. Recent substantial evidence indicates that postmenopausal HRT can reduce CHD risk, morbidity, and mortality (from CHD and all causes) in postmenopausal women.[61-67] The CHD risk reductions and mortality reductions are significant—50% and 40%, respectively—and larger than those afforded by other conventional medical treatments for CHD. In one study,[68] estrogen use was associated with an 80% reduction in the prevalence of CHD at angiography. Duration of HRT use appears to be an important factor in risk and mortality reduction, with current users benefiting more than past users, who in turn show greater benefits than nonusers.[64] It is unclear whether HRT is associated with greater benefits

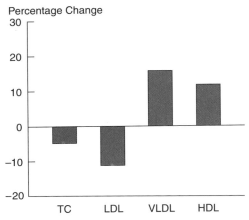

Figure 23.7. Effects of estrogen on lipid parameters. Source: Adapted from Paganini-Hill et al. (1988 [69]). Abbreviations: TC, total cholesterol; LDL, low-density lipoprotein; VLDL, very low density lipoprotein; HDL, high-density lipoprotein.

in the presence of CHD than in its absence. Whereas it is as yet unclear whether stroke risk is unaffected by HRT, mortality from stroke has been demonstrated to be reduced with HRT.[69] Therefore, HRT appears to be an important therapy to prevent cardiovascular disease and prolong life in postmenopausal women.

The mechanisms by which estrogen affords cardioprotection are multifactorial. In addition to benefits from chronic use, estrogen has been demonstrated to have acute effects on the vasculature.[70] Estrogen acts at several steps in the atherogenic process to prevent cardiovascular disease. Some of the benefits of estrogen (approximately one-fourth to one-half of the CHD risk reduction) are ascribed to its ability to favorably alter the lipoprotein profile (see Figure 23.7).[71] Oral conjugated estrogens are associated with the greatest benefit on the lipid profile, resulting in approximately 15% reductions in LDL cholesterol (from accelerated LDL catabolism) and a similar rise in HDL cholesterol levels.[71] Lipid benefits of lesser magnitude have been reported with the use of other formulations and delivery routes. Estrogen replacement is associated with a significant, though highly variable, rise in VLDL triglyceride levels[72] (resulting from increased production of large, triglyceride-rich VLDL).[71] The significance of hypertriglyceridemia as a consequence of HRT on CHD risk is unclear when compared to that of endogenous hypertryglyceridemia. Lastly, recent studies indicate that HRT use in post-menopausal women results in reductions in levels of lipoprotein(a).[73,74]

Despite the currently known benefits of HRT, estimates of noncompliance range from 15% to 41%.[75] The figures are particularly significant given the extent of cardiovascular risk and mortality reductions afforded by HRT, as demonstrated by studies to date. Elderly women, the highest-risk group for CHD, may face conflicts relating to the perception that CHD is a natural consequence of aging. Compliance is also affected by uncertainty regarding the risks of HRT.

The major well-established deleterious effect of unopposed estrogen therapy in women with a uterus is a three- to fourfold increase in the risk of endometrial cancer.[72,76,77] The rationale for combination therapy with estrogen and progestins in women with a uterus is that the addition of progestin protects the endometrium from prolonged stimulation with unopposed estrogen, thereby reducing the risk of endometrial cancer. In general, progestins alone attenuate the lipid effects of estrogen. However, as clearly demonstrated by the recent Postmenopausal Estrogen and Progesterone Intervention (PEPI) Trial,[72] if progestins are given in combination with estrogen, favorable effects on lipid parameters continue to be evident. Whether progestins attenuate the cardioprotective effects of estrogens is unclear at this time, as the effects on CHD risk and mortality resulting from combined estrogen and progesterone HRT have not been conclusively evaluated by studies to date. Data on the potential increase in risk for breast cancer from HRT remain inconclusive and will have to await clarification from future studies.[78–82]

Cardioprotective effects of estrogen cannot be explained solely on the basis of lipid changes, however. Recent studies indicate that a number of additional mechanisms are of significance. It appears that a substantial portion of the cardioprotective effects of estrogen may be mediated by direct effects on the vessel wall, leading to an attenuation of aortic cholesterol accumulation.[83–85] Estrogens have also been demonstrated to prevent oxidative modification of LDL cholesterol.[86] Other beneficial effects of estrogen include direct actions in decreased expression of adhesion molecules involved in monocyte adhesion to endothelium and in altering vasoreactivity of atherosclerotic vessels and thereby promoting vasodilation.[87] Furthermore, reductions in fibrinogen levels have also been reported with HRT in postmenopausal women (PEPI trial). Despite mounting evidence on the benefits of HRT, relatively few physicians prescribe hormonal therapy to their patients with CHD or lipid abnormalities, and many women are reluctant to accept such therapy.

This reality stems in part from the lack of physician and patient awareness of the known risks and benefits of HRT and from persistent unanswered questions regarding the optimal administration of HRT (e.g., long-term safety, dosing, use duration, side effects, and preferred formulations). The answers to these and other questions await the results of currently ongoing and future studies (see Table 23.6).

CONTROVERSIES

The relatively recent and rapid explosion of interest in cardiovascular disease in women has brought to the forefront the available epidemiological, clinical, and basic science information from studies on the topic to date. Simultaneously, there is heightened awareness of the inadequacies and lack of completeness of available data. This has in turn led to both excitement and a general sense of discomfort with this emerging medical discipline. Furthermore, when placed in the context of existing psychosocial structures, attitudes, and the impact of health care reform, controversies in the field are sure to emerge. This section focuses on a discussion of current controversies from three perspectives relating to women's misperceptions about cardiovascular risks; the impact of physician attitudes, behaviors, and psychosocial perspectives; and the gender gap in medical research.

Patient Perspectives

Opinion polls[88] indicate that women of all ages overwhelmingly (76%) identify cancer, particularly breast cancer, as their most serious health threat. Heart disease is very infrequently, if ever, cited as a significant health problem by women, who mistakenly believe that only men are affected. Because of this lack of awareness, women often minimize or misinterpret symptoms of heart disease, even if they have a known diagnosis of CHD. To the extent that risk-related behaviors are influenced by the perceived benefits or perceived consequences of those behaviors, women, and particularly younger women, are not focused on the prevention of CHD but rather approach their lives with the misbelief that CHD is a remote health concern that will not require attention until a very advanced age. For example, young women are more likely to initiate smoking and less likely to stop smoking than young men, despite men and women being equally aware of the health threats of smoking.[89] Therefore, the

TABLE 23.6 RECENTLY COMPLETED OR ONGOING WOMEN'S HEALTH STUDIES PERTAINING TO CORONARY HEART DISEASE

The Women's Health Initiative (WHI) Clinical Trial—(Assaf and Carleton, 1994)[a]

The Heart and Estrogen Progesterone Replacement Study (HERS)—(Schrott et al., 1997)[b]

Postmenopausal Estrogen/Progestin Intervention Trial (PEPI—JAMA, 1996)[c]

Women's Health Trial: Minority Feasibility Study—(Bowen et al., 1996)[d]

Cardiovascular Risk Factors and The Menopause—(Davis et al., 1994)[e]

Tamoxifen in Postmenopausal Women Trial: Cardiovascular Risk and Events—(Grey et al., 1995)[f]

Calciuim for Preeclampsia Prevention (CPEP) Trial—(Levine et al., 1996)[g]

The Women's Antioxidant and Cardiovascular Study (WACS)—(Manson et al., 1995)[h]

Systolic Hypertension in the Elderly Program (SHEP)—(Bearden et al., 1994)[i]

Asymptomatic Carotid Artery Plaque Study—(Espeland et al., 1996)[j]

Stress Reduction in Elderly Blacks with Hypertension—(Schneider et al., 1995)[k]

Trial of Nonpharmacologic Intervention in the Elderly (TONE)—(Appel et al., 1995)[l]

---

[a] A. Assaf and R. A. Carleton, The Women's Health Initiative Clinical Trial and Observational Study: History and Overview, *R I Med* 77, no. 12(1994), 424–427. Pawtucket Heart Health Program, Brown University, Providence, Rhode Island.

[b] H. G. Schrott et al., Adherence to National Cholesterol Education Program Treatment goals in postmenopausal women with heart disease: The Heart and Estrogen/Progestin Replacement Study (HERS), *Journal of the American Medical Association* 277, no. 16(1997), 1281–1286. Department of Preventive Medicine, University of Iowa, Iowa City.

[c] The Writing Group for the PEPI Trial, Effects of estrogen or estrogen/progestin regimens on heart disease risk factors in postmenopausal women: The postmenopausal Estrogen/Progestin Interventions (PEPI) Trial, *Journal of the American Medical Association* 273, no. 3(1995), 199–208.

[d] D. Bowen et al., The Women's Health Trial Feasibility Study in Minority Populations: Design and baseline descriptions, *Annals of Epidemiology* 6, no. 6(1996), 507–519. Emory School of Medicine, Atlanta, Georgia.

[e] C. E. Davis et al., Natural menopause and cardiovascular disease risk factors: The Poland and US Collaborative Study on Cardiovascular Disease Epidemiology, *Annals of Epidemiology* 4, no. 6(1994), 445–448. School of Public Health, Department of Biostatistics, University of North Carolina, Chapel Hill.

[f] A. B. Grey et al., The effect of the anti-estrogen tamoxifen on cardiovascular risk factors in normal postmenopausal women, *Journal of Clinical Endocrinology and Metabolism* 80, no. 11(1995), 3191–3195. Department of Medicine, University of Auckland, New Zealand.

[g] R. J. Levine et al., Trial of Calcium for Preeclampsia Prevention (CPEP): Rationale, design, and methods, *Controlled Clinical Trials* 17, no. 5(1996), 442–469. National Institute of Child Health and Human Development, Division of Epidemiology, Statistics, and Prevention Research, Bethesda, Maryland.

[h] J. E. Manson et al., A secondary prevention trial of antioxidant vitamins and cardiovascular disease in women: Rationale, design, and methods, *Annals of Epidemiology* 5, no. 4(1995), 261–269. Department of Medicine, Harvard Medical School, Boston, Massachusetts.

[i] D. Bearden et al., Age, race, and gender variation in the utilization of coronary artery bypass surgery and angioplasty in SHEP, *Journal of the American Geriatrics Society* 42, no. 11(1994), 1143–1149. Division of Geriatrics, University of Alabama at Birmingham.

[j] M. A. Espeland et al., Reliability of longitudinal ultrasonographic measurements of carotid intimal-medial thicknesses, *Stroke* 27. no. 3(1996), 480–485. Department of Public Health Sciences, Bowman Gray School of Medicine, Wake Forest University, Winston-Salem, North Carolina.

[k] R. H. Schneider et al., A randomised controlled trial of stress reduction for hypertension in older African Americans, *Hypertension* 26, no. 5(1995), 820–827. Department of Physiological and Biological Sciences, Maharishi University of Management, Fairfield, Iowa.

[l] L. J. Appel et al., Trial of Nonpharmacologic Intervention in the Elderly (TONE): Design and rationale of a blood pressure control trial, *Annals of Epidemiology* 5, no. 2(1995), 119–129. Welch Center for Prevention, Epidemiology and Clincal Research, Johns Hopkins Health Institutions, Baltimore, Maryland.

fear of weight gain with smoking cessation and the unaltered concern for increased breast cancer risk from smoking outweigh concerns for CHD risk despite smoking's known deleterious cardiovascular health consequences. Unfortunately, smoking has other potential deleterious effects on women that may impact CHD risk further, including its known antiestrogenic effect[90] and association with natural menopause at a younger age.[91]

Women's perceptions about their vulnerability to cardiovascular disease influence their approach to risk behaviors and to symptom recognition and labeling. Given that the recognition of symptoms of a disease is influenced by beliefs about their significance, it is not surprising that women delay reporting symptoms of CHD, minimize symptoms, and are more likely to attribute symptoms to noncardiac etiologies. For example, women with acute MI have been shown to have longer prehospital presentation delays than men.[92] This is particularly significant given the critical nature of the timing of thrombolysis administration in acute MI.

Coronary heart disease risk is also influenced by psychosocial factors, including socioeconomic and occupational status. A marked gradient in death rates from heart disease has been reported for women as a function of years of education completed.[93] In addition, with increasingly greater numbers of women entering the workforce (80% of women ages 20–64 are in the labor force), concerns about competing priorities and increasing demands on women become important. Interestingly, according to several health indicators, working women appear to be healthier overall than nonworking women.[94] However, as has been demonstrated in men, women who experience depression, repressed hostility, and anger have significantly increased risk of CHD[95]—these conditions can be more prevalent in female-dominated occupations characterized by low control and high demand.

Physician Attitudes and Perspectives

Gender differences in the diagnostic and treatment approach of physicians toward women with CHD have been well documented. In general, physicians are significantly less aggressive in the diagnostic evaluation and follow-up of women with suspected CHD. Sixty-two percent of women with a positive exercise treadmill test had no further diagnostic workup as compared to 38% of men.[96] In addition, only 4% of women with abnormal nuclear scans (vs. 40% of men) were referred for diagnostic cardiac catheterization.[97] The differences have been attributed to a number of possible factors, including gender bias,[97,98] the lower number of diagnostic predictors of CHD in women, and an overall lower rate of abnormal exercise studies in women.[96] Similarly, there has been a decline in the number of physicians prescribing HRT[99] in response to women's poor compliance.

There appear to be no gender differences in the physiologic perception of angina. Nonetheless, important differences exist in the etiology of angina in men and women. Although angina is more common in women than in men, it is also more commonly associated with normal coronary arteries,[54] microvascular angina,[100] and other noncoronary causes of chest pain, such as mitral valve prolapse.[101] This is in contradistinction to angina in men, which more commonly is associated with coronary artery disease. In addition, chest pain syndromes in women are more likely to be attributed to noncardiac (and possibly psychogenic) etiologies by physicians, as related diagnoses (e.g., depression and panic attacks) are more common in women.[102] These circumstances in turn may lead physicians to less aggressively pursue the evaluation of complaints of chest pain by women. Women's interpretation of physician behavior may in turn lead to a belief that anginal symptoms are unimportant or not serious and result in less diligence in symptom reporting.

Physicians may also be less inclined to recommend higher-risk invasive procedures to their female patients with CHD, as these patients tend to be older and sicker and have poorer procedure-related outcomes than male counterparts, as discussed earlier. In addition, a less invasive approach to evaluating patients with suspected CHD may be a consequence of the relative paucity of research data for women as a consequence of the fewer studies that have been done on women as research subjects. The larger body of knowledge on cardiovascular disease in men may serve to further reinforce the belief that it is a disease affecting primarily men.

Gender Gap in Biomedical Research

Until recently, women have been largely excluded as subjects in many cardiovascular research studies. This has resulted in inadequate information in nearly every aspect of the field and a poor understanding of the best approaches to the prevention and treatment of cardiovascular disease in women. It is largely this gender gap in research that has resulted in promoting many of the myths that have been discussed and that has led to controversies in the field. Furthermore, as a significant proportion of the elderly population in the United States is comprised of women, the underrepresentation of the elderly in research studies disproportionately excludes women from studies. However, progress has recently been made in this direction with the NIH and other funding agencies, encouraging and requiring the inclusion of women in research studies.

Finally, studies on women of ethnicity are sorely lacking in the field, resulting in a near information void in this subgroup of women. In general, cardiovascular disease risk among Latino women and Asian women is low, partly because of their lower rates of hypertension and lower levels of smoking. However, the higher incidence of diabetes mellitus in Latino women is not consistent with their heart disease advantage. Evaluation of gender-ethnicity interactions in the San Antonio Heart Study[103] clearly demonstrated a lower cardiovascular mortality in Mexican-American men than in non-Hispanic Caucasian men. In contrast, no ethnic differences in mortality were observed in Mexican-American women. The reasons for the gender-ethnicity differences in mortality are not well understood but may relate to lifestyle or cultural differences in disease perception. These factors may be very important in modifying cardiovascular risk and outcomes and are examples of critical information that can be derived by having a better understanding of the role of sociocultural factors on cardiovascular disease and including women of diverse ethnic backgrounds in ongoing and future research trials.

CONCLUSION AND FUTURE DIRECTIONS

Heart disease, the leading killer of American women, is underrecognized and frequently underdiagnosed. In addition, women have greater morbidity and higher mortality from heart disease than men. Furthermore, significant differences exist in the presentation, diagnosis, and treatment of CHD in men and women. It is therefore necessary to (1) identify approaches for promoting appropriate clinical services for women at risk for and with established cardiovascular disease, (2) develop educational programs for the public and health care providers, (3) focus research efforts on cardiovascular disease in women, and (4) guide public health care policy to address women's cardiovascular health issues.

The following section outlines a series of recommendations for action in each of these four areas.

Clinical Care

• Establish women's health or cardiovascular health clinics, programs, and/or centers in communities and academic institutions.

• Recruit more health care providers with an interest in women's health and create linkages among providers with knowledge and expertise in women's cardiovascular health.

• Educate physicians to recognize, aggressively pursue, and adequately manage chest pain or other potentially CHD-related symptoms and signs in women.

• Emphasize multidisciplinary and multicultural approaches to health care delivery in women's health, including cardiovascular health.

Education

• Educate physicians and health care providers on women's health issues and cardiovascular disease in women by sponsoring continuing medical education programs, specialty publications, case-based learning, telemedicine conferences, didactic teaching session, grand rounds presentations, women's health conferences, and so on.

• Develop and enrich women's health curricula for medical graduates and undergraduates in cardiovascular disease and integrate existing fragmented curricula. Pursue curricular approaches that strive for vertical integration through medical education and horizontal integration across disciplines.

• Increase public health education efforts to raise awareness of cardiovascular disease in women.

• Create linkages with and among existing educational venues, such as the National Office of Women's Health, the American Heart Association (AHA), the American Medical Association, the American Medical Women's Association (AMWA), and state health departments. Ongoing educational and awareness campaigns include AMWA's "Advanced Curriculum on Women's Health" and AHA's public education pamphlet "Heart Disease in Women: The Silent Epidemic."

• Raise awareness of cardiovascular disease in women by innovative public education campaigns at local or regional levels by creating partnerships with the media, holding public education forums and cardiovascular health fairs for women, and so on.

Research

• Enhance inclusion and participation of women (including elderly women and women of ethnicity) as subjects in cardiovascular research trials and studies.

• Fund and foster research that has as its focus cardiovascular disease in women and other understudied areas.

• Identify and support national agencies with women's health agendas, such as the U.S. Public Health Service Office of Research on Women's Health, Women's Health Collaboratives, the American Association of Medical Colleges, and others.

• Develop academic research consortiums that foster and support gender-specific research and research by women academicians.

• Establish a national registry of clinical trials that include women or include gender-specific analyses.

• Focus research efforts on cardiovascular disease in women and related topics and fields, including studies on gender differences in disease epidemiology, pharmacotherapy, risk factor stratification, pathogenic mechanisms, biobehavioral and psychosocial variables, and outcomes.

Public Policy

• Encourage women to become more active participants in formulating public health care policy.

• Establish an Office of Women's Health within state health departments.

• Support funding and legislative initiatives that address women's health issues.

• Initiate aggressive public health campaigns and programs aimed at preventing cardiovascular disease and modifying cardiac risk factors to include early detection and treatment of hypertension, smoking cessation, exercise, and control of dietary fat and cholesterol.

By working together and focusing attention on cardiovascular health and wellness in women as a common goal, health care consumers, providers, educators, researchers, and policy makers can make a significant impact to improve understanding, prevention, and treatment of cardiovascular disease—the leading killer of American men *and* women.

NOTE

The author wishes to acknowledge Rhonda McBride for secretarial assistance. This work was supported by an award from the UC/Health Net Wellness Lecture Series.

REFERENCES

1. Wenger, N. K., Speroff, L., and Packard, B., eds. 1993. *Proceedings of a National Heart, Blood, and Lung Disease Conference: Cardiovascular Health and Disease in Women.* Greenwich, Conn.: LeJacq Communications, Inc.
2. Lerner, D. J., and Kannel, W. B. 1986. Patterns of coronary heart disease morbidity and mortality in the sexes: A 26-year follow-up of the Framingham population. *American Heart Journal* 111, 383.
3. Goldberg, R. J., Gorak, E. J., Yarzebski, J., and Gore, J. M. 1994. Sex differences in postinfarction survival rates. *Cardiology Board Review* 11(5), 19-26.
4. Fiebach, N. H., Viscoli, C. M., and Horwitz, R. I. 1990. Differences between women and men in survival after myocardial infarction. *Journal of the American Medical Association* 263(8), 1082-1086.
5. Greenland, P., Reicher-Reiss, H., Goldbourt, U., and Behar, S. 1991. Israeli SPRINT Investigators: In-hospital and 1-year mortality in 1,524 women after myocardial infarction. *Circulation* 83, 484-491.
6. Tofler, G. H., Stone, P. H., Muller, J. E., et al. 1987. Effects of gender and race on prognosis after myocardial infarction: Adverse prognosis for women, particularly black women. *Journal of the American College of Cardiology* 9, 473.
7. Barnett, H. J. M. 1990. Stroke in women. *Canadian Journal of Cardiology* 6(Suppl. B), 11B-17B.
8. Cooper, R., Sempos, C., Hsieh, S. C., and Kovar, M. G. 1990. Slowdown in the decline of stroke mortality in the United States. *Stroke* 21, 1274-1279.
9. Wong, M. C. W., Giuliani, M. J., and Haley, C. 1990. Cerebrovascular disease and stroke in women. *Cardiology* 77(Suppl. 2), 80-90.
10. U.S. Public Health Service, Centers for Disease Control. 1991. *Health United States 1990.* Washington, D.C.: U.S. Government Printing Office, 85.
11. Kittner, S. J., White, L. R., Losonczy, K. G., et al. 1990. Black-white differences in stroke incidence in a national sample. *Journal of the American Medical Association* 264, 1267-1270.
12. National Center for Health Statistics. 1989. The National Nursing Home Survey: 1985. *Vital Health Statistics* [13]97, 43.
13. Broderick, J. P., Phillips, S. J., Whisnant, J. P., et al. 1988. Incidence rates of stroke in the eighties: The end of the decline in stroke? *Stroke* 19, 598-603.
14. Expert Panel on Detection Evaluation and Treatment of High Blood Cholesterol in Adults. 1993. Summary of the Second Report of the National Cholesterol Education Program (NECP) Expert Panel on Detection, Evaluation, and Treatment of High Blood Cholesterol in Adults (Adult Treatment Panel II). *Journal of the American Medical Association* 269(23), 3015-3023.
15. Arnold, A. Z., and Underwood, D. A. 1993. Coronary artery disease in women: A risk-factor analysis. *Cleveland Clinic Journal of Medicine* 60, 387-392.
16. Haurg, M. R., and Folmar, S. J. 1986. Longevity, gender and life quality. *Journal of Health and Social Behavior* 27, 332-345.
17. Williams, R. B., Barefoot, J. C., Califf, R. H., et al. 1992. Prognostic impor-

tance of social and economic resources among medically treated patients with angiographical documented coronary artery disease. *Journal of the American Medical Association* 267, 520–524.

18. Barrett-Conner, E., and Wingard, D. L. 1983. Sex differential in ischemic heart disease mortality in diabetics: A prospective population-based study. *American Journal of Epidemiology* 118, 489–496.

19. Barrett-Conner, E., and Wingard, D. L. 1984. Sex differences in diabetes mellitus. In E. Gold, ed., *The Changing Risk of Diseases in Women: An Epidemiologic Approach*. Lexington, Ky.: D. C. Heath, 257–286.

20. Maynard, C., and Weaver, W. D. 1992. Treatment of women with acute MI: New findings from the Miti registry. *Journal of Myocardial Ischemia* 4(8), 27–38.

21. Tansey, M. J. B., Opie, L. H., and Kennelly, B. M. 1977. High mortality in obese women diabetics with acute myocardial infarction. *British Medical Journal* 1, 1624–1626.

22. Philips, G. B. 1984. Evidence for hyperestrogenemia as the link between diabetes mellitus and myocardial infarction. *American Journal of Medicine* 76, 1041–1048.

23. Pyörälä, K., Laakso, M., and Uusitupa, M. 1987. Diabetes and atherosclerosis: An epidemiologic view. *Diabetes Metabolism Reviews* 3, 463–524.

24. Rowland, M., and Roberts, J. 1982. Blood pressure levels and hypertension in persons ages 6–74: United States, 1976–1980. *NCHS Advance Data from Vital and Health Statistics* 84, 1–11.

25. Frohlich, E. D. 1993. Cardiovascular health and disease in women. In N. K. Wenger, L. Speroff, and B. Packard, eds., *Proceedings of a National Heart, Lung, and Blood Disease Conference: Cardiovascular Health and Disease in Women*. Pp. 145–148. Greenwich, Conn.: LeJacq Communications Inc.

26. Macmahon, S. W., Furberg, C. D., and Cutler, J. A. 1987. Women as participants in trials of the primary and secondary prevention of cardiovascular disease: Part I. Primary Prevention: The hypertension trials. In E. D. Eaker, B. Packard, N. Kass-Wenger, et al., eds., *Coronary Heart Disease in Women: Proceedings of an NIH Workshop*. Pp. 233–240. New York: Haymarket Doyma Inc.

27. Anastos, K., Charney, P., Charon, R. A., et al. 1991. Hypertension in women: What is really known? *Annals of Internal Medicine* 115, 287–293.

28. Cornoni-Huntly, J., Lacroix, A. Z., and Havlik, R. J. 1989. Race and sex differentials in the impact of hypertension in the United States: The National Health and Nutrition Examination Survey I Epidemiologic Follow-Up Study. *Archives of Internal Medicine* 149, 780–788.

29. Deubner, D. C., Tyroler, H. A., Cassel, J. C., et al. 1975. Attributable risk, population attributable risk, and population attributable fraction of death associated with hypertension in a biracial population. *Circulation* 52, 901–908.

30. Castelli, W. P., Garrison, R. J., Wilson, P. W., et al. 1986. Incidence of coronary heart disease and lipoprotein cholesterol levels: The Framingham Study. *Journal of the American Medical Association* 256(20), 2835–2838.

31. Eaker, E. D., and Castelli, W. P. 1987. Coronary heart disease and its risk factors among women in the Framingham Study. In E. D. Eaker, B. Packard,

N. Kass-Wenger, et al., eds., *Coronary Heart Disease in Women: Proceedings of an NIH Workshop.* Pp. 122–130. New York: Haymarket Doyma Inc.

32. Gordon, D. J., Probstfield, J. L., Garrison, R. F., et al. 1989. High-density lipoprotein cholesterol and cardiovascular disease: Four prospective studies. *Circulation* 798, 8–15.

33. Kannel, W. B. 1988. Nutrition and the occurrence and prevention of cardiovascular disease in the elderly. *Nutrition Review* 48, 68–78.

34. Sandkamp, M., and Assmann, G. 1990. Lipoprotein(a) in PRO-CAM participants and young myocardial infarction survivors. In A. M. Scanu, ed., *Lipoprotein(a).* Pp. 205–209. New York: Academic Press.

35. Dahlen, G. H. 1990. Incidence of Lp(a) lipoprotein among populations. In A. M. Scanu, ed., *Lipoprotein(a).* Pp. 151–173. New York: Academic Press.

36. Austin, M. A. 1988. Epidemiologic associations between hypertriglyceridemia and coronary heart disease. *Seminars in Thrombosis and Hemostasis* 14, 137–142.

37. NIH Consensus Development Panel. 1993. Triglyceride, high-density lipoprotein, and coronary heart disease. *Journal of the American Medical Association* 269(4), 505–510.

38. Castelli, W. P. 1989. Cardiac risk in women. *The Female Patient* 14, 54–66.

39. Castelli, W. P. 1986. The triglyceride issue: A view from Framingham. *American Heart Journal* 112, 432–437.

40. Hill, J. O., Thiel, J., Heller, P. A., et al. 1989. Differences in effect of aerobic exercise training on blood lipids in men and women. *American Journal of Cardiology* 63, 254–256.

41. Gordon, T., Kannel, W. B., Hjortland, M. C., and McNamara, P. M. 1978. Menopause and coronary heart disease: The Framingham Study. *Annals of Internal Medicine* 89, 157–161.

42. Colditz, G. A., Willett, W. C., Stampfer, M. J., et al. 1987. Menopause and the risk of coronary heart disease in women. *New England Journal of Medicine* 316(18), 1105–1110.

43. Rosenberg, L., Hennekens, C. H., Rosner, B., et al. 1981. Early menopause and the risk of myocardial infarction. *American Journal of Obstetrics and Gynecology* 139, 47.

44. Centerwall, B. S. 1981. Premenopausal hysterectomy and cardiovascular disease. *American Journal of Obstetrics and Gynecology* 139, 58.

45. Wittels, E. H., Hay, J. W., and Gotto, A. M., Jr. 1990. Medical costs of coronary artery disease in the United States. *American Journal of Cardiology* 65, 432–440.

46. Sullivan, J. M., and Fowlkes, L. 1994. Estrogen replacement therapy and the cardiovascular system. *Journal of Myocardial Ischemia* 6(3), 10–14.

47. Sawada, S. G. 1992. How to test women for CAD. *Internal Medicine* 13(4), 34–42.

48. Wackers, F. J. T. 1992. Diagnostic pitfalls of myocardial perfusion imaging in women. *Journal of Myocardial Ischemia* 4(10), 23–37.

49. Ayanian, J. Z., and Epstein, A. M. 1991. Differences in the use of procedures between women and men hospitalized for coronary heart disease. *New England Journal of Medicine* 325, 221.

50. Chiriboga, D. E., Yarzebski, J., Goldberg, R. J., et al. 1993. A community-wide perspective of gender differences and temporal trends in the use of diagnostic and revascularization procedures for acute myocardial infarction. *American Journal of Cardiology* 71, 268–273.

51. Davis, K. B. 1987. Coronary artery bypass graft surgery in women. In E. D. Eaker, B. Packard, N. Kass-Wenger, et al., eds., *Coronary Heart Disease in Women: Proceedings of an NIH Workshop*. New York: Haymarket Doyma Inc., 249.

52. Eysmann, S. B., and Douglas, P. S. 1992. Women respond differently from men to reperfusion, revascularization. *Journal of the American Medical Association* 268, 1903–1907.

53. Gambino, A., and Steingart, R. M. 1994. Differences in managing coronary disease in men and women. *Choices in Cardiology* 7(9), 318–320.

54. Weiner, D. A., Ryan, T. J., McCabe, C. H., et al. 1979. Exercise stress testing: Correlations among history of angina, ST-segment response and prevalence of coronary-artery disease in the Coronary Artery Surgery Study (CASS). *New England Journal of Medicine* 301, 230–235.

55. Greenberg, M. A., and Mueller, H. S. 1993. Why the excess mortality in women after PTCA? *Circulation* 87(3), 1030–1032.

56. Manson, J. E., Stampfer, M. J., Colditz, G. Z., et al. 1991. A prospective study of aspirin use and primary prevention of cardiovascular disease in women. *Journal of the American Medical Association* 266(4), 521–527.

57. Wiseman, R. A., and MacRae, K. D. 1981. Oral contraceptives and the decline in mortality from circulatory disease. *Fertility and Sterility* 35, 277.

58. Stampfer, M. J., Willett, W. C., Colditz, G. A., et al. 1990. Past use of oral contraceptives and cardiovascular disease: A meta-analysis in the context of the Nurse's Health Study. *American Journal of Obstetrics and Gynecology* 163, 285.

59. Testeson, H., Buring, J., Jonas, M., and Hennekens, C. 1992. Risks and benefits of OCs and estrogen replacement in coronary heart disease. *Journal of Myocardial Ischemia* 4(5), 41–53.

60. Mileikowsky, G. N., Nadler, J. L., Huey, F., et al. 1988. Evidence that smoking alters prostacyclin formation and platelet aggregation in women who use oral contraceptives. *American Journal of Obstetrics and Gynecology* 159, 1547.

61. Henderson, B. E., Ross, R. K., Paganini-Hill, A., and Mack, T. M. 1986. Estrogen use and cardiovascular disease. *American Journal of Obstetrics and Gynecology* 154, 1181.

62. Henderson, B. E., Paganini-Hill, A., and Ross, R. K. 1992. The effect of estrogen replacement therapy on mortality. *Primary Cardiology* 18(6), 56–64.

63. Bush, T. L. 1990. The epidemiology of cardiovascular disease in postmenopausal women. *Annals of the New York Academy of Sciences* 592, 263–271.

64. Henderson, B. E., Paganini-Hill, A., and Ross, R. K. 1991. Decreased mortality in users of estrogen replacement therapy. *Archives of Internal Medicine* 151, 75.

65. Barrett-Connor, E. 1991. Postmenopausal estrogen and prevention bias. *Annals of Internal Medicine* 115(6), 455–456.
66. Grady, D., Rubin, S. M., Petitti, D. B., et al. 1992. Hormone therapy to prevent disease and prolong life in postmenopausal women. *Annals of Internal Medicine* 117(12), 1016–1038.
67. Limacher, M. C. 1993. Estrogen replacement in the management of coronary heart disease. *Journal of Myocardial Ischemia* 5(1), 36–48.
68. Hong, M. K., Romm, P. A., Reagan, K., et al. 1992. Effects of estrogen replacement therapy on serum lipid values and angiographically defined coronary artery disease in postmenopausal women. *American Journal of Cardiology* 69, 176–178.
69. Paganini-Hill, A., Ross, R. K., and Henderson, B. E. 1988. Post-menopausal oestrogen treatment and stroke: A prospective study. *British Medical Journal* 297, 519.
70. Williams, J. K., Adams, M. R., Herrington, D. M., and Clarkson, T. B. 1992. Short-term administration of estrogen and vascular responses of atherosclerotic coronary arteries. *Journal of the American College of Cardiology* 20(2), 452–457.
71. Walsh, B. W., Schiff, I., Rosner, B., et al. 1991. Effects of postmenopausal estrogen replacement on the concentrations and metabolism of plasma lipoproteins. *New England Journal of Medicine* 325(17), 1196–1204.
72. Writing Group for the PEPI Trial. 1994. Effects of estrogen or estrogen/progestin regimens on heart disease risk factors in postmenopausal women: The postmenopausal Estrogen/Progestin Interventions (PEPI) Trial. *Journal of the American Medical Association* 273(3), 199–208.
73. Taskinen, M. R., Puolakka, J., Pyörälä, T., et al. 1996. Hormone replacement therapy lowers plasma Lp(a) concentrations. *Arteriosclerosis, Thrombosis, and Vascular Biology* 16(10), 1215–1221.
74. Kim, C. J., Min, Y. K., Ryu, W. S., et al. 1996. Effect of hormone replacement therapy on lipoprotein(a) and lipid levels in postmenopausal women: Influence of various progestogens and duration of therapy. *Arch f Intl Mede* 156(15), 1693–1700.
75. Ravnikar, V. A. 1987. Compliance with hormone therapy. *American Journal of Obstetrics and Gynecology* 156, 1332–1334.
76. Mathews, K. A., Meilahn, E., Kuller, L. H., et al. 1989. Menopause and risk factors for coronary heart disease. *New England Journal of Medicine* 321, 641–646.
77. Briton, L. A., and Hoover, R. N. 1993. Estrogen replacement therapy and endometrial cancer risk: Unresolved issues. *Obstetrics and Gynecology* 81, 265.
78. Nachtigall, M. J., Smilen, S. W., Nachtigall, R. A. D., et al. 1992. Incidence of breast cancer in a 22-year study of women receiving estrogen-progestin replacement therapy. *Obstetrics and Gynecology* 80, 827.
79. Dupont, W. D., and Page, D. L. 1991. Menopausal estrogen replacement therapy and breast cancer. *Archives of Internal Medicine* 151, 67.
80. Steinberg, K. K., Thacker, S. B., Smith, S. J., et al. 1991. A meta-analysis of

the effect of estrogen replacement therapy on the risk of breast cancer. *Journal of the American Medical Association* 265, 1985

81. Colditz, G. A., Egan, K. M., and Stampfer, M. J. 1993. Hormone replacement therapy and risk of breast cancer: Results from epidemiologic studies. *American Journal of Obstetrics and Gynecology* 168, 1473.

82. Sillero-Arenas, M., Delgado-Rodriguez, M., Rodigues-Canteras, R., et al. 1992. Menopausal hormone replacement therapy and breast cancer: A met-analysis. *Obstetrics and Gynecology* 79, 286.

83. Wagner, J. D., St. Clair, R. W., Schwenke, D. C., et al. 1992. Regional differences in arterial low density lipoprotein metabolism in surgically post-menopausal cynomolgus monkeys. *Arteriosclerosis and Thrombosis* 12, 717–726.

84. Williams, J. K., Adams, M. R., and Klopfenstein, H. S. 1990. Estrogen modulates responses of atherosclerotic coronary arteries. *Circulation* 81, 1680.

85. Haarbo, J., Leth-Espensen, P., Stender, S., and Christiansen, C. 1991. Estrogen monotherapy and combined estrogen-progestogen replacement therapy attenuate aortic accumulation of cholesterol in ovariectomized cholesterol-fed rabbits. *Journal of Clinical Investigation* 87, 1274–1279.

86. Sugioka, K., Shimosegawa, Y., and Nakano, M. 1987. Estrogens as natural antioxidants of membrane phospholipid peroxidation. *FEBS Letters* 210(1), 37–39.

87. Nathan, L., and Chaudhuri, G. 1997. Estrogens and atherosclerosis. *Annual Review of Pharmacology and Toxicology* 37, 477–515.

88. Roper Center for Public Opinion Research. 1980. *Breast Cancer: Public Understanding.* Storrs: University of Connecticut.

89. Office of the Surgeon General. 1989. *Reducing the Health Consequences of Smoking: Twenty-Five Years of Progress: A Report of the Surgeon General.* Publication CDC. Washington, D.C.: U.S. Government Printing Office, 89.

90. Michnovicz, J. J., Hershcopf, R. J., Naganuma, H., et al. 1986. Increased 2-hydroxylation of estradiol as a possible mechanism for the anti-estrogenic effect of cigarette smoking. *New England Journal of Medicine* 315(21), 1305–1310.

91. Kaufman, D. W., Slone, D., Rosenberg, L., et al. 1980. Cigarette smoking and age at natural menopause. *American Journal of Public Health* 70(4), 420–422.

92. Moser, D. K., and Dracup, K. 1993. Gender differences in treatment-seeking delay in acute myocardial infarction. *Progress in Cardiovascular Nursing* 8(1), 6–12.

93. Feldman, J. J., Makuc, D. M., Kleinman, J. C., and Cornoni-Huntley, J. 1989. National trends in educational differentials in mortality. *American Journal of Epidemiology* 129, 919–933.

94. Lacroix, A. Z., and Haynes, S. G. 1987. Gender differences in the stressfulness of workplace roles: A focus on work and health. In R. C. Barnett, G. K. Baruch, and L. Beiner, eds., *Gender and Stress.* Pp. 96–121. New York: The Free Press.

95. Carney, R. M., Freedland, K. E., Smith, L. J., et al. 1991. Depression and anxiety as risk factors for coronary heart disease in women. Paper presented

at the Conference on Women, Behavior and Cardiovascular Disease, National Heart, Lung, and Blood Institute, Chevy Chase, Maryland, September 25–27.

96. Mark, D. B., Shaw, L. K., DeLong, E. R., et al. 1994. Absence of sex bias in the referral of patients for cardiac catheterization. *New England Journal of Medicine* 330(16), 1101–1106.

97. Tobin, J. N., Wassertheil-Smoller, S., Wexler, J. P., et al. 1987. Sex bias in considering coronary bypass surgery. *Annals of Internal Medicine* 107, 19–25.

98. Douglas, P. S. 1994. Is cardiac care biased in favor of men? *Choices in Cardiology* 7(4), 152–154.

99. Lieblum, S. R., and Swartzman, L. C. 1986. Women's attitudes toward menopause: An update. *Maturitas* 8, 47–56.

100. Cannon, R. O., III. 1991. Microvascular angina: Pathophysiology, diagnostic techniques, and interventions. In E. Braunwald, ed., *Heart Disease Update*. Pp. 343–350. Philadelphia: W. B. Saunders.

101. Devereux, R. B., and Kramer-Fox, R. 1988. Gender differences in mitral valve prolapse. In P. S. Douglas, ed., *Cardiovascular Health and Disease in Women*. Pp. 243–258. Philadelphia: F. A. Davis.

102. Dimsdale, J. E. 1993. Influences of personality and stress-induced biological processes on etiology and treatment of cardiovascular disease in women. In *Proceedings of a National Heart, Lung, and Blood Disease Conference: Cardiovascular Health and Disease in Women*. Pp. 225–230. Greenwich, Conn.: LeJacq Communications Inc.

103. Mitchell, B. D., Stern, M. P., Haffner, S. M., et al. 1990. Risk factors for cardiovascular mortality in Mexican Americans and non-Hispanic whites. *American Journal of Epidemiology* 131, 423–433.

24

Craig R. Waldo and
Thomas J. Coates

HIV/AIDS PREVENTION

Successes and Challenges

HIV prevention science is comprised of a variety of disciplines, including psychology, medicine, law, sociology, anthropology, statistics, epidemiology, economics, political science, and communications. Scientists from these disciplines have worked together to provide an impressive convergence of scientific evidence that demonstrates that the HIV epidemic can be controlled. In this chapter, we demonstrate that the failure to contain HIV and AIDS has not been because of a lack of know-how. Rather, we argue that the problem has been primarily in finding ways to apply the knowledge that scientists have accumulated. The application of this knowledge has been thwarted by forces other than scientific ones. Among these are political opposition, the inadequate allocation of resources to prevention, a failure to target interventions to those at risk for HIV, and a failure to address larger social problems that contribute to the transmission of HIV. To support this argument, we first present examples of successful HIV and AIDS prevention and then discuss how and why the clear implications of this research have not been pursued.

DO WE KNOW HOW TO PREVENT HIV AND AIDS?

Worldwide, the total numbers of AIDS cases reported as of June 30, 1997, was 1,644,183, with 576,972 cases in Africa and 797,227 cases in the Americas (World Health Organization, 1997). In the United States, as of June 30, 1997, the cumulative number of AIDS cases reported to the Centers for Disease Control and Prevention (CDC) was 612,078, with 72,868 incident cases in the previous year (Centers for Disease Control and Prevention, 1997). Adult and adolescent AIDS cases totaled 604,176, with 511,934 cases in males and 92,242 cases in females; 7,902 AIDS cases were reported in children (defined as persons under age 13 at the time of diagnosis). Total cumulative deaths of persons reported with AIDS were 379,258 by June 1997, including 374,656 adults and adolescents and 4,602 children. All these numbers of cases reported probably underestimate the actual number of cases because many cases are never reported to agencies such as the WHO and CDC. In addition, these numbers do not reflect the number of *HIV infections* because it takes several years for someone with HIV to develop AIDS. The actual number of HIV infections has, for example, been estimated to be one million in the U.S. alone (Centers for Disease Control and Prevention, 1995), and 40,000 new infections are estimated to occur annually (Holmberg, 1996).

According to the CDC (1997), most (49.4%, or 298,699) of the total reported U.S. adult and adolescent AIDS diagnoses have been among "men who have sex with men" (i.e., men who identify as gay or bisexual or who are homosexually active). The second-largest group has been injection drug users (IDUs), who represent 25.6% (154,664) of all adolescent and adult cases of AIDS. An additional 6.4% of cases are accounted for by men who both have sex with men and inject drugs (38,923 cases). Thus, over 80% of cases are accounted for by men who have sex with men and IDUs. AIDS has also been disproportionately distributed among U.S. racial/ethnic groups: 35.2% (212,394) of adolescent and adult cases have been among African Americans, 17.8% (107,419) have been among Hispanics, and 46.0% (277,672) have been among Whites. Among women, these rates are especially unevenly distributed, with 55.7% of cases represented by African Americans, 20.2% by Hispanics, and 23.1% by Whites.

Despite these alarmingly high incidence and prevalence rates, a large prevention science literature provides evidence that HIV and AIDS can be prevented through behavioral and social changes. Coates (1990) distinguished between two forms of HIV prevention. *Primary prevention* refers to preventing individuals from becoming infected with HIV, and *secondary prevention* refers to the prevention of disease progression in those already infected with HIV. Important scientific studies have been conducted for both kinds of prevention, demonstrating the feasibility of behavior change to prevent the spread of HIV and the development of AIDS.

Elsewhere (Coates and Collins, 1998; Waldo and Coates, in press), we have conceptualized HIV prevention at multiple levels of analysis. We have theorized that HIV and AIDS prevention can focus on different social units to promote behavioral changes. In our view, these are the individual, dyadic/small group, organizational, community, and societal/cultural levels of analysis. A comprehensive approach to HIV and AIDS prevention includes interventions at all these levels. To demonstrate how behavior change can occur at each level, we present exemplars of research here. Taken together, these demonstrate that HIV prevention can be successful in multiple ways.

Individual-Level Change

The overwhelming majority of HIV prevention research has occurred at the level of the individual. In their comprehensive review of HIV preventive interventions, Choi and Coates (1994) found that most interventions were individual-level interventions, such as HIV testing and counseling and skills training, or small-group interventions designed to alter individual's knowledge, attitudes, and beliefs. The purpose of such interventions is to motivate individuals and to teach skills to reduce or eliminate HIV risk behaviors, such as anal or vaginal intercourse without condoms or the sharing of syringes during drug use.

A good example of an intervention that targets individuals is Project Respect, a large longitudinal study of heterosexual sexually transmitted disease (STD) clinic patients conducted by the CDC. The intervention incorporated elements of Social Learning Theory, the Theory of Reasoned Action, and the Health Belief Model in a randomized controlled trial of HIV testing and counseling (Kamb et al., 1996). Kamb et al. (1997) reported the results of the intervention with 5,758 HIV-negative heterosexual participants. The study involved three face-to-face intervention conditions: (1) two brief informational educational messages, (2) HIV prevention counseling with two client-centered sessions based on CDC guidelines, and (3) enhanced counseling with four sessions based on the three theories. All participants were followed up at three and six months with assessments of risk behavior as well as blood tests for STDs. Those in both conditions 2 and 3 were significantly more likely than those in condition 1 to use condoms 100% of the time at three-month follow-up and significantly less likely than those in condition 1 to have another STD at six-month follow-up.

Another exemplar of individual-level change is found in Peterson et al.

(1996), who evaluated a randomized controlled HIV risk reduction intervention with 318 African-American gay and bisexual men. Two intervention groups, one involving a single three-hour session and the other having three three-hour sessions, were compared to a wait-list control group before and after the interventions. Both the three-session and the one-session interventions were designed to be culturally appropriate and involved education about HIV transmission, cognitive-behavioral self-management training, assertion training, and efforts to develop personal identity and social support. Results of the study indicated that the prevalence of unprotected anal intercourse (based on the six months previous to assessment) among those receiving the three-session intervention was reduced one year following the intervention (46% baseline decreased to 20%) and that this change was maintained at 18-month follow-up (18%). In contrast, those in the wait-list control group did not demonstrate any such behavior change at either the 12- or the 18-month follow-up, and the prevalence of unprotected anal intercourse among those receiving the single-session intervention was reduced only modestly (from 47% baseline to 38% at both one-year and 18-month follow-ups). Importantly, this study targeted African-American gay and bisexual men, who have been underrepresented in research on HIV preventive interventions even though they are at higher risk for HIV infection (Peterson et al., 1992). Most studies have been done with largely White gay and bisexual men, and those that included randomized designs have also found successful results (e.g., Kelly et al., 1989; Valdiserri et al., 1989).

Dyadic/Small-Group Change

An example of an intervention at the dyadic/small-group level is found in Allen et al.'s (1992) study of confidential HIV testing of women in Rwanda. In this study, all women received educational information and were tested for HIV antibodies; the male partners of 26% of these women also received the education and testing with their female partners. The results at one-year follow-up indicated that women whose male partners had received the intervention were twice as likely to use condoms as the women whose partners had not received the intervention. Such results strongly suggest that the efficacy of the intervention was strengthened by engaging both partners in the intervention. HIV/AIDS prevention strategies may, therefore, be especially effective when they capitalize on relationships that are significant for individuals. A similar process exists for small-group interventions that utilize peer and family relationships to promote HIV risk reduction. For example, Dolcini (1997) has shown that peer group membership is a strong predictor of sexual and health risk behaviors among young adolescents. Interventions, therefore, may benefit from promoting peer influences that advocate the reduction or elimination of HIV risk behaviors.

Organizational Change

Examples of organizations where HIV preventive interventions can occur include schools, bathhouses or sex clubs, injection drug user shooting galleries, workplaces, and prisons. The focus of these interventions is on changing the organizations to which individuals belong, thereby promoting an environment that supports healthy behaviors. Dolan et al. (1995) discussed strategies for reducing HIV incidence among incarcerated drug injectors. Their review highlights the utility of performing interventions at an organizational level. As Dolan et al. point out, correctional facilities have many characteristics that make them likely to increase rates of HIV transmission, including the higher prevalence of both HIV and IDUs as well as situational male homosexuality. In addition, the lack of availability of condoms and clean syringes as well as the presence of boredom heighten the potential for HIV transmission. Brewer and Derrickson (1992) also note that prisons tend to contain more people of color and those from lower socioeconomic strata, groups that are at higher risk for HIV infection. Thus, prisons can be considered organizations that contain high levels of HIV risk. Dolan et al. (1995) discuss possible interventions directed at prisons, including condom distribution, methadone treatment availability, needle exchange, bleach distribution, education, compulsory testing, and segregation of HIV-positive prisoners. Where it has been implemented, Dolan et al. (1995) report that there is some indication that prison-based methadone treatment has been effective in reducing HIV risk behaviors. Nelles and Harding (1996) discuss the fact that since Switzerland has implemented needle exchange programs in its prisons, the rate of needle sharing among injecting prisoners has dropped from approximately half to virtually none. In addition, although 5,335 syringes were exchanged during an experimental period, the rate of injection drug use did not increase during the same period.

An additional example of HIV/AIDS prevention at the organizational level is provided by sex clubs in San Francisco. Before the onset of the

AIDS epidemic, there were a large number of bathhouses in the city, the majority of which had private rooms where gay men engaged in sex. Bathhouses with private spaces were ultimately closed, however, because of the perception that they adding fuel to the burning epidemic fire. Sex clubs with no private spaces were eventually introduced as their replacement. The new generation of public sexual spaces all belong to a community coalition of similar organizations that mandates that they have only well-lit space that can be monitored for unprotected sexual activity. Some clubs go further and have an "oral sex only" policy to prevent higher-risk sexual activity in their establishments. Many of these sex clubs also provide educational materials and condoms, but the most significant interventions in these settings are the architectural and policy changes that they have introduced. Woods et al. (1997) performed a systematic observational study of four such spaces in San Francisco and concluded that little anal intercourse occurs in these settings, and, when it does, condoms are used the majority of the time.

Community-Level Change

Interventions performed at the community level attempt to change social norms in communities to encourage individuals within those communities to reduce their risk behaviors. Kegeles et al. (1996) implemented a community-wide HIV primary prevention program for young gay and bisexual men in a multiple baseline design. The peer-led intervention consisted of community outreach, small groups, community organizing, and a publicity campaign and was successful in reducing the amount of unprotected anal intercourse with both primary and nonprimary sexual partners. The intervention was based largely on empowerment (Rappaport, 1981) and Diffusion of Innovations theories (Rogers, 1983) and involved young gay and bisexual men in important aspects of the intervention implementation. The results of the study showed a decrease in prevalence of reported unprotected anal intercourse from a baseline of 41% to 30% after the intervention, including a decrease from 20.2% to 11.1% with nonprimary sexual partners. In contrast, a comparison community that was randomized to not receive the intervention demonstrated no such change. Given that gay bars are often the most typical gay community settings and that there is an association between substance use and HIV sexual risk taking (Leigh and Stall, 1993), it is important to note that the intervention may have decreased risk taking not simply because it promoted safer sex and condom use but also because it provided an alcohol-free community space for gay men called the Mpowerment Center.

The most widely implemented successful community-level intervention is needle exchange programs for IDUs. Watters et al. (1994) surveyed a large sample of IDUs (N = 5,644) in San Francisco and found that 61% had obtained syringes from needle exchange sites in the previous year and that 45% had "usually" used the program to obtain syringes. The number of syringes exchanged in the program escalated from 7,821 in the spring of 1989 to 343,883 during the spring of 1992 as the program was implemented more widely in the community. In addition, they found that those who had used the needle exchange program frequently were significantly less likely to report having shared syringes than those who had used the program infrequently or not at all. Thus, this community-level intervention reached a large number of individuals and was related to a reduction in parenteral risk taking. Lurie and Drucker (1997) reviewed the studies to date on needle exchange programs and concluded not only that these programs are highly effective in reducing HIV risk behaviors but also that they do not lead to an increase in drug use, an outcome that many fear these interventions will produce.

Societal/Cultural Level

Interventions at the societal/cultural level change social structures to provide individuals access to resources that enable behavior change. Examples of societal/cultural interventions include local and national policy changes, widespread mass-media campaigns, altering living conditions, social movements, and working to decrease homophobia, racism, sexism, and poverty. Policy changes are often effective and efficient modes of HIV prevention at the societal/cultural level. Perhaps the most significant policy change came when the U.S. blood supply began to be screened for HIV in March 1985. Before that time, many individuals (particularly hemophiliacs) were infected with HIV because of the presence of HIV in the blood supply; currently, however, it is estimated that only 1 in 450,000 to 1 in 660,000 donations per year (18 to 27 total donations) are infectious for HIV but are not detected by currently available screening tests (Centers for Disease Control and Prevention, 1996).

In Thailand, the government enacted a policy of mandatory condom use in brothels in 1990 (The 100% Condom Program). The policy was implemented through a collaboration between brothel owners, police, and public health clinics. The brothel owners ensure that customers use condoms, the police threaten brothel closure if the policy is not followed, and the clinics track STD infections in sex workers as an indicator of policy adherence. The results of this policy change indicate that consistent condom use has escalated to over 90% among sex workers, while diagnosable STDs have declined by more than three-quarters (Hanenberg et al., 1994). Although it is possible that these changes were not caused by the policy change per se, the evidence strongly rules out any other causal explanation (Rojanapithayakorn and Hanenberg, 1996).

An example of a *negative* impact of policy on HIV prevention can be found in sub-Saharan Africa, which receives only 2.8% of global expenditures for HIV prevention even though this area contains 10% of the world's population and *two-thirds* of the world's HIV infections; in addition, sub-Saharan African countries spend $0.07 per capita on HIV prevention, whereas the United States spends $2.95 (Lurie et al., 1995). It can be logically argued that this relative lack of spending has contributed to the high prevalence of HIV infection in these countries.

A final illustration the impact of policy occurred in the state of Connecticut in 1992. Although almost all developed countries have made access to sterile syringes legal, the U.S. government continues to maintain a federal ban on their sale over-the-counter or distribution at needle exchanges sites (DesJarlais et al., 1995). In July 1992, however, the Connecticut state laws changed to allow the purchase of nonprescription syringes in pharmacies and for individuals to possess up to 10 such syringes. Since this policy change, surveys indicate that more IDUs reported purchasing syringes at pharmacies (19% before, 78% after) and that fewer reported sharing needles (52% before, 31% after; Groseclose et al., 1995). In addition, a stratified random sample of pharmacies showed that those in neighborhoods with a higher prevalence of IDUs saw a significant increase in nonprescription syringe sales after the policy was implemented, whereas those in other neighborhoods experienced no such change. Results of this study demonstrated that the total number of nonprescription syringes sold per month in the IDU-prevalent neighborhoods increased steadily from 460 in July 1992 to 2,482 in June 1993, while sales remained stable at the other pharmacies (Valleroy et al., 1995).

A study by Hogg et al. (1994) demonstrates the influence of societal/cultural variables in HIV/AIDS prevention. They studied the association between socioeconomic status and AIDS mortality, providing implications for interventions. Their longitudinal cohort study of 364 HIV-positive Canadian gay men demonstrated that men from lower socioeconomic classes (defined as earning less than $10,000 per year in 1984) died significantly faster than men from higher socioeconomic classes. They found that lower-income men had a 60% higher mortality risk after controlling for the effects of age, initial CD4 count, use of antiretroviral therapies, PCP prophylaxis, and year of infection. They argued that socioeconomic class itself caused mortality more quickly rather than other factors, such as greater access to health care, because of the equitable distribution of medical services to all men in the study as well as the presence of universal health care insurance in Canada. The findings of this study suggest that preventing poverty can be a form of secondary HIV prevention, an implication that is particularly relevant because HIV and AIDS have become more prevalent among those of lower socioeconomic status (Hogg et al., 1994). This finding, along with similar ones (see Lurie et al., 1995; Tawil et al., 1995), indicates that prevention of poverty should be a part of the HIV/AIDS prevention arsenal.

WITH ALL THE EVIDENCE SHOWING THAT HIV AND AIDS CAN BE PREVENTED, WHY DOES THE EPIDEMIC CONTINUE TO SPREAD?

Political Opposition: Sex-, Homo-, and Junky-Phobias

Political opposition is perhaps the most outstanding reason why successful HIV/AIDS prevention has not been widely implemented, particularly in the United States. When AIDS first began to appear clinically in the United States, it was dubbed gay-related immune deficiency (GRID). This "gay cancer" was labeled as such because it was believed that it was somehow uniquely associated with gay men. Although gay and bisexual men continue to make up the majority of U.S. AIDS cases, it is of course not true that AIDS is confined solely to gay men. The impact of the initial (and continued) association of the disease with gay men has, however, irrevocably shaped the historical response to it. Political opposition to funding for HIV and AIDS research has been prevalent because of the perception (and reality) that gay men are most affected by the disease. The epidemiological facts of AIDS set up a political war of "pro-AIDS" liberals versus "anti-AIDS" conservatives, with homophobia as the inspiration for the conservative army.

Many scientists believe that HIV prevention science is not as advanced today as it could be because of this history. That the disease is associated with (homo)sexuality and drug use has made many uneasy in discussing it, and conservative political forces have been especially reluctant to support funding for HIV/AIDS research because of beliefs that AIDS is associated with "immoral" behavior. For example, in 1987 a congressional amendment sponsored by Senator Jesse Helms prohibited federal funding of educational projects that "promote homosexuality" (i.e., discuss homosexual acts) despite the fact that the majority of AIDS cases were appearing in gay men.

More recently, President Clinton signed into law a congressional bill that provided $50 million per year for the next five years for "abstinence only" education to be taught in American schools. All 50 states applied for these block grant funds (Associated Press, 1997) despite empirical evidence indicating that comprehensive sexuality education (that explores abstinence as well as issues such as contraception, homosexuality, abortion, and condom use) does not increase sexual activity in teenagers (the outcome that conservative forces fear these programs will produce) and may increase condom use and delay the onset of sexual intercourse (Collins, 1997). Moreover, it is extremely unlikely that the two-thirds of American teenagers who report having engaged in sexual intercourse are likely to all be dissuaded by abstinence only education, making such education seem of little utility to them (Collins, 1997). Political decisions like these, based in ideology rather than scientific data, are detrimental to HIV/AIDS prevention efforts because without discussion of sexuality—especially homosexuality—HIV education and prevention are impossibilities.

Another glaring example of politics being chosen over science can be found in the resistance to more wide implementation of needle exchange programs, including the U.S. government's ban on federal funds for needle exchange programs. Such opposition is also based in politics rather than empirical data. Ironically, the U.S. government itself has funded several studies to evaluate the impact of needle exchange programs, and all have found similar results: These programs serve to reduce needle sharing but do not increase drug use (Lurie and Drucker, 1997). Lurie and Drucker (1997) used mathematical models and estimated that thousands of lives could have been saved in the United States if needle exchange programs were not banned by the U.S. government.

All this political opposition stems from phobias common to the United States: sexphobia, homophobia, and junky-phobia. The discomfort that sexuality, homosexuality, and drug use engenders has led to many backs being turned to HIV and AIDS prevention. If prevention is to be successful, these attitudes must be overcome in favor of more open discourses. In countries that have approached these issues head-on, the HIV epidemic has virtually been averted. In Australia, for example, the number of new HIV infections among men who have sex with men decreased from a peak of 2,284 in 1987 to 772 in 1994, and in New Zealand the number of total cases of AIDS has declined sharply to 511 by September 1995 (Sharples et al., 1996). In addition, neither country has experienced an epidemic among IDUs. DesJarlais et al. (1995) further demonstrated that HIV can be controlled among IDUs if aggressive prevention strategies are implemented early. As a result of such aggressive efforts, cities like Glasgow (Scotland), Sydney (Australia), Lund (Sweden), Toronto (Canada), and San Francisco have stabilized HIV prevalence at low levels among IDUs.

Failure to Target Interventions
to Those at Risk for HIV

The Advent of the HIV Antibody Test The lack of targeted interventions has also led to a diminution of the efficacy of HIV prevention efforts. A major turning point in the history of AIDS that contributed to this lack of focus was the identification of the virus associated with AIDS and the subsequent development of a test for its antibodies. Making a test for the AIDS virus widely accessible quickly became a priority for government agencies (Shilts, 1987). Gay men, in general, reacted to the availability of the test with skepticism, and community-based groups in cities such as New York and Chicago advised gay men not to take it. Instead, these groups emphasized the importance of practicing "safe sex" regardless of serostatus, the dominant view being that everyone was affected by AIDS regardless of their actual HIV status and that identifying those who tested seropositive would lead to increased discrimination or possibly even the quarantine of those particular people (Patton, 1990). In addition, few promising treatments for HIV disease were available, leaving people to question the utility of knowing one's HIV status.

The sentiment changed in urban gay communities, however, as some activists began to argue that test taking could promote behavior change and as some treatments became available to prevent AIDS-related opportunistic infections. The importance of testing also became further emphasized outside of gay communities with the disclosure that Rock Hudson, a Hollywood icon of heterosexuality (although a homosexually active man in the real world), had died of AIDS, inspiring the realization that White middle-class heterosexuals might be at risk for what had been constructed as a "gay disease." Fear became rampant in the "general population" and testing sites saw large increases in White middle-class heterosexual clients (Patton, 1990), a trend that continues to the present time (Bennett and Sharpe, 1996; King, 1993).

Test taking thus became the centerpiece of AIDS "prevention" because it was believed that if victims could be identified, the spread of the virus could be halted by containing it within those individuals. In addition, people who got tested received counseling and information on how HIV is transmitted, a process that presumably would lead to a substantial decrease in risky behaviors. The advent of the HIV antibody test thereby inspired an epistemology of *individual responsibility* for HIV transmission with the complementary focus of HIV prevention on educating people about HIV transmission "facts" as the linchpin of prevention. It then became important for "everyone" to be tested, not just those groups at high risk. Once everyone knew the transmission facts, it was presumed that the spread of AIDS could be stopped.

In a bitter irony, the attempt to make AIDS "everyone's problem" woefully backfired in that because so much effort was put into generalizing the threat of AIDS, prevention efforts, including HIV testing and counseling, were not targeted to those really at risk. AIDS had become "de-gayed" to prevent AIDS-related prejudice and stigma (King, 1993), but the cost was profound: Prevention dollars and resources were not directed at gay men or IDUs for fear that funding agents and charitable donors would not empty their pockets for sexual and drug-using outcasts. In addition, testing was seen as "everyone's right," not to be reserved for any special class of persons. Prevention efforts attempted to be nonspecific and diffuse, choosing to believe that everyone is at equal risk of contracting HIV. Such an ethos, although apparently well intentioned, was an epidemiological disaster. Instead of focusing prevention on the groups that needed it most, programs were made available to "everyone" and were not targeted to risk groups. For example, HIV testing and counseling, the largest federally funded prevention approach, does not adequately reach men who have sex with men and IDUs and their sexual partners. Rather, these programs are disproportionately utilized by other groups that are at much lower risk: Of the 2.4 million HIV antibody tests conducted in 1994, only 13% were administered to gay and bisexual men and IDUs (Bennett and Sharpe, 1996). This misguided approach has led to a need to refocus prevention to target those groups most at risk of HIV infection: gay and bisexual men, IDUs, and their sexual partners.

High-Risk Individuals within High-Risk Populations

Even when targeted to high-risk populations, however, researchers have reported difficulty in reaching the most at-risk members within those populations (Kegeles et al., 1996). For example, Kelly (1995) discusses the difficulty in recruiting high-risk men who have sex with men to individual and small-group interventions. In particular, men who have sex with men but who do not necessarily identify as "gay" or "bisexual" are less likely to attend such programs despite evidence that such "closeted" men are more likely to engage in risky sexual behaviors (Heckman et al., 1995). Similarly, Hoff et al. (1997) reported that in a sample of 1,001 gay and bisexual men, only 6% of the 142 who had engaged in unprotected anal intercourse in the previous month had been reached by an intervention consisting of counseling and testing (although 58% of this same group was reached by a community-level intervention consisting of volunteer outreach in multiple venues). Even though they are at higher risk for HIV, racial and ethnic minority gay and bisexual men are also less likely to attend intervention program sessions (Stokes et al., 1996).

Lack of Primary Prevention
with HIV-Positive Individuals

A curious, yet understandable, phenomenon also represents a portion of the failure to reach high-risk individuals with preventive interventions: Few primary prevention efforts are targeted to HIV-positive individuals. This issue is just now being seriously confronted among primary educators and prevention scientists. The lack of targeted interventions to HIV-infected individuals is attributable mostly to an entrenched fear of exacerbating the stigma that HIV-positive individuals already face. By targeting interventions toward people with HIV, educators and others involved with prevention have feared that the overwhelming message of such approaches would be branding HIV-positive people as purveyors of disease. This view has coincided with the "individual responsibility" theme that has historically surrounded AIDS discourse. Individuals are thought to be solely responsible for themselves, and if they choose to have unprotected sexual contact or share needles with an HIV-infected person, it is their fault for choosing to do so.

This view needs to be reconsidered. Although it is undeniably true that HIV-infected persons face considerable stigma, it is a mistake to forgo them as agents of interventions simply because they are HIV infected. Much altruism and care for others could be capitalized on if interventions were targeted to HIV-positive people. Moreover, the possibility that HIV-positive people may become infected with different (and perhaps drug-resistant) forms of HIV as well as other STDs provides an incentive for HIV-positive people to engage in safer sexual and needle-sharing behaviors. It also makes epidemiological sense because targeting interventions to those who have HIV necessarily reaches individuals who are likely to transmit the virus. Yet HIV-positive people have rarely been targeted for interventions.

In sum, interventions need to be targeted to high-risk groups if they are to be successful. Among those who should be targeted are men who have sex with men, IDUs, and the sexual partners of both of these groups. In addition, the most high risk individuals within these groups need to be reached by preventive interventions, and primary prevention with HIV-infected persons needs to be undertaken seriously. By focusing interventions to these populations, scarce resources will be better utilized (DesJarlais et al., 1994).

INADEQUATE ALLOCATION OF RESOURCES TO PREVENTION

HIV prevention has also not been more successful because of a lack of funding and resources for HIV prevention efforts. The previously mentioned emphasis on *individual responsibility* as well as a privileging of medical "cures" over behavioral preventive strategies have contributed to this failure to allocate adequate resources to prevention.

Individual Responsibility

Emphasizing individual responsibility has led to deemphasizing prevention programs. Because individuals are believed to be solely accountable for their behaviors, prevention programs are deemed unimportant. This discourse boils down to something like this: Everyone should know how to avoid HIV, so why do we need prevention? Among the many problems with this view is the fact that *knowledge does not equal prevention*. Although it may be true that most individuals in American society are aware of HIV transmission knowledge, such knowledge does not necessarily lead to an enactment of risk reduction or elimination. Certain situational variables—such as the presence of alcohol or drugs; a partner who is controlling, powerful or abusive; or the need to feel close and intimate with a partner—may all contribute to engaging in risky behaviors. HIV prevention programs can address these issues, but programs need to be funded and widely available if they are to do so.

Biomedicine as the Popular Science

Prevention is unpopular in American culture. Medical cures are looked to instead. Case in point: Even though there is an effective vaccine for hepatitis B, few take advantage of it. Most believe that medicine will cure them once they are sick. Most STDs can also be avoided through the use of condoms, but many people choose to take antibiotics after they are infected rather than change their behavior first. As another example, the risk of heart disease and lung cancer can be severely reduced through diet, exercise, and quitting smoking, but many hope for medical cures once they become sick rather than preventing these diseases in the first place through behavior changes. Few people get flu shots even though they may help to avert serious discomfort down the road. The point is that prevention is less popular because the threat of disease is less proximal and that this unpopularity translates into the lack of energy supporting prevention research and programming.

Relatedly, within the scientific communities, biomedical research is often viewed as supreme. Behavioral research is the ugly stepsister of "real" medical research conducted with the gold standard of research: the randomized clinical trial design. Without "hard" outcomes such as blood test results, behavioral research is sometimes viewed as "soft" (as in the "soft sciences"). These perceptions come into play when research dollars are at stake and when value is placed on scientific findings. Should the study with blood draws and DNA testing be funded, or the one with only self-report outcome measures? Which study's results are more believable? Unfortunately, the process surrounding research often plays out in this manner.

Prevention has to date, however, without question been more successful than biomedical science in saving lives from HIV disease. Although new medical therapies show promise, many more lives are saved by primary prevention than by biomedical science. This is not to say that both approaches should not be encouraged but rather that prevention has done a great deal, and it is illogical to privilege biomedical research over prevention science. In fact, the ideal approach would be to combine these approaches in multidisciplinary research that studies prevention in an era of increasingly successful medical treatments. More effective treatments undoubtedly have an impact on people's risk behavior, and preliminary data indicate that this is the case (Dilley et al., 1997). In addition, the success of biomedical treatments may rest largely on behavior, such as adherence to drug regimens (Vanhove et al., 1996). Thus, a comprehensive and more successful approach to preventing HIV and AIDS incorporates biomedical and behavioral research in a complementary manner rather than pitting them against each other.

FAILURE TO ADDRESS LARGER SOCIAL PROBLEMS THAT CONTRIBUTE TO THE TRANSMISSION OF HIV

A final reason for prevention of HIV and AIDS not being more successful is found in the lack of attention to social problems that contribute to the spread of HIV and the rapid progression of AIDS. Issues such as homophobia, racism, poverty, sexism, substance use, and homelessness are all important to consider in HIV and AIDS prevention. Although addressing these issues is daunting, it is necessary if the epidemic is to be controlled.

For example, gender roles and sexism are at play when one is attempting to prevent HIV and AIDS. Paying attention to gender roles and working to challenge sexism should be components of HIV prevention. Because the disease has been more prevalent in men, women's HIV and AIDS prevention and treatment needs have often been overlooked. Prevention programs based largely on models developed by grassroots gay male community organizations may not be as successful for women because they do not incorporate explicit attention to gender roles in their content. Women in heterosexual relationships may, for example, be in abusive relationships or be economically dependent on their male partners, thus making it more difficult to be assertive about condom use (Amaro, 1995). Women with children may be additionally concerned about their children's welfare if they are not sexually cooperative. Given that the use of condoms makes sex less pleasurable, it is difficult to ask a partner to wear one. Although the "female" condom has been developed as a female-controlled prevention device, many women have reported not liking it (Moore, 1997). Alternatives to these barriers are microbisides, which are less intrusive and can even be used by women without their male partners' knowledge. These products need to be better developed, however, because they have not been successful to date in reducing HIV transmission (Reuters, 1997).

It may seem idealistic to say that attention to social issues is important in HIV and AIDS prevention. It may even appear unrealistic to argue that it is possible to challenge these entrenched social problems. It is undeniable, however, that these problems are forces that contribute to the proliferation of HIV and AIDS. Although it certainly may be difficult to eradicate things such as sexism, racism, and homophobia quickly, it is quite possible to be aware of these issues when creating research protocols or prevention programs. The very attention to these matters in every step of these processes reduces their presence.

CONCLUSION

HIV/AIDS prevention science has written many success stories. Good stories, however, need be read. HIV and AIDS prevention will be more successful in the future if obstacles to it are addressed. These include political opposition and the failure to allocate ample resources to prevention, to target interventions to those most at risk for HIV, and to confront social problems that contribute to the transmission of HIV. The knowledge that scientists have worked diligently to produce will be most useful if these barriers to success are challenged.

REFERENCES

Allen, S., Serufilira, A., Bogaerts, J., et al. (1992). Confidential HIV testing and condom promotion in Africa: Impact on HIV and gonorrhea rates. *Journal of the American Medical Association, 268,* 3338–3343.

Amaro, H. (1995). Love, sex and power: Considering women's realities in HIV prevention. *American Psychologist, 50*(6), 437–447.

Associated Press. (1997). Sex education that teaches abstinence wins support. *New York Times,* July 23, A19.

Bennett, A., and Sharpe, A. (1996). AIDS fight is skewed by federal campaign exaggerating risks: Most heterosexuals face scant peril but receive large portion of funds, less goes to gays, addicts. *Wall Street Journal,* May 1, A1.

Brewer, T. F., and Derrickson, J. (1992). AIDS in prison: A review of epidemiology and preventive policy. *AIDS, 6,* 623–628.

Centers for Disease Control and Prevention (1995). *HIV/AIDS Surveillance Report.* Vol. 7, No. 2. Atlanta: Centers for Disease Control and Prevention.

————. (1996, March 1). *U.S. Public Health Service Guidelines for Testing and Counseling Blood and Plasma Donors for Human Immunodeficiency Virus Type 1 Antigen*. Vol. 45, No. RR-2. Washington, D.C.: U.S. Department of Health and Human Services, Public Health Service.

————. (1997). *HIV/AIDS Surveillance Report*. Vol. 9 No. 1. Atlanta: Centers for Disease Control and Prevention.

Choi, K. H., and Coates, T. J. (1994). Prevention of HIV infection. *AIDS, 8,* 1371–1389.

Coates, T. J. (1990). Strategies for modifying sexual behavior for primary and secondary prevention of HIV disease. *Journal of Consulting and Clinical Psychology, 58*(1), 57–69.

Coates, T. J., and Collins, C. (1998). Preventing HIV infection. *Scientific American, 279*(1), 76–77.

Collins, C. (1997). *Do as I Say . . . Should We Teach Only Abstinence in Sex Education?* San Francisco: University of California San Francisco Center for AIDS Prevention Studies.

DesJarlais, D. C., Hagan, H., Friedman, S. R., et al. (1995). Maintaining low HIV seroprevalence in populations of injecting drug users. *Journal of the American Medical Association, 274,* 1226–1231.

DesJarlais, D. C., and Padian, N. S., and Winkelstein, W., Jr. (1994). Targeted HIV-prevention programs. *New England Journal of Medicine, 331*(21), 1451–1453.

Dilley, J. W., Woods, W. J., and McFarland, W. (1997). Are advances in treatment changing views about high-risk sex? *New England Journal of Medicine, 227*(7), 501–502.

Dolan, K., Wodak, A., and Penny, R. (1995). AIDS behind bars: Preventing HIV spread among incarcerated drug injectors. *AIDS, 9,* 825–832.

Dolcini, M. M. (1997). Young adolescent crowds and risk behavior: A longitudinal study. Paper presented at the annual meeting of the American Psychological Association, Chicago, August.

Groseclose, S. L., Weinstein, B., Jones, T. S., et al. (1995). Impact of increased legal access to needles and syringes on practices of injecting drug-users and police officers—Connecticut, 1992–1993. *Journal of Acquired Immune Deficiency Syndromes and Human Retrovirology, 10*(1), 82–89.

Hanenberg, R. S., Rojanapithayakorn, W., Kunasol, P., and Sokal, D. C. (1994). Impact of Thailand's HIV-control programme as indicated by the decline of sexually transmitted diseases. *The Lancet, 344,* 243–245.

Heckman, T. G., Kelly, J. A., Sikkema, K. J., et al. (1995). Differences in HIV risk characteristics between bisexual and exclusively gay men. *AIDS Education and Prevention, 7*(6), 504–512.

Hoff, C. C., Kegeles, S. M., Acree, M., et al. (1997). Looking for men in all the wrong places . . . : HIV prevention small-group programs do not reach high risk gay men. *AIDS, 11*(6), 829–831.

Hogg, R. S., Strathdee, S. A., Craib, K. J. P., et al. (1994). Lower socioeconomic status and shorter survival following HIV infection. *The Lancet, 344,* 1120–1124.

Holmberg, S. D. (1996). The estimated prevalence and incidence of HIV in 96 large U.S. metropolitan areas. *American Journal of Public Health, 86,* 642–654.

Kamb, M. L., Bolan, G., Zenilman, J., et al. (1997). Does HIV prevention counseling work? Results from a multi-center randomized trial (Project Respect). Paper presented at the 12th meeting of the International Society of Sexually Transmitted Diseases Research, Seville, Spain, October.

Kamb, M. L., Dillon, B., Fishbein, M., and Willis, K. L. (1996). Quality assurance of HIV prevention counseling in a multi-center randomized controlled trial. *Public Health Reports, 111*(Suppl. 1), 99–107.

Kegeles, S. M., Hays, R. B., and Coates, T. J. (1996). The Mpowerment Project: A community-level HIV prevention intervention for gay men. *American Journal of Public Health, 86*(8), 1129–1136.

Kelly, J. A. (1995). *Changing HIV Risk Behavior: Practical Strategies.* New York: Guilford Press.

Kelly, J. A., St. Lawrence, J. S., Hood, H. V., and Brasfield, T. L. (1989). Behavioral intervention to reduce AIDS risk activities. *Journal of Consulting and Clinical Psychology, 57*(1), 60–67.

King, E. (1993). *Safety in Numbers: Safer Sex and Gay Men.* New York: Routledge.

Leigh, B. C., and Stall, R. (1993). Substance use and risky sexual behavior for exposure to HIV: Issues in methodology, interpretation, and prevention. *American Psychologist, 48*(10), 1035–1045.

Lurie, P., and Drucker, E. (1997). An opportunity lost: HIV infections associated with lack of a national needle-exchange programme in the USA. *The Lancet, 349,* 604–608.

Lurie, P., Hintzen, P., and Lowe, R. A. (1995). Socioeconomic obstacles to HIV prevention and treatment in developing countries: The roles of the International Monetary Fund and the World Bank. *AIDS, 9,* 539–546.

Moore, L. J. (1997). "It's like you use pots and pans to cook. It's the tool": The technologies of safer sex. *Science, Technology, and Human Values, 22*(4), 434–471.

Nelles, J., and Harding, T. (1996). Preventing HIV transmission in prison: A tale of medical disobedience and Swiss pragmatism. *The Lancet, 346,* 1507–1508.

Patton, C. (1990). *Inventing AIDS.* New York: Routledge.

Peterson, J. L., Coates, T. J., Catania, J. A., et al. (1992). High-risk sexual behavior and condom use among gay and bisexual African American men. *American Journal of Public Health, 8,* 1490–1494.

Peterson, J. L., Coates, T. J., Catania, J., et al. (1996). Evaluation of an HIV risk reduction intervention among African-American homosexual and bisexual men. *AIDS, 10,* 319–325.

Rappaport, J. (1981). In praise of paradox: A social policy of empowerment over prevention. *American Journal of Community Psychology, 9*(1), 1–25.

Reuters. (1997). Spermicide films does not halt AIDS, study finds. *Washington Post,* April 3, A3.

Rogers, E. M. (1983). *Diffusion of Innovations.* New York: The Free Press.

Rojanapithayakorn, W., and Hanenberg, R. (1996). The 100% Condom Program in Thailand. *AIDS, 10,* 1–7.

Sharples, K. J., Dickson, N. P., Paul, C., and Skegg, D. C. G. (1996). HIV/AIDS in New Zealand: An epidemic in decline? *AIDS, 10,* 1273–1278.

Shilts, R. (1987). *And the Band Played On: Politics, People and the AIDS Epidemic.* New York: Penguin Books.

Stokes, J. P., McKirnan, D. J., Doll, L., and Burzette, R. G. (1996). Female partners of bisexual men: What they don't know might hurt them. *Psychology of Women Quarterly, 20,* 267–284.

Tawil, O., Verster, A., and O'Reilly, K. R. (1995). Enabling approaches for HIV/AIDS prevention: Can we modify the environment and minimize the risk? *AIDS, 9,* 1299–1306.

Valdiserri, R. O., Lyter, D., Leviton, L., et al. (1989). AIDS prevention in homosexual and bisexual men: Results of a randomized trial evaluating two risk reduction interventions. *AIDS, 3,* 21–26.

Valleroy, L. A., Weinstein, B., Jones, T. S., et al. (1995). Impact of increased legal access to needles and syringes on community pharmacies' needle and syringe sales—Connecticut, 1992–1993. *Journal of Acquired Immune Deficiency Syndromes and Human Retrovirology, 10*(1), 73–81.

Vanhove, G. F., Schapiro, J. M., Winters, M. A., et al. (1996). Patient compliance and drug failure in protease inhibitor monotherapy. *Journal of the American Medical Association, 276*(24), 1955–1956.

Waldo, C. R., and Coates, T. J. (In press). Multiple levels of analysis and intervention in HIV prevention science: Exemplars and directions for new research. *AIDS.*

Watters, J. K., Estilo, M. J., Clark, G. L., and Lorvick, J. (1994). Syringe and needle exchange as HIV/AIDS prevention for injection drug users. *Journal of the American Medical Association, 271*(2), 115–120.

Woods, W. J., Mayne, T., and Kegeles, S. (1997). Few men at sex clubs and cruising areas have unprotected anal intercourse. Paper presented at the International AIDS Conference, Vancouver, British Columbia, Canada, June.

World Health Organization. (1997). *Weekly Epidemiological Record, 72*(27), 197–204.

.

**Sheldon Margen and
Joyce C. Lashof**

AFTERWORD

The collective chapters in this volume clearly demonstrate the great breadth and diversity of the issues addressed by public health today. Notwithstanding their differences in modality and approach, what they all have in common is the societal context in which each of the various health problems occur. Recent research on the etiology of chronic diseases has stressed the multifactorial nature of disease causation and identified genetics, environmental factors, and individual behavior as the three major areas involved. Although many investigators do emphasize the importance of the interrelationship between these factors, each area continues to be researched separately, and interventions end up being directed exclusively toward one or the other of these domains. What is particularly clear, however, is that the variables examined in each of the models can account for only a small percentage of the variance in each problem under consideration because the "root causes" of the individual and environmental factors are not being addressed. And what are these "root causes"? First and foremost, they are poverty and inequality, accompanied either causally or by association with such conditions as racism, discrimination, hunger, gender inequality, and lack of education.

What, then, can we do about this? How useful is the public health model? In attempting to deal with concepts like poverty, we have tended to simplify (and often oversimplify). As our society has become increasingly dominated by money, it is the absence of money that ends up defining poverty. But is this simplistic definition of poverty adequate, or, as we suspect, is the concept of poverty much more complex?

According to well-known social critic and philosopher Majid Rahnema,[1]

> In vernacular societies, poverty was not a stereotyped condition defined primarily by a set of economic factors. Neither were all the riches the same. Attitudes toward both the poor and the rich were ambiguous. They depended not only on people's material possessions but also on the ways they each related to their condition, on a certain quality of their desire to possess or to earn money, and on the impacts of that desire on the moral and human dimensions of their being. As such, there were both noble and despicable "poor." It was nonetheless believed that money and possessions had a generally corruptive influence on their holders, a fact that made them unwelcome to the Kingdom of Heavens. There were as many forms of poverty and riches as humans and communities.

Is it possible, in a society such as ours, where the economic model dominates and the discrepancy between rich and poor is increasing at a dramatic rate, to create some sense of equality? Since we tend to disassociate economic elements from the political and social issues, can we possibly address social and economic injustices by denying their existence or assuming they are self-correcting?

Being wealthy means having power over others and controlling their access to goods and services while limiting their ability to make choices or change. This is a condition that many social psychologists, sociologists, and now epidemiologists suggest is one of the principle determinants of health. In this respect, it is helpful to recall John Stuart Mill:[2]

> One of the greatest dangers, therefore, of democracy, as of all other forms of government, lies in the sinister interest of the holders of power: it is the danger of class legislation; of government intended for (whether really effecting it or not) the immediate benefit of the dominant class, to the lasting detriment of the whole. And one of the most important questions demanding consideration, in determining the best constitution of a representative government, is how to provide efficacious securities against this evil.

This volume is filled with demonstrations of how the public health model can be used to analyze and solve societal problems that only recently have been recognized as impinging on health. Many remain categorical and segmented, but once we realize that the basic causes are the same, it will be possible to progress in more holistic and multidisciplinary ways by dealing with both poverty and inequality in concert with communities and community health problems. Obviously, public health professionals cannot solve the problem of poverty alone, but we can and must continue to explore and clarify the complex relationship between poverty and health. We must also rethink the approach that we have taken in developing programs designed to deal with individual health problems and find new ways to work with and empower communities to address not only specific health problems but also the root causes of these problems. This will require not only partnerships between governmental agencies and educational, business, and social agencies but also the necessary human and financial resources that will allow communities to provide leadership and set priorities.

As public health professionals, we must not isolate ourselves from society; rather, we must become activists for social change that will result in equity for all while still acknowledging the uniqueness of each individual. This must be our goal for the millennium. How far we can progress depends on how well we learn to work together.

REFERENCES

1. Rahnema, Majhid. 1995. "Dann stürzen sie ins Elend." *Der Überblick,* January, 5–8.
2. Mill, John Stuart. 1873. *Considerations on representative government.* New York: Henry Holt, 141.

Christopher M. Anderson is project director for the California Smokers' Helpline, a statewide program funded by the California Department of Health Services, Tobacco Control Section, and operated by the University of California, San Diego. He has taken a leading role in the development and implementation of counseling protocols and measurement instruments used for adult and adolescent smokers enrolled in the program.

John C. Beck, M.D., Ph.D. (honoris causa), D.Sc. (honoris causa), was born in the United States and lived a large portion of his life in Canada, returning to the United States in 1974. He was educated at McGill University and had extensive postgraduate training in Europe and the United States. He has held senior academic positions at McGill University; the University of California, San Francisco; and the University of California, Los Angeles. In 1993, he became emeritus professor of medicine (recalled) and now spends full time in research with projects in Switzerland, Germany, and the United States. His major research interests include risk factor identification for functional decline, prevention of disability, health risk appraisal in the elderly, alcohol use in the elderly, and quality-of-care indicators in nursing homes.

Lester Breslow, M.D., M.P.H., Sc.D. (honoris causa), is a professor and dean emeritus at the UCLA School of Public Health. He also serves as chair of the Los Angeles County Public Health Commission, is a fellow of the American College of Physicians, and is a member of the UCLA Jonsson Comprehensive Cancer Center as well as the Institute of Medicine of the National Academy of Sciences. He has held numerous other professional positions, including director of the California State Department of Health, director of the UCLA Health Promotion/Disease Prevention Center, president of the American Public Health Association, president of the International Epidemiology Association, and chairman of the National Committee on Vital and Health Statistics. He received both his M.D. and his M.P.H. from the University of Minnesota. His many awards include the Lienhard Award from the Institute of Medicine of the National Academy of Sciences, the Healthtrac Award for Health Improvement, the Charles A. Dana Award for Outstanding Achievement in Health, the American Public Health Association Sedgwick Medal for Distinguished Service, and the Lasker Award. He was founding editor of the *Annual Review of Public Health* and has published a large number of scholarly articles.

Johanna Birckmayer holds a Ph.D. in health policy from Harvard University. She received a master's degree in public health from the Department of Health Behavior and Health Education at the University of North Carolina. She has extensive work experience in Africa in the design, implementation, and evaluation of health programs and now serves as an evaluator for a public health organization in Colorado.

Thomas J. Coates, Ph.D., director and principal investigator on the University of California, San Francisco (UCSF), Center for AIDS Prevention Studies and director of the UCSF AIDS Research Institute, is a professor of medicine and epidemiology and biostatistics at UCSF. He received his Ph.D. in psychology from Stanford University. He was among the first behavioral scientists to conduct research on HIV primary and secondary prevention. During the last 10 years, he has worked to keep the AIDS research agenda abreast of new challenges that emerge as the epidemic unfolds. He has recruited biomedical, social, and behavioral scientists to address these challenges at the Center for AIDS Prevention Studies (CAPS) and elsewhere. His advice on AIDS is sought by the Office of AIDS Research at the National Institutes of Health, Family Health International's AIDS Prevention Project, the World Health Organization, the U.S. Congress, and other important policy-making bodies. Throughout his career, he has conducted theory-based research on health-related behavior, with an emphasis on interventions to prevent disease and promote health. His research ranges from studies on individual determinants of behavior to community-based interventions.

Sharon Danoff-Burg is an assistant professor of psychology at the State University of New York at Albany. Her interests are in the area of psychosocial aspects of women's health and chronic illness. Currently, she is conducting research on interpersonal stress and coping with rheumatoid arthritis.

Andrew Duxbury, M.D., received his M.D. from the University of Washington. He completed his residency in internal medicine and a fellowship in geriatrics at the University of California, Davis (UCD), Medical Center and joined the faculty of the UCD School of Medicine in 1993. There he was director of community-based programs for the Section of Geriatrics, including the Geriatrics Clinics, the House Call Program, and the Sacramento County Multipurpose Senior Services Program. In 1998, he joined the faculty of the University of Alabama, Birmingham, in gerontology and geriatric medicine, where he combines a busy clinical practice caring for the frail elderly in the community with both professional and community teaching.

Patricia L. East is an associate research scientist in the Department of Pediatrics at the University of California, San Diego, School of Medicine. She has published extensively on teenage sexuality, pregnancy, and parenting and is author of *Adolescent Pregnancy and Parenting: Findings from a Racially Diverse Sample* (with Marianne Felice; Lawrence Erlbaum Associates, 1996). She has served on the editorial board of *Developmental Psychology, Journal of Research on Adolescence,* and *The International Journal of Behavioral Development* and is editor of *The Society for Research on Adolescence Newsletter.* She is also on the National Institutes of Health's grant review study section for social sciences and population, has regularly reviewed grant applications for the National Science Foundation, and was part of the San Diego Task Force on Adolescent Pregnancy for the American Academy of Pediatrics. Currently, she is conducting an evaluation of the Adolescent Sibling Pregnancy Prevention Program, a $3 million annual statewide teenage pregnancy prevention program administered through the California Department of Health Services, Maternal and Child Health Branch.

Sheryle J. Gallant is an associate professor of psychology at the University of Kansas. She was chair of the American Psychological Association's 1994 conference "Psychosocial and Behavioral Factors in Women's Health: Creating an Agenda for the 21st Century." Her research has focused on conceptual and methodological issues in the assessment of mood and behavior changes during the menstrual cycle and biopsychosocial correlates of premenstrual syndrome.

Theodore G. Ganiats, M.D., is associate professor and vice chair of the Department of Family and Preventive Medicine at the University of California, San Diego (UCSD), School of Medicine. He received both his medical school and his family medicine residency training at UCSD. Ganiats is currently the program director for the UCSD Health Outcomes Assessment Program. His research often combines his experience in national clinical guideline development with his interest in health outcomes assessment and health policy.

Sylvia Guendelman is an associate professor in the Division of Health Policy and Administration and the Maternal and Child Health Program at the University of California, Berkeley, School of Public Health. She holds the Sweezey-Womack Endowed Chair in Medical Research. Several of her research studies focus on the health effects of immigration and on United States–Mexico border health issues. She often combines qualitative and quantitative methodologies to analyze policy-relevant questions.

Adele Dellenbaugh Hofmann, M.D., is a clinical professor of pediatrics at the University of California, Irvine (UCI) and a subspecialist in adolescent medicine. At the time of this paper's original writing in 1993, she was adjunct professor of pediatrics and director of adolescent medicine at UCI. Prior to coming to UCI, she was, first, associate director of the Teen Clinic at Beth Israel Hospital and, subsequently, director of the Adolescent Medical Unit at Bellevue Hospital–New York University Medical Center, both in New York City. Among many honors and distinctions, Dr. Hofmann has served as a president of the Society for Adolescent Medicine, chairperson of the Section on Adolescent Health of the American Academy of Pediatrics, and consultant to the World Health Organization. She also is a recipient of the Outstanding Achievement in Adolescent Medicine Award of the Society for Adolescent Medicine and the Distinguished Service in Adolescent Health Award of the American Academy of Pediatrics (subsequently renamed the Adele Dellenbaugh Hofmann Award in her honor). Dr. Hofmann has authored four books and has over 100 publications. She also has been a frequent visiting professor and lecturer throughout the United States and abroad.

Robert M. Kaplan is professor and chair of the Department of Family and Preventive Medicine at the University of California, San Diego. He has been a recipient of an NHLBI Lung Division Research Career Development Award. He is a past president of several organizations, including the American Psychological Association Division of Health Psychology, Section J of the American Association for the Advancement of Science (Pacific), the International Society for Quality of Life Research, and the Society for Behavioral Medicine. He is editor-in-chief of the *Annals of Behavioral Medicine* and consulting or associate editor of five other academic journals. Selected additional honors include the following: APA Division of Health Psychology Annual Award for Outstanding Scientific Contribution, 1987; Distinguished Research Lecturer, 1988; Health Net Distinguished Lecturer, 1991; University of California 125th Anniversary Award for Most Distinguished Alumnus, University of California, Riverside; American Psychological Association Distinguished Lecturer; and Distinguished Scientific Contribution Award from the American Association of Medical School Psychologists.

Joyce C. Lashof is currently professor emerita of public health at the University of California, Berkeley (UCB). She was dean of the School of Public Health at UCB from 1981 to 1991. She has combined a career in academic medicine with a career in public service. She has published in the area of public health policy, technology assessment, and the interface of public health and primary care. She was elected to the Institute of Medicine, National Academy of Sciences, in 1981 and was awarded the Sedgewick Medal for distinguished service in public health by the American Public Health Association in 1995 and the Henrik Blum Award by the Northern California Public Health Association in 1998. She served as president-elect (1990–91) and as president of the American Public Health Association (1991–92).

Sheldon Margen received his medical degree from the University of California, San Francisco, Medical School, in 1943. He practiced internal medicine in Berkeley, California, until 1962, when he joined the faculty of the University of California, Berkeley. He has served as an adviser to many national and international agencies. He has published approximately 150 scientific articles in the area of nutrition and public health and has coauthored two medical books: a nutrition encyclopedia and a self-help handbook. He is currently an emeritus professor of public health and chairman of the editorial board of advisers of the University of California, Berkeley, *Wellness Letter.*

Meredith Minkler is professor and chair of health and social behavior in the School of Public Health at the University of California, Berkeley (UCB), where she received her Dr.PH in 1975. She was founding director of the UCB Center on Aging and a cofounder of the San Francisco–based Tenderloin Senior Organizing Project (TSOP). A Kellogg National Fellow, she has served as a consultant to groups and organizations, including the U.S. Congress Office of Technology Assessment, the White House Conference on Aging, the Ford Foundation, and the Health Promotion Directorates of several Canadian provinces. Her more than 100 publications include the coauthored book *Grandmothers as Caregivers: Raising Children of the Crack Cocaine Epidemic* (Sage 1993), the co-edited volume *Critical Perspectives on Aging* (Baywood Publishing, 1998), and an edited book, *Community Organizing and Community Building for Health* (Rutgers University Press, 1997).

Philip R. Nader is professor of pediatrics and chief of the Division of Community Pediatrics at the University of California, San Diego. His expertise in health and educational services for school-age children has resulted in extension of his leadership in child health policy at the state and national levels to the international level, with the awarding of a Fogarty Senior International Fellowship to New Zealand and Australia from 1995 to 2001. His research has concentrated on systems influencing children's health behaviors, specifically dietary and physical activity, with a view toward reducing childhood risk factors of adult cardiovascular disease. A majority of his research has been on the evaluation of educational interventions taking place in and through schools.

Mack Roach III, M.D., is an associate professor of radiation oncology at the University of California, San Francisco (UCSF). He also holds a position as an associate professor in the Department of Medicine, the Division of Medical Oncology, and the Department of Urology. He is a diploma-certified internist and medical oncologist, as well as a board-certified radiation oncologist. He is a member of the American College of Radiology's Appropriateness Criteria Task Force for Prostate Cancer, which defines appropriateness guidelines for staging and treatment of prostate cancer. Dr. Roach is the lead author of the section on *Guidelines* *for Treatment Planning.* He also currently serves on the task forces of the National Cancer Institute's Concept Evaluation Panel Committee for Prostate Cancer, as well as the NCI-sponsored Intensity Modulated Radiation Therapy Working Group. He is the chief editor of the InterNet Journal Club section on Genitourinary Topics, and is active on the editorial boards of *The Prostate Journal* and the *International Journal Radiation Oncology Biology Physics.* He serves as a reviewer for *Cancer,* the *Journal of Clinical Oncology,* and *Urology.* Dr. Roach has received significant grants from the National Institutes of Health for prostate cancer radiotherapy trials and from the American Cancer Society for clinical oncology, and was recently recognized for his work by the Best Doctors in the Bay Area and Best Doctors in America awards program. He has authored more than 60 peer-reviewed articles on the topics of radiation therapy, prostate cancer, and lung cancer. He has published extensively on the topic of race and survival from cancer, and currently chairs the Special Populations Sub-committee of the Radiation Therapy Oncology Group (RTOG).

Kathy Sanders-Phillips, Ph.D., a pediatric psychologist, is an associate professor at the University of California, Los Angeles (UCLA), School of Medicine and an associate member of the Jonsson Comprehensive Cancer Center within the UCLA School of Health. As a result of her interest in factors affecting development and health in ethnic minority children, she began to identify and explore barriers to healthy behaviors in ethnic minority families. Her research in this area, funded by the Henry J. Kaiser Family Foundation, assessed perceptions regarding health promotion behaviors among low-income, Black, and Latino women. The findings from this study subsequently provided a foundation for a health promotion program funded by the National Cancer Institute and implemented in 16 Head Start sites in South Central Los Angeles.

Marc B. Schenker is professor and chair of the Department of Epidemiology and Preventive Medicine, School of Medicine, University of California, Davis. He is also director of the University of California Agricultural Health and Safety Center at Davis. His training is in internal medicine (pulmonary disease), preventive medicine (occupational), and epidemiology. His research has focused on risk factors and prevention of occupational disease and on occupational cancer. His work has addressed hazards in a wide range of workplaces, from agriculture to semiconductor manufacturing.

Margaret Schneider Jamner, Ph.D., is an assistant researcher in the School of Social Ecology at the University of California, Irvine. She is a health psychologist whose research focuses on the cognitive, social, and environmental factors influencing health behavior change. She has used a social-ecological approach to explore the processes underlying the adoption of health promotion practices, such as engaging in regular physical activity, and the initiation of health protective practices, such as using condoms to prevent infection with HIV. Her research supports the use of community-based interventions that combine innovative educational interventions with environmental facilitation to bring about behavior change.

William J. Sieber, Ph.D., earned his doctorate degree in clinical psychology from Yale University and completed his clinical training at the Palo Alto Veterans Affairs Medical Center. He has published in the areas of chronic pain management, psychoneuroimmunology, and the assessment of the mind-body relationship. He currently holds an appointment as assistant adjunct professor in the Department of Family and Preventive Medicine, University of California, San Diego, School of Medicine. As a senior research manager with the Lewin Group, he serves as a consultant to pharmaceutical and biotechnology companies assisting in the design and analysis of studies determining the effectiveness of a variety of health care interventions. His current research interests include the effect of mood on the perception and reporting of health, the direct physiological impact of perceived control on health, and the development of quality-of-life measures that are useful to both clinician and researcher. His clinical activities focus on marital and family therapy for the chronically ill.

Stuart J. Slavin, M.D., M.Ed., is associate professor of pediatrics in the Division of General Pediatrics of the University of California, Los Angeles, School of Medicine. Since 1989, he has served as director of the Pediatric Residency Program. He is also director of undergraduate education for the department. He serves as cochair of the Medical Education Committee for the School of Medicine.

Annette L. Stanton is a professor and director of the graduate specialty in clinical health psychology at the University of Kansas. She also serves as associate editor for *Health Psychology*. Her edited books are *Infertility: Perspectives in Stress and Coping Research* (with C. Dunkel-Schetter; Plenum, 1991) and *The Psychology of Women's Health: Prog-*

ress and Challenges in Research and Application (with S. J. Gallant; American Psychological Association, 1995). She has focused on stress and coping theory in her research, particularly as applied to individuals and couples coping with cancer or infertility.

Daniel Stokols, Ph.D., is professor of social ecology and dean emeritus of the School of Social Ecology at the University of California, Irvine. He is past president of the Division of Population and Environmental Psychology of the American Psychological Association, serves as a section editor of the *American Journal of Health Promotion,* and is a member of the editorial boards of the *Health Education and Behavior* and the *Journal of Architectural and Planning Research.* He also received the Annual Career Award from the Environmental Design Research Association in 1991. His current research examines the effects of physical and social conditions within work environments on employees' health, performance, and social behavior. Additional areas of his research include the design and evaluation of community and work-site health promotion programs, transdisciplinary approaches to the prevention of tobacco use, the health and behavioral impacts of environmental stressors such as traffic congestion and overcrowding, and the application of environmental design research to urban planning and facilities management.

Richard C. Strohman, having done research into molecular and cellular aspects of development, is now emeritus professor of Molecular and Cell Biology at the University of California, Berkeley (UCB). He has been chair of the UCB Zoology Department (1973–76) and director of Berkeley's Health and Medical Sciences Program (1976–79). While on leave from UCB in 1990, he was research director for the Muscular Dystrophy Association's international effort to combat genetic neuromuscular diseases. His recent writing that deals with the limits of genetic reductionism in biology and medicine has received wide acclaim and has identified him as one of the leading figures thinking and writing on current changes in the structure of modern biology.

S. Leonard Syme is a professor emeritus of epidemiology and a professor in the Graduate School at the University of California, Berkeley. His research has focused on social and psychological risk factors for disease. In this work, he has studied Japanese migrants to Hawaii and California, British civil servants in London, bus drivers in San Francisco, and residents of Alameda County. He has done research on social mobility, acculturation, social support, social class, and empowerment. In recent years, he has increasingly turned his attention to community interventions to prevent disease. He is the principal investigator of The Wellness Guide Project.

Amparo C. Villablanca is an associate professor of cardiovascular medicine and founder and director of the Women's Cardiovascular Health Program and Clinic in the Department of Internal Medicine at the University of California, Davis (UCD). She has been interested in all aspects of preventive cardiology and has become a recognized expert in heart disease in women. She currently serves on the advisory boards for the UCD site of the NIH-sponsored Women's Health Initiative Study, the Consortium for Women and Research at UCD, and the Executive Steering Committee of the UCD Health System Center of Excellence in Women's Health. In 1994, she was appointed to the advisory council of the California Department of Health Services' Office of Women's Health, where she is chair of its Cardiovascular Health Technical Advisory Group. Her research in basic science utilizes cellular and molecular biology techniques to study the way in which female hormones regulate the function of blood vessels and the expression of genes in vascular cells.

Craig R. Waldo, Ph.D., is a research psychologist at the University of California, San Francisco (UCSF), Center for AIDS Prevention Studies in the Department of Medicine. He received his Ph.D. in clinical/community psychology at the University of Illinois at Urbana-Champaign, where his work focused mainly on minority stress related to sexual and antigay harassment in the workplace. At UCSF, he continues his theoretical interest in organizational and community settings as contexts that can shape behavior by studying the influence of these settings on HIV risk-taking behavior. He is also interested in evaluating HIV preventive interventions, particularly those that rely on empowerment theory and that take community-based approaches with gay and bisexual men.

Lawrence Wallack is currently professor and director, School of Community Health, Portland State University. This work was done when he was professor of public health at the University of California, Berkeley. He is the founding director of the Berkeley Media Studies Group, which worked on the Violence Prevention Initiative described in his chapter. He writes and lectures extensively on issues related to public health and mass media.

Carol Hirschon Weiss is a professor in the Harvard University Graduate School of Education. She has published 11 books, including *Evaluation: Methods of Studying Programs and Policies* (Prentice Hall, 1998). She pioneered the concept of theory-based evaluation in her best-selling book *Evaluation Research* (Prentice Hall, 1972). She is the author of scores of journal articles on evaluation, the uses of research and evaluation, and methods for improving the use of research evidence in policy and programs. She has been a consultant to such organizations as the U.S. Department of Education, the National Institutes of Health, the National Science Foundation, the Rockefeller Foundation, the Aspen Institute, and the Rand Corporation.

Michael S. Wilkes, M.D., Ph.D., is an associate professor of medicine in the Division of General Internal Medicine and Health Services Research in the University of California, Los Angeles, School of Medicine. He is the associate director of the Center for Educational Development and Research. In 1997, he was the recipient of the Alpha Omega Alpha Distinguished Teacher Award.

Shu-Hong Zhu is an associate professor of family and preventive medicine at the University of California, San Diego. As principal investigator of the California Smokers' Helpline, which enrolls a large number of smokers and other tobacco users from the general community on an ongoing basis, he is able to test clinical hypotheses with large subject samples that are usually not available to clinical researchers. His recent work has focused on developing effective brief interventions for smoking cessation for adolescents and pregnant women.

Index

AADLs (advanced activities of daily living), 40, 41, 425, 448
AAMC. *See* Association of American Medical Colleges (AAMC)
AARP. *See* American Association of Retired Persons (AARP)
Abortion, 193, 550, 551, 553–55
Abrams, A., 234–35, 236, 237, 241–42
Abstinence-only approach to sex education, 4, 541–42, 545, 562–63
Accessibility: of health care, 13, 45, 74, 488, 596–97; of smoking cessation programs, 380–82
Accidents: and farmworkers, 591–95; mortality from, 487, 646, 647
Accountability in health care, 46, 74
Acculturation: and pregnancy outcomes, 246–49. *See also* Immigrants
ACE inhibitors, 113
ACE mutation, 112–14, 122
ACS. *See* American Cancer Society (ACS)
Activities of daily living (ADLs), 40, 41, 425, 428–29, 441–42, 448
ADLs (activities of daily living), 40, 41, 425, 428–29, 441–42, 448
Adolescent Family Life case management services, 213
Adolescent medical clinics, 565–66
Adolescent pregnancy. *See* Pregnancy; Pregnancy prevention
Adolescent Social Action Program (ASAP), 352, 356
Adolescents: and abortion, 550, 551, 553–

55; accidents as cause of deaths of, 487; and agricultural fatalities, 592; alcohol use by, 489, 513, 516; biological predispositions of sisters for pregnancy, 195–96; and cardiovascular health, 493–95; cigarette smoking by, 82, 364, 490; clothing for, 542–43; concluding comments on adolescent sexuality, 575–78; and confidentiality issues, 568–69, 575; contraceptive and condom use by, 490, 559–61, 563–65, 566, 567, 573; and depression, 489–90, 543; diet of, 490, 494; and divorce of parents, 544–45; as dropouts, 488–89, 498, 544; drug use by, 489; economic impact of teen childbearing on family of origin, 197, 198, 202–3; and exercise, 490; and exposure to violence, 298, 300, 305–6; financing of health care for, 570–71; group discussions with, on health topics, 212, 495–96; health care for, 566–78; health habits and behaviors of, 489–90; hearing loss among, on farms, 601; and HIV/AIDS, 487, 495, 541, 557–59, 567, 677, 680; and hopelessness, 305–6; modeling by younger sisters of older sisters' early childbearing, 197, 198–99; modifying sexual risk taking by, 561–66; mortality and morbidity in, 358, 359, 476, 487; optimal health services for, 572–75; parenting influences on, and early child bearing, 192–93, 197, 198, 201–

Compositor:	G & S Typesetters, Inc.
Text:	10/13 Sabon
Display:	Franklin Gothic
Printer:	Sheridan Books, Inc.
Binder:	Sheridan Books, Inc.